Calorie, Fat & Carbohydrate Counter

Diet Guides & Counters

Weight Control Tips

✔ Eat Sensibly
- Avoid fad diets. Eat 3 sensible meals daily.
- Limit fats and fatty foods, sugar, soda and alcohol.

(Sample Diet Plan, Page 9)

✔ Exercise Daily
- Get active and exercise every day!
- Include muscle-strengthening exercises. You'll lose more fat and keep it off. You'll also feel and look better, and you can eat a little more food. *(Exercise Guide, Page 10)*

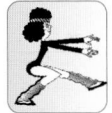

✔ Reshape Eating Behaviors
- Be aware of eating and shopping behaviors that lead to overeating.
- Also focus on social and emotional situations that make you snack compulsively.

(Extra notes - Page 12)

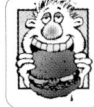

✔ Keep a Food & Exercise Diary
- A diary helps you see exactly what you eat and drink, and how much you really exercise.
- An excellent motivator.
- Keeps you honest! *(Page 13)*

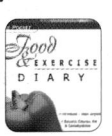

✔ Arrange Moral Support
Gain the support of family and friends. Get extra professional help if required, from your doctor, dietitian, psychologist, exercise trainer, or slimming group. Beware of family saboteurs who discourage you from adopting a healthier lifestyle!

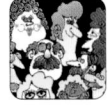

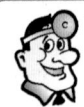

DOCTOR CHECK-UP
Ask your doctor to check you for high blood pressure, diabetes, and high blood cholesterol.

HEALTHY WEIGHTS
for Men & Women
(Over 18 years)

Based on weights with least risk of disease or death from heart disease, diabetes, stroke and cancer.

Based on Body Mass Index - range 20-25.

BMI calculated as: $\dfrac{\text{Weight (kg)}}{\text{Height (m)}^2}$

Height (No Shoes)	Healthy Weight Range
Ft Ins	**Pounds**
4'7"	86-108
4'8"	88-110
4'9"	92-114
4'10"	97-121
4'11"	99-123
5'0"	101-127
5'1"	105-132
5'2"	110-136
5'3"	112-140
5'4"	114-145
5'5"	119-149
5'6"	123-156
5'7"	127-158
5'8"	129-162
5'9"	134-167
5'10"	138-173
5'11"	143-178
6'0"	145-182
6'1"	149-187
6"2"	156-193
6'3"	158-198
6'4"	162-202
6'5'	170-211
6'6"	172-215
6'7"	175-220

Body Fat Distribution & Health

Fat above the hips carries a far greater health risk than fat on or below the hips - better to be a **'pear-shape'** than an **'apple-shape'**.

Abdominal obesity greatly increases the risk of developing diabetes, heart disease, high blood fats, hypertension, stroke and some cancers. So-called **'cellulite'** carries no extra health risk.

Waist Measurement (High Health Risk)

Men: Over 39 inches **Women:** Over 34 inches

Women who become obsessed with dieting away their thighs and buttocks on an otherwise lean body, are fighting mother nature and may well be inviting health problems.

If you are within a healthy weight range, it is better to exercise regularly to maintain body shape, rather than to be constantly dieting and lacking in energy. Accept your body shape and focus on other pursuits and enjoying life!

> Abdominal obesity greatly increases the risk of ill-health and earlier death.

Estimating Body Fat Percentage

Body fat percentage is a better indicator of health than total weight.

Bioelectric impedance analysis (BIA) is gaining support as a practical and economical method for estimating body fat in both clinical and home settings.

BIA measures the resistance of a weak electrical current that is passed through the body. A computer within the body fat analyzer calculates the amount of body water, fat and muscle.

More Information: www.calorieking.com

BODY FAT & OBESITY

Men:	Above 25% body fat
Women:	Above 32% body fat

TANITA

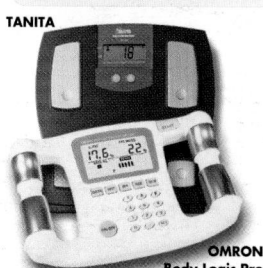

OMRON
Body Logic Pro

**Easy-to-use
body fat monitors for home
and professional use.**

HEALTHY BODY FAT RANGES

Men:	Under 30 years	~	14 - 20%
	Over 30 years	~	17 - 23%
Women:	Under 30 years	~	17 - 24%
	Over 30 years	~	20 - 27%

Note: Less than 13% body fat in women can be unhealthy.

Calories & Weight Loss

Calories in Food

Calories in food are derived from protein, fat and carbohydrate. Alcohol also provides calories. Vitamins, minerals and water provide no calories.

Calorie Values Per Gram

Fat/Oil	~	9 Calories
Carbohydrate	~	4 Calories
Protein	~	4 Calories
Alcohol	~	7 Calories

Note that fats have over double the calories of protein and carbohydrate. The higher the fat content of food, the higher the calories.

Sample Calculation

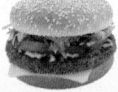

QUARTER POUNDER® WITH CHEESE has 534 calories derived from:

30g Fat (x 9 cals/gram)	=	270
38g Carbohyd.(x 4 cals/gram)	=	152
28g Protein (x 4 cals/gram)	=	112
Total Calories	**=**	**534**

Calorie Levels for Weight Loss

Commence with a calorie-controlled diet that allows a moderate weight loss of $1/2$ - 1 pound per week. Weight loss is usually much larger in the first few weeks due to extra fluid losses.

Note: It is better to increase exercise rather than lessen food calories too drastically.

Suggested Calories for Weight Loss

Women:	Non-active	1000 - 1200
	Active	1200 - 1500
Men:	Non-active	1200 - 1500
	Active	1500 - 1800
Teenagers:		1200 - 1800

The Food Guide Pyramid emphasizes eating a wide variety of foods from the 5 major food groups. For weight loss, make lowfat choices and eat the lower number of servings.

Food Guide Pyramid:
- Fats Sweets — ◄ Use Sparingly
- Milk Soy — 2-3 Servings ►
- Meat Beans Nuts — ◄ 2-3 Servings
- Vegetables — 3-5 Servings
- Fruit — 2-4 Servings
- Bread, Cereals, Rice, Pasta — 6-11 Servings (4-6 Servings For Weight Loss)

Examples of Serving Size

Bread & Cereal Group:
- 1 slice bread
- $1/2$ bun, bagel or English muffin
- 4 small crackers or 1 tortilla
- 1 oz ready-to-eat cereal
- $1/2$ cup cooked cereal, rice, pasta

Fruit Group:
- 1 medium apple, orange, banana
- $1/2$ cup canned fruit
- $1/4$ cup dried fruit
- $3/4$ cup fruit juice
- $1/4$ medium avocado

Vegetable Group:
- 1 cup raw leafy vegetables
- $1 1/2$ oz raw chopped vegetables
- $1/2$ cup cooked vegetables
- $1/2$ - $3/4$ cup vegetable juice

Meat & Alternatives Group:
- 2-3oz (cooked) lean meat/poultry/fish
- 2 eggs **or** 7oz tofu **or** $1/2$ cup nuts
- 1 cup (cooked) dried beans or chickpeas
- 4 Tbsp peanut butter

Milk & Alternatives Group:
- 1 cup (8 fl.oz) milk, soy drink, yogurt
- $1 1/2$ oz cheese or $1/2$ cup cottage cheese

Portion Size Counts!

Food portion size is critical to controling calorie intake for weight control.

Super-sized food servings have become more common when eating out and in the home. This can mean a day's worth of calories being consumed in one meal; or a snack being equivalent to a full meal.

It is easy to underestimate portion size of foods and drinks, and unwittingly consume excess calories – even if the fat content is low or even zero!

To more accurately estimate portion size of different foods, weigh and measure your food with food scales, measuring spoons and cups. Better control of calories will result.

For a visual idea of portion sizes, visit www.CalorieKing.com. See examples (fries and cola) on this page.

Allow for Extra Calories in Packaged Food

The actual weight of packaged foods is usually 5-10% more than the label net weight (the minimum legal weight) - and in some cases up to 50% more. However, manufacturers calculate the calories based on the net weight. For actual calories, weigh the product and calculate the extra calories. **For extra details see www.CalorieKing.com**

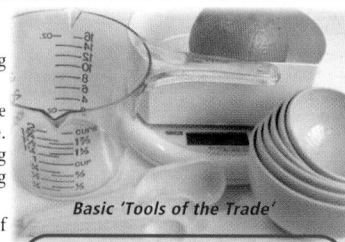

Basic 'Tools of the Trade'

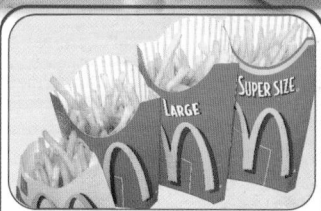

Fries

	Cal	Fat	Carb
Small	210	10	26
Medium	450	22	57
Large	540	26	68
Super Size	610	29	77

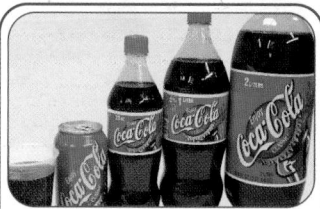

Cola

	Cal	Fat	Carb
8 fl.oz Cup	100	0	25
12 fl.oz Can	150	0	37
20 fl.oz Bottle	250	0	63
1 Liter Bottle	400	0	100
2 Liter Bottle	800	0	200

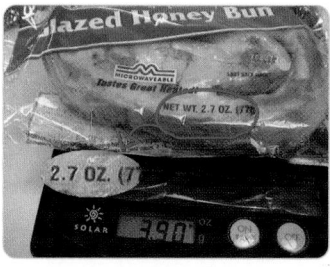

Fat Percentages Explained

Percent Fat Calories
(Percentage of Calories from Fat)

While health authorities recommend that not more than 30% of our total food calories should come from fat, it is not implied nor even recommended that you eat only those foods with less than 30% calories from fat.

Our normal diet is made up of foods that are either well above or below 30%. Only on average should the total diet be less than 30% calories from fat.

Some higher fat foods such as avocados, nuts and seeds, are highly nutritious and favor lower blood cholesterol levels. **Moderation is the aim . . . not elimination.**

Nevertheless, knowing the percentage of calories from fat can be useful in spotting high-fat foods and drinks.

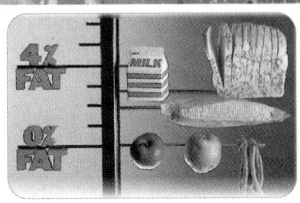

Fat Percentage Content
(Percentage of Fat in Food)

Don't be fooled by promotion of foods claiming to have a low percentage of fat. It's **serving size and total grams of fat that count.**

For example, whole milk with 3.5% fat sounds low (3.5g fat/100ml) but an 8fl.oz cup contains 8g fat (and 2 cups contain 16g fat).

Icecream with 10% fat seems high, yet a large scoop (3fl.oz) has only 5g fat. (Low-fat icecream has less than 2g fat/serve.)

❖   ❖   ❖

Also note that the percentage of fat in a food is not the same as the percentage of calories derived from fat.

Foods with a low percentage of fat can still have a high percentage of calories derived from fat - as shown below.

For example, around 50% of total calories in whole milk comes from fat - yet whole milk has less than 4% fat. Low fat/light milk with less than 1% fat has only 18% of total calories from fat - a much better choice.

FORMULA FOR CALCULATING PERCENTAGE CALORIES FROM FAT

$$\frac{\text{Grams of Fat/Serve} \times 9}{\text{Total Calories/Serve}} \times \frac{100}{1}$$

EXAMPLE:

Mars Bar (11g fat, 240 cals)

Percentage Calories from Fat

$$= \frac{11 \times 9}{265} \times \frac{100}{1} = 37\%$$

FAT CONTENT & PERCENTAGES OF MILK

	Whole Milk	Reduced Fat	Low-Fat (light)	Non-Fat Skim
Percentage Fat	3.5%	2%	1%	0%
Fat (Grams) in 8 fl.oz Cup	8g	5g	2g	0g
Calories	150	120	100	95
Percent Calories From Fat	48%	38%	18%	0%

Recommended Fat Intake

Americans consume too much fat with many having over 40% of total calories from fat - either as fat or oil, or as fat in foods and drinks. A range of 20-30% is healthier.

Fat Intake - Healthy Ranges

Children	30-60g
Teenagers (Active)	40-80g
Women	30-60g
Men: Active	40-80g
Heavy Activity/Athlete	80-120g

The chart below recommends maximum fat intake for different calorie levels.

MAXIMUM DESIRABLE FAT INTAKE (Daily)

Calories	Fat	% Fat Cals
1200 cals	30g fat	23%
1500 cals	40g fat	24%
1800 cals	50g fat	25%
2000 cals	60g fat	27%
2200 cals	70g fat	28%
2500 cals	80g fat	29%
2800 cals	90g fat	29%
3000 cals	100g fat	30%
3500 cals	117g fat	30%
4000 cals	135g fat	30%

Infants Fat Intake

Infants and toddlers under 3 years should not be restricted in their fat intake because much larger volumes of food would be required to guarantee adequate calorie intake and growth. Whole milk should be used rather than light milk (1%) or nonfat milk. Similarly, a high fiber diet is also not suitable for infants.

Calories Versus Fats

For successful weight control it is important to be aware of both fats and calories in foods. It widens your choices at the supermarket and when eating out.

While choosing more lowfat foods is wise, it does not guarantee that total calories will be reduced, particularly if portion size is not limited.

It is a mistake to think that eating lowfat or fat-free foods allows you to eat double the quantity.

Be aware that lowfat and fat-free cakes, cookies and ice cream are **not calorie-free.** Nor are soda drinks, fruit juices, beer, alcoholic spirits, sugar and sugar candy which are also fat-free. Bread, rice and pasta also have negligble fat.

Carbohydrate Calories Count

It is also a fallacy that carbohydrate calories don't count. Carbohydrates in excess of body needs can still be converted to and stored as body fat - particularly in women in their child-bearing years.

Total Calories Count!

Ultimately, it is food portion size and total calories that count whether from fat, carbohydrate or protein. Remember, cows get fat on grass!

FOOD LABEL MEANINGS
FDA Nutrition Claim Definitions
(All are on a Per Serving Basis.)

Low Calorie: 40 calories or less
Light or Lite: One third fewer calories or, 50% or less fat than regular product
Fat-Free: Less than half a gram of fat
Low-Fat: 3 grams or less of fat
Reduced-Fat: 25% less fat than regular product
Fewer or Less Calories: At least 25% fewer calories than regular product

Hints to Reduce Fat

Meats & Poultry

- **Choose lean cuts** of meat with little marbling. Choose the white meat of chicken and turkey, and extra lean ground beef.
- **Trim all visible fat** from meat and remove the skin from poultry. Removal of fat after cooking is okay (to prevent dryness).
- **Eat modest portions** (3-4 oz cooked weight) of meat, poultry or fish. **Add extra** beans, lentils, tofu, tempeh, vegetables, potatoes, rice, pasta, bread, or tortillas.
- **Avoid high-fat meat products** such as salami, bacon, sausage and franks. Choose lowfat and fat-free brands. Choose lean luncheon meats (90% or more fat-free).
- **Broil or bake. Avoid frying.** Allow casseroles to cool and skim off surface fat.

Fish & Seafood

- **Choose fresh or frozen fillets**, and canned fish (in water pack).
- **Avoid fried fish**, frozen fish in batter, canned fish in oil.

Fats & Oils

- **Use minimal amounts** of all types of fat and oil. All are high in calories.
- **Choose** 'light' and 'reduced fat' spreads but still use sparingly. Check the Fats and Spreads section of this book for lower fat brands.
- **Use** minimal amounts of oil when stir-frying. Use no-stick sprays like *Pam*.

Salad Dressings & Sauces

- **Avoid regular mayonnaise and oil dressings.** Choose 'light', 'reduced fat' or 'fat-free' brands (Check salad dressings section of this book).
- **Choose** lowfat or fat-free sauces. Most tomato-based pasta sauces are lowfat but avoid 'pesto', 'alfredo', cheese and 'creamy' sauces.

Milk, Dairy, Soy Drinks

- **Choose** lowfat or skim milks and yogurts. **Avoid** full-cream milk, cream, *Half & Half* coffee creamers.
- **Soy Drinks:** Choose lowfat brands.
- **Cheese:** Choose fat-free, lowfat and fat-reduced (e.g. cottage, part-skim ricotta). Cheese substitutes can still be high in fat.
- **Icecream:** Choose lowfat and fat-free brands, frozen yogurt, sorbet, sherbet and ices. Limit regular icecream to a small serving. Avoid rich high-fat icecreams.

Frozen Meals & Entrees

- **Choose lowfat varieties** such as *Lean Cuisine, Healthy Choice* and *Weight Watchers*. Add extra vegetables.

Soups

- **Choose lowfat brands.** Avoid high-fat ramen noodle blocks/soup.

FRYING ADDS FAT!

The greater the surface area of potato exposed to fat or oil, the higher the fat content.

Whole Potato (3 oz)
Nil Fat, 65 Cals

Roast Potato (3 oz)
5g Fat, 155 Cals
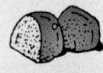

Fries (Large, 3 oz)
12g Fat, 220 Cals
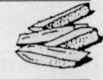

Fries (Small, 3 oz)
15g Fat, 265 Cals
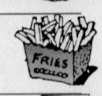

Potato Chips (3 oz)
30g Fat, 450 Cals

Bread, Bagels, Crackers

- **All breads are suitable** as well as pita, bagels, English muffins and rice cakes. Avoid croissants, sweet rolls, danish pastry and doughnuts. **Avoid** fat-soaked toast and garlic bread.
- **Choose lowfat crackers** such as graham, saltines, matzo, bread sticks, crispbreads. **Avoid** regular cheese or butter crackers.

Cereals, Pasta, Noodles, Rice

- Most cold and hot cereals are low in fat and nil in cholesterol. Avoid granola made with hydrogenated oils.
- **Choose** plain pasta or rice. Avoid dishes made with cream, butter or cheese sauces. **Avoid** high-fat ramen noodle blocks/soups.

Fruits & Vegetables

- **Choose all types.** (Note: Avocados contain no cholesterol. Their fat and fiber can help lower blood cholesterol). Use mashed avocado on bread in place of fat.
- **Choose** dried beans, lentils, chick peas, baked beans.
- **Avoid** french-fried potatoes and regular potato salad. Avoid vegetables made in butter, cream or sauce.
- **Avoid** deli-style salads made with high fat dressings. Choose lowfat brands. Use lowfat and fat-free salad dressings.

Snacks, Cookies, Candy

- **Avoid** high-fat snacks such as potato chips, corn/tortilla chips, cheesy balls, buttered popcorn, chocolate and carob bars.
- **Choose** fat-free potato chips and tortilla chips made with *olestra* (such as *Wow!* brand) but still limit quantity.
- **Choose** plain popcorn, lowfat cookies and muffins, hard candy, jelly beans, fruit rolls and frozen fruit bars and popsicles.
- **Choose** fresh and dried fruits, vegetables. Limit nuts and seeds if overweight.

Desserts/Sweets

- **Avoid high-fat desserts**, such as fruit pies, pastries, cheesecake, cheese board.
- **Choose** fresh fruits, fresh fruit salad, lowfat custard and lowfat yogurt. Use yogurt in place of cream or ice cream.
- **Avoid** regular icecream. *Choose* lowfat brands but still limit quantity.
- **Choose** sugar-free gelatin desserts such as *Jell-O* (sugar-free package).

Fast-Foods & Take-Out

Check the Fast-Foods Section of this book for actual fat counts and wise selections.

- **Delis:** Choose sandwiches/bread rolls, pitas with lowfat fillings and plain salad. Limit meat/cheese to small portions. Request half quantities.
- **Avoid high-fat deli salads.** Choose plain salads and add your own lowfat dressing. Eat more fruit.
- **Chicken & Fish:** Avoid deep-fried chicken or fish, BBQ chicken with fat or skin, chicken nuggets. Choose broiled or baked chicken breast without fat or skin.
- **Hamburgers:** Choose medium size, lower fat burgers. Avoid bacon. Have a side salad (without dressing).
- **Pizzas:** Avoid sausage/pepperoni. Choose vegetarian topping and modest quantity of cheese. Eat a moderate serving. Eat extra salad and fruit.
- **Desserts:** Avoid apple pie, danish, choc chip cookies. Choose lowfat muffins (e.g. *McDonald's*), fresh fruit or fruit salad.
- **Avoid regular shakes and sundaes.** Choose lowfat milk, lower fat shakes (such as *McDonald's*), and orange juice, but choose smaller sizes.

Hints to Reduce Sugar

- While reducing the amount of fat is an important dietary focus for weight control, sugar intake also needs to be watched.

- Most overweight, inactive persons consume over 500 calories of refined sugars per day (equivalent to over 30 level teaspoons) - a significant amount in weight control terms. Halving this amount would be reasonable and worthwhile.

Note: Naturally occurring sugars in fruits, vegetables and milk are fine when consumed in normal recommended amounts.

- Most sugar in our diet is 'hidden' in processed foods such as soft drinks, fruit drinks, candy, cookies, cake, jam, sauces, icecream, desserts, canned foods, and breakfast cereals.

Certainly enjoy moderate quantities of these foods, but for serious weight control, look for 'low calorie', 'diet' or sugar-free alternatives. Be careful not to substitute sugar-rich foods with high-fat foods which might boost calories even more!

- Sweeteners such as *DiabetiSweet*, *Equal*, *NutraSweet*, *Splenda*, *Sweet'n Low* and *Stevia* make it easy to reduce sugar in drinks and recipes. (Most recipes can be adapted to contain less sugar with little effect on taste or quality.)

- The body can obtain sufficient sugar for its needs from carbohydrate-rich foods such as bread, rice, spaghetti and other pasta, potatoes, corn, fruit, vegetables, beans, nuts, seeds and lactose in milk.

These foods are also rich in other nutrients. Refined sugar is referred to as 'empty calorie' because it supplies calories but negligible nutrients and no fiber.

DIFFERENT FORMS OF SUGAR

Be aware that sugar comes in different forms. Check the label.

- Sugar
- Brown Sugar
- Dextrose
- Fructose
- Corn Syrup
- Honey
- Maple Syrup
- Sucrose
- Confectioners' Sugar
- Glucose
- Malt, Maltose
- High-Fructose Corn Syrup
- Molasses
- Turbinado Sugar

SUGAR CONTENT OF SOME COMMON FOODS

	Teaspoons of Sugar
Coca Cola or *Pepsi*, 12 oz	10
20 oz size	17
Iced tea, sweetened, 12 oz	8
Choc malted Milk, 12 oz	4.5
Honey Smacks Cereal, 1 oz	4
Popcorn, caramel, 1 cup	3.5
Chocolate Bar, 1.5 oz	6
M&M's, 1.7 oz pkg	7
Cake, sponge, jam-filled	8
Choc Chip Cookie, 1 oz	2
Donut, iced	6
Apple Pie, 1 piece	7
Jell-O, 1/2 cup	4.5
Jam, 1 Tbsp, 20g	2.5
Syrup, maple, 1 Tbsp	3

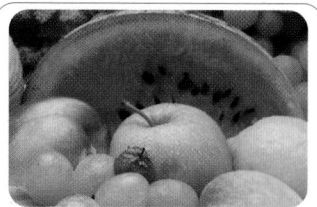

Reach for fresh fruit when you want to snack instead of candy or snack products rich in sugar and fat.

Sample Diet Plan - 1200 Calories

For Overweight Persons. Please Check With Your Doctor.
(Menu contains approximately 30-35 Grams Fat)

 Breakfast (approx. 250 cal)
1 Small Fruit or 1/2 oz Dried Fruit

Plus Cereal: 1 1/2 oz Dry (high fiber)
or 1 cup cooked Oatmeal

Plus Milk (from daily allowance)

 Breakfast ~ Choice 2
1 Small Fruit

Plus 1 Toast (no added fat)

or 3/4 oz Cheese
or 2 oz Cottage Cheese
or 1/4 cup Baked Beans

Plus 1 Toast or 1/2 Muffin (English)

Milk Allowance (160 calories)
2 cups Skim Milk or 1 1/2 cups LowFat Milk
or equivalent Soy Drink, Yogurt, Cheese, Tofu

Fat Allowance (140 calories; 15g Fat)
4 tsp Fat or 6-8 tsp Diet Margarine or 3 tsp Oil
or 1 1/2 Tbsp Mayonnaise or 1/2 medium Avocado
or 1 1/2 Tbsp Peanut Butter or 30g Nuts/Seeds

 Lunch (approx. 440 calories)
2 slices Bread (2 oz) or 1 medium Roll or Bagel
or 4 Crispbreads/Crackers or 6" Pita

Plus 2 oz lean Meat, Chicken or Turkey
or 3 1/2 oz Tuna (in water) or 2 1/2 oz Salmon
or 1 oz Cheese or 3 oz Cottage Cheese
or 2 1/2 oz Ricotta Cheese
or 1/2 cup, 4 oz Fruit Yogurt (lowfat)
or 1/2 cup (4 oz) Baked Beans or Bean Salad

Plus Large Salad (Oil-free dressing)
Plus 1 small Fruit or 1/2 oz Dried Fruit

 Dinner (approx. 360 Calories)
Soup (fat-free)

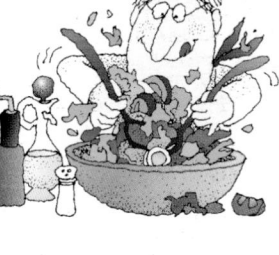

Plus 3 oz lean Meat (cooked weight)
or 4 oz Chicken Breast (no skin)
or 3 oz Chicken Thigh/Leg (no skin)
or 5 oz Fish (grilled, no fat)
or 3/4 cup (6 oz) Beans (Soy, Baked, Haricot etc)/Lentils
or LowFat Recipe Dish (e.g. Lean Cuisine)

Plus 1 small Potato or 1/2 cup Rice/Pasta or 1 slice Bread
Plus 2-3 servings Vegetables/Salad
Plus 1 small Fruit + Diet Gelatin Dessert

 Between Meals: Water, Coffee, Tea, Diet drinks,
Fruit from main meals; Raw vegetable pieces, Milk from Allowance
Note: Take a multivitamin/mineral supplement daily while dieting.

Reshape Eating Behaviors

- Persons who exercise regularly **lose more weight** and keep it off longer than non-exercisers.

- Exercise also improves general health and well-being. **Mood, confidence and self-esteem** are enhanced by a sense of control and accomplishment.

- **Exercise increases the metabolic rate** of the body even for hours after exercise - a good way to 'wake up' a sluggish metabolism and burn extra fat.

  Exercise compensates for any decrease in metabolic rate with increasing age and also in some heavy smokers who stop smoking.

- **Strength training** further builds muscle and aids body reshaping. You can also eat more food!

Note: It is muscle which burns fat. Each extra pound of muscle burns an extra 100 calories daily ~ even while you sleep! Weight from exercised muscles is okay. It is surplus fat that is potentially harmful.

- **Avoid injury** by beginning with walking, low impact aerobics, or weight-supported exercise (e.g. swimming, cycling). Avoid competitive sports.

- **How Much?** Start with 10 - 20 minutes/day and progress to 30-45minutes/day - even if broken into 5-10 minute lots. It all adds up! **Aim to achieve 250-500 calories of exercise daily.**

  Also walk up stairs instead of using lifts. Take a brisk walk at lunch. Use an exercise bike, treadmill or stair machine while watching TV.

- **How Often?** While aerobic fitness requires only 3 - 4 sessions weekly, **weight control is a daily event which requires daily exercise.**

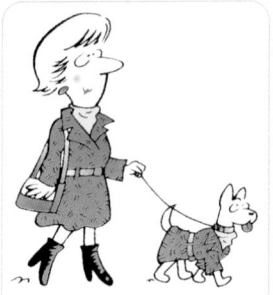

Brisk walking each day is a safe and effective way to keep trim and fit. Try it - you'll like it!"

Strength-training with light weights helps to retain or rebuild muscle tissue and enhances weight control.

TV CAN BE FATTENING!

Many adults and children watch over 20 hours of television per week and indulge in high-fat snacks at the same time - potent contributors to obesity.

Are you a TV couch potato? Limit your TV hours and plan healthy physical activities. At least use an exercise bike or treadmill while watching TV!

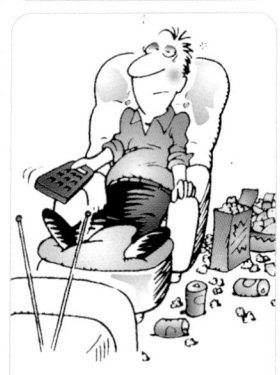

Middle-age spread has little to do with getting older. Too little exercise is the main culprit.

Daily exercise and sensible eating can minimize middle-age spread.

LIGHT	MODERATE	HEAVY
4 Calories/Minute	**7 Calories/Minute**	**10 Calories/Minute**
Walking, slow	Walking, brisk	Walking (power), Jogging
Cycling, light	Cycling, moderate	Cycling (vigorous), Spinning
Gardening light	Swimming, crawl	Swimming, strenuous
Golf, social	Weight-training, light	Weight-training, heavy
Tennis, doubles	Tennis, singles	Wrestling/Judo, advanced
Housework, cleaning	Racquetball, beginners	Racquetball, advanced
Callisthenics, Yoga	Aerobics, light	Tae Bo, Kick Boxing
Ten Pin Bowls	Football, Grid Iron	Football, training
Ping-pong, social	Basketball, Baseball	Basketball (Pro)
Ice Skating	Walking Downstairs	Climbing Stairs, Skipping
Aquarobics	Snow Skiing (downhill)	Skiing (cross country)
Skate Boarding	Shoveling snow	Aquarobics, advanced
Line/Square Dancing	Dancing (vigorous)	Dancing (strenuous), Zumba

Note: Only those sports or activities that are sustained over a period of time (e.g running) qualify for heavy exercise. Stop-start sports such as tennis are considered 'moderate'.

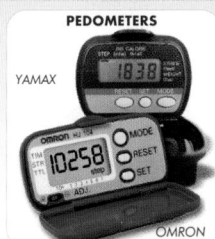

PEDOMETERS

YAMAX

OMRON

10,000 STEPS PER DAY

A pedometer can motivate you to be more active every day.

Different models count steps, miles and even calories used. It clips to your belt or waist band and registers each step.

Aim for 8,000 - 10,000 steps per day, instead of an average of only 3,000 - 4,000 steps.

Extra information: www.CalorieKing.com
Ordering Details ~ Page 287

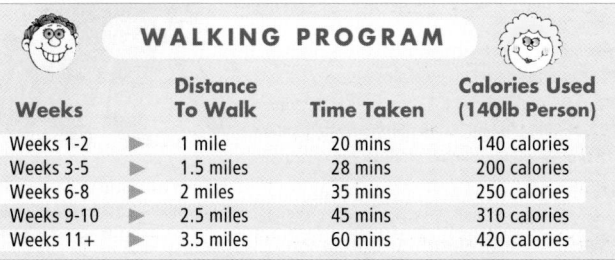

WALKING PROGRAM

Weeks	Distance To Walk	Time Taken	Calories Used (140lb Person)
Weeks 1-2 ▶	1 mile	20 mins	140 calories
Weeks 3-5 ▶	1.5 miles	28 mins	200 calories
Weeks 6-8 ▶	2 miles	35 mins	250 calories
Weeks 9-10 ▶	2.5 miles	45 mins	310 calories
Weeks 11+ ▶	3.5 miles	60 mins	420 calories

Reshaping Eating Behaviors

- Eating is a behavior that is largely controlled by people with whom we live or socialize, places in which we carry out our lives, and our emotions. Become aware of those situations that commonly lead to extra food being eaten.

- We may also be unaware of 'bad' eating habits that can lead to excess calorie intake; e.g. eating quickly, large mouthsful, eating when tense or bored, finishing a large serving of food when not hungry.

Hints to help uncover and correct those 'bad' eating habits include:

- **Don't eat while engaged in other activities;** for example, watching TV, reading. Eat only at the table, not at the fridge or while standing.

- **Don't eat quickly.** Chewing slowly allows time to register a feeling of fullness. Don't use fingers, only utensils. Cut food into smaller pieces. Don't load your fork until the previous mouthful is finished.

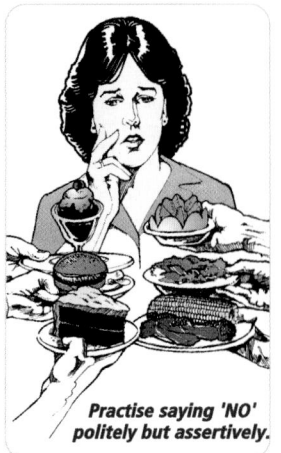

Practise saying 'NO' politely but assertively.

- **Don't purchase problem high calorie foods.** Shop from a set list to prevent impulse buying. Avoid shopping with children.

- **Buy snack foods** in the smallest package. The larger the serving size or package, the more you are likely to eat or drink.

- **Plan meals in advance.** Stick to a set menu.

- **Plan a strategy to avoid uncontrolled eating** and drinking at social events, or when your emotions urge you to binge.

  Rehearse repeatedly in your mind exactly what you will do in such situations. Remind yourself several times each day that you are in charge of your actions and that you can be strong-willed. Seek counseling or coaching on various strategies.

- **Promise yourself** that when you feel the urge to snack, you will engage in some activity that will distract you away from food (e.g. go for a walk, brush your teeth, phone a friend.)

  If you eat out of boredom, find some new hobby or interest that gets you out of the house. Even enrol in an adult education class.

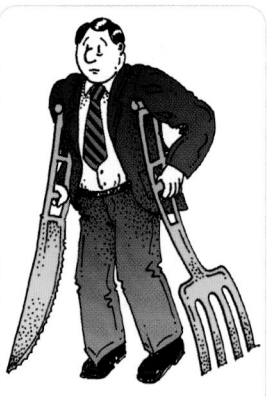

Do you use food as an emotional crutch? If so, professional counseling may be helpful.

The Value of a Food Diary

The food diary is the most powerful proven aid for dieters. Persons who keep a food and exercise diary not only lose more weight they also keep it off. Here are some of the reasons:

- Recording your eating and exercise habits jolts you into realizing just what you do eat and drink each day; and also whether you exercise sufficiently.

- **Helps you identify problem foods** and drinks with excessive calories and fat.

- **Helps identify moods**, situations and events that lead to excessive eating of unwanted calories. You can then plan to overcome or avoid them.

- **Prevents 'calorie amnesia'**, the forgetfulness that leads to rebound weight gain after successful weight loss. Recording puts you back on the right track.

- **Helps you develop greater self- discipline.** You will think twice about over indulging if you have to record it - especially if someone checks your diary regularly. It certainly keeps you honest!

- **Motivates you** to carefully plan your meals and to exercise each day.

- **Serves as a check system** for your doctor, dietitian or counselor to assess your progress and make recommendations.

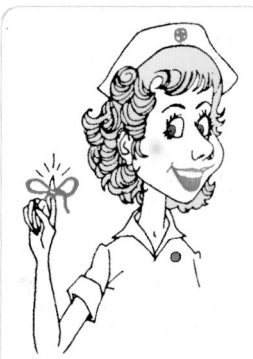

"Keeping a diary gives me feedback on exactly what I eat each day.
It helps prevent 'calorie amnesia' and reminds me to exercise each day.
It's a must for successful weight control!"

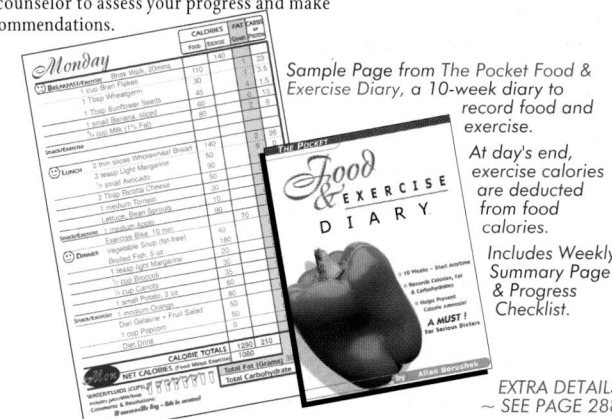

Sample Page from The Pocket Food & Exercise Diary, a 10-week diary to record food and exercise.

At day's end, exercise calories are deducted from food calories.

Includes Weekly Summary Page & Progress Checklist.

EXTRA DETAILS ~ SEE PAGE 288

Diabetes Guide

What is Diabetes?

Diabetes is a disorder in which the body cannot make proper use of carbohydrates (sugar and starches).

- After digestion, sugar and starches are changed into **glucose** - the simplest form of sugar that is vital to body cells for energy and growth.

- **Insulin** is the hormone which acts like a key that opens the door to body cells and allows glucose to enter.

- **Without sufficient insulin**, unused glucose builds up in the blood and passes into the urine. This produces symptoms of frequent urination, continual thirst and tiredness.

- **Untreated diabetes** increases the risk of damage to nerves and blood vessels. This, in turn, increases the risk of heart disease, stroke, blindness, kidney damage, foot ulcers and gangrene, impotence and other complications.

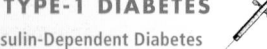

*Insulin acts like a key.
It opens the door to body cells
and allows glucose to enter.*

Some persons with diabetes (Type 1) have too few or no keys and require insulin injections.

Others (Type 2) have ample keys but 'mis-shapen' key holes (insulin resistant) - particularly if obese and inactive.

TYPE-1 DIABETES

Insulin-Dependent Diabetes

- Occurs in 10% of diabetes cases.

- Usually children and young adults.

- Pancreas gland produces little or no insulin. Daily insulin injections are necessary, plus:

- Regular meals with even carbohydrate distribution to match insulin dosage. Regular exercise and weight control are also important.

WARNING SIGNALS

- Frequent urination
- Continual thirst
- Rapid weight loss
- Unusual hunger
- Extreme weakness/fatigue
- Nausea, vomiting, irritability

TYPE-2 DIABETES

Non-Insulin Dependent

- Occurs in 90% of diabetes cases.

- Occurs mainly in adults - particularly in overweight and inactive persons.

- Insulin is produced but body cells resist its action and glucose cannot enter cells.

- Usually treated with diet and exercise. Sometimes requires medication (pills or insulin injections).

WARNING SIGNALS

- Any Type-1 symptom
- Blurred vision
- Excessive itching
- Skin infections with slow healing
- Tingling/numbness in feet

Importance of Weight Control

- **Type-2 diabetes** occurs 2-3 times more often in overweight persons - particularly if inactive.

- Such persons do not usually lack insulin. Rather, their insulin is less effective. As obesity develops, muscle and other body cells may resist insulin in varying degrees. The resultant build-up of blood glucose may lead to diabetic symptoms.

- **Weight loss alone** often corrects this condition in Type-2 diabetes. If overweight, try a moderate diet of 1200-1500 calories **plus daily exercise**.

Within several weeks, body cells can lose their resistance and become sensitive once again to the effects of insulin. Insulin and blood glucose levels may normalise, and symptoms may disappear.

Further, the need for oral antidiabetic drugs might be prevented or much lessened in dosage. **So, give diet and exercise a fair go** - and maintain them to keep symptoms under control.

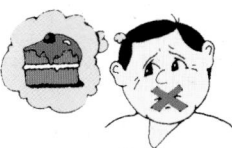

Modest weight loss and daily exercise can greatly improve control of Type-2 diabetes.

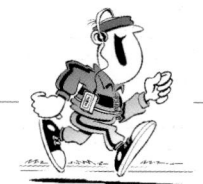

Get Moving! Everyday, do at least 30 minutes of moderate intensity exercise. It's the key to improving insulin sensitivity.

Add strength-training 3-4 times a week to double the benefits.

Managing Diabetes

Don't battle diabetes alone. Establish a partnership with your doctor, dietitian, nurse educator and pharmacist. For extra support, contact the *American Diabetes Association* 1-800-342-2383.

Hints to keep blood glucose within safe limits:

- **Control your diet.** Know what and when you will eat. Seek referral to a dietitian for expert advice.

- **Exercise regularly.** It assists weight control and can improve sensitivity of body cells to insulin. Plan exercise into your daily routine.

- **Monitor your blood glucose** at home and work - ideally with a portable blood glucose meter. It will help you become familiar with your blood glucose patterns, and the effects of diet, exercise and medication. **Insulin pumps** can also help control blood glucose levels around the clock.

- **Don't skip prescribed insulin or oral medication.** If on insulin, know what action to take if hypoglycaemia (low blood glucose) occurs. Also educate family and friends.

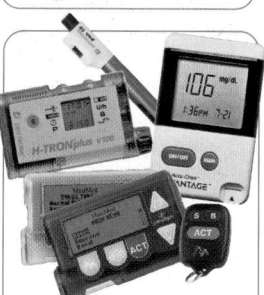

Blood glucose meters, insulin pumps and pens can greatly improve control of diabetes and lifestyle choices.

Diabetes ~ Diet Hints

Guidelines for choosing a healthy diet apply equally to persons with or without diabetes. Eating a wide variety of foods with the emphasis on low-fat, high fiber and low in refined sugars, is recommended.

However, actual food quantities, as well as when you eat, will also influence control of blood glucose. Your dietitian will individualize a diet plan to suit your food preferences, lifestyle and medical status. Here are a few hints:

- **Maintain a healthy weight.** If overweight, even a modest weight loss plus daily exercise can help to normalise blood glucose in Type-2 diabetes.

- **Don't skip meals.** If you take insulin or an oral hypoglycemic agent, regular meals are important.

- **If on insulin**, eat meals at the same time each day. Eat a similar amount of food at each meal. An even distribution of carbohydrate over the day will make best use of the available insulin and prevent wide fluctuations in blood glucose levels. Leave an interval of about 30 minutes between insulin injection and breakfast.

- **Avoid sugars and foods high in added sugar** particularly if overweight. Small amounts of sugar as part of a meal may occasionally be okay. Check with your dietitian. Use *Equal*, *Splenda* and *NutraSweet*-sweetened foods and drinks.

- **Choose wholegrain breads, cereals and pasta.** Eat fresh fruits, vegetables and legumes. These foods contain more fiber and slow the release of glucose into your blood after a meal.

- **Limit foods high in saturated fat and cholesterol.** Enjoy fish, soy foods, and other foods rich in omega-3 fats. *(See Fats & Cholesterol Guide, Pages 251-255)*

- **Foods (and supplements) rich in antioxidant vitamins** C, E and beta-carotene, as well as omega-3 fats, magnesium, zinc and chromium may help prevent long-term complications of diabetes (such as damage to small blood vessels and nerves). Be sure to check with your doctor.

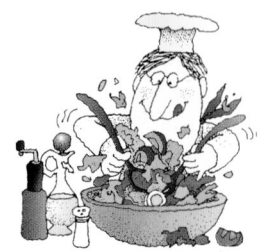

Eat a well-balanced diet, high in fiber-containing foods and low in fat.

NEW BLOOD SUGAR LEVEL FOR DIAGNOSING DIABETES
(Adopted by American Diabetes Assoc.)

Blood Sugar Levels
Previously: 140 mg/dL
New: 126 mg/dL

Everyone 45 and older should have a blood test every 3 years.

Excess Alcohol contributes to obesity, diabetes, and high blood pressure.

The risk of hypoglycemia (low blood sugar) and drug interactions with alcohol is also increased.

Carbohydrates & Diabetes

- Carbohydrate foods in their more natural forms are an important part of a healthy diet. They provide energy, fiber, vitamins, minerals, protein and water.

  Carbohydrates are found mainly in cereal grains, fruit, vegetables and milk. Animal flesh foods contain negligible amounts. A healthy diet of at least 2000 calories is based around carbohydrate foods and should provide over 50% of total calories - whether or not we have diabetes. Lower calorie diets for weight control will have as little as 40% carbohydrate calories.

- Carbohydrates include sugars, starches and fibers. Sugars and starch provide energy to body cells. Even though fiber is not digested, it benefits the body - more so in diabetes. *(See Fiber Guide ~ Page 262)*

  The **various forms of carbohydrate** affect blood glucose levels in different ways; and it is difficult to predict the effect of particular foods, sugars or meals, simply by their actual carbohydrate content. Thus, the **same amount** of carbohydrate from different foods may affect blood sugar differently. It depends on many factors.

  For example, fiber can slow digestion and absorption of sugars by acting as a physical barrier or by forming a gel. Both fiber and fat also slow the emptying rate of the stomach into the intestines where further digestion and absorption takes place. The physical form of food (solid, puree, liquid) also matters - the more natural the better.

  Generally, raw foods rather than cooked foods, and whole-foods rather than ground-up foods, are more slowly absorbed.

- **Sugar: Small amounts** eaten as part of a meal, may not adversely affect blood glucose in persons with good blood glucose control. Nevertheless, minimal amounts of sugar are encouraged for nutritional and weight control reasons.

Glycemic Index

- Glycemic index (GI) indicates how fast a carbohydrate-containing food is digested and how much it causes blood glucose to rise (glycemic response).

Slower Acting Carbohydrates

These foods are more slowly digested and absorbed. They help maintain more even blood glucose levels. Use these foods regularly but still limit quantities for weight control. Examples:

- Dried beans, peas, lentils
- Nuts and seeds
- Wholegrain breads, pita
- Bran cereals, oats
- Barley, buckwheat, bulgur
- Spaghetti, pasta, Basmati Rice
- Fresh fruit: apples, avocados, bananas (firm), cherries, grapefruit, grapes, olives, oranges, peaches, pears, plums
- Vegetables: sweet corn, yam
- Milk, yogurt, soy drinks

Quicker Acting Carbohydrates

These foods more rapidly raise blood glucose levels. Eat in moderation.

- White bread, rice cakes, bagels, croissants, doughnuts
- Low fiber cereals: Cornflakes, *Rice Krispies, Froot Loops*
- White potato, white rice
- Watermelon, ripe bananas, cantaloupe, pineapple
- Glucose drinks and candy

(See Carbohydrate Distribution next page)

Diabetes & Carbohydrate Distribution

- **For people with diabetes**, regular meals with even distribution of carbohydrate over the day are important for good control of blood sugar levels.
- **Smaller amounts of food** eaten more frequently result in steadier, more even blood glucose levels. (Be sure to control your weight.)

Recommended daily eating patterns for good blood glucose control:

1. **Three Meals & Three Snacks ~**
   Best for persons on insulin (Type-1 diabetes) with normal blood glucose variations.

2. **Three Meals ~**
   Best for Type-2 diabetes (especially if overweight).

Note: If blood sugar levels show excessive variations see doctor and dietitian.

- **Your doctor or dietitian** will select the level of calories and carbohydrate most appropriate to your weight, medication and activity. (Regular blood glucose checks will provide feedback on the level of control.)

- **Amounts of carbohydrate** in the guide below provide an average of 50% of total calories. **A rough rule of thumb is:** 13 grams of carbohydrate per 100 calories.

At calorie levels above 2000, carbohydrates approach 50-60% of total calories.

At lower calorie levels used for weight loss (1200-1500 calories), carbohydrates account for as little as 40% of total calories. This is because protein has nutritional priority.

These carbohydrate quantities (and percentages) apply equally to persons with or without diabetes.

IDEAL CARBOHYDRATE DISTRIBUTION
For Type-1 Diabetes (Insulin Dependent)

3 MEALS & 3 SNACKS
Balanced Blood Sugar Levels

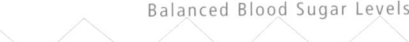

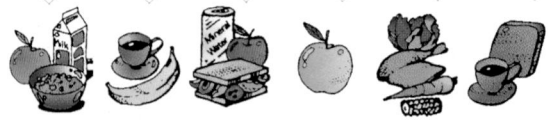

GUIDE TO CARBOHYDRATE DISTRIBUTION

Daily Total Calories		Daily Total Carbohyd.	Percent Carbohyd. Cals	Each Main Meal (3)	Between Meals (3)
1200 Cals	~	120g	40%	30g	10g
1500 Cals	~	170g	45%	40g	15g
2000 Cals	~	250g	50%	60g	25g
2500 Cals	~	345g	55%	70g	45g
3000 Cals	~	450g	60%	90g	60g

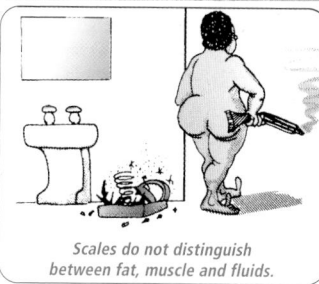

Scales do not distinguish between fat, muscle and fluids.

Body Fluid Changes

Body weight fluctuates from day to day. This is mainly due to changes in body fluids which make up around 70% of total body weight. It can be affected by changes in hormone levels, dietary factors such as salt and carbohydrate, and even exercise.

Weight change over several weeks is more likely to reflect changes in levels of fat and muscle rather than fluid. Unfortunately, the scales do not distinguish between weight changes due to water, fat or muscle. This is why we shouldn't allow every fluctuation in weight to rule our lives.

To limit fluid retention, avoid salty foods and go easy on the salt shaker. Eating sufficient fruit and vegetables supplies extra potassium which counteracts sodium and encourages fluid loss. However, do not limit water intake. Be sure to drink at least 6-8 glasses of water and other fluids per day.

When dining out, be aware that the extra pound or two that might show on the scales the next morning is not the result of a small dietary indiscretion. It is more likely due to fluid retention resulting from more highly seasoned and salty food.

Monthly hormonal changes in women can also account for a build-up of fluids of several pounds prior to menstruation.

Menopausal Weight Gains

Most women gain an average of 4-5 pounds in the years leading up to the menopause - usually in their middle to late 40's. This can occur even when exercise and eating habits have not changed significantly.

With hormonal changes occurring at that time, body fat also tends to be redistributed from thighs, buttocks and hips to the breast and stomach areas (a greater health risk).

Be sure to eat wisely and continue daily physical activity including strength-training to maintain or build muscles - and to boost metabolism and self-esteem.

Underactive Thyroid

Thyroid hormone is secreted into the bloodstream by the thyroid gland in the neck. When insufficient thyroid hormone is made, metabolism and body processes slow down and weight gain can occur.

Symptoms of hypothyroidism can be subtle and easily overlooked as signs of normal aging. Early symptoms may include fatigue, muscle weakness, sluggishness, a swollen tongue that you keep biting, and a puffy face. As metabolism continues to slow, further signs can include chronically cold hands and feet, slow reflexes, constipation, dry skin and coarse hair, brittle nails, heavy menstrual periods, slower pulse, and a husky voice. Depression-like symptoms may also develop such as forgetfulness, loss of interest, mood swings and irritability.

Weight gains of as much as 10-20 pounds (mainly fluid) can occur, as well as a raised blood cholesterol level.

The condition is more common in women, especially following pregnancy, around menopause, or after age 60.

A simple blood test through your doctor can detect hypothyroidism. It is easily treated in most cases with thyroid hormone pills.

Adults 35 and older should have a TSH (thyroid stimulating hormone) test every 5 years. Testing when pregnant is also wise.

Notes, Abbreviations, Measures

- Calorie and fat values have been rounded off.
  Calories - to the nearest 5 or 10 calories.
  Fat - to the nearest half gram.
  Note: Trace amounts of fat (less than 0.3 grams per serving) have been treated as zero.

- Because manufacturer's figures on labels are rounded off, figures in this book may differ slightly from the label. Serving sizes may also vary.

- Food product formulations change from time to time, and hence the need to regularly update this type of publication. Many products also come and go. Check the food label for any changes.

- **Seek Professional Advice:** This book is intended for educational purposes only. It is not a substitute for professional advice.

- **Feedback Welcome:** Please contact the author directly with your queries, and suggestions for foods to be included in future editions.

  Write to: Allan Borushek (Dietitian)
  PO Box 1616, Costa Mesa CA 92628
  Email: allan@calorieking.com

- **Free Information Service:** Check the author's website for new food product updates.

  www.calorieking.com

C ~ **Calories**
F ~ **Fat (grams)**
Cb ~ **Carbohydrate (grams)**

Abbreviations

tsp	= teaspoon
Tbsp	= Tablespoon
oz	= ounce(s)
c	= cup
fl.oz	= fluid ounce(s)
g	= gram(s)
<1	= less than 1

Volume Measures

3 tsp	= 1 Tbsp
2 Tbsp	= 1 fl.oz
½ cup	= 4 fl.oz
1 cup	= 8 fl.oz or 16 Tbsp
2 cups	= 1 Pint
2 Pints	= 1 Quart

(All measures are level)

Note: 8 oz weight is not the same as 8 fl.oz volume (space occupied). Dense foods weigh more per set volume. Examples:
1 cup popcorn weighs ½ oz
1 cup milk weighs 8½ oz
1 cup pudding weighs 10 oz

Metric Conversion

½ oz	= 14 grams
1 oz	= 28.4 grams
2 oz	= 57 grams
3½ oz	= 100 grams
1 fl.oz	= 30 mls
1 cup (8 fl.oz)	= 240 mls
33 fl.oz	= 1 liter (volume)

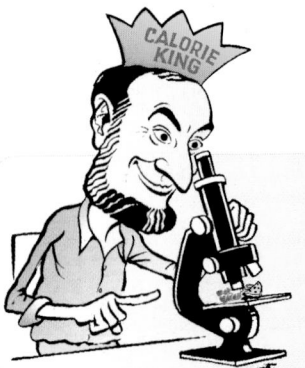

SOURCES OF INFORMATION

- U.S. Dept. of Agriculture
- Food Manufacturers
- Food Industry Boards & Councils
- Independent laboratory analysis
- Scientific publications
- Overseas food composition tables
- Author extrapolations

Quick Guide   **C**   **F**   **Cb**

Cow Milk
Average All Brands

Whole (3.5% fat):

	C	F	Cb
2 Tbsp, 1 fl.oz	20	1	1.5
1 Glass, 6 fl.oz	110	6	8.5
1 Cup, 8 fl.oz	150	8	12
1 Pint, 16 fl.oz	300	16	23
1 Quart, 946 ml	600	32	46

Reduced-fat (2% fat):

2 Tbsp, 1 fl.oz	15	0.5	1.5
1 Glass, 6 fl.oz	90	4	8.5
1 Cup, 8 fl.oz	130	5	13
1 Pint, 16 fl.oz	260	10	26
1 Quart, 946 ml	520	20	52

Light/Lowfat (1% fat):

2 Tbsp, 1 fl.oz	12	0.3	1.5
1 Glass, 6 fl.oz	75	2	8.5
1 Cup, 8 fl.oz	120	2.5	14
1 Pint, 16 fl.oz	240	5	28
1 Quart, 946 ml	480	10	56

Fat Free/Skim:

2 Tbsp, 1 fl.oz	10	0	1.5
1 Cup, 8 fl.oz	90	0.5	13
1 Pint, 16 fl.oz	180	1	26
w. Replace (Oatrim Fiber): 1 cup	85	0	12

Protein-Fortified:

2% fat, 1 cup	140	5	14
1% fat, 1 cup	120	3	14
Skim, 1 cup	100	0.5	14

Acidophilus: *Average All Brands*

Reduced Fat (2%), 1 cup	130	5	13
Lowfat (1%), 1 cup	100	2	13

Buttermilk: *Average All Brands*

Reduced Fat (2%), 1 cup	120	5	10
Low Fat (1%), 1 cup	100	2.5	12
Oak Farms (1%), 1 cup	100	2.5	12

Lactose-Reduced:

Reduced Fat: *Lactaid*, 1 cup	130	5	12
Dairy Ease 100, 1 cup	130	5	12
Lowfat, *Lactaid*, 1 cup	110	2.5	13
Fat Free *Lactaid/Lucerne*, 1 cup	80	0	13

Soy & Non-Dairy Drinks
~ See Page 25 ~

Goat/Sheep Milk, Kefir

Goat's Milk *(Meyenberg):*

	C	F	Cb
Whole, 1 cup, 8 fl.oz	140	7	11
Light/Lowfat (1%), 8 fl.oz	90	2.5	9
Evaporated, reconst., 8 fl.oz	145	8	11
Kefir: *Alta Dena*, 1 cup, 8 fl.oz	240	4.5	41
Nancy's, fruit flavors, avg, 1 cup	200	8	25
Steve's Kefir Peach, 1 cup	220	9	25
Sheep's Milk: Whole, 1 cup	265	17	13

Canned & Dried Milk

	C	F	Cb
Condensed: Reg. 2 Tbsp, 1 fl.oz	130	3	22
Lowfat *(Eagle)*, 2 Tbsp	120	1.5	23
Fat Free *(Eagle)*, 2 Tbsp	110	0	24
Evaporated: Whole, 2 Tbsp	40	3	3
Whole, 1 cup	170	10	13
Lowfat *(Carnation)*, 2 Tbsp	25	1	3
¹/₂ cup	110	3	12
Light/Skim, ¹/₂ cup	100	0.5	14
Dried: Whole, ¹/₄ cup, 1 oz	150	8	11
Skim/Nonfat, ¹/₃ cup	80	0	12
Made-up, 1 cup, 8 fl.oz	80	0	12
Buttermilk, sweetcream, 1 oz	110	2	3
Nonfat, 1 Tbsp	25	0	3

Whey Drink

	C	F	Cb
Acid: Dry, 1 Tbsp, 3g	10	0	2
Fluid, 1 cup, 8 fl.oz	60	0	13
Sweet: Dry, 1 Tbsp, 8g	25	0	6
Fluid, 1 cup, 8 fl.oz	65	1	13
Nutri Mil: Orig./Low Fat 8 fl.oz	80	3	11
Chocolate, 8 fl.oz	110	3	19
Fat Free (Calcium Enriched)	60	0	11

Flavored Milk Drinks

Quick Guide   C   F   Cb

Chocolate Milk
Average All Brands: Per Cup, 8 fl.oz

	C	F	Cb
Whole Milk (3.3%): 1 cup	225	9	26
1 Pint	450	18	52
Reduced Fat (2%), 1 cup	190	5	26
Lowfat (1%), 1 cup	160	3	26

Brands ~ Chocolate Milk

Ready-To-Drink: Per 8 fl.oz Cup

	C	F	Cb
Albertson's, lowfat	170	2.5	30
Bodywise, nonfat	180	0	35
Borden: Dutch Choc., 1 cup	220	8	28
Bosco	230	8	33
Brown Cow Farm, 1 cup	250	8	39
Deans'Chug': Regular	220	9	26
Lowfat, 1 cup	160	2.5	27
Dominick's Lowfat, 1 cup	170	2.5	28
Golden Guernsey, 1 cup	130	2.5	15
Grocers Pride Choc D'Lite, 1 cup	120	3	22
Hershey's: Lowfat (2%) Choc Milk	190	5	25
Whole Choc., 1 cup, 240ml	230	9	28
Hood, Lowfat (1%)	150	2	27
Horizon Organic	160	2.5	27
Knudsen	200	3	32
Kroger (3.25% milk)	220	9	28
Lactaid (1%)	160	3	26
Land O'Lakes, lowfat (0.5%)	150	1.5	35
Meadow Gold (3.5%)	210	8	25
Nesquik Chocolate:			
Regular, 1 cup, 8 fl.oz	230	8	31
16 fl.oz bottle	460	16	62
Fat Free, 1 cup, 8 fl.oz	160	0	31
16 fl.oz bottle	320	0	62
Double Chocolate, 1 cup, 8 fl.oz	230	9	30
16 fl.oz bottle	460	18	60
Oak Farms, 1 cup	210	8	26
Parmalat (2%)	180	5	28
Quik: (Nestle) Chocolate Milk	230	8	30
Strawberry Milk	220	9	31
Ralph's	240	3	34
Sobe Love Bus Chocolate, 8 fl.oz	140	1	28
Yoo Hoo Choc Drink, 9 fl.oz	150	1	33

Bottled Coffee

See Coffee Section: Page 159

Shakes & Smoothies   C   F   Cb

Smoothies
Made Up Ready-To-Drink
(8 fl. oz Milk/Soy + Fruit): *Per 12 fl.oz*

	C	F	Cb
Average all types: w. Whole Milk	300	8	50
+ Icecream, 1 scoop	400	13	62
with Nonfat Milk	240	0	50
Langers: 8 fl.oz, all flavors	135	0	34
Shakes			
Regular: Chocolate, 10 fl.oz	360	11	58
Vanilla/Strawberry, 10 fl.oz	320	9	53
McDonald's Thick Creamy Shakes,			
16 fl.oz, all flavors, average	570	16	92
Burger King: Vanilla, medium	720	41	73
Chocolate w. Syrup, medium	790	42	89
Killer Shake (14oz): Choc./Van., 1 c.	210	5	36

Cocoa-Chocolate Mixes

Add extra cals/fat/carbohydrate for milk

	C	F	Cb
Alba '66 Milk Choc, 1 pkt	60	0	14
Carnation Cocoa Mixes:			
Chocolate Rich, 3 Tbsp/1 pkt	110	1	24
Milk Chocolate, 3 Tbsp	110	1	24
w. Mini Marshmallows, 1 oz pkt	110	1	24
Malted Milk Original, 3 Tbsp	90	2	15
70 Calorie Cocoa Mix, 3 tsp	70	0.5	15
Fat-Free, 2 Tbsp/1 pkt	25	0	4
No Sugar, 1 pkt	50	0.5	8
Land O' Lakes: *Per 1 1/4 oz Pkt*			
Choc.Mint/Raspb./Supreme	160	5	25
Nestle Hot Cocoa Mix, 1 oz	110	1	23
w. Marshmallows, 1 oz	120	1	23
French Vanilla	120	3	22
Ghirardelli: *Per 2 heaping tsp*			
Choc. Mocha/Hazelnut/Dble Choc	80	1.5	21
Pralines & Creme, 2 Tbsp	90	0	23
Ovaltine Cocoa Mixes, 4 tsp	80	0	20
Swiss Miss Cocoa Mixes:			
Milk Chocolate, 1 oz pkt	110	1.5	22
w. Marshmallows, 1.2 oz pkt	140	3	22
Choc. Sensation, 1.25 oz pkt	150	4	27
Lite, 1 pkt	70	0	18
Diet Cocoa Mix, 1 pkt	20	0	4
Sugar Free	60	0	10
Fat Free, 0.53 oz	50	0	9
Vending Machine, 1.34 oz pkt	145	2	24
Weight Watchers: Hot Cocoa Mix	70	0	10

Soy & Non-Dairy Drinks

Soy ~ Ready-To-Drink

Per 1 Cup Serving (8 fl.oz)

	C	F	Cb
Cereal Match, 1 cup	100	3	17
Eden Blend: 1 cup	120	3	18
Edensoy: Original, 1 cup	130	5	13
Extra, Vanilla	150	3	23
Carob	170	4	27
Light: Original, 1 cup	95	2	14
Vanilla	120	2	21
8th Continent: Chocolate (lowfat)	140	3	23
Original, Lowfat	80	3	8
Vanilla, Lowfat	90	3	11
Hain Soy Supreme: Original	80	3	9
Vanilla, 1 cup	100	3	12
Harmony Farms: Regular, 1 cup	80	3	10
Enriched; Vanilla, 1 cup	100	3	14
Health Source: All flavors	150	1.5	23
Health Source Plus	160	1	17
Soy Protein Shake	100	1	4
Health Valley: Soy Moo	110	0	21
It's Soy Delicious: Vanilla	110	1	22
Awesome; Chocolate	120	2	22
Lifeway: Soy Treat, Apple; Caramel	160	4	23
Naked Juice: Choc Soy Shake	210	2	38
Vanilla Soy Shake	170	1	33
Odwalla Future Shake: Chocolate	160	3	27
Vanilla al'monde	190	6	24
Pacific: Ultra, Plain/Vanilla	150	5	20
Original unsweetened	100	5	5
Enriched (Soy Isoflavin): Plain	90	2.5	14
Vanilla, 1 cup	110	2.5	16
Fat Free: Plain	70	0	14
Vanilla	90	0	17
Select (Soy Isoflavin), Plain	100	2.5	13
PowerDream: Mango Passion	320	5	65
Java Jolt, Chai, Vanilla Blast	250	5	42
X-treme Chocolate	260	5	48
Silk (White Wave): Plain, regular	100	4	8
Plain, unsweetened	90	4	5
Chai, Mocha	140	3	20
Chocolate	140	3.5	23
Coffee Soylatte, 1 cup	170	3.5	29
11 oz Bottle	220	5	38
Spice Soylatte, 11 oz bottle	200	6	27
Vanilla	100	3.5	10
Silk Creamer, 1 Tbsp	15	1	1
SoyDream: Orig./Enriched 8 fl.oz	130	4	17
Carob/Chocolate Enriched	210	4	37
Vanilla; Vanilla Enriched	150	4	22
Soy Fusion: Berry, 1 cup	120	1.5	24

Soy Nice:	C	F	Cb
Natural, 8 fl.oz	70	3.5	2
Original	80	3	6
Chocolate, 1 cup	110	3	17
Vanilla	100	3	11
SunSoy: Chocolate, 1 cup	140	3	23
Creamy Original	80	3	5
Vanilla	110	3	15
Ultra Slim-Fast: Juice based			
With Soy, all flavors, 11 oz can	220	1	46
Vitasoy: Refrigerated, Crmy Orig.	110	4	12
Rich Chocolate	160	4	24
Low Fat Vanilla Delite	90	2	13
Long Life: Creamy Original	110	5	9
Creamy Unsweetened	80	5	5
Carob Supreme; Rich Cocoa	150	4.5	20
Vanilla Delite	120	4	14
Light: Original	60	2	7
Cocoa	110	2.5	18
Vanilla	90	2	14
Enriched: Original	90	4	9
Light Original	60	2	7
Vanilla	110	4	14
Light Vanilla	90	2	13
WestSoy: Plus, Plain	130	3.5	18
Plus, Vanilla	140	3.5	19
100% Organic: Original (2% fat)	140	5	18
Unsweetened, Plain	90	4.5	4
Unsweetened, Vanilla	100	4.5	5
Nonfat: Plain	80	0	16
Vanilla	90	0	17
Lite: Plain, 1 cup	100	2	15
Cocoa	120	2.5	28
Vanilla	120	2.5	21
Lowfat: Plain	90	1.5	14
Chocolate	180	3	32
Vanilla	110	1.5	20
Smart Lite: Plain	120	2	19
Vanilla	150	2	25
Café: Coffee; Mocha; Fr. Vanilla	130	2.5	24
Chai: Orig./Green Tea, avg	140	3	26
Smoothies, all flavors	140	1.5	28
Soy Shakes: Choc; Vanilla	170	3.5	30
Vigor Aid: French Vanilla	260	6	44
Choc Mocha, Creamy Choc.	240	6	38
Juice Bar, average all flavors	120	1.5	24
Vitamite 100: 1 cup, 8 fl.oz	110	5	14
Wild Oats: Original, 1 cup, 8 fl.oz	100	3.5	12

Rice & Cereal Drinks • Yogurt

Soy Powder Mix   C   F   Cb

(1 oz (1/4 cup) mix makes 1 cup, 8 fl.oz)

	C	F	Cb
Better Than Milk: Original, 1 oz	100	2.5	16
Light, 1 oz	80	0.5	13
Joy Soy: Extra (Carob/Van.), 2 T.	80	3	11
Revival Soy: Plain, 1 oz pkt	110	1.5	2
Vanilla w/Fructose, 2 oz pkt	220	2	31
Unsweetened/Aspartame, 35g	120	2	6
Soyagen: Reg./No Sugar, 1 oz dry	130	6	12
Carob, 1 oz dry	130	6	13
Soy Protein Isolate, 1 oz dry	95	1	0
Soy Quik *(Ener-g),* 1 oz dry	100	4.5	8

Rice & Cereal Drinks

	C	F	Cb
Almond Breeze: Original, 8 fl.oz	60	3	8
Vanilla, 8 fl.oz	90	3	16
Amazake: Almond Light, 8 fl.oz	110	2	20
Horchata (Don José), 8 fl.oz	140	4	25
Eden Blend: Rice & Soy, 1 cup	120	3	18
Eden Rice: 1 cup, 8 fl.oz	110	3	21
Hain Rice Supreme: Lowfat Orig.	100	3	16
Lowfat Cinnamon, 8 fl.oz	130	3	22
Pacific Foods: Multigrain, 8 fl.oz	150	2	31
Naturally Oat: Original, 1 cup	110	1.5	21
Vanilla, 1 cup, 8 fl.oz	130	1.5	24
Naturally Almond: Original, 1 cup	70	2.5	10
Vanilla, 1 cup, 8 fl.oz	90	2.5	15
Pacific Rice: Lowfat, Plain, 1 cup	90	2	18
Fat Free: Plain, 8 fl.oz	80	0	18
Cocoa, 8 fl.oz	100	0	21
Vanilla, 8 fl.oz	110	0	24
Rice Dream: Carob, 1 cup	150	2.5	32
Chocolate: Enriched, 1 cup	170	3	36
Vanilla/Vanilla Enriched, 1 cup	130	2	28
Original/Original Enriched, 1 cup	120	2	25
Westbrae: Oat Plus, 1 cup	150	3	26
Original Vanilla, 1 cup, 8 fl.oz	150	3	20
Rice: Plain, 1 cup, 8 fl.oz	100	2.5	18
Vanilla, 1 cup, 8 fl.oz	120	2.5	22
Wild Oats: Vanilla, 1 cup, 8 floz	120	2	26
Original, 1 cup, 8 fl.oz	100	2	20

Rice/Nut Drink Mixes

	C	F	Cb
Better Than Milk: Light, 19g	70	0.5	14
Original, 23g	100	2.5	16
Nut Quik, 2 Tbsp powder, 18g	110	9	3
Rice Moo, 2 Tbsp powder, 19g	72	0	17
Solait, 3 Tbsp powder, 22g	80	1.5	13
Sun's Up, 2 scoops, 40g powder	160	2	36

Quick Guide   C   F   Cb

Yogurt
Average All Brands: Per 8 oz Cup

	C	F	Cb
Plain Yogurt: Whole, 8 oz	180	7	11
Lowfat	140	4	16
Nonfat	110	0	18
Fruit Flavored: Whole, 8 oz	250	6	38
Lowfat	230	3	32
Nonfat, regular	150	0	32
Nonfat, no sugar added	120	0	32
Goat's Milk Yogurt-Same as Regular Yogurt			

Yogurt ~ Brands

	C	F	Cb
Alex Rod: Fat Free, all flav., 8 oz	70	0	12
Albertson's: Plain, lowfat, 8 oz	140	2.5	17
Fruit on the Bottom (lowfat):			
Average all flavors, 8 oz	220	2	42
Swiss (Nonfat), average, 6 oz	90	0	14
Indulgents (Lowfat), 6 oz	180	2	35
Alta Dena: Lowfat: Plain, 8 oz	170	4.5	20
Vanilla, 8 oz	260	3.5	44
Nonfat: Plain, 8 oz	110	0	17
Flavors, average	190	0	39
America's Choice: Swiss Style	210	2.5	41
Fruit on the Bottom: Cherry Van.	270	2.5	55
Other flavors, average	220	2.5	40
Nonfat, all flavors, average	100	0	15
Berkeley Farms (8 oz Cup)			
Lowfat: Boysenberry/Cherry	230	2.5	46
Raspberry	220	2.5	43
Strawberry, Lemon, Vanilla	270	2.5	52
Nonfat: Average all flavors	100	0	16
Breyers: Light n' Lively: 125g	130	1	25
Lowfat: 1% fat, all flavors, 8 oz	250	2.5	48
1.5% fat, plain	130	3	15
Flavors, average	220	3	38
Smooth & Creamy: 125g	130	1	25
Brown Cow Farm (Fat Free): Plain	80	0	11
Cappuccino/Maple Alm./Vanilla	170	0	33
Cherry Vanilla/Strawberry, 8 oz	190	0	39
Chocolate, 8 oz	220	0	45
Whole Milk, 8 oz	210	8	30
Plain, 8 oz	170	9	13
Cabot: Plain, 8 oz	140	4	16
Flavors, 8 oz	220	3	42
Cascade Fresh: Lowfat, 6 oz	140	2	23
Fat Free: All flavors, 6 oz ctn	110	0	20
(32 oz ctn) 1 cup, 8 oz	160	0	27

Yogurt ~ Brands (Cont)

Colombo

	C	F	Cb
Light, all flavors, 8 oz	120	0	22
Classic (Fruit on the Bottom), 8 oz	200	4	43
Non Fat: Plain, 8 oz	110	0	17
Continental: Nonfat, 8 oz	200	0	38
Nonfat Fruit on the Bottom, 8 oz	190	0	38
Crowley: Lowfat Blueberry, 8 oz	240	2.5	43
Dannon: Plain (Natural), 8 oz	170	8	14
Light: All flavors, 8 oz	100	0	16
w. Crunchy Toppings, aver. 8 oz	170	0	28
Nonfat: Snackpack, 4 oz	60	0	11
Light 'n Fit: 8 oz	120	0	21
Light n' Fit Creamy: 6 oz ctn	100	0	16
Multipack, 4 oz ctn	70	0	11
Fruit on the Bottom (99% FF):8 oz	230	2.5	40
Minipack, 4 oz	110	1	20
Nonfat: Plain, 8 oz	130	0	19
Blended, 4 oz	100	0	21
Chunky Fruit (Nonfat), avg, 6 oz	160	0	32
Low Fat: All types, 8 oz	220	3.5	36
Double Delights Lowfat:			
w. Fruit Topping, avg, 6 oz	170	1	34
w. Choc. Topping, 6 oz	220	1	46
La Creme, all flavors, 4 oz cup	140	5	20
Light Duets: w. fruit topping, 6 oz	90	0	34
Danimals: Lowfat, 4 oz	120	1.5	20
Super Creamy, avg, 4 oz	130	3	20
Sprinkl'ins: All types, 4 oz	125	1	23
Whipped (lowfat), avg, 4 oz	120	2.5	20
Dominick's: Lowfat, 8 oz	230	2	40
Fruit on the Bottom, avg, 8 oz	230	2	40
Fat Free 80 Calories, 8 oz	80	0	13
Plain: Lowfat, 8 oz	130	2.5	15
Nonfat, 8 oz	120	0	17
Friendship: Regular type, 6 oz	190	5	31
Grocer's Pride: Lowfat, 4.4 oz	140	1.5	28
Hood: Fat Free, Plain, 8 oz	130	0	18
Average all flavors, 8 oz	190	0	40

Horizon Organic

	C	F	Cb
Whole Milk: Vanilla, 8 oz	220	6	32
Lowfat, fruits, avg, 6 oz	160	2	30
Fat Free: Plain and Simple, 6 oz	80	0	13
Vanilla, 6 oz	130	0	24
Fruit On The Bottom, avg, 6 oz	140	0	27
Fruit, Blended, 6 oz	160	0	30
32 oz Ctn: Plain, 1 cup, 8 oz	105	0	17
Vanilla, 1 cup, 8 oz	170	0	33

Imperial Supreme	C	F	Cb
Lowfat, 6 oz	140	1.5	26

Jerseymaid (Vons)

	C	F	Cb
Fruit on the Bottom, 8 oz	240	2.5	46
Prestirred (lowfat), average	240	2.5	46
Plain, lowfat, 8 oz	140	3.5	18
Jell-O: Kid Pack, all flavors, 125g	130	1	25
Hellios: Kefir Organic, 1 cup,	120	5	13
Jewel: Lowfat, average, 8 oz	250	2.5	48
Knudsen: 70 Calories, 6 oz	70	0	11
Free, average, 6 oz	170	0	33
Cottage Doubles, 5.5 oz	140	2.5	18
Kroger: Lite, avg all flav., 8 oz	100	0	14
Lowfat, average all flavors, 8 oz	210	1.5	40
Health Indulgence (Nonfat):			
Fruit on the Bottom, avg	170	0	35
Fat Free: Plain, 8 oz	120	0	30
Vanilla, 8 oz	190	0	36
98% Fat Free: Plain, 8 oz	140	4	16
Vanilla, 8 oz	240	4	42
Lactaid: Lowfat Vanilla, 8 oz	240	2.5	45

La Yogurt

	C	F	Cb
Fruit Flavors, average, 6 oz	170	2	32
Light, average all flavors, 6 oz	70	0	12
Fruit La More, average, 6 oz	160	0	32

Light n' Lively

	C	F	Cb
Free 50 Calories, 4 oz	50	0	8
Free 70 Calories, 6 oz	70	0	13
Free (Regular) 6 oz: Vanilla	160	0	32
Strawb. Fruit/Peach/Lem./Berry	170	0	34
Strawberry/Raspberry	180	0	36
Kidpack/Multipack, avg 4.4 oz	140	1	28

Lucerne

	C	F	Cb
Low Fat: Plain, 8 oz	150	3.5	18
Fruit flavors, avg, 8 oz	240	2.5	47
Vanilla	230	2.5	43
Fat Free: Plain, 8 oz	130	0	19
Light Fat Free, fruit, 8 oz	120	0	22
YoCups, avg all flavors, 4 oz	130	1	27
Yo On The Go, 2.25 oz tube	80	2	13
Meadow Gold: Plain, 8 oz	160	5	16
Flavors, average, 8 oz	250	4	42

Mountain High

	C	F	Cb
Original: Plain, 8 oz	190	8	18
Fat Free Plain, 8 oz	120	0	20
Fat Free: Plain, 8 oz	110	0	19
Flavors, average, 8 oz	170	0	33
Low Fat: Plain/Vanilla, 8 oz	150	2	22

Yogurt (Cont)

Brands (Cont)

	C	F	Cb
Mystic Lake Dairy (Goat Milk Yogurt)			
Plain, 1 cup, 8 oz	120	6	9
Nancy's: *Per 8 oz Serving*			
Whole Milk: Plain, regular	180	8	16
Honey, plain	180	8	17
w. Fruit Cup, avg, 9.5 oz	225	8	29
Low Fat: Plain/Lemon/Vanilla, avg	140	3	16
Other flavors, average	180	3	28
Nonfat: Plain, 8 oz	120	0	17
Maple, Vanilla (8 oz ctn)	160	0	27
w. Fruit Cup, avg, 9.5 oz	165	0	29
Vanilla (32 oz ctn), swtn'd, 8 oz	220	0	40
Soy Cultured: Vanilla, 8 oz	170	4	25
Kiwi-Lime; Mango, avg	240	4	43
Other flavors, average	190	4.5	32
Pavel's: Original Russian, 8 oz	140	8	10
Lowfat Vanilla, 8 oz	120	4	12
Nonfat Russian, 8 oz	110	0	15
Private Selection (Ralph's)			
Lowfat, average all flavors, 8 oz	220	2	43
Fat Free: Coconut Cream Pie, 6 oz	130	0	23
Other flavors, average, 6 oz	100	0	16
Mountain Dairy, 6 oz	150	1.5	27
Publix: Light, average, 8 oz	130	0	21
Fruit on the Bottom, avg, 8 oz	250	2.5	43
Fat Free: Plain, 8 oz	140	0	23
Swiss Style (lowfat), 8 oz	240	2.5	41
Ralphs: Lite, Lemon, 8 oz	100	0	15
Lowfat: Plain, 8 oz	150	4	17
Fruit on Bottom: Spiced Apple	250	2.5	47
Strawberry Banana, 8 oz	220	3	41
Redwood Hill Farm (Goat Milk Yogurt)			
Fruit flavors, average, 8 oz	180	5	28
Vanilla, 8 oz	190	6	28
Plain, 8 oz	120	6	9
Silk (Soy): Plain, 1 cup, 8 oz	120	2.5	22
Vanilla, 6 oz ctn	120	2	23
Other flavors, average, 6 oz	170	2	31
Sky Hill Napa Valley: Plain, 8 oz	130	8	8
Snackwell's: Nonfat, 6 oz	160	0	36
Stonyfield Farm (Organic)			
Whole Milk: Plain, 1 cup, 8 oz	180	9	16
French Vanilla, 8 oz	250	8	36
6 oz Cups: Vanilla, Mocha	190	6	27
Other flavors, avg	170	6	24
Nonfat: Plain, 8 oz cup	100	0	15
Chocolate; Caramel, avg	220	0	46
Other flavors, avg	160	0	32

	C	F	Cb
O'Soy: 4 oz Multipack, avg			
Fruit On Bottom (6 oz), Vanilla	150	2	26
Other flavors, 6 oz, avg	170	2	33
YoSqueeze, 2 oz tube	60	1	11
Stop & Shop: Blended Lite, 8 oz	120	0	20
"TCBY" Fat Free (Fantasies):			
Banana Creme Pie, 6 oz	110	0	18
White Chocolate, 6 oz	90	0	12
Trader Joe's			
Nonfat: Regular 8 oz	190	0	40
French Village, Vanilla, 8 oz	170	0	32
Organic Vanilla, 8 oz	160	0	27
Lowfat, average, 8 oz	230	2.5	43
Organic Low Fat, average, 6 oz	150	2.5	24
Cultured Soy, all varieties, 6 oz	140	2.5	28
YoFarm: All flavors, avg, 8 oz	220	6	37
YoCrunch: Lowfat w. Toppings, 6.5 oz cup			
Oreo Cookies	190	4	35
Peach/Strawb./Rasp. w. Granola	220	2	46
Strawberry w. Nestlé Crunch	240	6	41
Vanilla w. Choc Crunch/Reese's	240	7	39
Yoplait			
Light: All flavors, 6 oz	90	0	16
Light, Fat Free: Average, 4 oz	70	0	13
Original Lowfat: C'nut Creme, 6oz	200	3	35
99% Fat Free: All flavors, 6 oz	170	1.5	33
Multipack, 4 oz	110	1	22
Exprèsse: All flavors, 2.25 oz tube	70	1.5	11
Go-Gurt: 2.25 oz tube	70	2	11
Custard Style: All flavors, 6 oz	190	3.5	32
Trix: Multipack, 4 oz	120	1.5	23
Whips!: All flavors, 4 oz ctn	140	2.5	26
Yumsters, 4 oz	120	2	21
WholeSoy			
Plain, 6 oz ctn	140	2.5	24
Other flavors, avg, 6 oz ctn	150	2.5	27

Yogurt Drinks & Probiotics

	C	F	Cb
Actimel (Dannon) Probiotic, 3.3 fl.oz	90	2	16
Alta Dena, Drinkables, 1 cup	220	0	46
Dannon, Danimals, 3.3 oz box	100	1.5	18
Glen Oaks, all flavors, avg, 1 cup	250	4	46
Nouriche, all flavors, 11 fl.oz	290	0	60
Stonyfield Farm, 10 fl.oz	240	3	44
WholeSoy, 12 fl.oz bottle	210	3	35
Yonique, 6 fl.oz: Pina Colada	190	4	30
Peach; Banana; Guava	170	2	30
Yo Soy, 8 fl.oz	80	4	4

Icecream & Frozen Yogurt

Quick Guide — C F Cb

Icecream

Vanilla: *Average All Brands*

Other flavors ~ See Brand Listings.

Regular Icecream (10% fat):
(Examples: *Borden/Hood*)

	C	F	Cb
3 fl.oz scoop	100	5	12
1/2 cup, 4 fl.oz	130	7	16
1 Pint, 16 fl.oz	520	28	62
1/2 Gallon (4 Pints)	2100	112	248

Rich (16% fat):

3 fl.oz scoop	130	8	12
1/2 cup, 4 fl.oz	170	10	17
1 Pint	690	40	68

Super-Rich (20% fat): (*Haagen-Dazs/Ben & Jerry's*)

3 fl.oz scoop	200	14	16
1/2 cup, 4 fl.oz	270	18	21
1 Pint	1100	72	84

Reduced Fat/Light (6% fat):
(*Breyer's Light/Hood Light*)

3 fl.oz scoop	100	3	14
1/2 cup, 4 fl.oz	140	4	18
1 Pint	560	16	72

Low Fat (less than 4% fat):
(*Healthy Choice/Weight Watchers/Snackwell's*)

3 fl.oz scoop	90	2	17
1/2 cup, 4 fl.oz	120	2.5	22
1 Pint	480	10	88

Fat Free: (*Baskin-Robbins FF/Borden FF/ Breyers FF/Dreyers FF/Hood FF)*)

3 fl.oz scoop	75	0	17
1/2 cup, 4 fl.oz	100	0	22
1 Pint	400	0	88

Soft Serve: Regular, 1/2 cup

Regular, 1/2 cup	140	5	20
1 cup	280	10	40
Nonfat, 1/2 cup	90	0	23
1 cup	180	0	46

Quick Guide — C F Cb

Frozen Yogurt

Average All Brands

	C	F	Cb
Hard: Lowfat, 1/2 cup	140	3	26
Nonfat, 1/2 cup	110	0	29
Soft: Lowfat, 1/2 cup	120	2.5	28
Nonfat, 1/2 cup	100	0	30

Brands: *See Icecream & Ices Section*

Quick Guide — C F Cb

Gelato/Ices

Gelato: *Per 1/2 Cup*

	C	F	Cb
Milk base: Vanilla	200	15	18
Choc. Hazelnut	370	29	26
Water base: 1/2 cup	100	0	25
Ice (Milk base): *Average all flavors*			
Hard (4% fat), 1/2 cup	100	3	15
Soft Serve (3% fat), 1/2 cup	110	2	19
Shaved Ice: Average, 12 fl. oz	160	0	40
Sherbet: Average, 1/2 cup	120	2	28
Sorbet: Fruit (no fat), 1/2 cup	120	0	30
Fruit Ice Pops	80	0	20

Tofu Frozen Desserts: *Page 34*

Sundaes

Denny's Sundaes:

	C	F	Cb
Single Scoop, no topping	190	14	14
Double Scoop, no topping	375	27	29
Banana Split	895	43	112
Butterfinger® Hot Fudge	780	38	106
Toppings:			
Blueberry, 2 oz	70	0	17
Chocolate, 2 oz	320	25	27
Fudge, 2 oz	200	10	30
Strawberry, 2 oz	80	1	17
McDonald's Sundaes:			
Hot Fudge Sundae, 6.3 oz	340	12	52
Oreo® Cookie McFlurry™	570	20	82
Toppings: Nut/Sundae, 1/4 oz	40	3.5	2

Icecream Bars & Pops

See Pages 34-36

Icecream Cones & Cups

	C	F	Cb
Wafer Cone/Cup, average	20	0	4
Sugar Cone, average	40	0	9
Waffle Cone:			
Small	60	0	11
Large	100	1	22
Brands:			
Oreo Chocolate Cone	50	1	10
Comet Sugar Cone	50	0	11
Keebler Sugar Cone	45	0	11

Icecream & Frozen Yogurt (Cont)

Brands	C	F	Cb
Alta Dena: Per 1/2 Cup			
Golden Honey Vanilla	160	10	17
Honey Chocolate	160	9	19
Baskin-Robbins: *See Page 182 (Fast-Foods)*			
Ben & Jerry's: Per 1/2 Cup			
Apple Crumble	280	14	33
Butter Pecan	290	21	20
Cherry Garcia; Vanilla	260	16	26
Choc. Chip Cookie Dough	270	15	31
Choc. Fudge Brownie	280	14	33
Chubby Hubby	330	21	32
Chunky Monkey; Coffee Heath	310	19	32
Concession Obsession	310	19	32
Fudge Central	300	18	31
Honey, I'm Home!	260	15	29
Karamel Sutra	280	15	32
Makin' Whoopie Pie	270	14	33
Mint Chocolate Cookie	270	17	28
New York Super Fudge Chunk	310	20	30
Nutty Waffle Cone	310	19	31
One Sweet Whirled	280	15	33
Peanut Butter Cup	310	18	32
Peanut Butter Me Up	330	21	25
Peanut Butter Truffle	300	17	30
Phish Food	280	13	38
Pistachio Pistachio	280	19	21
S'mores	260	12	34
The Full Vermonty	260	16	27
Triple Caramel Chunk	290	17	32
World's Best Chocolate	280	17	27
World's Best Vanilla	250	16	21
2-Twisted: Half Baked	280	15	33
Everything But The . . .	320	19	30
From Russia With Buzz	270	17	26
Jerry's Jubilee	260	14	29
S.N.A.F.U.	250	14	28
Vanilla Caramel Fudge	280	16	32
Vanilla Heath Bar Crunch	300	19	29
Frozen Yogurt: Per 1/2 Cup			
Cherry Garcia Yogurt	170	3	32
Choc. Fudge Brownie Yogurt	190	3	36
Half Baked Yogurt	210	4	39
Phish Food Yogurt	230	5	42
Sorbet: Average all flavors	120	0	30
Bars/Pops: *See Page 34*			

Ben & Jerry's (Cont)	C	F	Cb
Scoop Shop: Per 1/2 Cup			
Coconut Almond Fudge	260	18	20
Coffee Buzz; Marble Mint Chip	240	15	22
Mint Chocolate Chunk	240	16	23
S'Mores	180	2	34
Southern Peach; Strawberry	180	10	20
Sweet Cream & Cookie	230	14	23
White Russian	200	13	18
Bon Bon's			
Vanilla w. choc. coating, 5 pieces	200	14	17
8 pieces	330	23	27
Bresler's: Per 1/2 Cup			
All Flavors Icecream: average	230	12	23
Royal Cremes, average	260	16	24
Royal Lites, average	220	0	49
Breyers: Per 1/2 Cup			
Dulche de Leche	160	7	21
Extra Creamy Chocolate	160	8	19
Extra Creamy Vanilla	150	8	17
Peanut Butter & Fudge	180	10	17
Vanilla & Choc Fudge Checks	150	9	17
Wild Berry Swirl	140	8	16
Fat Free: Average	110	0	2
Lactose-Free: Vanilla du Cream	130	7	14
Reduced Fat: Average	160	6	19
All Natural: Butter Pecan	180	12	15
Cherry Vanilla; Coffee	150	7	17
Chocolate; French Vanilla	160	10	15
Choc. Chip; Mint Choc. Chip	170	10	17
Cookies 'n Cream	170	9	19
Peach; Strawberry	130	6	18
Vanilla; Van./Choc./Strawberry	150	8	16
Van. & Choc.; Van. Fudge Twirl	160	8	18
Light: Average all flav., 1/2 cup	140	4	19
Icecream Parlor: Almond Joy	170	9	20
Chips Ahoy	160	8	19
Candy Bar Sundae	170	8	21
Double Choc Malt	160	7	21
English Toffee	180	8	23
Heath Toffee	180	9	22
Hershey's Choc. w. Almonds	170	8	21
Icecream Sandwich	160	7	21
Mint w. Oreos	160	7	22
Oreo	160	8	19
Reese's Peanut Butter Cup	180	9	22

Icecream & Frozen Yogurt (Cont)

Brands (Cont)

	C	F	Cb
Breyers (Cont): *Per ¹/₂ Cup*			
Homemade: Double Choc Fudge	180	9	23
Butter Pecan; Van.; Neopolitan	150	8	16
Vienetta: All flavors, 1 slice	190	11	17
No Sugar Added: Vanilla	80	4	11
Vanilla Fudge Twirl	90	3.5	11
Vanilla Chocolate Strawberry	90	4	11
Mint Chocolate Chip	100	5	21
Frozen Yogurt: Average, ¹/₂ cup	140	3	25

Carvel Icecream ~ *See Page 186*

Colombo: *Per ¹/₂ Cup*

	C	F	Cb
Frozen, Soft Serve: Nonfat var.	100	0	22
Slender Sensations varieties	65	0	11
Lowfat: Old Worlde; P'nut Butter	120	2.5	20
Vanilla varieties	110	1.5	21

CremaLita (Soft Serve)
Calories will vary with density (air in product) and serving size.
Best to weigh product and calculate on 25 cals per 1 oz weight.

	C	F	Cb
Vanilla: Small (4 fl.oz cup),			
If 2¹/₂ oz weight	60	0	14
If 4 oz weight*	100	0.5	23
If 6 oz weight*	150	1	35
(*) Most common weights			
Medium (8 fl.oz cup), 11 oz wt	275	1.5	63
Chocolate: Small, 6 oz weight	160	1	36

Dairy Queen/Brazier ~ *See Page 190*

Dannon Frozen Yogurt: *Per ¹/₂ Cup (4 fl.oz)*

	C	F	Cb
Light Soft, all flavors, average	90	1	21
Light 'N Crunchy, all flavors, aver.	110	1	23
Pure Indulgence, all flavors, aver.	150	3	25

Dolewhip (Soft Serve): *Per 4 fl.oz, ¹/₂ Cup*

	C	F	Cb
Chocolate; Vanilla	100	3	18
Fruit flavors, average	80	0.5	16

Dreyers: *Per ¹/₂ Cup*

	C	F	Cb
No Sugar Added: Aver. all flavors	90	3	12
Fat Free: Average all flavors	110	0	25
No Sugar Added	95	0	20
Grand: Cracker Jack	170	9	20
Scooby Doo!	160	8	16
Dexter's Lab., Amazing Creation	160	7	21
Grand Light: Vanilla	100	3	15
Cookie Dough; P'nut Butter Cup	130	5	17
Other varieties, average	120	4	18

Dreyers (Cont): *Per ¹/₂ Cup*

	C	F	Cb
Candy Bar: Twix	190	9	23
Snickers; M&M's Vanilla	180	9	22
M&M's Chocolate	170	8	22
Milky Way; 3 Musketeers	160	7	22
Dreamery: Banana Boogie	290	17	27
Black Raspberry Avalanche	270	16	27
Caramel Toffee Bar: Heaven	290	16	32
Vanilla	260	15	25
Cashew Praline Parfait	260	13	30
Cherry Chip ba da Bing	280	15	33
Chocolate Almond Bar	300	17	32
Choc P'nut Butter Chunk	310	18	29
Choc Truffle; Nuts About Malt	280	15	30
Cool Mint	300	17	32
Coney Island Waffle	300	18	31
Dulce de Leche, Caramel	270	14	32
Galactic Choc Swirl	280	12	37
Grandma's Cookie Dough	300	17	32
Strawberry Fields	220	12	26
New York Strawb. Cheesecake	260	15	27
Nothing But Chocolate	280	14	34
Raspberry Brownie a la Mode	270	14	33
Tiramisu	270	14	33
Homemade: Butter Pecan, 71g	160	9	16
Banana Crunch; Strawb. & Crm	130	6	17
Chocolate Peanut Butter, 71g	200	12	18
Cracker Jack; Scooby Snack	170	9	20
Orbit City Swirl	160	8	19
Peaches & Cream, 65g	120	5	16
Vanilla, ¹/₂ cup, 71g	140	7	16
Frozen Yogurt: Vanilla	90	0	19
Chips Supreme, ¹/₂ cup	120	4	19
Fat Free, average all flavors	90	0	20
Starburst Sherbet: Avg all flav.	150	2.5	30
Whole Fruit Sorbet: Boysenberry	150	0	37
Strawberry, Peach; Raspberry	130	0	33

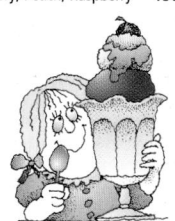

31

Icecream & Frozen Yogurt (Cont)

Brands (Cont)

	C	F	Cb
Edys: Per 1/2 Cup			
Banana Split; Choc. Fudge Mousse	160	8	19
Cherry Choc; Van./Choc.; Espresso	150	8	17
Choc. Fudge Sundae; Dble Fudge	170	9	19
Ice Cream Sandwich	140	8	14
Grand Light: Vanilla	100	3	15
Butter Pecan; Choc. Almond	120	5	16
Chiquita 'N Chocolate	110	5	13
Choc. Fudge Mousse	110	3	17
Cookie Dough; P'nut Butter Cups	130	5	18
Cookies 'n Cream; Rocky Road	110	4	16
French Silk	120	4	18
Fat Free: Average all flavors	115	0	25
Eskimo Pie: Per 1/2 Cup			
Reduced Fat: Butter Pecan	140	7	16
Choc. Marshmallow	130	4	23
Neopolitan; Vanilla	110	4	18
Fudge Ripple	120	4	19
Bars: See Page 35			
Friendly's: Per 1/2 Cup			
Icecream: Chocolate Almd Chip	170	10	18
Forbidden Chocolate	150	9	14
Fudge Nut Brownie	200	11	23
Vanilla Choc. Strawb.; Vanilla	150	8	16
Vienna Mocha Chunk	180	11	19
Frozen Yogurt: Lowfat flav., avg	120	3	20
Regular flavors, average	150	4	24
Frostline (Soft Serve): Chocolate	90	2	20
Vanilla, 1/2 cup	90	3	18
Frusen Gladje: Per 1/2 Cup			
Butter Pecan	280	21	16
Chocolate	240	17	17
Chocolate Choc. Chip	270	18	21
Mocha Chip; Praline & Cream	280	18	22
Strawberry	230	15	20
Swiss Choc. Candy Almond	270	19	18
Vanilla	230	17	16
Vanilla Swiss Almond	270	19	18
Godiva: Per 1/2 Cup			
Belgian Dark Chocolate	280	17	26
Choc Hazelnut Truffle	350	23	31
Choc Raspberry Truffle	290	16	32
Chocolate Cheesecake	310	17	36
Chocolate w. Choc Hearts	330	20	32
Classic Milk Chocolate	290	18	28

	C	F	Cb
Godiva (Cont): Per 1/2 Cup			
Pecan Caramel Truffle	320	19	32
Vanilla Caramel Pecan	290	16	33
Vanilla w. Choc. Caramel Hearts	310	18	32
White Choc. Raspberry	260	12	32
Good Humor: Per 1/2 Cup			
Light: Coffee	110	3	18
Choc. Chip, Toffee Bar Crunch	130	4	20
Cookies n' Crm; Praline Alm. Crnch	130	3	21
Vanilla, Vanilla Choc. Strawb.	110	3	19
Haagen-Dazs			
Icecream, Sorbet, Frozen Yogurt: See Pg 203			
Bars: See Page 35			
Healthy Choice: Per 1/2 Cup			
Brownie Bliss	130	2	25
Cookies 'N Cream	130	2	24
Double Karma	140	2	28
Happy Together	150	2	29
Jumpin' Java	140	2	25
Peanut Butter	110	2	19
Praline & Caramel	130	2	25
Rocky Road	130	2	25
Vanilla; Mint Choc Chip	100	2	18
Other flavors, average	120	2	22
Lowfat, No Sugar Added: Vanilla	90	2	16
No Sugar Add: Coffee Almd Fudge	110	2	20
Chocolate Fudge Brownie	110	2	20
In the Beginning	110	2	21
Mint Chocolate Chip	100	2	28
Hood: Per 1/2 Cup Serving			
Icecream:			
Regular: Average all flavors	150	8	17
Light: Creamy Vanilla	110	3.5	18
Raspb. Swirl; Heavenly Hash, avg	130	3.5	22
Other flavors, average	140	5	22
No Sugar Added, Lowfat Icecream:			
Vanilla Dream; Classic Trio	100	2.5	14
Choc Frenzy; Mocha Madness, avg	120	2.5	19
Chocolate Chip	120	4	16
Fat Free: Average all flavors	100	0	23
Dble Brownie; Heavenly Hash	120	0	27
Frozen Yogurt:			
Nonfat: Strawb., Old Fashion. Van.	110	0	24
Other flavors, average	120	0	27
Regular: Average all flavors	150	8	17
Icecream Bars: See Page 35			

Brands (Cont)

	C	F	Cb

I Can't Believe It's Yogurt: *See Page 204*

Jerseymaid (Vons): *Per 1/2 Cup*

	C	F	Cb
After Dinner Mint; Cookies & Crm	170	9	19
Choc Chip; Mint Choc Chip	160	9	17
Heavenly Hash; Nut Chunky Choc.	170	8	22
Mocha Almd Fudge; Rocky Road	160	7	20
Neopolitan; Vanilla	140	7	16
Strawberry	140	6	18

Kilwin's: *Per 1/2 Cup*

	C	F	Cb
Black Cherry; Caramel Revel	90	0	22
Butter Pecan	190	13	16
Butter Pecan Yogurt	130	6	17
Chocolate	170	10	17
Chocolate Chip Cookie Dough	190	10	22
Chocolate Ripple	100	0	23
French Silk; Mud	190	11	20
Lemon/Raspberry Sorbetto	100	0	25
Old Fashioned Vanilla	180	9	20
Topping: Caramel	160	4.5	31
Fudge	110	6	28

Luigi's Real Italian Ice

	C	F	Cb
Squeeze-Up Tube: 8 fl.oz each	150	0	37

Rice Dream *(Non Dairy): Per 1/2 Cup*

	C	F	Cb
Vanilla Carob/Choc/Cappuccino	150	6	23
ChocChip/Cookies/Carob Chip	170	8	26
Supreme, average all flavors	170	8	24

Sealtest: *Per 1/2 Cup*

	C	F	Cb
Butter Pecan	160	9	16
Choc. Chip Cookie Dough	160	8	20
Fudge Royal; Heavenly Hash	150	7	20
Vanilla/Choc. Strawberry	140	7	16

Snackwell's: *Per 1/2 Cup*

	C	F	Cb
Brownie; Rocky Road	130	2	26
Praline Caramel	140	2	28
Vanilla	100	2	18

Soy Delicious (Organic): *Per 1/2 Cup*

	C	F	Cb
Quarts: Twisted Vanilla Orange	120	2	24
Choc Peanut Butter	150	5	23
Mocha Fudge	150	3.5	27
Other flavors, avg	140	4	23
It's Soy Delicious (Pints): *Per 1/2 Cup*			
Almond Pecan	160	5	24
Choc Almond/P'Nut Butter	150	5	24
Other flavors, average	130	3	25

Soy Dream *(Non-Dairy): Per 1/2 Cup*

	C	F	Cb
Butter Pecan	160	10	17
Chocolate Fudge Brownie	150	8	20
Mint Chocolate Chip	150	9	19
Average other flavors	140	6	20
Rocket Bars: Choc/Vanilla	220	12	29
Heavenly Pies: Mocha/Van	290	14	40

Starbucks: *Per 1/2 Cup*

	C	F	Cb
Biscotti Bliss	240	12	30
Brownies & Caramel; Van. Mocha	270	14	31
Chocolate Chocolate Fudge	290	17	28
Classic Coffee; Italian Roast	230	12	26
Coffee Almond Fudge	250	13	28
Espresso Swirl	220	10	29
Java Chip	250	13	29
Java Toffee	260	14	30
Mud Pie	240	11	32
Lowfat: Mocha Mambo; Latte	170	3	30
Bars: *See Icecream Bars & Pops Section*			

Stonyfield Farm (Organic): *Per 1/2 Cup*

	C	F	Cb
Icecream: Chocolate	265	18	22
Decaf Coffee; Vanilla, avg	260	18	21
Other flavors, average	260	16	26
Frozen Yogurt: Nonfat Choc.; Raspb.	100	0	21
Nonfat Vanilla; Decaf Coffee	90	0	19
Nonfat Vanilla Fudge Swirl	110	0	23
Lowfat: Creme Caramel	120	1.5	23
Choc Mint; Mocha Almond	130	3	22

Sweet Nothings *(Non-Dairy/Fat Free)*

	C	F	Cb
Average all flavors, 1/2 cup, 3 oz	120	0	28

TCBY: *Per 1/2 Cup*

	C	F	Cb
Paradise Ice: Medium	430	0	110
Large	550	0	140
Froz. Yogurt Family Style: Peach	110	1	21
Dutch Choc;.Summertime Strwb	100	1.5	20
Other flavors, average	110	1.5	23
Hand-Dipped: Medium	310	6.5	57
Large	390	8.5	73
No Sugar Add. Non Fat: Med.	175	0	44
Large	225	0	56
Non Fat: Medium	240	0	51
Large	310	0	64
Regular, all flavors: Medium	285	6.5	51
Large	365	8.5	64

Icecream Bars & Pops

Brands (Cont) — C F Cb

TCBY: Per 1/2 Cup

	C	F	Cb
Hand-Dipped Icecream: Small	320	19	37
Medium	440	26	50
Large	560	34	64
Sorbet: Medium	220	0	53
Large	280	0	67

Tasti D-Lite (Soft Serve)
Calories will vary with density (air in product) and serving size.
Best to weigh product and calculate on 25 cals per 1 oz weight.

	C	F	Cb
Vanilla: Small (4 fl.oz cup), 6 oz wt	180	4	35
Medium (8 fl.oz cup), 11 oz wt	330	7	64

Tofutti Non-Dairy Dessert: Per 1/2 Cup

	C	F	Cb
Premium: Vanilla	190	11	20
Better Pecan; Alm. Bark	220	13	22
Choc. Cookie Crunch	210	11	26
Chocolate Supreme	180	11	18
Van. Fudge; Wildberry	190	9	24
Low Fat Supreme: Average	110	2	25
Cutie Pies: Average, 67g bar	250	19	18
Too Toos: Vanilla S'wich	215	10	28
Van. Choc. Swirl/Chip S'wich	230	11	30
Teddy Fudge: 52g bar	70	1	19

Turkey Hill: Per 1/2 Cup

	C	F	Cb
Black Cherry	140	7	18
Butter Pecan	170	11	16
Choco. Mint Chip, Cookies 'n Crm	160	10	17
Neapolitan, Vanilla & Choc.	150	8	18
Rocky Road	170	8	23
Vanilla, Vanilla Bean	140	8	16
Lite: Choco Mint Chip	140	5	19
Cookies 'n Cream	130	5	21
Vanilla & Choc., Van. Bean	110	3	18

Weight Watchers: Per 1/2 Cup

	C	F	Cb
Cookie Dough Craze	140	3.5	24
Oh! So Very Vanilla	120	2.5	20
Positively Praline Crunch	140	3	25
Reckless Rocky Road	140	3	23
Triple Chocolate Tornado	150	3.5	26
Bars: Smart Ones, See Page 36			

WholeSoy Glace: Per 1/2 Cup, 70g

	C	F	Cb
Mocha Fudge	130	4	21
Swiss Chocolate	180	9	21
Strawberry	150	6	20
Vanilla Bean	190	9	25

Bars & Pops — C F Cb

Per Bar/Serving

	C	F	Cb
Baby Ruth (Nestlé)	180	12	15
Baskin Robbins: Tiny Toons	140	17	20
Cappuccino Blast, average	120	4	20
Sundae Bar, Pralines 'n Cream	280	17	28
Ben & Jerry's:			
Cherry Garcia: Icecream Bar	240	16	23
Yogurt Bar	250	11	35
Chocolate Fudge Brownie	230	11	28
Cookie Dough: 89ml Bar	330	19	36
110ml Bar	410	24	45
Cookie Dough Pop	410	24	45
One Sweet Whirled	260	16	27
Phish Stick: 89ml Bar	260	16	29
110ml Bar	290	17	33
Vanilla Heath Crunch	320	21	32
Big Bear: See Klondike			
Big Ed's Super Saucer: 10 fl.oz	420	28	32
1/2 Sandwich, 5 fl.oz	210	14	16
Borden: Sundae Cone	210	10	27
Twin Pops	60	0	14
Bon Bons (Nestlé): Milk Choc., (8)	330	23	27
Dark Chocolate, 8 pces	310	21	26
Bounty: all varieties	70	5	7
Butterfinger: Bar, 2.5 oz	190	13	16
Breyers: Vanilla Bar	250	17	21
w. Chocolate coating	230	15	20
Sandwich (Vanilla)	250	11	32
Carnation: Orange Sherbet, 3 oz	90	1	19
Icecream Cup: Choc., 3 fl.oz	140	8	16
Strawb., Vanilla, 3 fl.oz	100	6	12
Choc./Vanilla Malt, 12 oz	270	6	48
Sundae Cup, all types, 5 fl.oz	210	9	30
Chipwich Jr: Choc. Chip S'wich	240	10	35
Chiquita: Swirls, all flavors	80	3	12
Cool Creations: Mini Sandwich	110	5	16
Cookies & Cream Sandwich	240	11	34
Pops, all types, 2 oz	60	0	14
Mickey Mouse: 2.5 oz Bar	120	8	10
4 oz Bar	170	11	17
Creamsicle: Sugar-free pops	25	0	15
Orange, 2.8 fl.oz	110	3	20
Crunch (Nestlé): King, 4 oz	270	19	21
Reduced Fat, 2.5 oz	130	7	14
Regular Icecream Bar, 3 oz	200	14	16
Crystal Light: Cool 'n Creamy	50	2	7

Icecream Bars & Pops (Cont)

Per Bar/Serving	C	F	Cb
Dole Bars: Coconut, 4 oz	210	7	33
Fruit Juice, reg., 1.75 oz	45	0	11
No Added Sugar, 1.75 oz	25	0	6
Fruit 'n Juice: Small, 2.5 oz	70	0	16
Pine-Coconut, 4 oz	150	4	27
Other flavors, 4 oz	120	0	28
Dove Bar: Almond	340	22	30
Bite Size, 5 pces, average	350	22	36
Caramel Pecan	350	35	35
Mocha Cashew	260	17	25
Peppermint	390	17	31
Vanilla Dark Choc; Cookie	340	21	35
Single Vanilla Dark	200	12	24
Vanilla Milk Chocolate	350	24	29
Dreyers: Icecream Bars, average	250	17	22
Fruit Bars, 3 fl.oz	90	9	23
Smoothie Bars, average	95	0	23
Sundae Cone, 4 fl.oz	240	11	31
Whole Fruit Bars, 1.75 fl.oz	60	0	14
Drumstick *(Nestlé):* Chocolate	320	17	36
Choc. Dipped	320	16	40
Original Vanilla	340	19	35
Vanilla Caramel/Fudge	360	20	39
Eskimo Pie: Arctic Madness, 2.5 oz	230	15	23
Bars: Milk/Dark Choc, 50g	160	11	15
Fudge Bar, 55g	60	1	11
Reduced Fat varieties	120	8	13
Crispy Bar, 47g	130	8	13
Pecan, 51g	190	15	12
Big Bar, 99g	300	20	26
Icecream Sandwich, 65 g	160	4	27
Cones, 74g	210	12	24
No Sugar Added: Bar, 49g	120	8	13
Pudding Bar, 59g	90	1.5	16
Flintstones: Push Up Sherbet	100	2	20
Push Up Pebbles, 2.75 oz	120	6	15
Cool Cream, 2.75 oz	90	2	14
Frosty Dreams *(Nestlé)*	100	2	19
Frosty Pops *(Nestlé)*	40	0	11
Froz-Fruit: Cherry	60	0	15
Strawberry	80	0	20
Fruit A Freeze: Coconut	130	5	20
Lime	65	0	16
Banana; Strawberry	90	1.5	19
Dark Choc-Dipped Strawberry	90	3.5	14
Fudge Bar *(Nestlé)*	110	1	23

Per Bar/Serving	C	F	Cb
Fudgesicle: Fudge Bar (1)	45	0.5	9
Fat Free (1)	60	0	13
Fudgetastics: Sticks Sundae	220	15	37
Godiva: Pecan Caramel Bar	380	23	39
Good Humor: Candy Crunch	280	21	21
Chocolate Eclair; Colonel Crunch	170	9	21
Chocolate Taco	320	17	38
Classic Almond	210	12	21
Dinosaur	110	2	25
Giant Sandwich, 5 fl.oz	240	10	35
Icecream Sandwich	190	8	28
King Cone, 8 fl.oz	390	21	42
Mississippi Mud (Giant), 6 fl.oz	310	15	39
Reese's Peanut Butter, 1 bar	250	16	24
Shots Popsicle, 3.2 fl.oz	25	1.5	3
Strawberry Shortcake, 4 fl.oz	230	12	30
Cups: Sundae Twist	160	3	33
Combo, 6 fl.oz	200	10	25
Haagen-Dazs: *Per Bar*			
Caramel & Almond Crunch	310	21	27
Caramel Pecan Nut Cluster	420	31	31
Chocolate & Dark Chocolate	350	24	28
Chocolate Fudge & Almonds	330	23	25
Coffee & Almond Crunch	370	27	27
Cookies & Cream Crunch	370	26	30
Dulce De Leche (Caramel)	300	19	28
Vanilla & Almonds	380	28	26
Vanilla Caramel & Pecans	350	25	27
Vanilla & Dark Chocolate	280	20	22
Vanilla & Milk Chocolate	340	24	25
Sorbet & Yogurt, Raspb. & Vanilla	90	0	20
Chocolate Sorbet	80	0	21
Hood: Chocolate Eclair, 1 bar	150	10	14
Cooler Cup, 2.1 oz	80	1	18
Crispy Bar	180	13	15
Fabukous Fudgies, 1 bar	100	3	19
Fabulous Fudge P'nut Butter	110	4	17
Fudge Bar	100	1	21
Hendrie's Cherry Choc. Dips	120	9	11
Hoodsie Cup Van./Choc.	100	5	12
Orange Cream Bar	90	2	18
Rockets, each	120	5	18
Vanilla Bar	160	12	11
Icecream Sandwich *(Nestle)*	170	6	26
Jell-O: Pop Bars	31	0	7
Jigglers, all varieties, 6 oz	215	1.5	50
Pudding Bars	80	2	13

Icecream Bars & Pops (Cont)

Per Bar/Serving	C	F	Cb
Klondike: Almond Bar	310	21	26
Big Bear Van. Icecream S'wich	290	10	46
Neopolitan	300	12	42
Caramel & Peanut	300	20	28
Choc Chip Cookie Sandwich	520	21	77
Giant Cookies Sandwich			
w. Hershey's Choc Chips	470	20	66
Gold Bar	340	23	30
Heath Toffee	300	20	27
Krunch	270	17	26
Lite Bar	110	6	14
No Sugar Added	190	10	19
Oreo Cookie Sandwich	230	9	34
Sandwich: Chocolate	270	10	41
Lite	100	2	18
Vanilla	250	9	37
The Original (Vanilla), 5 fl.oz	280	19	24
York Peppermint Patty	290	20	24
Kool-Aid Pops	40	0	10
Krispy Frostick:	150	10	13
Juice Flavored Sticks	50	0	13
M&Ms: Cookie Icecream S'wich	240	12	32
Mars Almond Bar	210	14	20
Matterhorn: Cone, 10 fl.oz	510	38	19
Milky Way: Choc, Reduced Fat	140	7	19
Caramel Swirl, 1 bar	180	10	21
Snack Bar, Vanilla/Chocolate	70	4	9
Minute Maid: Fruit Juice Pops	60	0	15
Nestlé Icescreamers: Push Up Pop	90	1.5	19
Shock Tarts, 1 pop	45	0	11
Tiger Tails, 1 pop	60	0	15
Drumstick: S'Mores	290	16	33
Strawberry Cheesecake	260	12	34
Oreo: Choc; Vanilla	160	9	19
Big Stuf, 1 sandwich	240	10	33
Cookies n' Cream, 1 bar, 59g	180	12	18
Pathmark: Vanilla w. choc. coat.	150	10	14
Polar Bar: Vanilla w. choc. coat.	240	18	15
Choc. Chip Cookie Dough	450	28	48
Pops (water/juice), average	60	0	14
Popsicles: Fudgesicle Fudge Pop	90	1.5	16
Scribblers Icecream: 2 pces	130	7	15
Juice Pops, 2 pces	60	0	16
Sprinklers Icecream, 1 bar	130	6	18
Pokémon Ice w. Candy, 1 pce	80	0	19
Rugrats Cookie S'wich, 1 pce	150	7	20
Wildlife Icecream, 1 piece	110	6	14

Per Bar/Serving	C	F	Cb
Popsicles (Cont): Ice Pops, 1 pce	45	0	11
Sugar-Free, 1 pce	15	0	3
Reece's: Peanut Butter Icecream	160	11	22
Rice Dream: Pies, all flavors	320	18	40
Bars: Stawbery	250	13	31
Chocolate, Vanilla	270	15	32
Choc/Vanilla Nutty	270	18	23
Silhouette (Skinny Cow) Lowfat			
Icecream Sandwich, Van./Choc.	130	2	23
Smart Ones (Weight Watchers):			
Chocolate Mousse	40	1	9
Chocolate Treat	100	0.5	20
English Toffee Crunch	110	6	12
Mocha Java	80	1.5	15
Orange Vanilla Treat	40	0.5	10
Vanilla Lowfat Sandwich	150	3	28
Snackwell: Icecream Sandwich	90	1.5	18
Yogurt Bars, 1 bar, 80g	120	2	22
Snickers: Pralines n' Creme	220	13	22
Icecream Bar (The Big One)	250	15	25
Snack, 4 bars	390	25	38
Soy Delicious: Big Buddy	240	8	42
s/w Li'l Buddy, Vanilla	265	14	32
Mocha Mania (choc coated)	265	14	32
Mint Choc Chips	260	10	41
Bars: Creamy Fudge	140	4	25
Creamy Vanilla	250	13	31
Vanilla & Almond	300	17	32
Soy Dream (Non-Dairy):			
Dreamwich Vanilla	130	6	15
Heavenly Pies: Mocha; Vanilla	290	14	40
Lil' Dreamers: Choc; Vanilla	60	3	7
Rocket Bars: Choc; Vanilla	220	12	29
Starbuck's: Java Ice Cream Bar	270	16	29
Coffee & Almond Bars, 81g	280	18	26
Coffee Frappuccino Bar	110	2	20
Mocha Frappuccino Bar	120	2	21
Starburst: Juice Bars	20	0	5
Super Sundae Bar, 86g	310	20	29
3 Musketeers: 2 fl.oz bars	170	10	21
Snack Bars, regular	60	4	16
Tandem (Nestlé): Sandwich	380	21	39
Twin Pop (Nestlé)	60	0	14
Vitari: soft serve, 4 fl.oz, average	80	0	20
Welch's: Fruit Juice Bars, 92g	80	0	19
Tropical Coolers, 92 bar	45	0	11
No Sugar Added, 1 bar	25	0	4
Fruit Smoothie, 1 ctn	240	0	59

Quick Guide

Cream

	C	F	Cb
Average All Brands			
Half & Half Cream: 1 Tbsp, 0.5 oz	20	2	0.5
2 Tbsp, 1 oz	40	4	1
Light, coffee/table (20% fat): 1 T.	30	3	0.5
2 Tbsp, 1 oz	60	6	1
Medium (25% fat), 2 Tbsp, 1 oz	40	4	0.5
Sour Cream:			
Regular, 1 Tbsp, 0.5 oz	30	3	0.5
1 cup, 8 oz	490	48	8
Lowfat/Light, 1 Tbsp, 0.5 oz	20	2	1.5
2 Tbsp, 1 oz	40	2.5	2
Half & Half, 1 Tbsp, 0.5 oz	20	2.5	0.5
Fat Free, 2 Tbsp, 1 oz	20	0	3
Fat Free: (HeluvaGood), 2 Tbsp	20	0	6
(Kroger), 2 Tbsp, 1 oz	25	0	5
(Naturally Yours; Oak Farm), 2 T.	20	0	3
(Knudsen), 2 Tbsp, 1 oz	35	0	6
Sour Cream Substitute:			
(Albertson's/ IMO), 2 T., 1 oz	60	5	2
(Tofutti) Sour Supreme, 1 oz	50	5	1
Whipping Cream:			
Heavy (37% fat):			
1 Tbsp fluid/2 Tbsp whipped	50	5	1
1/4 cup whipped	100	11	2
1/2 cup fluid/1 cup whipped	400	44	8
Light (30% fat):			
1 tbsp fluid/2 Tbsp whipped	45	5	0.5
1/2 cup fluid/1 cup whipped	350	37	4

Coconut Cream/Milk

	C	F	Cb
Coconut Cream (Canned),			
Plain/unsweetened, 2 Tbsp, 1 oz	70	6	4
1/2 cup, 4 oz	280	24	16
Sweetened: *Coco Lopez*, 1 oz	120	5	20
1/2 cup, 4 oz	480	20	80
Coconut Milk (Canned):			
Natural Value: Reg., 1/4 c., 2 fl.oz	90	9	1
Lite, 1/4 c., 2 fl.oz	55	5	1
Thai Kitchen: Reg., 1/4 c., 2 fl.oz	125	12	3
Lite, 1/4 cup, 2 fl.oz	50	4	2
Coconut Water (center), 1 cup	45	0.5	9

Whipped Toppings

	C	F	Cb
Average All Brands			
Cream (Pressurized): 2 Tbsp	20	2	1
1/4 cup	45	4	2
1/2 cup	90	8	4
Cream Toppings: *Jewel,* Lite, 2 T.	20	1	2
Cool Whip: Extra Creamy, 2 T.	25	1.5	2
Lite, 2 Tbsp, 9g	20	1	2
Free, 2 Tbsp, 9g	15	0	3
Non Dairy, 2 Tbsp	22	2	2
Kraft: Whipped, 2 Tbsp	20	2	1
Real Cream, 2 Tbsp	20	2	1
Reddi-Wip: Original, 2 T., 8g	20	2	0
Original Light, 2 T.	15	1	2
Non-Dairy, 2 T., 8g	20	1.5	2
Extra Creamy, 2 Tbsp, 8g	30	3	0.5
Fat Free, 2 Tbsp, 8g	10	0	2

Non-Dairy Coffee Creamers

	C	F	Cb
Powder *Coffee-Mate/Cremora/N-Rich:*			
Regular, 1 tsp	20	2	1
1 heaping tsp	25	2	2
Fat Free, 1 tsp	10	0	2
Lite, 1 tsp	10	0.5	2
Flavors: 1 1/3 Tbsp	60	3	9
Fat Free: Average, 1 1/3 Tbsp	50	0	11
Liquid/Refrigerated: *Per Tbsp*			
Coffee-Mate Non-Dairy Creamer:			
Plain: Regular/Plain, 1 Tbsp	20	1	2
Fat Free, 1 Tbsp	10	0	2
Lite, 1 Tbsp	10	0.5	1
Flavors: All flavors, 1 Tbsp	40	2	5
Fat Free, all flavors, 1 Tbsp	25	0	5
Crème de la Soy (Westsoy):			
Original, 1 Tbsp	20	1.5	2
Amaretto; French Vanilla, 1 T.	25	1	4
Hood (Non Dairy), 1 Tbsp	25	0	5
International Delight: 1 Tbsp	35	1.5	6
Fat Free flavors, 1 Tbsp	30	0	7
Mocha Mix: Original, 1 Tbsp	20	1.5	1
Fat Free, 1 Tbsp	10	0	1
Lite, 1 Tbsp	10	0.5	1
Rich's Coffee Rich: Regular, 1 T.	25	1	2
Light	15	0.5	0.5
Rich's Farm Rich: Regular, 1 Tbsp	20	1	2
Light/Fat Free	10	0	0.5
Silk (White Wave) Creamer, 1Tbsp	15	1	1
French Vanilla, 1 Tbsp	20	1	3

Fats, Spreads & Oils

Butter & Margarine

Average All Brands

	C	F	Cb
Regular: 1 tsp (5g)	35	4	0
1 Pat (5g)	35	4	0
1 Tbsp, approx. ¹/₂ oz	100	11	0
2 Tbsp, 1 oz	205	23	0
1 Stick, ¹/₂ cup, 4 oz	810	92	0
1 Pound, 2 cups, 16 oz	3240	368	0
Light (Regular) 40% Fat:			
1 tsp, 5g	17	2	0
1 Tbsp, ¹/₂ oz	50	6	0
2 Tbsp, 1 oz	100	11	0
Whipped Butter (Regular):			
1 tsp (4 g)	27	3	0
1 Tbsp (10g)	70	7.5	0
1 Stick, ¹/₂ cup, 2²/₃ oz	570	60	0
Whipped Light Butter 40% Fat:			
1 tsp, 5g	10	1	0
1 Tbsp, 9g	35	3.5	0
2 Tbsp, 18g	70	7	0
Unsalted: Same as Regular			

Clarified Butter

	C	F	Cb
100% Fat: 1 Tbsp, ¹/₂ oz	130	15	0
2 Tbsp, 1 oz	260	30	0

Flavored Butter/Spread

Average All Brands

	C	F	Cb
Honey Butter (60% Fat):			
1 Tbsp, ¹/₂ oz	90	7	4
Downey's, 1 Tbsp, ¹/₂ oz	60	1	11
Garlic Butter (80% Fat):			
1 Tbsp, ¹/₂ oz	100	11	0
Sweet Cream Butter:			
Regular, 1 Tbsp	100	11	0
Stick (70% Fat), 1 Tbsp	90	10	0
Tub (60% Fat), 1 Tbsp	80	9	0

Other Spreads & Fats

	C	F	Cb
Copha, Dripping, Lard, Suet, Shortening:			
1 Tbsp, ¹/₂ oz	120	13	0
Chicken, Duck, Goose Fat:			
1 Tbsp, ¹/₂ oz	115	13	0

Light & Reduced Fat Spreads **C** **F** **Cb**

Per 1 Tbsp, ¹/₂ oz (Unless Stated)

	C	F	Cb
Benecol: Spread, 1 Tbsp, 14g	80	9	0
Light, Spread, 1 Tbsp, 14g	45	5	0
Blue Bonnet Homestyle (48% Veg Oil)	60	7	0
Breakstone's Whipped Butter	60	7	0
Brummel & Brown: Spread	45	5	0
Chiffon: Whipped, 1 Tbsp	70	7	0
Country Crock (Shedd's): Regular	60	7	0
Light; Calcium & Vitamins	50	5	0
Country's Delight (70% Veg.)	90	10	0
Country Morning: Light	50	6	0
Downey's Honey Butter	60	1	0
Dutch Farms: 52% Veg. Spread	70	7	0
Fleischmann's: Soft Spread	80	9	0
Original	80	9	0
Fat Free Spread	5	0	0
'I Can't Believe It's Not Butter': Reg.	90	10	0
Light; Sweet Cream	50	6	0
Imperial: Diet, 1 Tbsp	50	6	0
Jewel: Soft Spread	60	7	0
Unbelievably Butter	90	9	0
Kraft: 'Touch of Butter' (bowl)	50	6	0
Land O'Lakes: Fresh Buttery Taste	80	8	0
Honey Butter	90	7	4
Light Butter Whipped	35	3.5	0
Light Butter	50	6	0
Mazola: Diet	50	6	0
Mother's; Mrs Filbert's, 1 Tbsp	70	8	0
Miracle: Soft	60	7	0
Stick	70	7	0
Nucoa: HeartBeat Margarine	25	3	0
Olivio: Vegetable Spread	80	8	0
Parkay: Squeeze, 1 Tbsp	80	9	0
Stick, ¹/₃ Less Fat	70	7	0
Tub, Light/Soft Diet	60	7	0
Tub, Light/Soft Diet	50	6	0
Whipped	70	7	0
Promise: Regular	90	10	0
Extra Light	50	6	0
Buttery Light	45	5	0
Ultra, w. Canola Oil	35	4	0
Smart Balance: Regular, 1 Tbsp	80	9	0
Light, 1 Tbsp	45	5	0
Smart Beat: Fat Free	10	0	3
Take Control: Regular Spread	80	8	0
Light Spread	45	5	0
Weight Watcher's: Light, all types	45	4	2

Fats, Spreads & Oils

Butter Substitutes

	C	F	Cb
Bake It Perfect (Fat Free Spread), 1 T.	5	0	0
Best O'Butter, 1/2 tsp	4	0	0
Butter Buds: 1 serving, 1/2 tsp	4	0	0
Butterlike Saute Butter, 1 Tbsp	35	2	0
Butter Sprinkles (Watkins): 1 tsp	5	0	0
Earth Balance, Non GMO,1 tsp	35	3.5	0
Molly McButter: 1/2 tsp	5	0	0
Mrs Bateman's Baking Butter, 1 T.	35	1	0

Spreads Comparison

	C	F	Cb
Mayonnaise: Regular, 1 Tbsp	100	11	0.5
Light, average, 1 Tbsp	50	5	1
Fat Free (e.g. *Wt. Watcher's*), 1 T.	12	0	3
Miracle Whip (*Kraft*):			
Regular, 1 Tbsp	70	7	2
Light, 1 Tbsp	40	3	3
Free, 1 Tbsp	15	0	3
SmartBeat Dressing: 1 Tbsp	12	0	2
Extra Listings for Mayonnaise & Dressings			
~ See Page 90 ~			
Peanut Butter, 1 Tbsp	100	8	3.5
Avocado, mashed, 1 Tbsp	25	2.5	2
Birdseye:			
No Fat Veggie Dip, 2 T., 1.1 oz	25	0	5

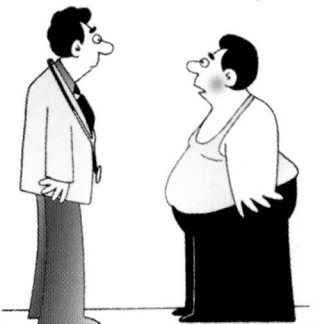

"I push myself away from the table but my wife's good cooking pulls me right back."

Animal Fats/Lards

Average All Types

	C	F	Cb
Beef Tallow/Drippings, Lard (Pork), Chicken, Duck, Goose, Turkey.			
1 Tbsp (13g)	115	13	0
2 1/4 Tbsp, 1 oz	255	28	0
1 cup, 7 1/4 oz	1850	205	0
1/2 pound, 8 oz	2040	227	0
Ghee/Butter Oil: 1 Tbsp, 13g	110	13	0
2 1/4 Tbsp, 1 oz	250	28	0

Vegetable Shortening

Average All Types (example, *Crisco*)

	C	F	Cb
1 Tbsp, 0.44 oz	113	13	0
2 1/4 Tbsp, 1 oz	250	28	0
1 cup, 7 1/4 oz	1810	205	0

Vegetable Oils

Includes almond, avocado, canola, corn, coconut, flaxseed, grapeseed, linseed, mustard, olive, palm, peanut, rice-bran, safflower, sesame, sunflower, soybean, wheatgerm. Note: Oil is 100% fat.

	C	F	Cb
1 tsp, 5g	45	5	0
1 Tbsp, 1/2 oz	120	14	0
2 Tbsp, 1 oz	250	28	0
1 cup, 7 3/4 oz	1930	205	0

Fish Oils

Average All Types (Includes cod liver, herring, salmon, sardine):

	C	F	Cb
1 Tbsp, 1/2 oz	125	14	0

Cooking Sprays / Squeezes

	C	F	Cb
Cooking Sprays (*Pam, Mazola, Weight Watchers, Wesson*):			
Per serving	2	0	0
2-3 second spray	6	1	0
I Can't Believe It's Not Butter	0	0	0
Parkay Buttery Spray	0	0	0
Squeeze (*Parkay*), 1 Tbsp, 0.5 oz	70	8	0

Olestra (Olean)

	C	F	Cb
Olestra (*Olean*)	0	0	0

Olean is *Proctor & Gamble's* brand name for olestra - a no-calorie cooking oil that gives snacks (like potato chips, tortilla chips and crackers) taste and texture without adding fat or calories.

Cheeses

Firm/Hard Cheeses
(American, Cheddar, Colby, Coon, Swiss)

Regular Cheese:	C	F	Cb
1 oz slice/piece	110	9	0.5
8 oz package	880	72	4
16 oz (1lb) package	1760	144	8
Cubes: 1" cube, 3/4 oz	55	5	0.5
1 1/4" cube, 1 oz slice	110	9	0.5
Diced: 1 cup, 4 1/2 oz	500	40	2
Grated: 1 Tbsp, 1/4 oz	27	2	0
Shredded:			
1/4 cup, 1 oz	110	9	0.5
1 cup, 4 oz	440	36	4
Sliced: 1 thin (3 1/2" sq.), 3/4 oz	85	7	0.5
Rectangular (7"x 4"x 1/8"), 1 1/2 oz	165	14	1
Round (3 1/4" diam. x 1/8"), 3/4 oz	85	7	0.5
Semi-circular, 1 1/4" oz			
(5 1/2" long, 3 1/2" radius, 1/8"thick)	140	11	0.5
Light: Average All Brands, oz	80	5	0.5
Fat Free: Average All Brands, 1 oz	50	0	2
Lowfat: Average All Brands, 1 oz	50	1.5	1

Cheese
Per 1 oz Unless Indicated

American:	C	F	Cb
Regular, 1 slice, 1 oz	110	9	1
Kraft Deluxe, 0.7 oz slice	70	6	0.5
Grated, 1 Tbsp, 1/4 oz	23	2	0
Light *(Borden)*, 1 oz	70	4	0.5
Land O'Lakes, 1 oz	70	5	0.5
Smart Beat, 0.6 oz slice	35	2	0
Fat Free: Single, 0.75 oz	30	0	3
Alpine Lace, 1 oz	45	0	2
HealthyChoice, Singles, 0.7 oz	25	0	2
Weight Watchers, all types, 3/4 oz	30	0	3
Babybel (Laughing Cow), 1 oz	90	7	0
Crumbled, 1/2 cup, 2 1/2 oz	250	20	2
Dorman's Castello, 1 oz	135	12	1
Bonbel (Laughing Cow), 1 oz	100	8	0
Mini, 3/4 oz	75	6	0
Brick, 1 oz	100	8	0
Brie, 1 oz	95	8	1
Camembert, 1 oz	90	7	1
Caraway, 1 oz	105	8	1

Cheddar: (Also see 'Quick Guide')	C	F	Cb
Regular, 1 oz	110	9	0.5
Reduced Fat/Light, 1 oz	80	5	0.5
Weight Watchers, 1 oz	80	5	1
Fat Free: *Alpine Lace*, 1 oz	45	0	2
Weight Watchers, 1 sl., 3/4 oz	30	0	3
Cheese Balls *(Kaukauna)*, 1 oz	100	7	0.5
Cheese Nut, Average, 1 oz	100	7	2
Cheese Logs, Average, 1 oz	100	7	0.5
Cheshire, 1 oz	110	9	1.5
Colby, Regular, 1 oz	110	9	0.5
Reduced Fat *(Alpine Lace)*, 1 oz	80	5	1
Colby-Jack, 1 oz	110	9	0.5
Cottage Cheese: *Average All Brands*			
Creamed (4% milk fat): 2 Tbsp, 1 oz	30	1	1
1/2 cup, 4 oz	120	5	4
w. fruit, 1/2 cup, 4 oz	130	4	15
Reduced Fat (2%), 2 T., 1 oz	25	<1	1
1/2 cup, 4 oz	100	2	4
Low Fat (1%), 2 Tbsp, 1 oz	20	<1	1
1/2 cup, 4 oz	80	1	3
Fat Free/Non Fat, 2 Tbsp, 1 oz	20	0	1
1/2 cup, 4 oz	80	0	3
Borden Dry Curd (0.5%), 1/2 c., 4 oz	80	0	0
Cottage Doubles, avg, 5.5 oz ctn	150	2.5	18
Friendship: Low Fat P'apple, 4 oz	120	1	17
Non Fat Plus Peach, 1/2 c., 4 oz	110	0	15
Pot Style, 1/2 cup, 4 oz	90	3	3
w. Pineapple, 4 oz	140	4	16
Hood Fruit Stirs, avg, 110g ctn	200	2.5	24
Knudsen: 1.5% Fruit, 4 oz	110	2	12
Free, Non Fat, 1/2 cup, 4.3 oz	80	0	7
Low Fat, 2% Milk Fat, 1/2 c., 4.3 oz	100	2.5	5
4% Milk Fat, 1/2 cup, 4.3 oz	120	5	5
Light N' Lively: Garden Salad, 4 oz	90	2	5
Peach and Pineapple,			
1/2 cup, 4.3 oz	120	1	14
Cream Cheese: See Page 43			
Edam, Regular, 1 oz	100	8	0
Farmer *(Friendship)*, 2 Tbsp, 1 oz	50	3	0
Feta: Regular, *Frigo*, 1 oz	100	8	1
Crumbled, 1/2 cup, 2 1/2 oz	190	15	2.5
Reduced Fat *(Alpine Lace)*,	60	4	1
Fontina *(Sargento/Classica)*, 1 oz	110	9	0.5
Gjetost (Goat's Milk, fresh), 1 oz	85	7	0.5
Sargento, 1 oz	130	8	12
Goat's Milk: Soft: *Chevre*, 1 oz	70	6	0.5
Chavril, 3 Tbsp, 1 oz	60	4.5	0.5

Goat's Milk Cheese (Cont)	C	F	Cb
Semi-Soft: 1 oz	100	8.5	1
Hard: Sargento, 1 oz	130	10	0.5
Gorgonzola: 1 oz	110	9	0.5
Galbani Dolcelatte: 1 oz	95	8	1
Gouda: 1 oz	100	8	0.5
Gruyere, 1 oz	115	9	0
Havarti, 1 oz	120	11	0
Italian (Classica Italiano), 1 oz	110	10	1
Jarlsberg, 1 oz	100	7	1
Jarlsberg Lite shredded, 1 oz	70	4	1
Kefir, 2 Tbsp, 1 oz	60	4	1
Limburger, 1 oz	90	8	0
Mascarpone, 1 oz	130	13	1
Mexican (Sargento Recipe Blend), Shredded, 1/4 cup, 1 oz	110	9	0.5
Monterey, 1 oz	105	8.5	0
Monterey Jack: regular, 1 oz	110	9	0
Light Naturals (Kraft), 1 oz	80	5	0
Alpine Lace, Monti-Jack Lo, 1 oz	80	5	0
Weight Watchers, 1 oz	90	6	1
Mozzarella:			
Regular: Kraft/Dorman's, 1 oz	90	7	0.5
Land O'Lakes/Polly-O, 1 oz	80	6	0.5
Shredded, 1/4 cup, 1 oz	80	6	0.5
Light: Polly-O Lite, 1 oz	60	2.5	0.5
Kraft Light Naturals, 1 oz	80	5	0.5
Sorrento Lite, 1 oz	60	3	0.5
Part Skim (Alpine Lace), 1 oz	70	5	0.5
Polly-O, 1 oz	90	6	0.5
Fat Free: Healthy Choice, 1/4 c.,1oz	45	0	1
Polly-O, 1 oz	35	0	1
Kraft, shredded, 1/4 cup, 1 oz	50	0	2
Muenster: regular, 1 oz	110	9	0
Reduced Fat: Dorman's, 1 oz	80	5	0
Neufchatel: Dominick's, 1 oz	70	6	2
Philadelphia, 1 oz	70	6	0.5
Flavored: Fruit/Herbs	80	7	1
Chocolate (Hickory Farms), 1 oz	110	8	1
Parmesan: Fresh/Block, 1 oz	110	7	1
Shredded/Grated, 1 Tbsp	22	1.5	0
Grated (Packaged): 1 Tbsp	26	2	0
1oz quantity	130	9	2
1/2 cup, 1-3/4 oz	230	16	2
w. Romano (Frigo), grated, 1 oz	130	9	1

Note: Packaged grated and shredded Parmesan have more calories (per unit weight) than block Parmesan due to a lower moisture content.

	C	F	Cb
Pizza, shredded:			
Frigo, 1/4 cup, 1 oz	90	7	1
1 cup, 4 oz	360	28	4
Lowfat (Frigo), 1 oz	65	3	1
Port Du Salut, 1 oz	100	8	0.5
Port Wine (Hickory Farms), 1 oz	100	7	2.5
Pot (Sargento), 1 oz	25	0	1
Provolone: Regular, 1 oz	100	8	1
Reduced Fat, Alpine Lace, 1 oz	70	5	1
Pub (Hickory Farms), 1 oz	95	7	1
Quark: 40% fat, 1 oz	47	3	1
20% fat, 1 oz	32	1.5	1
Skim, 1 oz	22	0	1.5
Queso: Anego/Asadero/Blanco	105	9	1
Queso Chichuahua/De Papa	110	9	2
Queso De Taco, 1 oz	105	9	1
Ricotta Cheese:			
Whole Milk, 2 Tbsp, 1 oz	50	3.5	1
1/2 cup, 4-1/2 oz	225	16	4.5
Part Skim, 2 Tbsp, 1 oz	40	2.5	1
1/2 cup, 4-1/2 oz	180	12	4.5
Light/Low Fat, 2 Tbsp, 1 oz	30	1.5	1.5
1/2 cup, 4-1/2 oz	140	6	6
Fat Free (Polly-O), 1/2 c., 4-1/2 oz	100	0	4
Baked Ricotta, 2 oz portion	130	9	3
Romano: Block/Loaf, 1 oz	110	8	1
Grated (Pkg), 1 oz	120	9	1
1 Tbsp	26	2	0.5
Roquefort, 1 oz	105	9	0.5
Slim Jack (Dorman's), 1 oz	90	7	1
Sheep's Milk (Hollow Rd Farm)	45	3	1
Smoked: Sargents Smokestick	100	7	1
Hickory Farm, Smoky Lyte, 1 oz	80	6	1
Stilton, 1 oz	118	10	1
String (Frigo/Kraft/Sargento), 1 oz	80	5	1
String Lite (Frigo), 1 oz	60	2	1
Mootown Light (Sargento), 1 stick	50	2.5	1
Swiss: Regular, 1 oz	110	9	1
Reduced Fat: Alpine Lace, 1 oz	90	6	1
Dorman's/Kraft Light Naturals, 1oz	90	5	1
Weight Watchers, 3/4 oz slice	30	0	2
Taco, shredded, 1/4 cup (Frigo/Kraft/Sargents)	110	9	1
Tilsit (Sargents), 1 oz	100	7	0.5
Tybo (Dorman's/Sargents), 1 oz	100	7	0.5
Vermont (Churny), 1 oz	100	9	1
Wensleydale, 1 oz	108	9	1
Whey Cheese, 1 oz	125	8	9

Cheese (Cont)

Cheese Products

	C	F	Cb
Cheese Food:			
Average all flavors, 3/4 oz slice	70	5	1.5
1 oz slice	90	6	2
Alouette: Fr. Onion/Garl.,2 T., 0.8oz	70	7	1
Light Garlic, 2 Tbsp, 0.8 oz	50	4	1
Cracker Barrel, Cheddar, 1.1 oz	100	8	4
Delico: Alouette Cajun, 2 T, 0.8 oz	70	7	1
Garden Vegetable, 2 T, 0.8 oz	60	6	1
Handi-Snacks:			
Cheez 'n Breadsticks, 1 pkg	130	7	11
Cheez'n Pretzels, 1 oz pkg	110	6	11
Cheez'n Crackers, 1.1 oz pkg	130	8	10
Mozzarella Stringchse Stick, each	80	6	0.5
Healthy Choice: Amer. Singles, 1 sl.	30	0	2
Heluva Good Cheese:			
American, 1 slice	45	5	2
Cheddar w. H/radish, 2 Tbsp, 1oz	90	7	3
Jalapeno: Aver., all brands, 1 oz	90	7	2
Kraft: American grated, 1T., 0.2 oz	25	2	1
Singles, 1 slice, 3/4 oz	70	6	1
Free Singles, 1 slice, 0.7 oz	40	3	3
Pimento Spread, 2 Tbsp, 1.1 oz	80	6	3
Velveeta (Process Cheese Spread)			
Regular, 3/8" slice, 1 oz	100	6	3
Light, 3/8" slice, 1 oz	60	3	3
Rip-Ums, 1 strip, 0.75 oz	80	7	0.5
Lifeway: Farmers Cheese, 2 oz	75	5	2.5
Precious: String Chse Stuffsters, 1 oz	70	4.5	1
Roka Blue, 2 Tbsp, 1.1 oz	80	7	2
Rondele: Soft Spread., 2 T, 1 oz	100	9	1
Light, 2 Tbsp, 0.9 oz	60	4	2
SmartBalance: Crmy Cheddar, 1 sl.	40	2	2
SmartBeat: All flav., 1 sl., 0.6 oz	35	2	2
Spreadery: Vermont, 2 Tbsp, 1 oz	80	5	3
Neufchatel, all flavors, 2 T, 1 oz	80	7	1
Velveeta: Cheese, 1 slice, 1 oz	100	6	3
Light, 1 oz	60	3	3
Shredded, 1/4 cup, 1.3 oz	130	9	3
WisPride: Hickory Smoked Cup;			
Port Wine Ball/Cup, 2 T., 1.1 oz	100	7	4
Light, 2 T., 1.1 oz	80	3	5

Cheese Whiz (Sauce)

	C	F	Cb
Regular, 2 Tbsp, 33g	90	7	2
Light, 2 Tbsp, 33g	80	3	6
Squeezable, 2 Tbsp, 33g	100	8	4

Cheese Substitutes

Per 1 oz Unless Indicated

	C	F	Cb
Almond Rella (Nu Soya):			
Cheddar; Garlic & Herb, 1 oz	60	3	3
Borden: Taco-Mate, 1 oz	100	7	2
Delicia: American Colby	80	6	1
Dorman's Lo Chol: All types	100	7	1
Formagg:			
American Wh./Yellow, 1 sl. 0.7oz	60	4	0.5
Cheddar, 1 slice, 0.7 oz	60	4	0.5
Mozzarella (Old World), 1 oz	60	3	1
Parmesan Grated, 1 Tbsp, 1/4 oz	22	1.5	1.5
Provolone (Vintage), 1 oz	60	3	1
Swiss White, 1 slice, 0.7 oz	60	4	0.5
Frigo: Cheddar; Mozzarella, 1 oz	90	7	1
Georgio's: Imitation Cheddar;			
Mozzarella., shredded, 1/4 c., 1 oz	90	7	1
Golden Image: American 1 slice, 0.7 oz			
Mild Cheddar, 1 slice, 0.7 oz	70	5	1
Harvest Moon : *Per 1/4 Cup, 1.3 oz*			
Shredded: American; Cheddar	120	9	3
Mozzarella	110	9	3
Nu Tofu: Mozzarella, 1 oz	70	4	2
Fat Free: Mozz./Ched./Jack, 1 oz	40	0	2
Sargento Classic Supreme:			
Cheddar, shredded, 1 oz	90	6	2
Mozzarella, shrd, 1/4 cup	80	6	0.5
Smart Beat, all varieties, 0.6 oz sl.	35	2	2
Soya Kaas: Regular, 1 oz	70	5	1
Fat Free, all varieties, 1 oz	40	2	1
Soyco: Almond/Oat/Rice Slices,			
1 slice, 0.7 oz	40	2	1
Veggy Singles, 1 slice, 0.7 oz	40	2	1
Grated Parmesan, 2 tsp, 5g	15	0.5	0
Tofu Rella: Per 1 oz			
Tofu Rella, average all varieties	180	2	39
Zero-Fat Rella, all varieties	45	0	3
Almond/Hemp/Rice Rella,			
average all varieties	70	3.5	3
Tofutti Better Than Cream Cheese	80	8	1
Weight Watchers: Fat Free Slices,			
All varieties, 3/4 oz slice	30	0	3
Grated Italian Topping, 1 Tbsp	20	0	2
White Wave, Soy A Melt:			
Cheddar/Mozz./Mont. Jack, 1 oz	80	5	1
Fat Free, 1 oz	40	0	3
Singles: Amer./Mozzrlla, 3/4 oz sl.	60	4	1
Yves Good Slice, 3/4 oz slice, aver.	35	2	1

Snack & Cheese Dips, Spreads

Cream Cheese	C	F	Cb
Regular/Soft: 2 Tbsp, 1 oz	100	10	1
3 oz pkg	300	30	2
w. Chives/Herbs/Pimento, 1 oz	90	9	0.5
w. Fruit/Strawb./P'apple, 1 oz	90	8	5
Lox, 1 oz	90	9	0.5
Philadelphia Brand:			
Plain/Soft, 2 Tbsp, 1 oz	100	10	1
1/3 Less Fat, 1 oz	70	6	1
Light, 1 oz	70	5	2
Fat Free, 2 Tbsp, 1 oz	30	0	3
Flavor./Herbs/Fruit/Salmon, 1 oz	100	10	2
w. Smoked Salmon 1 oz	100	9	1
Light Blueberry, 2 Tbsp	70	4.5	5
Snack Bars: avg, all types (1)	190	11	20
Whipped, 3 Tbsp, 1 oz	110	11	4
Alpine Lace: Fat Free, 2 T., 1 oz	30	0	1
Weight Watchers, 2 Tbsp, 1 oz	40	2.5	1

Dips/Spreads ~ Per 2 Tbsp (1 oz)

	C	F	Cb
Avocado/Guacomole	50	4	4
Baba Ghannoush (Eggplant/Sesame)	70	6	2
Birdseye: No Fat Veggie Dip, 1.1 oz	25	0	5
Breakstone's: Sour Cream, all flav.	50	4	4
Chalco: Quéso Quesadilla; Cotija	120	10	0
Fresco, 2 Tbsp, 1 oz	70	8	0
Chi-Chi's: Con Quéso, 2 Tbsp	90	7	4
Hot/Medium/Mild/Acante, 2 T.	10	0	2
Cool Cuts: Carrot & Ranch	60	4	5
Celery & Peanut Butter	170	14	9
French Onion Dip, aver. all brands	60	6	3
Frito Lay: Chili Cheese; Jalapeno	50	3	4
French Onion	60	5	4
Bean/Jalapeno Bean	40	1	6
Guacamole, 2 Tbsp, 1 oz	50	4	4
Guiltless Gourmet: Nacho Dip	25	0	5
Other varieties	30	0	5
Heluva Good Cheese: Chse 'N Salsa	80	3	3
Clam/French Onion	50	5	2
Bacon/Homestyle/Ranch	60	5	2
Light Fr. Onion/Jalapeno Cheddar	40	2	3
Hummus, 2 Tbsp, 1 oz	50	1	5
1/2 cup, 4.5 oz	220	4.5	23
Hy-Top: Pimiento, 1 oz	90	8	3
Kaukauna: Nacho Cheese	90	7	4
Knudsen: Nacho Cheese	60	4	3
Sour Cream Bacon & Onion	60	5	2
Sour Cream French Onion	50	4	2

Dips/Spreads (Cont)
Per 2 Tbsp (1 oz)

	C	F	Cb
Kroger: The Big Dipper; all flavors	60	5	2
Kraft: Average all flavors, 2 Tbsp	60	5	4
Premium: Bac. & On./Nacho Ch.	60	5	2
Other flavors	50	4	2
Philly flavors: Pineapple	100	9	1
Chive & Onion; Salmon	110	10	2
Cheesecake; Strawberry	110	9	5
Fat Free: Strawberry	45	0	6
Garden Veges	30	0	2
Lay's: Lowfat Sr. Cream, Onion	40	1	0
Louise's: (Fat Free) Honey Mustard	40	0	0
Sour Cream & Onion/Wh. Cheese	25	0	0
Luisa's Fiesta Dip, 2 Tbsp	35	2	3
Marie's: Reg, all types	90	9	2
Lite, 2 Tbsp, 1 oz	60	4	4
Nalley's: All flavors, average	120	12	3
Naturally Fresh: All flavors, 1 oz	80	5	19
Old Dutch: Cheddar, Nacho	35	3	3
Old El Paso: Black Bean	25	0	5
Cheese'n Salsa: Mild; Medium	40	3	3
Lowfat, medium	30	1.5	3
Chunky Salsa varieties	15	0	3
Jalapeno Dip	30	1	4
Olys Bagel Spread: Berry	100	8	3
Honey Cinnamon; Raisin	100	8	6
Garden Veg; Garlic & Herb	90	9	1
Prices: Orig. Pimiento Cheese Spr.	80	7	2
Rite: Cream Cheese & Lox Spread	90	8	1
Ruffles: French Onion; Ranch	70	6	4
Sealtest: French Onion	50	4	2
Snyder's Mustard Pretzel	90	4	13
Stop & Shop: Veggie Dip, 2 Tbsp	110	10	3
Sour Crm French Onion, 2 T.	60	5	2
Supremo Chihuaha: Quéso Bianco	100	8	0
Quéso Fresco; Rancherito	80	6	0
TGI Fridays: Spinach,Chse,Artichoke	45	3.5	2
Black Bean & Cheese Dip	50	2.5	5
T. Marzetti: Blue Cheese	200	21	3
Light Ranch Veggie	70	6	3
Other flavors, average	130	13	2
Tostitos Dip: Con Quéso	40	2	5
Medium/Mild/Hot	15	0	3
Tzatziki (Cucumber/Yoghurt Dip)	40	3	1
Wise: Jalapeno Bean	25	0	5
Taco	12	0	3

Salsa – See Page 86

Egg & Egg Dishes

Chicken Eggs | C | F | Cb |

Fresh Eggs
Raw (weight with shell):	C	F	Cb
Small, 40g	65	4	0
Medium, 44g	70	4	0
Large, 50g	75	4.5	0
Extra Large, 56g	80	5	0
Jumbo, 63g	90	5.5	0
Egg Yolk, 1 extra large	63	5	0
Egg White, 1 extra large	16	0	0

Dried Egg Powder
	C	F	Cb
Whole Egg: 1/4 cup, 1 oz	170	12	0
1 Tbsp	30	2	0
Egg White, 1/4 cup, 1 oz	105	0	0
Egg Yolk, 1/4 cup, 1 oz	195	18	0

Egg Substitutes

1/4 Cup (Equivalent to 1 Egg) ~ Zero Cholesterol.

	C	F	Cb
Better 'n Eggs (Papetti), 1/4 cup, 2 oz	30	0	0
Egg Beaters (Fleischmann's):			
Regular, 1/4 cup	30	0	1
Cheese Omelete, 1/2 cup	110	5	2
Vegetable Omelete, 1/2 cup	50	0	5
Egg Watchers (Tofutti), 2 oz	30	0	1
Eggstra, 1/2 envelope	50	2	0
Healthy Choice, 1/4 cup, 2 oz	25	0	0
Egg Substitute (Jewel), 1/4 cup	30	0	1
Scramblers (Morn Star), 1/4 cup	35	0	4
Second Nature: Regular, 1/4 cup	60	2	3
Fat Free, 1/4 cup, 60ml	30	0	1
Simply Eggs, 1/4 cup	35	1	1

Other Eggs

	C	F	Cb
Duck, 1 large, 2 1/2 oz	130	9.5	0
Goose, 1 large, 5 oz	280	19	0
Quail, 3 eggs, 1 oz	42	3	0
Turkey, 1 large, 3 oz	135	9.5	0
Turtle, 1 egg, 1 3/4 oz	75	5	0

Omega-3 Fat Enriched

	C	F	Cb
Eggs Land's Best, 1 large	70	4.5	0
Eggs Plus (Pilgrim's Pride), 1 large	70	4.5	0

Note: Cholesterol content same as regular eggs, but Omega-3 fats inhibit blood cholesterol increase.
(Also see Cholesterol ~ Page 253)

Cooked Eggs | C | F | Cb |

	C	F	Cb
Boiled Egg: Same as raw egg			
Fried Egg:			
With fat: 1 large egg	100	8	0.5
2 small eggs	175	13	0.5
No fat/nonstick pan, 1 large	80	5.5	0
Deviled Egg, 2 halves	145	13	0.5
Eggs Benedict (2) on toast			
or English muffin	860	56	25
Eggs Florentine (2) on toast			
or English muffin	890	59	25
Pickled Egg, 1 large	80	5.5	0
Poached Egg: 1 large	80	5.5	0
Scotch Egg, 1 egg	300	21	16
Scrambled Eggs: 1 large egg:			
w. 1 Tbsp milk + 1 tsp fat	120	9	1
w. 1 Tbsp skim milk/no fat	85	5.5	1
2 large eggs:			
w. 2 Tbsp milk + 2 tsp fat	260	20	2
w. 2 Tbsp skim milk/no fat	180	11	2

Omelets

	C	F	Cb
1 Egg: Plain (w. 1 tsp fat)	125	10	0.5
with 1/2 oz cheese	175	15	0.5
w. 1/2 oz cheese + 1/2 oz ham	200	16	0.5
2 Eggs: Plain (w. 2 tsp fat)	250	20	1
with 1 oz cheese	360	29	2
w. 1 oz cheese + 1 oz ham	410	32	2
3 Eggs: Plain (w. 1 Tbsp fat)	360	29	1.5
w. 2 oz cheese	580	47	2.5
w. 2 oz cheese + 2 oz ham	680	53	2.5
Extras: Tomato/Onion/Veges	20	0	4.5
Egg Substitute (Eggbeaters):			
2 eggs (1/2 cup) + 1 tsp fat	100	4	2
3 eggs (3/4 cup) + 2 tsp fat	160	8	3
Extras: 1 oz cheese	110	9	1
1 oz ham	50	3	1
Tom./Onion/Veges	20	0	4.5

Egg Nog ~ *Per 1/2 Cup (4 fl.oz)*

	C	F	Cb
Regular: Borden	160	9	16
Crowley	190	9	23
Hood (Golden)	180	8	22
Light/Lowfat: Borden	120	2	23
Horizon; Hood	140	3	23
Fat Free: Hood	100	0	21

Breakfast Sides	C	F	Cb
Toast: Plain, 1 thick slice	85	1	13
with 2 tsp butter/marg.	155	9	13
with 3 tsp/1Tbsp fat	190	13	13
English Muffin: Plain, 2 oz	130	1	26
with 3 tsp fat	230	12	26
Bacon, 2 strips	70	5	0
Ham: Lean, 2 oz	100	3	0
Hash Browns: $^1/_2$ cup	125	6.5	14
1 cup serving	250	13	28
Sausages, 2 links (1 oz ea.)	180	16	1.5

Frozen Egg Dishes

	C	F	Cb
Pillsbury Toaster Scrambles, 1			
Cheese, Egg & Bacon/Ham	180	12	14
Cheese, Egg & Sausage	180	12	14
Swanson Great Starts: *Per Package*			
Breakfast Wrap w/Bacon	270	11	30
Cinn. Roll, French Toast & Saus.	410	20	47
Croissant Sandwich, 5 oz	470	33	27
Egg, Sausage & Cheese	510	34	35
French Toast & Sausage	430	25	38
Muffin Sandwich	290	11	26
Pancakes w. Sausage	490	25	52
Scrambled Eggs: w. Burrito	200	8	17
w. Bacon & Home Fries	290	19	17
w. Sausage & Hash Browns	360	26	21
Uncle Ben's Breakfast Bowls: See Page 68			
Weight Watchers: Omelet	220	5	30

Frozen Egg Rolls

	C	F	Cb
Chun King/La Choy: *Average All Brands*			
Chicken Egg Rolls: Mini, 6 rolls	210	9	25
Restaurant Style, 1 roll, 3 oz	210	9	25
Pork & Shrimp Egg Rolls:			
Mini, 6 rolls, 3 oz	210	9	27
Shrimp Egg Rolls: Mini, 6 rolls	190	6	28
Restaurant Style, 1 roll, 3 oz	180	7	25
Lotus: Pork, 3 oz	180	7	18
Vegetable, 3 oz	70	1.5	13
Kahiki: Pork, 3 oz	190	6	25
Chicken, 3 oz	120	2	16
Vegetable, 3 oz	120	2	23

Fast Food/Restaurants	C	F	Cb
Bojangles:			
Bacon/Egg/Chse S'wich	550	42	27
Burger King:			
Egg'wich Bacon/Egg/Cheese	420	23	36
Croissan'wich Saus./Egg/Chse	520	39	24
Carl's Jr: Scrambled Eggs	180	14	1
Denny's: Two Egg Breakfast	825	67	24
Omelette: Ham 'n Cheddar	580	45	4
Veggie-Cheese	480	39	9
Sirloin Steak & Eggs	620	49	1
Hardees: Bacon Egg, Chse Bisc.	520	30	45
Sausage & Egg Biscuit	620	40	45
Ultimate Omelet	550	32	45
McDonald's: Egg McMuffin®	300	12	29
Bacon, Egg & Cheese Biscuit	480	31	31
Scrambled Eggs (2)	160	11	1
Perkins: Country Club Omelet	930	79	6
Roy Rogers: Ham & Egg Bisc.	470	26	44
Sausage & Egg Biscuit	560	35	44

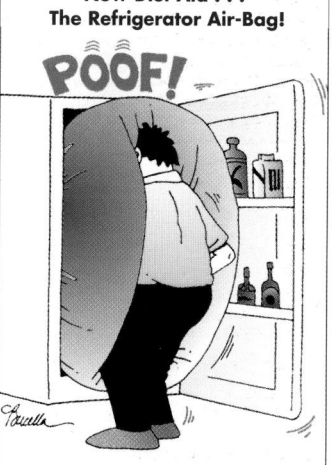

New Diet Aid . . .
The Refrigerator Air-Bag!

POOF!

Meat & Beef

Note: Cooking reduces weight of meat by 20-45% due to water and fat losses. Average weight loss is 30%. Actual loss depends on cooking method and cooking time. Examples:
- 4 oz raw wt. = approx. 3 oz cooked wt.
- 4 oz cooked wt. = approx. $5^{1}/2$ oz raw wt.

What 3 oz Cooked Meat Looks Like
- Half the size of this book ($4^{1}/4$" x 3" x $3/8$" thick)
- Rectangular piece (4" x $2^{1}/2$" x $1/2$" thick)
- Pack of cards ($3^{1}/2$" x $2^{1}/2$" x $5/8$" thick)

Quick Guide

	C	F	Cb

Steak

Sirloin (Choice Grade)
External fat trimmed to $1/4$"
Broiled, Edible Portion (no bone)

Small Serving, 3 oz
(3 oz cooked, from 4-$4^{1}/2$ oz raw)

	C	F	Cb
Lean + fat ($1/4$"), 3 oz	230	14	0
Lean + marbling, 3 oz	195	10	0
(External fat trimmed **before** cooking)			
Lean only, 3 oz	170	7	0
(No external fat or marbling)			

Medium/Regular Serving, 5 oz
(from approx. 7 oz raw)

	C	F	Cb
Lean + fat ($1/4$"), 5 oz	470	29	0
Lean + marbling, 5 oz	400	20	0
Lean only, 5 oz	350	14	0

Large Serving, 8 oz
(from 11-12 oz raw)

	C	F	Cb
Lean + fat, 8 oz	610	38	0
Lean + marbling, 8 oz	520	26	0
Lean only, 8 oz	454	18	0

Extra Large Serving, 12 oz
(from approx. 16-17 oz raw)

	C	F	Cb
Lean + fat, 12 oz	915	57	0
Lean + marbling, 12 oz	780	39	0
Lean only, 12 oz	680	27	0

Pan Fried
Sirloin (choice), medium serving:

	C	F	Cb
Lean + fat ($1/4$"), 5 oz	450	32	0
Lean only, 5 oz	330	15	0

Other Steaks

	C	F	Cb

Filet Mignon (Tenderloin):
1 medium steak, 6 oz raw wt.
Broiled, with $1/4$" fat trim

	C	F	Cb
Lean + fat ($1/4$"), 4 oz	340	24	0
Lean only, $3^{1}/2$ oz	210	10	0

Broiled, ($1/4$" fat removed before cooking)

	C	F	Cb
Lean + marbling, $3^{1}/4$ oz	220	12	0
Lean only, 3 oz	180	8	0

New York/Club Steak:
Top Loin/Short Loin
1 steak, regular ($9^{1}/4$ raw, $1/4$" fat)
Broiled:

	C	F	Cb
Lean + fat ($1/4$"), $6^{1}/4$ oz	510	35	0
Lean + marbling, $5^{1}/2$ oz	330	16	0
Lean only, $5^{1}/4$ oz	310	14	0

Porterhouse Steak:
1 medium, 6 oz raw wt. (no bone)
Broiled:

	C	F	Cb
Lean + fat ($1/4$"), $4^{1}/4$ oz	370	27	0
Lean only, $3^{1}/2$ oz	220	11	0

T-Bone Steak:
1 medium, 8 oz raw wt.

	C	F	Cb
Broiled: Lean + fat	380	27	0
Lean only	220	10	0

Beef - Average All Cuts

Average All Retail Cuts
Edible weight (no bone)

	C	F	Cb

Raw
(1 lb raw yields approx. 11-12 oz cooked)

	C	F	Cb
Lean + fat ($1/4$" trim), 1 oz	70	5.5	0
$1/2$ Pound, 8 oz	560	44	0
Lean only, 1 oz	40	2	0
$1/2$ Pound, 8 oz	320	16	0
Fat only, 1 oz	190	20	0

Cooked (No Added Fat)

	C	F	Cb
Lean + fat ($1/4$"), 1 oz	86	6	0
Small serving, 3 oz	260	18	0
Lean + marbling, (no ext. fat), 1 oz	78	5	0
Small serving, 3 oz	235	15	0
Lean only, 1 oz	60	3	0
Small serving, 3 oz	180	9	0
Fat only, 1 oz	193	20	0

Beef - Individual Cuts

Average All Grades
Edible Weight (no bone)

	C	**F**	**Cb**
Brisket, whole, braised:			
Lean + fat ($1/4$"), 3 oz	330	27	0
Lean + marbling, 3 oz	250	17	0
Lean only, 3 oz	205	11	0
Chuck, blade, braised:			
Lean + fat ($1/4$"), 3 oz	290	22	0
Lean + marbling, 3 oz	285	20	0
Lean only, 3 oz	210	11	0
Flank: Raw, 4 oz	200	12	0
Braised, 3 oz	225	14	0
Broiled, 3 oz	190	11	0
Ribs, whole (ribs 6-12):			
Average all grades, roasted			
(1 lb raw yields $10^{1}/4$ oz roasted)			
Lean + fat ($1/4$")			
(3.6 oz w. bone, 3 oz no bone)	300	25	0
Lean only, 3 oz (no bone)	200	11	0
Round, bottom, braised:			
Lean + fat ($1/4$"), 3 oz	235	14	0
Lean only, 3 oz	180	7	0
Round, eye/tip, roasted:			
Lean + fat ($1/4$"), 3 oz	200	11	0
Lean, 3 oz	150	5	0
Round, top: *Per 3 oz*			
Braised, Lean + fat	210	10	0
Lean only	175	5	0
Broiled, Lean + fat	185	8	0
Lean only	155	4	0
Pan-fried, Lean + fat	235	13	0
Lean only	190	7	0

Ground Beef

	C	**F**	**Cb**
Raw: Regular (73% fat free), 4 oz	350	30	0
Lean (80% fat free), 4 oz	300	24	0
Extra lean (85% fat free), 4 oz	250	17	0
Healthy Choice (97% lean), 4 oz	130	4	0
Baked/Broiled: Reg., 3 oz	250	18	0
Lean, 3 oz	230	16	0
Extra lean, 3 oz	200	12	0
Pan-fried: Regular, 3 oz	260	19	0
Lean, 3 oz	230	16	0
Extra lean, 3 oz	200	12	0
Ground Beef Patties: Average			
Frozen, raw, 4 oz	320	26	0
Broiled, 3 oz	240	17	0

Quick Guide

Roast Beef

Round (Eye/Tip, average)
Average All Cuts

	C	**F**	**Cb**
Small Serving, 3 oz			
(2 thin slices/1 thick slice)			
Lean + fat ($1/4$"), 3 oz	200	11	0
Lean only, 3 oz	150	5	0
Medium Serving, 5 oz, (3-4 thin slices)			
Lean + fat, 5 oz	330	18	0
Lean only, 5 oz	250	8	0
Large Serving, 8 oz, (3 thick slices)			
Lean + fat, 8 oz	530	29	0
Lean only, 8 oz	400	13	0

Roast Dinner Extras

	C	**F**	**Cb**
Gravy: Thin, 2 Tbsp	20	1	0.5
Thick, 2 Tbsp	50	2	0.5
1 Ladle/4 Tbsp	100	4	1
Veges: Beans, green, $1/2$ cup	20	0	5
Cauliflower w. cheese sauce, 4 oz	135	9	15
Corn, kernels, $1/4$ cup	35	0	9
Carrots, $1/4$ cup	20	0	3
Peas, $1/4$ cup	35	0	6
Pumpkin baked: w.fat, 4 oz	90	7	5
No added fat, 2 pces, 4 oz	25	0	5
Potato:			
Roasted w. fat, 1 small	155	8	30
Baked in Jacket, 1 large	220	0	50
with 1 Tbsp whipped butter	295	8	50
with Sour Cream, 2 Tbsp	270	6	51
Sweet Potato/Yam, 1 medium	80	0	20

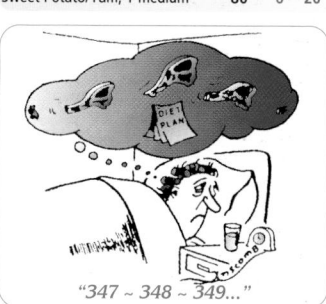

"347 ~ 348 ~ 349..."

Meat • Lamb, Veal, Pork

Lamb

	C	F	Cb
Choice Grade			
Leg (Whole), roasted:			
Lean + fat, 3 oz	220	14	0
Lean only, 3 oz	160	7	0
Leg (Sirloin Half), roasted:			
Lean + fat, 3 oz	250	18	0
Lean only, 3 oz	175	8	0
Leg (Shank Half), roasted:			
Lean + fat, 3 oz	190	11	0
Lean only, 3 oz	155	6	0
Loin Chop, broiled:			
1 chop (raw wt., 4 1/4 oz):			
Lean + fat (2 1/4 oz edible)	200	15	0
Lean only (1.6 oz edible)	100	5	0
Rib Chop, broiled/roasted:			
1 chop (raw wt., 3 1/2 oz):			
Lean + fat (2 1/2 oz edible)	255	21	0
Lean only (1 3/4 oz edible)	120	7	0
Shoulder (Arm/Blade):			
Braised: Lean + fat, 3 oz	290	21	0
Lean only, 3 oz	240	14	0
Broiled: Lean + fat, 3 oz	240	16	0
Lean only, 3 oz	180	9	0
Roasted: Similar to Broiled			
Cubed Lamb (Leg/Shoulder):			
For stew or kabob			
Raw, lean only, 8 oz	310	12	0
Braised, lean only, 3 oz	190	8	0
Broiled, lean only, 3 oz	160	6	0
New Zealand Lamb (Imported):			
Similar calories and fat to domestic.			

Veal

	C	F	Cb
Edible Weights			
Leg (Top Round):			
Braised: Lean + fat, 3 oz	180	6	0
Lean only, 3 oz	170	5	0
Pan-fried, breaded:			
Lean + fat, 3 oz	195	8	9
Lean only, 3 oz	175	6	9
Pan-fried, not breaded:			
Lean + fat, 3 oz	180	7	0
Lean only, 3 oz	155	4	0
Roasted: Lean + fat, 3 oz	135	4	0
Lean only, 3 oz	130	3	0

Veal (Cont)

	C	F	Cb
Loin Chop: 1 chop, 7 oz raw wt.			
Braised: Lean + fat	230	14	0
Lean only	155	6	0
Roasted: Lean + fat	175	10	0
Lean only	125	5	0
Rib, roasted: Lean + fat, 3 oz	195	12	0
Lean only, 3 oz	150	7	0
Shoulder, Arm/Blade, roasted:			
Lean + fat, 3 oz	155	7	0
Lean only, 3 oz	145	6	0
Sirloin, roasted:			
Lean + fat, 3 oz	170	9	0
Lean only, 3 oz	145	6	0
Cubed for Stew, braised:			
Leg/Shoulder, lean only, 3 oz	160	4	0
(1 lb raw yields approx. 9 1/4 oz cooked)			

Pork

	C	F	Cb
Figures based on NLMB data (1990)			
Fresh Pork (Cooked Wt., no bone)			
(4 oz raw wt. = approx. 3 oz cooked wt.)			
Blade Steak, broiled:			
Lean + fat, 3 oz	220	15	0
Lean only, 3 oz	190	11	0
Country Style Ribs, broiled:			
Lean + fat, 3 oz	270	22	0
Lean only, 3 oz	205	13	0
Leg (Ham), roasted:			
Lean + fat, 3 oz	250	18	0
Lean only, 3 oz	180	9	0
(Ham, cured ~ See Cold Meats)			
Loin Chops, broiled: Average			
(From 1 chop: 5 oz raw wt. w.bone			
or 4 oz raw wt., no bone)			
Lean + fat, 3 oz	200	11	0
Lean only, 3 oz	165	7	0
Rib Chops, broiled:			
Lean + fat, 3 oz	215	13	0
Lean only, 3 oz	180	7	0
Rib Roast, roasted:			
Lean + fat, 3 oz	210	13	0
Lean only, 3 oz	175	9	0
Loin Roast, roasted:			
Lean + fat, 3 oz	190	10	0
Lean only, 3 oz	160	7	0

Meat • Bacon, Ham, Game

Pork (Cont)

	C	F	Cb
Sirloin Chop, broiled:			
Lean + fat, 3 oz	175	8	0
Lean only, 3 oz	155	6	0
Sirloin Roast, roasted:			
Lean + fat, 3 oz	215	14	0
Lean only, 3 oz	180	9	0
Tenderloin, roasted:			
Lean + fat, 3 oz	147	5	0
Lean only, 3 oz	140	4	0
Ground Pork			
Raw: Average, 1/4 lb, 4 oz	300	24	0
Broiled, 3 oz	245	18	0
Pan-fried, drained, 3 oz	250	19	0

Bacon

	C	F	Cb
Raw: 1 med. slice (20 lb), 3/4 oz	125	13	0
1 thick slice (12 lb), 1 1/3 oz	210	22	0
(1 lb raw yields approx. 5 oz cooked)			
Broiled/Pan-Fried: 1 med. sl., 6 g	36	3	0
3 medium slices, 18g	110	9	0
2 thin slices, 1/2 g	80	7	0
1 thick slice, 12g	70	6	0
Canadian-style: Cooked, 1 slice	43	4	0
As purchased, 1 slice, 1 oz	45	4	1
Bacon Bits, 1 Tbsp, 1/4 oz	20	1	0
Breakfast Strips: Broil., 1 sl, 12 g	50	4	0

Ham

	C	F	Cb
Boneless Ham, cooked:			
Regular, (approx. 11% fat):			
Unheated (as purch.), 1 oz	52	3	0
Roasted, 3 oz	150	8	0
Extra Lean (5% fat):			
Unheated, 1 oz	37	2	0
Roasted, 3 oz	125	5	0
Whole Ham, cooked:			
Lean + fat (as purchased)			
Unheated, 1 oz	70	5	0
Roasted, 3 oz	345	26	0
Lean only, unheated, 1 oz	40	2	0
Roasted, 3 oz	135	5	0
Canned Ham: Similar to boneless ham			
Chopped, canned, 3 oz	260	21	0
Ham Patties, ckd, 1 pty, 2 1/4 oz	205	18	1
Ham Steak, extra lean, 2 oz	70	2	0
Luncheon Slices: See Deli Meats, Page 52			

Game & Other Meats

	C	F	Cb
Bison Steak,			
lean, 6 oz (raw)	210	4	0
Boar (wild), roasted, 3 oz	140	4	0
Buffalo Steak (New West Foods), 4 oz	70	3	0
Caribou, roasted, 3 oz	140	4	0
Deer/Venison, roasted 3 oz	135	3	0
Goat (Capretto): Raw, 3 oz	110	2.5	0
Roasted, 3 oz	150	3	0
Ostrich: Blackwing Ostrich Meats,			
Sport Jerky, 1/2 oz pce	25	0	0
Sausage Patties, (2) 2 oz	60	0.5	0
New West Foods:			
Ground Ostrich, 4 oz	110	2	0
Ostrich Steak, 4 oz steak	130	2.5	0
Rabbit: Roasted, 3 oz	130	6	0
Stewed, 1 cup, diced, 5 oz	300	14	0

Variety & Organ Meats

	C	F	Cb
Brains: Braised, 3 oz	130	9	0
Pan-fried, 3 oz	200	14	0
Chitterlings, pork, simmered, 3oz	260	25	0
Ears, pork, simmered, 1 ear	180	12	0
Feet, pork: Simmered, 3 oz	165	11	0
Cured, pickled, 3 oz	170	14	0
Hormel, 2 oz	80	6	0
Head Cheese (Pork Snouts/Ears/Vinegar/Spices):			
1 oz slice	50	4	0
Heart: Average, braised, 3 oz	140	5	0
Jowl, pork, raw, 4 oz	750	80	0
Kidneys, simmered, 3 oz	130	4	0
Liver: Raw, 4 oz	160	5	3
Braised, 3 oz	140	4	3
Pan-fried, 3 oz	200	9	3
Pancreas, braised, 3 oz	200	13	0
Pork Cracklins, 0.5 oz	80	6	0
Pork Hocks, 1 piece, 6 oz	340	23	0
Scrapple, pork, 1 oz	60	4	4
Spleen, braised, 3 oz	130	4	0
Stomach, pork, raw, 4 oz	180	11	0
Sweetbreads: Beef, ckd., 3 oz	270	20	0
Lamb, cooked, 3 oz	150	5	0
Tail, pork, simmered, 3 oz	340	31	0
Tongue, braised, 3 oz: Veal	170	9	0
Beef/Lamb/Pork, average	240	17	0
Tripe, beef, raw, 4 oz	110	5	0
Lean + fat	310	25	0

49

Sausages, Franks

Quick Guide　C F Cb

Franks & Weiners

Beef: *Average All Brands*
Regular/Smoked: *Per Frank*

	C	F	Cb
4 oz link	280	22	5
2.6 oz link	240	19	2
2 oz link (8/16 oz pkg)	180	17	2
1.6 oz link (10/16 oz pkg)	140	13	1
1.5 oz link (8/12 oz pkg)	135	12	1
1.2 oz link (10/12 oz pkg)	110	10	1
1 oz link (16/16 oz pkg)	90	8	0.5
Small/Cocktail (50/lb), each	30	3	0.5

Beef Light/Reduced Fat Franks:

	C	F	Cb
Best's Kosher	50	1	5
Oscar Mayer, 2 oz link	110	8	2
Hebrew National: 97% Fat Free	50	1.5	2
Reduced Fat, 1	120	10	0
Healthy Choice, lowfat, 1.75 oz	70	2.5	6

Beef Fat-Free Franks:

	C	F	Cb
Ball Park (1),1.76 oz	50	0	5
Oscar Mayer (1)	40	0	3

Pork Franks:

	C	F	Cb
Country Style, 2 oz panfried	240	22	1
Chorizo, 5 sausages, 2 oz	280	26	3
El Popular, 2 oz cooked	210	17	3
Jimmy Dean, cooked, 2 oz	240	21	0
Oscar Mayer (2), 1.7 oz, ckd	170	15	1
Light, 2 oz link	110	8	2

Turkey Franks:

	C	F	Cb
Ball Park, Smkd White, fat free, 1	45	0	5
Butterball, 1 frank, 1.75 oz	45	5	7
Empire Kosher, 2 oz	90	6	1
Foster Farms, 2 oz	130	11	0
Louis Rich: Orig., Lower Fat (1)	100	8	2
Bun Length (1)	120	10	3
Mr Turkey, smoked, 2 oz	90	5	3
Shelton's: 1 frank, 1.2 oz	80	6	1

Chicken Franks:

	C	F	Cb
Empire Kosher, 2 oz	100	7	1
Foster Farms, 2 oz	140	12	0
Scott Petersen, 1.2 oz	80	6	1
Shelton's, 1.2 oz	95	8	1
Zacky Farms, 2 oz	150	13	0

Vegetarian Sausages

See Frozen/Canned & Packaged Meals

Quick Guide　C F Cb

Fresh Sausages

Pork/Beef: *Average All Types*

	C	F	Cb
Small: Raw, 4" link, 1 oz	120	12	1.5
Broiled/Pan-fried	50	4	1.5
Medium: Raw, 2 oz	235	23	2.5
Broiled/Pan-fried	100	8	2.5
Large: Raw, 3 oz	360	36	3.5
Broiled/Pan-fried	150	12	3.5
Italian: Raw, 3.2 oz	315	28	1.5
Cooked, 2.4 oz	215	17	1.5

Note: Fat is lost in broiling/pan frying.
(Cooked wt. = approx. 60-70% raw wt.)

Smoked Sausages

	C	F	Cb
Ball Park: Knockwurst(1) 4 oz	360	33	4
Beef Corn Dog(1) 2.6 oz	220	12	21
Butterball (w. Turkey), 2 oz	60	0	6
Eckrich, 2 oz	180	16	4
Healthy Choice, 2 oz	80	2.5	6
Lemington Foods: 2 oz link	180	15	3
Skinless, 3 oz link	250	21	5
Bacon & Cheddar, 3 oz pce	250	20	7
Scott Petersen: Skinless, 3 oz link	280	24	5

Breakfast Sausages/Biscuits

Healthy Choice

	C	F	Cb
Breakfast Sausage, 2 patties, 1.6 oz	50	1.5	3
Breakfast Sausage Links, (3) 1.6 oz	50	1.5	3
Jimmy Dean: Sausage Biscuit, 2	400	27	29
Pancakes 'n Sausage, 2 sticks	340	21	42
Saus. Egg & Cheese, Biscuit, 1	380	23	29
Minyard: Pork Sausage Biscuit, 1	200	12	16

Owens Border Breakfast

	C	F	Cb
2 Sausages, Egg, Cheese, Tacos	330	11	42
2 Hot Sausages, Biscuits	370	23	26
Knob Sausages, 2 oz, ckd	210	18	0

Swift Premium *Morning Makers: Per 3.5 oz*

	C	F	Cb
Egg & Cheese, 1 pce	240	8	30
Ham, Egg & Cheese	250	10	31
Sausage, Egg & Cheese	250	8	32

Chorizo - Reynaldo's

	C	F	Cb
Beef Chorizo, 2.5 oz piece	320	31	3
Pork Chorizo, 2.5 oz	250	22	4

Bagel, Corn & Hot Dogs

Hot Dogs, Ready-To-Go	C	F	Cb
(Includes Ketchup/Relish; No Mayo)			
Small (1 oz frank/ 1 oz roll)	200	8	24
Regular (1½ oz frank/ 2 oz roll)	310	13	39
Large (2 oz frank/ 2 oz roll)	360	18	40
Super/Giant (3 oz frank/3 oz roll)	540	26	59
Weinerschnitzel: See Fast-Foods			

Corn Dogs

	C	F	Cb
Beef/Pork Frank: Average, 2.6 oz	250	17	21
Mini, each	65	4.5	5
Foster Farms Chicken Franks:			
1 dog, 2.6 oz (75g)	180	10	15
Chili Cheese, 1 dog, 2.6 oz (75g)	200	9	24
Mini Corn Dogs, (4) 2.68 oz	210	12	18
State Fair w. Ball Park Franks,			
Corn Dogs, 1 dog, 2.68 oz (76g)	170	10	16
Beef, 1 dog, 2.68 oz (76g)	180	12	15
Mini Corn Dogs, (4) 2.68 oz (76g)	230	13	22
Turkey: *Gobblers! (Shelton's)*	220	11	27

Bagel Dogs

	C	F	Cb
Best's Kosher: 1 dog, 1 oz	320	11	43
Mini, piece, 0.8 oz	60	2	8
Vienna Beef: 1 piece, 1 oz	85	3.5	7

Toppings/Extras

	C	F	Cb
American Chse, 1 slice, 1 oz	110	9	1
Catsup, 1 Tbsp	16	0	4
Chili (w. Beans), ¼ cup	70	3.5	9
Mustard, 1 Tbsp	20	0	1
Pickle Relish, 1 Tbsp	20	0	5
Sauerkraut, ½ cup	20	0	5

WILL-POWER TONIC
~ RECIPE ~

- 1 Cup of Desire
- 1 Quart of Determination
- 1 Tbsp of Common Sense
- 1 Tbsp of Stick-to-itiveness
- 1 Tbsp of Foresight
- 1 Cup of Energy

Deli & Luncheon Meats

Beef Jerky:	C	F	Cb
Bridgeford Beef Jerky, 1 oz	50	1	3
Beef Stick (5.5 oz stick), 1 oz	140	12	0
Beef Steak, 1 oz	50	1	0
Beef & Cheese (Giant Size),			
½ pkg, 1.5 oz	170	14	1
Pepperoni Sticks, 2, 1 oz	140	12	1
Pepperoni (1" diam.), 1 oz	130	12	0
Teriyaki, 1.25 oz pkg	80	1	5
Original; Hot 'n Spicy	70	1	5
Berliner (pork/beef), 1 oz	65	4	0.5
Beerwurst (Beef):			
Small (2.75"diam), 1/16" slice	20	2	0
Large (4"diam), 1/8" slice	75	7	0.5
Beerwurst (Pork):			
Small (2.75"diam), 1/16" slice	15	1	0
Large (4"diam), 1/8" slice	55	4	0.5
Bologna, Beef & Pork:			
Regular: 1 thin slice, 1 oz	90	8	1
1 thick slice, 1.6 oz	145	13	1
Light *(Oscar Mayer)*, 1 sl., 1 oz	60	4	2
Red. Fat *(Hebrew Nat.)*,1 oz	65	6	0
Fat Free *(Osc. M.)*, 2 sl., 1.6 oz	40	0	1
Healthy Choice, 1 oz	35	1	3
Weight Watchers, 2 sl., ¾ oz	35	2	0
Turkey, average, 1 oz	60	5	0.5
Chicken *(Tyson)*, 1 slice	45	4	0.5
Ring *(Boar's Head)*, 2 oz	160	13	0.5
Blood Sausage, 1 oz	100	9	0.5
Bratwurst:			
Average, 1 oz	90	8	0.5
Boar's Head, cook., 1 wurst, 4 oz	300	25	0
Bob Evan's, Beer, 2.6 oz link	270	21	1
Braunschweiger (Pork/Liver/Sausage),			
Oscar Mayer, 1 oz slice	100	9	1
Chicken, *Average All Brands*			
1 thick or 2 thin slices, 1 oz	30	1	1
Chicken Roll, 1 slice, 1 oz	90	4	1.5
Corned Beef:			
Average, full fat, 1 oz	70	5	1.5
*Healthy Choice, Hillshire Farm,*1oz	30	1	0.5
Hebrew National, 4 slices, 2 oz	90	4.5	1
Loaf, jellied, 1 oz	45	2	1
Hash, canned, average, 1 oz	50	3	2
Dutch Brand Loaf, average, 1 oz	70	5	1.5

Continued Next Page

Deli & Luncheon Meats

Ham, Luncheon:	C	F	Cb
Baked/Boiled, sliced, 1 oz	30	1	0.5
Chopped: *Eckrich* (97% FF), 1 oz	25	1	1
Armour, canned, 1 oz	35	1.5	0.5
97% Fat Free, 1 oz	25	1	1.5
Healthy Choice Deli Traditions:			
Baked, 2 sl., 2 oz	60	1.5	4
Larger Slice, 1 slice, 1 oz	30	1	1
Hormel (Black Label), 1 oz	70	6	0
Oscar Mayer, 1 oz slice	60	3	1
Honey/Brown Sugar, aver., 1 oz	30	1	0.5
Healthy Choice Deli Traditions:			
2 slices, 2 oz	60	1.5	2
Prosciutto, average, 1 oz	70	5	1
Ham & Cheese Loaf, aver., 1 oz	70	5	0.5
Head Cheese (Osc. Mayer), 1 oz sl.	50	4	0
Honey Loaf (Osc. Mayer), 1 oz sl.	35	1	2
Italian Sausage, 2.6 oz	270	21	1
Kielbasa (Polish Sausage), 1 oz	85	7	0.5
Scott Petersen, 3.4 oz link	320	27	4
Beef, 2.8 oz link	290	25	4
Boar's Head, 1 oz	60	5	0
Kippered Beefsteak:			
(Hickory Farms), 3 slices, 0.75 oz	50	1	1
Knackwurst, 1 oz	90	8	0.5
Liverwurst, 1 oz	95	8	0.5
Liver Pate, fresh, average, 1 oz	110	10	3.5
Luncheon Loaf (Foods Co), 1 oz	80	7	2
Mortadella, 1 oz	90	7	0.5
Olive Loaf, average, 1 oz	70	5	3
Oscar Mayer, 1 oz slice	70	6	2
Pastrami (Beef), average, 1 oz	40	2	0.5
Healthy Deli, 1 oz	34	1	0.5
Hillshire (DeliSelect), 6 sl., 2 oz	60	1	1
Turkey Pastrami, 1 slice, 1 oz	30	1	1
Peppered Beef, 1 oz slice	40	2	1
Pepperoni, 5 slices, 1 oz	135	12	0
Pickle Loaf, average, 1 oz	80	6	2
Pickle & Pimiento Loaf			
(Oscar Mayer), 1 oz	80	6	3
Polish Sausage: See Kielbasa			
Proscuitti, average, 1 oz	70	5	1
Hormel, 1 oz	90	7	1
Roast Beef, lean, 1 oz	40	1	0.5
Healthy Choice, all types, 2 oz	60	1	2
Salami: Beef, average, 1 oz	80	7	1
Beer, average, 1 oz	70	6	0.5
Cotto: *Oscar Mayer,* 1 slice, 1 oz	70	5	1

Salami (cont)	C	F	Cb
Dry: Hard, aver. 3 slices, 1 oz	110	10	0.5
Oscar Mayer, 2 slices, 1.6 oz	120	10	1
Genoa: Average, 1 oz	110	10	0
Stick (Best's Kosher), 2, 1.75 oz	180	15	2
Italian (Bridgeford), 1 oz	120	11	0
Turkey, average, 1 oz	55	4	1
Spam (Hormel):			
Regular: $1/4$" slice, 1 oz	90	8	0
$1/2$" slice, 2 oz	180	16	1
Lite: $1/4$" slice, 1 oz	55	4	0
$1/2$" slice, 2 oz	110	8	1
Turkey: $1/4$" slice, 1 oz	40	2	0.5
$1/2$" slice, 2 oz	80	4	1
Summer Sausage:			
Bridgeford, 1 oz	100	9	0
Oscar Mayer, 1 slice, 0.8 oz	70	7	0
Treet (Armour), canned, 1 oz	100	9	1.5
Turkey: Average, 1 oz slice	30	1	0.5
$3/4$ oz slice	22	0.5	1
Turkey Breast:			
Butterball Fat Free, 4 sl., 2 oz	50	0	2
Deli Thin Smoked, 1 sl., 2 oz	30	5	1
Hillshire Deli Select, 6 sl., 2 oz	60	0.5	2
Louis Rich Carvery Board,			
2 slices, 1.8 oz (52g)	50	2	2
Free, 2 slices, 2 oz	50	0	2
Healthy Choice, 2 slices, 2 oz	60	2	2
Hearty Deli Rst'd, 2 sl., 2 oz	50	0.5	1
Honey Roasted, 2 sl., 2 oz	70	2	2
Oven Roasted, 2 sl., 2oz	45	0	2
Honey Rst & Smoked, 2 oz	60	0	2
Salsa Turkey Breast, 2 oz	60	1	1
Turkey Ham, 1 slice, 1 oz	35	1.5	0.5
Turkey Pastrami, 1 oz	35	1.5	0.5
Turkey Roll, 1 oz	40	2	0.5
Turkey Loaf, 1 oz	30	1	0.5
Vegetarian Deli:			
Worthington, Yves: Page 77			

Worthington, Yves: Page 77

Meat Spreads	C	F	Cb
Average All Brands: Per $1/4$ Cup (2 oz)			
Chicken	120	8	2
Ham, deviled	160	14	0
Liverwurst	170	14	3
Roast Beef	140	11	0
Sandwich Spread	140	10	8
Turkey	110	7	2

Paté | | C | F | Cb |

		C	F	Cb
Canned: *Average All Brands*				
Chicken Liver, 1 Tbsp, $^1/2$ oz		30	2	1
2 Tbsp, 1 oz		60	4	2
Foie Gras, goose liver, 1 oz		130	12	2
Sells, liverpate, $2^1/8$ oz		190	16	3
Fresh (Refrigerated):				
Average all types, 1 oz		110	10	4
Marcel Henri, 2 oz serving		220	20	1
Pate de Campagne, 1 oz		105	9	1
Chicken Liver w. Port Wine, 1 oz		105	9	1
Duck Truffle w. Port Wine, 1 oz		120	12	1
Coeur de France:				
Smoked Salmon Pate, 1 oz		45	3.5	1
Spinach Pate w. Roquefort, 1 oz		50	4	1
Garden Fresh Vegetable Pate:				
Spinach, Cauliflower & Carrot				
in Puff Pastry, 2 oz		110	7	10
Trois Petit Cochons:				
MousseTruffee, $^1/4$ pkg, 2 oz		170	15	2
Paté w. mushrooms, 2 oz		190	17	2

Lunch Packs | | C | F | Cb |

	C	F	Cb
Funny Bagels *(Stonyfield Farm):* Per Package			
Ham Sandwich, 2 bagels & juice	350	3.5	66
Pizza Bagel, 2 bagels & juice	420	8	71
P B & J, 2 bagels & juice	490	13	79
Turkey Bologna, 2 bagels & juice	370	6	66
Turkey Breast, 2 bagels & juice	400	10	67
Lunchables *(Oscar Mayer):* Per Package			
All-Star Burger/Juice/Candy	400	10	66
Ham & American Cheese	450	19	54
Ham & Chedder	360	20	21
Hot Dogs/Choc Balls/Drink	450	19	64
Lean Ham/Chedd./Crackers/Cookie	420	21	39
Lean Ham/Swiss Chse/Crackers	350	20	20
Turkey & Chedder	350	20	20
Cracker Stackers: *Per Package w. Drink, Dessert*			
Bologna & American Cheese	520	24	64
Ham & American Cheese	420	15	60
Ham & Chedder	390	20	21
Ham & Swiss	350	9	52
Turkey & American Cheese	420	14	60
Turkey & Chedder	420	14	61
Nachos: Cheese & Salsa	380	21	39
w. Capri Sun/Choc Fudge	540	26	70
w. Capri Sun/Nestle Crunch	570	29	70
Tacos: Beef Taco & Cheese	310	11	34
Beef Tortilla/Drink/Wonka Nerds	480	13	72
Mega Lunchables: *Per Package*			
2 Pepp. Pizza/Reese's P.B.Cup/Cola	760	28	105
2 Extra Cheesy Pizza/M&Ms/Drink	700	24	104
MEGA Cracker Combo	770	32	102
Soft Pizzastix + Twix	680	16	118
Ultimate Nachos	800	38	107
Sandwiches:			
Ham, Turkey, Chedder	470	22	47
Oven Rst. Turkey & Chse Sub	410	11	45
Smoked Ham & Chedder Sub	380	14	44
Smoked Turkey & Chedd. Bagel	380	4	63
Pizza: 3 Extra Cheesy	300	13	28
w. Fruit Punch, Crunch Bar	450	15	63
Pepperoni Flavored Sausage, 3	310	15	28
w. Capri Sun/Crunch	470	17	65
Munch-A-Bunch *(Jewel):* Per 4 oz Package			
Bologna/Chse/Crackers/Cookies	430	29	27
Other varieities, average	350	19	29
Smuckers: Snackers, 3.96 oz pkg	610	24	88
StarKist: Tuna Salad & Crackers	190	6	25
Chunk White Tuna w.Mayo	230	9	17

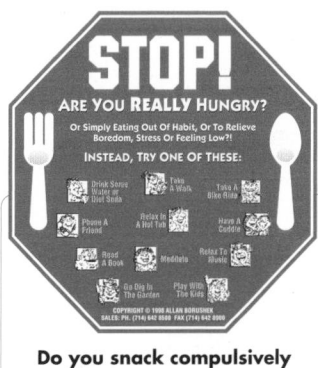

Chicken

Quick Guide

Chicken | C | F | Cb

From 3lb ready-to-cook chicken

Breast/Wing Quarter	C	F	Cb
Roasted: With skin	300	15	0
Without skin	190	5	0
Fried, batter dipped	480	26	18
Leg Quarter: Thigh & Drumstick			
Roasted: With skin	265	15	0
Without skin	180	8	0
Fried, batter dipped	430	26	16

KFC ~ See Fast-Foods Section

Average - All Meats

Average of Light & Dark Meats
Per 4 oz Serving (no bone)

	C	F	Cb
Roasted: With skin	270	15	0
Without skin	215	8	0
Stewed: With skin	250	14	0
Without skin	200	8	0
Fried: Batter-dipped	330	20	11
Flour coated	305	17	3.5

Chicken Parts

Broilers or Fryers: Edible Weights (no bone)

Breast: *Per 1/2 Breast*

	C	F	Cb
Raw: With skin, 5 oz	245	13	0
Without skin, 4 1/4 oz	130	2	0
Roasted: With skin, 3 1/2 oz	195	8	0
Without skin, 3 oz	140	3	0
Stewed: With skin, 4 oz	210	8	0
Without skin, 3 1/4 oz	140	3	0
Fried: Batter-dipped, 5 oz	370	19	12
Flour coated, w. skin, 3 1/2 oz	220	9	7

Drumstick: *Per Drumstick*

	C	F	Cb
Roasted: With skin, 2 oz	125	6	0
Without skin, 1 1/2 oz	75	2	0
Fried: Batter-dipped, 2 1/2 oz	195	11	7
Flour coated, 1 3/4 oz	120	7	1
Stewed: With skin, 2 oz	115	6	0
Without skin, 1 1/2 oz	80	3	0

Thigh Portion: Edible Wt. (no bone)

	C	F	Cb
Raw: With skin, 3.3 oz			
(4 1/4 oz with bone)	200	14	0
Without skin, 2.4 oz	80	3	0
Roasted: With skin, 2 1/4 oz	155	10	0
Without skin, 2 oz	110	6	0

Thigh Portion (Cont)

	C	F	Cb
Stewed: With skin, 2 1/2 oz	160	10	0
Without skin, 2 oz	105	5	0
Fried: Batter-dipped, 3 oz	240	14	8
Flour coated, 2 1/4 oz	165	9	2

Wing: *Per Wing*
Raw Weight 3.2 oz (with bone)

	C	F	Cb
Raw: With skin	110	8	0
Without skin	35	1	0
Roasted: With skin	105	7	0
Without skin	45	2	0
Fried: Batter-dipped	160	11	5
Flour coated	105	7	1
Stewed: With skin, 4 oz	100	7	0
Neck: Simmered, with skin	95	7	0
Without skin	30	2	0

Skin Only: *Skin from 1/2 Chicken*

	C	F	Cb
Raw skin, 2 3/4 oz	275	26	0
Roasted skin, 2 oz	255	22	0
Stewed skin, 2 1/2 oz	260	24	0
Fried, Flour coated, 2 oz	280	24	5
Fried, Batter-dipped, 6 3/4 oz	750	55	45

Roasters

Average of Light & Dark Meat:

	C	F	Cb
Roasted: With skin, 4 oz	250	15	0
Without skin, 4 oz	190	8	0
Light Meat: Without skin, rst.	175	5	0
Dark Meat: Without skin, rst.	206	10	0

Stewing Chicken

Stewed: *Per 4 oz Serving*
Average of Light & Dark Meat:

	C	F	Cb
With skin	325	21	0
Without skin	270	14	0
Light Meat: Without skin	240	9	0
Dark Meat: Without skin	295	17	0

Capon Chicken

	C	F	Cb
Roasted: With skin, 4 oz	260	13	0
1/2 Chicken, with skin	1460	74	0

Chicken Offal & Stuffing

	C	F	Cb
Giblets, simmered, 1 cup	230	7	1.5
Fried, flour-coated, 1 cup	400	20	6
Gizzard, simmered, 1 cup	220	5	1.5
Heart, simmered, 1 cup	270	12	0.5
Liver: Raw, 4 oz	140	5	3.5
Simmered, 1 cup	220	8	7
Liver Pate Fresh, 1 Tbsp, 1/2 oz	60	8	1
Stuffing: Average, 1/2 cup	200	2	22

Chicken Products

Shop Stop	C	F	Cb
Blazing Chicken Wings, 3 oz	200	12	1
Breaded Tenderloins, (3) 4 oz	240	12	15
Boneless Skinless Breasts, (1) 8 oz	210	5	3
Tyson: Chick. Chunks: Reg., (6)	280	20	19
Breast, (6)	220	19	11
Southern Fried, (6)	260	19	11
Breast Patties: Regular, each	190	12	11
Chick 'n Quick/Chedd., 74g ea.	220	14	12
Crispy Baked, each	80	0	9
Thick 'n Crispy, each	200	19	10
Southern Fried, each	180	12	8
Nuggets: Breaded White Meat, (6)	250	18	12
Wings: Flavored, average, (3)	170	10	1
BBQ Style, (3)	200	13	2
Stir Fry Kit: Chicken, 2³/4 c. froz.	430	4.5	73
Wraps: Southwest Black, 1¹/2	560	12	82
Mandarin Sesame, 1¹/2 wraps	560	12	82
M/wave S/wiches: Breast, 119g	320	15	33
Stove Top: Per Serving			
Chicken Stuffing Mix: 1 oz	110	1	20
¹/2 cup prepared	170	9	20

Duck, Goose, Quail

	C	F	Cb
Duck: roasted, with skin, 3 oz	285	24	0
Without skin, 3 oz	170	10	0
¹/2 whole duck, with skin	1300	108	0
Goose: roast, with skin, 3 oz	260	19	0
Without skin, 3 oz	200	11	0
Pheasant: ¹/2 bird, raw	720	37	0
Quail: 1 whole, raw	210	13	0

Turkey

Fryer-Roasters: Per 3 oz Serving	C	F	Cb
Roasted: Light Meat, with skin	140	4	0
without skin	120	1	0
Dark Meat: with skin	155	6	0
without skin	140	4	0
¹/4 of Whole Turkey: (Approx. 3¹/4 lbs raw wt. w/out neck and giblets; 2 lb 6 oz cooked wt.)			
Roasted: With skin	1400	64	0
Without skin	1030	18	0
Ground Turkey, Raw: (4 oz raw wt. = 3 oz ckd wt.)			
Regular (85% lean), 4 oz	180	10	0
Lean (90% lean), 4 oz	160	8	0
Breast, no skin, 4 oz	115	1	0

Turkey Parts

Roasted, Edible Weights (no bone)	C	F	Cb
Breast (¹/4): (from 17¹/4 oz raw wt. w/bone)			
With skin, 12 oz (no bone)	525	11	0
Without skin, 10³/4 oz	415	2	0
Back (¹/2): With skin, 4¹/2 oz	265	13	0
Without skin, 3¹/2 oz	165	5	0
Leg (Thigh & Drumstick): (from 1 lb raw wt. w/bone)			
With skin, 8¹/2 oz (no bone)	420	13	0
Without skin, 7³/4 oz	355	8	0
Wing: (from 7¹/4 oz raw wt. w/bone)			
With skin, 3 oz (no bone)	185	9	0
Without skin, 2 oz	100	2	0
Neck: Simmered, 1 neck (9 oz w. bone)	275	11	0
Giblets, simm., 1 cup, 5 oz	240	7	3

Young Hens (Roasted)

	C	F	Cb
Light Meat: With skin, 3 oz	175	8	0
Without skin, 3 oz	135	3	0
Dark Meat: With skin, 3 oz	200	11	0
Without skin, 3 oz	165	7	0
Young Toms — Similar to Young Hens			

Turkey Products

	C	F	Cb
Banquet: See Frozen Meals, Page 59			
Circle L: Boneless Turk Bacon, 3 oz	120	9	1
Louis Rich			
Fat Free Breast of Turkey			
Rotiss'd/Smoked/Rstd, 2 oz	60	0	1
Turkey Ham & Chunks, cooked:			
Breast & White Turkey, 2 oz	60	1	2
Turkey Ham/Pastrami, 2 oz	70	3	1
Turkey Salami, 2 oz	100	8	0
Luncheon Slices: See Deli Meats, Page 52			
Franks: Medium, 1¹/2 oz	80	6	2
Large, 2 oz	110	8	3
Smoked Sausage/Kielbasa, 1 oz	45	2	2
Turkey Nuggets, cooked, each	65	4	4
Turkey Patties, cooked, each	220	13	13
Turkey Sticks, cooked, each	75	5	4
Swanson: Frozen Meals, Page 68			
Turkey Store			
Gobble Stix: Honey, each	25	0	6
Lean Burger Patties, 1 patty	180	8	5
Lean Italian Sausage, 1 link	190	8	2

Fish ~ Fresh & Canned

Fresh Fish

Low Oil (Less than 2.5% fat)
White/pale colored flesh. Examples:
Cod, Flounder, Haddock, Halibut, Monkfish
Perch, Pike, Pollock, Snapper, Sole, Whiting.

Per 4 oz Edible Portion	C	F	Cb
Raw, 4 oz (no bones)	90	1	0
Steamed, Broiled, Baked	130	1	0
Fried: Lightly Floured	210	8	3.5
Breaded	260	12	8
In Batter	320	16	27

Medium Oil (2.5-5% fat)
Pale colored flesh. Examples:
Bluefin Tuna, Catfish, Kingfish, Salmon (Pink),
Swordfish, Rainbow Trout, Yellowtail.

	C	F	Cb
Raw, 4 oz (no bones)	140	5	0
Baked, Broiled, 4 oz	175	6	0
Fried, 4 oz	230	11	8

High Oil (Over 5% fat)
Darker colored flesh. Examples:
Albacore Tuna, Bluefish, Herring, Mackerel,
Orange Roughy, Salmon (Atl./Chinook/Sockeye),
Sardines, Trout, Whitefish.

	C	F	Cb
Raw, 4 oz (no bones)	230	16	0

Cooking Yields (Fin Fish):
4 oz Raw wt. = 3 1/2 oz Cooked wt.
4 oz Cooked wt. = 5 oz Raw wt.

Calorie & Fat Variations
The amount of fat/oil in fish varies with the species, season and locality. Within the same fish, fat/oil content is generally higher towards the head.

Fish & Shellfish	C	F	Cb
Edible Weights: (no bones/shell)			
Abalone: Raw, 4 oz	120	1	7
Anchovy: Paste, 1 Tbsp, 1/4 oz	15	1	0.5
Cnd. in oil, drnd., 5 only, 3/4 oz	40	2	0
Pickled, 1 oz	50	3	0
Barracuda (Pacific), raw, 4 oz	130	3	0
Bass: Black, raw, 4 oz	105	1	0
Striped, raw, 1 fillet, 5 1/2 oz	150	4	0
Blue Fish, raw, 1 fillet, 5 1/4 oz	185	6	0
Butterfish, raw, 4 oz	165	9	0
Calamari, breaded/fried, 1 serve	360	21	10
Carp, raw, 4 oz	145	6	0
Catfish: Raw, 4 oz	130	5	0
Fried, breaded, 1 fillet, 3 oz	200	12	7
Caviar: black/red, 1 Tbsp, 16g	40	3	0.5
Clams: Raw, 3 oz (4 lge/9 small)	65	1	2
Fried, breaded, 3/4 cup, 4 oz	450	26	39
Canned, 3 oz	125	2	4
Minced, 1/4 cup, 2 oz	25	0	0.5
Cod, Atlantic/Pacific: Raw, 4 oz	95	1	0
Baked/Broiled, 1 fillet, 6 1/4 oz	135	2	0
Canned, 3 oz	90	1	0
Minced, 1/4 cup, 2 oz	25	0	0
Smoked, 3 oz	95	1	0
Crab: Alaska King, raw, 4 oz	95	1	0
1 leg, cooked, 4 3/4 oz	130	2	0
Blue, raw, 1 crab			
(1/3 lb whole crab, 3/4 oz flesh)	18	0.5	0
Canned, 1/2 cup, 2 1/2 oz	65	0.5	0
Dungeness, 1 crab, 5 3/4 oz edible			
(from 1 1/2 lb whole crab)	140	2	2
Imitation Crab Legs/Stix, 3oz	80	1	8.5
Crayfish, raw, 4 oz (edible)	100	1	0
Croaker, raw, 4 oz	120	3	0
Cuttlefish, raw, 4 oz	90	1	1
Dolphinfish, raw, 4 oz	95	1	0
Eel: Raw, 4 oz	210	13	0
Smoked, 2 oz	190	16	0
Flounder/Sole, raw, 4 oz	120	0.5	0
Gefilte Fish: *See Kosher Foods, Page 172*			
Grouper, raw, 4 oz	105	1	0
Haddock: Raw, 4 oz	100	0.5	0
Broiled, 1 fillet, 5 1/4 oz	170	1	0
Smoked, 2 oz	22	0.5	0
Halibut, raw, 4 oz	125	3	0
Herring: Atlantic, raw, 4 oz	180	10	0
Pickled, 2 pieces, 1 oz	60	4	2

	C	F	Cb
Herring (Cont): Pickled			
In Sour Cream, 1 oz	50	5	1
Party Snacks, 1/4 cup, dr., 2 oz	120	5	0
Rollmops, 1 1/2 oz	110	8	6
Canned: Plain w. liq., 4 oz	235	15	0
in Tomato Sauce, 4 oz	200	12	1
Smoked, kippered, 4 oz	245	14	0
Jellyfish, raw, 4 oz	30	0	0
Salted, 4 oz	40	0	0
Kingfish, raw, 4 oz	120	3.5	0
Ling, raw, 4 oz	100	0.5	0
Lobster, Northern: Raw, 4 oz	105	1	0.5
1 Lobster, 6 1/4 oz			
(from 1 1/2 lb whole lobster)	135	1.5	0.5
Cooked, 1 cup, 5 oz	140	1	2
Lobster Newberg, 3/4 cup	360	20	9
Lobster Thermidor, 1 serving	370	22	15
Lobster Salads, 1/2 cup	220	13	5
Lox, Regular/Nova, 2 oz	65	2.5	0
Mackerel: Atlantic, raw, 4 oz	235	16	0
Jack, can., 1/2 cup, 3 1/3 oz	150	6	0
King, raw, 4 oz	120	2	0
Pacific/Jack, raw, 4 oz	180	9	0
Spanish, raw, 4 oz	160	7	0
Mahi-Mahi, raw, 4 oz	140	5	0
Monkfish, raw, 4 oz	75	1	0
Mullet, striped, raw	135	4	0
Mussels: Raw, 4 oz (edible)	100	2	4
1 cup, 5 1/4 oz (edible)	130	3	5
Cooked, moist heat, 3 oz	150	4	6
Ocean Perch, raw, 4 oz	90	1.5	0
Octopus, common, raw, 4 oz	95	1	2
Orange Roughy, raw, 4 oz	145	9	0
(Cals may be much lower. Over 90% of total fat is waxester which may not be metabolized)			
Oysters: Common, raw, 3 oz	70	1	3.5
Eastern raw:			
6 medium, 3 oz	60	2	3
1 cup, 8 3/4 oz	170	6	8.5
Fried/bread., 6 medium, 3 oz	170	11	10
Pacific, raw, 1 med., 1 3/4 oz	40	1	2
Oysters Rockfeller, 3 oysters	220	13	12
Perch, average, raw, 4 oz	105	2	0
Pollock, raw, 4 oz	100	1	0
Pompano, Florida, raw, 4 oz	190	10	0
Porgy/Scup, raw, 4 oz	130	4	0
Quahogs ~ See Clams			
Rockfish, Pacific, raw, 4 oz	110	2	0
Roe, raw, 1 oz	40	2	0.5

	C	F	Cb
Sable: Raw, 4 oz	220	17	0
Smoked, 3 oz	220	17	0
Salmon:			
Raw: Chinook, 4 oz	205	7	0
Atlantic; Coho/Silver, 4 oz	160	7	0
Chum; Pink, 4 oz	135	4	0
Red/Sockeye, 4 oz	190	10	0
Smoked Salmon: Chinook, 3 oz	100	4	0
Pacific Supreme, 2 oz	100	4	0
Wild Oats, Pastrami Style, 2 oz	130	9	0
Canned Salmon: *Average All Brands*			
Pink: 1 oz	40	2	0
1/4 cup, 63g (2.2 oz)	90	5	0
3 3/4 oz can, whole	155	8.5	0
7 1/2 oz can, whole	300	17	0
Skinless/boneless, 1/4 c., 2 oz	70	2	0
Red Sockeye: 1 oz	50	3	0
1/4 cup, 63g (2.2 oz)	110	7	0
3 3/4 oz can, whole	190	12	0
Atlantic, 1/2 cup, 3 1/2 oz	230	14	0
Chinook/King, 1/2 cup	210	14	0
Chum, 1/2 cup, 3 1/2 oz	140	5	0
Coho/Silver, 1/2 cup	155	5	0
Atlantic Steaks: Small, 8 oz	320	14	0
Medium, 12 oz	480	21	0
Large, 16 oz	640	28	0
Salmon Cake, take-out, 4 oz	240	15	6
Sardines (Canned): *Average All Brands*			
In Oil, undrained, 1 oz	85	7	0
Drained of oil, 1 oz	60	3	0
3 3/4 oz can, drained, (3 1/4 oz)	190	11	0
1 lrg/2 med. 3"/5 small, 0.8 oz	50	3	0
In Tom./ Mustard Sce, 1 oz	45	3	0
3 3/4 oz can (8 sardines)	170	11	0
Sashimi ~ See Japanese Foods, Page 171			
Scallop: Raw, 6 lg./14 sm., 3 oz	75	0.5	2.5
Breaded/fried, 6 lge, 3 oz	200	10	9
Seabass, raw, 4 oz	110	2	0
Shark: Raw, 4 oz	150	6	0
Batter-dipped, fried, 4 oz	260	16	7
Shrimp: Raw, in shell, 1/2 lb	140	2	1.5
Raw, shelled, 4 oz (12 lge)	90	1.5	0.5
Breaded/fried, 3 oz (11 lge)	210	11	10
Canned, 2 oz	60	1	0.5
Smelt, Rainbow, raw, 4 oz	115	3	0
Snapper, raw, 4 oz	115	1.5	0
Sole, Lemon, raw, 4 oz	90	1	0

Fish (Cont) • Frozen Meals

Fish (Cont)

	C	F	Cb
Squid, raw, 4 oz	105	1	3.5
Surimi (Imitation Crab), 4 oz	110	1	7.5
Swordfish, raw, 4 oz	140	5	0
Trout, Rainbow, raw, 4 oz	135	4	0
Smoked, 2 oz	110	6	0
Tuna: Raw: Albacore, 4 oz	190	8	0
Bluefin, 4 oz	160	5.5	0
Skipjack, Yellowfin, 4 oz	120	1	0
Canned: *Average All Brands*			
In Water, drained:			
Chunk/Solid, 2 oz can	60	0.5	0
3 oz can	90	1	0
6 oz can	150	1.5	0
In Oil, drained:			
Chunk Light, 2 oz	110	5.5	0
6 oz can, drained	275	14	0
Solid White, 2 oz	90	2.5	0
6 oz can, drained	225	6.5	0
Tuna Salad: Deli Style, 1/2 c., 4oz	300	24	15
Whitefish: Raw, 4 oz	150	6.5	0
Smoked, 3 oz	90	1	0
Whiting, raw, 4 oz	100	1.5	0

Frozen Fish Products

Fisher Boy: *See Page 60*
Gorton's: *See Page 61*
Kroger Fish Portions: *See Page 63*
Louis Kemp: *See Page 64*
Mrs Paul's: *See Page 65*
SeaPak: *See Page 67*
Van De Kamp's: *See Page 68*

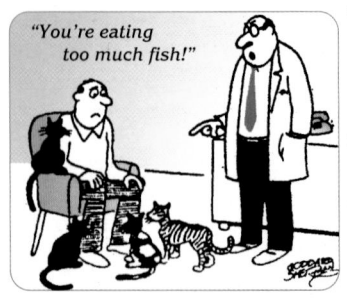

"You're eating too much fish!"

Amy's (Vegetarian)

Per Serving

	C	F	Cb
Pot Pies: Country Vege, 7 1/2 oz	370	16	47
Mexican Tamale, 8 oz	150	3	27
Shepherd's Pie, 8 oz	160	4	27
Vegetable (Non Dairy), 7 1/2 oz	420	19	54
Bowls: Brown Rice & Vegs, 10 oz	240	8	46
Santa Fe Enchilada, 10 oz	340	9	47
Stuffed Pasta Shell, 10 oz	300	12	30
Teriyaki w. Veges, Rice, 10 oz	300	12	59
Entrees: Chse Enchilada, 4.75 oz	210	12	13
Blk Bean Vege. Enchilada, 4.75 oz	170	5	26
Cheese Lasagna, 10.25 oz	330	12	36
Garden Vege./Tofu Lasagne, 9.5 oz	300	10	41
Macaroni & Cheese, 9 oz	410	16	47
Macaroni & Soy Cheeze, 9 oz	370	15	42
Pasta Primavera, 9 oz	300	11	37
Ravioli w. Sauce, 8 oz	340	12	43
Vegetable Lasagne, 9.5 oz	280	12	29
Burgers: Californian, 2 1/2 oz	100	3	17
Chicago Veggie, 2 1/2 oz pattie	160	5	20
Classic All-Amerian, 1 burger	120	3	15
Texas Veggie, 2 1/2 oz pattie	120	2.5	14
Burritos: Bean & Rice, 6 oz	280	8	49
w. Cheddar Cheese, 6 oz	270	6	48
Black Bean Vegetable, 6 oz	320	8	54
Breakfast Burrito, 6 oz	210	6	38
Burrito Especial, 6 oz	260	6	45
Asian Meals: Thai Stir Fry, 9.5 oz	270	11	36
Asian Noodle Stir Fry, 10 oz	240	4.5	41
Snacks: Cheese Pizza, 5-6 pc, 3 oz	180	6	22
Spinach & Fetta Mini Pockets, 3 oz	170	6	24
Whole Meals: Cannelloni, 9 oz	330	12	34
Black Bean Enchilada, 10 oz	320	6	55
Country Dinner, 11 oz	380	12	60
Cheese Enchilada, 9 oz	330	14	38
Chili & Cornbread, 10.5 oz	320	6	59
Veggie Loaf, 10 oz	280	7	47
Skillet Meals: Country Ched., 1 c.	250	11	27
Pasta & Veges Alfredo, 1 cup	220	8	27
Teriyaki Stir Fry, 1 cup	320	2.5	64
Pizza: Cheese; Spinach; Pesto, 1/3	300	12	38
Mushroom & Olive, 1/3 pizza	250	9	33
Roasted Vegetable, 1/3, 4 oz	260	8	43
No Cheese, 1/3 pizza	260	8	42
Soy Cheese, 1/3 pizza	280	10	37

Frozen Entrees & Meals (Cont)

Astrochef

	C	F	Cb
Cheese Puffs (Tyropita) 1 pce, 1 oz	70	4	5
Mushroom Puffs, 1 pce, 1 oz	37	2	5
Spinach Puffs, 1 pce, 1 oz	58	2	8
Sth Western Bean Rolls, 1 pce, 1 oz	66	3	8

Banquet

Per Meal

	C	F	Cb
BBQ Chicken	330	13	37
Boneless Pork Rib	400	20	39
Chicken Fried Beef Steak	420	23	38
Chicken Nugget	410	21	38
Corn Dog	490	19	68
Meat Loaf	240	16	23
Mexican Style Enchilada Combo	370	12	55
Our Original Fried Chicken	470	27	35
Salisbury Steak Meal, 9.5 oz	380	24	28
Sliced Beef, 9 oz	270	10	17
Spaghetti Meatballs	440	20	43
Swedish Meatballs	400	19	33
Turkey Mostly White Meat	270	13	30

Birds Eye – Voila!

Per Cup, Cooked (2 Cups Frozen)

	C	F	Cb
Chicken Voila!: Garden Herb	310	15	28
Alfredo; 3-Cheese Chicken	230	8	26
Grilled Salsa Chicken w/Rice	240	5	35
Italian Pesto; Teriyaki	240	9	24
Zesty Garlic Chicken	270	11	28
Steak Voila!: Beef Sirloin/Potato	240	9	26
Turkey Voila!: Turkey w. Potato	200	6	24
Birds Eye Hearty Spoonfuls Soup Bowls: See Page 79			

Boca (Vegetarian)

	C	F	Cb
Boca Burgers: Cheeseburger (1)	130	6	6
All American, 2.5 oz	110	3.5	6
Garden Vegetable	120	3	9
Original	90	1	7
Roasted Garlic	100	2	7
Roasted Onion	140	2.5	11
Sausages: Italian (1), 2.5 oz	130	7	7
Bratwurst	130	7	7
Smoked	130	5	7
Breakfast: Patties, (1), 1.4 oz	80	3	6
Bkfst Links, (2), 1.5 oz	90	3	8
Chik'n: Patties, (1), 2.5 oz	150	6	12
Chik'n Nuggets: (4), 3 oz	190	7	16

Budget Gourmet

	C	F	Cb
Classics: Per Serving			
Chinese Style Veg. & White Chick.	250	6	40
Escalloped Noodles & White Turkey in Sauce	320	15	35
Fettucini Alfredo w. Four Cheeses	310	11	49
Italian Style Veg. w. Cream Rice	250	6	39
Lasagna Alfredo w. Broccoli	290	10	36
Lasagna Mozzarella	280	8	39
Macaroni & Chse w. Cheddar	240	5	39
Penne Pasta w.Toms.& Ital.Saus.	270	6	46
Spaghetti Marinara	280	5	49
Spicy Szechuan Vege & Chicken	280	9	41
Stir Fry Rice & Vegetables	350	16	45
Ziti Parmesan	230	7	36
Dinner: Angel Hair Pasta w. Tom. Meat Sce, 8 oz	240	5	39
Italian Style Meatballs & Vege.	280	15	25
Premium: Beef Stroganoff	240	6	32
Beef Pepper Steak w. Rice	260	4	46
Chicken w. Fettucine	340	14	40
Fettuccine Primavera w. Chicken	230	7	30
Fried Chicken w. Pot. & Gravy	340	21	27
Glazed Turkey w. Stuff. & Potato	250	10	33
Linguini w. Clams & Shrimp	300	4	52
Orange Glazed Chicken	300	3.5	55
Pepper Steak w. Rice	260	4	44
Roast Beef Supreme	270	10	34
Three Cheese Lasagna	450	16	53
Bowls: Per Serving			
Potato Topped w. Baked Chicken	260	13	26
Shrimp & Vegetables	370	9	53
Shrimp Fried Rice	430	7	76
Spicy Beef & Broccoli	380	3	78
Sweet & Sour Chicken w. Rice	420	4	82
Teriyaki Chicken	420	3	80
Vegetable & Beef Stew	230	4.5	32
Vegetables & White Chicken	370	9	59

Cascadian Farm

	C	F	Cb
Per 9 oz Bowl: Pasta Primavera	280	8	41
Country Herb Chicken w. Veg Rice	250	3.5	38
Schechuan Rice Veggie	210	1.5	45
Teriyaki Rice Veggie	270	7	44
Per Tray: Chicken Fettuccine	380	12	43
Spinach Lasagne, 11 oz	330	10	39

Frozen Entrees & Meals (Cont)

Celentano

	C	F	Cb
Eggplant: Parmigiana, 10 oz pkg	350	28	17
Great Choice Rollettes, 10 oz pkg	290	20	17
Rollettes, 1.72 oz	230	18	11
Lasagne: Lasagne, 1/2 tray, 7 oz	270	12	29
Light Lasagne, 10 oz tray	290	6	40
Lasagne Primavera, 10 oz tray	260	4.5	39
Ravioli: Cheese	260	6	40
Light Cheese, 4.2 oz	280	3.5	46
Meat Ravioli	270	5	44
Stuffed Shells: Broccoli, 10 oz pkg	250	4	39
Tortellini: Cheese, 1 cup, 5 oz	420	8	68
Meat, 1 cup, 5 oz	340	4	55
Specialty Pastas: Baked Ziti, 9 oz	250	13	24
Cavatelli, 1 cup, 5 oz	400	1.5	77
Gnocchi, 1 cup, 5 oz	210	0.5	38

Croissant Pockets

	C	F	Cb
Italian Style Chicken Melt	380	20	37
Egg, Sausage & Cheese	350	18	38
Ham & Cheddar	340	16	36
Pepperoni Pizza	370	19	40
Philly Steak & Cheese	360	20	34

El Monterey

Family Classics: Per Serving

	C	F	Cb
Burritos: Chicken Fajita, 5 oz	250	6	40
Egg, Bacon, Chse & Salsa, 4.5 oz	270	12	33
Monterey Supreme, 5 oz	290	10	37
Sausage Breakfast, 4.5 oz	290	14	31
Steak Fajita, 5 oz	250	6	40
Ultimate Chicken, 5 oz	290	9	40
Chimichangas: Beef & Chse, 5 oz	310	13	35
Chicken & Cheese, 5 oz	320	13	38
Taquitos: Beef & Cheese, 4.5 oz	330	15	36
Chicken & Cheese, 4.5 oz	310	13	36
Egg, Bacon, Chse & Salsa, 4.5oz	290	11	38
Tacos: Soft Beef & Cheese, 5.5 oz	440	23	42
Beef & Pork, 4 oz	230	8	29
Spicy Chicken, 5.5 oz	320	9	46
Spicy Beef & Cheese, 5 oz	380	19	37
Spicy Beef & Cheese, 5.5 oz	420	21	40
Enchiladas: Beef w. Sauce, 4.5 oz	180	9	17
Cheese w. Sauce, 4.5 oz	210	13	15
Chicken w. Sauce, 4.5 oz	190	10	18
Tamales: Beef, 4.5oz	230	14	26
Chicken, 4.5 oz	250	11	27

El Monterey (Cont)

Regular: Per Serving

	C	F	Cb
Burritos: Beef & Bean (Reg./Green Chili/Spicy Red),			
5 oz Size	370	17	42
8 oz Size	580	27	68
10 oz Size	730	34	85
Bean & Cheese, 8 oz Size	470	14	70
Chicken, 4 oz	210	6	32
Tamales: Chicken, 4.5 oz	250	11	27
Beef, 4.5 oz	300	19	24

Empire Kosher

	C	F	Cb
Express Meal: Chicken Fajita, 1	130	2.5	15
Chicken w. Pasta, 1 cup	140	2	17
Chicken Stir-Fry, 1 cup	160	2.5	20
Pierogies: Potato Cheese, 5.3 oz	250	4	44
Potato Onion, 5.3 oz	245	4	47
Pies: Chicken Pie, 8 oz	440	21	41
Turkey Pie, 8 oz	470	23	45
Blintzes: Cheese, 2	200	6	29
Blueberry, 2	190	4	36
Potato Pancakes: Mini, 12, 3 oz	150	7	19

Ethnic Gourmet

	C	F	Cb
Vegetarian Teriyaki, 12 oz	350	3	73
Chicken Biryani, 12 oz	340	9	52
Kung Pao Chick. (Rice Bowl), 12 oz	340	6	56
Shrimp Fried Rice, 12 oz	400	10	64
Teriyaki Chicken, 11 oz	360	5	66
Thai Chef Ethnic Gourmet:			
Peanut Satay Chicken, 11 oz	400	14	50
Thai Sweet & Sour Veges, 12 oz	340	5	70
Veget'n Chkn w. Lemongrass, 11 oz	390	11	61
Lemongrass & Basil Chkn, 11 oz	390	10	55
Taj: Channa Bhaji, 12 oz	360	10	57
Shahi Paneer, 12 oz	400	15	59
Bean Masala, 12 oz	360	10	57
Tofu Samosa, 6 oz	160	5	23
Ethnic Wraps: Vege Paneer, 8 oz	320	10	50
Chicken Tikka Masala, 8 oz	320	7	47

Fisher Boy

	C	F	Cb
Quik Stix, 6 sticks, 3 oz	200	11	16
Quik Bake Crunchy Fish Portions,			
2 portions, 3 oz	200	10	19
Fish Rings, 7 rings, 3.2 oz	230	12	20
Salmon Fillet, 1 pce, 3.8 oz	100	2.5	1

Fortune Avenue	C	F	Cb
Chicken Won Ton, 15 Pce, 8 oz	310	7	39

Foster Farms			
Corn Dogs, 1 Dog, 2.6 oz	200	9	24

GardenBurger (Vegetarian)			
B'Fast Sausage, 1 patty 1.5 oz (43g)	50	3.5	2
Garden Vegan, 1 patty	110	1	17
Hamburger Style, Classic, 2.5 oz	90	1	8
Savory Portabello, 1 pce	120	2.5	18
The Original, 2.5 oz	110	3	16
Meatless: Meatballs, 6 balls, (25g)	110	4.5	8
Riblets w. BBQ Sce., 5 oz (142g)	210	5	10
Flame Grilled: Hamburger Style	120	4	7
Chik'n Grill, 2.5 oz	100	2.5	5
Gourmet Style: Santa Fe, 2.5 oz	130	2.5	20
Fire Rsted Vege, 2.5 oz	120	2.5	18
Veggie Medley, 2.5 oz	90	0	18

Gorton's			
Crunchy Fish Fillets: Breaded *(Per Fillet)*			
Lemon Pepper	135	9	9
Garlic & Herb; Hot & Spicy	125	7	10
Grilled: It. Herb; Lemon Pepper	130	6	2
Cajun Blackened; Lemon Butter	120	6	1
Battered: Parmesan, 1 fillet	130	7.5	10
Plain; Garlic & Herb, 1 fillet	125	6.5	11
Lemon Pepper, 1 fillet	135	9	9
Homestyle Baked: Au Gratin, 4.6 oz	230	12	14
Primavera, 1 fillet, 4.6 oz	120	5	4
Grilled Fillets: Garlic Butter (1)	100	3	1
Caesar Parmesan, 3.8 oz fillet	100	3	0.5
Cajun Blackened (1) 3.8 oz fillet	100	3	1
Lemon Butter/Pepper (1) 3.8 oz	100	3	0.5
Shrimp Bowl: Alfredo, 1 bowl	290	5	49
Fried Rice, 1 bowl	320	2	65
Garlic Butter, 1 bowl	280	5	46
Primavera, 1 bowl	270	6	41
Teriyaki, 1 bowl	320	6	57
Fish Portions: 1 portion, 2¹/2 oz	170	11	12
Fish Sticks: Breaded, 6, 3 oz	210	12	17
Popcorn Shrimp: 20 shrimp, 3 oz	240	12	26
Skillet Fillets: Traditional, 3.7 oz	200	11	14
Tenders: Extra Chunky, 3¹/2 pcs	260	12	29
Original, 3¹/2 pieces, 4 oz	260	15	22

Green Giant	C	F	Cb
Create A Meal: *Prepared with Meat & Oil*			
(Prepared Wt. ~ Approx 10 oz)			
Oven Roasted:			
Garlic Herb Chicken, 1³/4 cup	350	9	35
Lemon Pepper Chicken, 1²/3 cup	310	8	30
Parmesan Herb Chicken, 1³/4 cup	340	11	29
Pasta & Beef:			
Beefy Noodle, 1¹/4 cup	350	14	31
Cheesy Pasta & Veg, 1¹/4 cup	420	21	29
Chicken Alfredo, 1¹/4 cup	400	13	36
Homestyle Stew, 1 cup	340	16	24
Mushroom Wine Chicken, 1¹/4 c.	390	13	31
Skillet Lasagna, 1¹/4 cup	340	13	31
Stir Fry:			
Beef & Broccoli Stir Fry, 1¹/3 cup	290	13	15
Garlic & Ginger Stir Fry, 1¹/2 cup	270	7	25
Lo Mein Stir Fry, 1¹/4 cup	320	7	33
Sweet & Sour Stir Fry, 1¹/4 cup	340	7	43
Szechuan Stir Fry, 1¹/4 cup	310	14	20
Teriyaki Stir Fry, 1¹/4 cup	230	6	18
Complete Skillet Meal!:			
Per 8 ox (¹/4 Package) ~ Prepared			
Chicken Alfredo, 1¹/4 cup	270	7	37
Chicken & Cheesy Pasta, 1¹/4 cup	270	7	39
Chicken Lo Mein, 1¹/4 cup	250	7	30
Chicken Noodle, 1¹/4 cup	290	6	45
Chicken Teriyaki, 1¹/4 cup	250	1.5	45
Garlic Chicken Pasta, 1¹/4 cup	250	7	30
Sweet & Sour Chicken, 1¹/4 cup	320	1.5	62

Health is Wealth			
Buffalo Wings, Meatless (3) 2.2 oz	100	1.5	11
Chicken: Nuggets (4) 3 oz	150	6	9
Chicken Free (3) 2.25 oz	90	1	11
Patties (1) 3 oz	150	6	9
Chicken Free (1) 3 oz	120	1.5	15
Tenders (3) 3 oz	130	3	11
Munchies, average (2) 1 oz	60	1.5	10
Egg Rolls: Oriental Veg. (1) 3 oz	160	4	23
Oriental Chicken Free (1)	120	4	21
Spinach (1) 3 oz	180	8	20
Spring Rolls, 2 pce, 1.6 oz	70	2	10

Frozen Entrees & Meals (Cont)

Healthy Choice

	C	F	Cb
Bowl Creations: Beef Broccoli	300	8	41
Chicken Teriyaki w. Rice	300	6	50
Duos: Grilled Chick. Brst & Pasta	240	6	26
Grilled Chicken Breast w. Potato	190	4	19
Breaded Chicken & Macaroni Chse	270	6	34
Sirloin Beef Tips & Mushroom Rice	270	6	35
Salisbury Steak & Mashed Pot.	210	6	21
Turkey Breast w. Mash. Potatoes	200	5	19
Solos: Beef Macaroni	220	4	34
Cheese Rice & Chicken	230	4	33
Chicken Enchilada	310	7	46
Dinners: Beef Pot Roast	320	9	39
Beef Tips Portabello	280	8	28
Blackened Chicken	300	6	36
Boneless Beef Ribs w. BBQ Sauce	360	9	47
Chicken Broccoli Alfredo	300	7	34
Chicken Enchilada	360	7	59
Chicken Parmigiana	320	9	40
Chicken Teriyaki w. Rice	270	6	37
Country Herb Chicken	280	6	37
Herb Baked Fish	360	8	55
Lemon Pepper Fish	320	7	50
Mesquite Beef w. BBQ Sauce	340	9	40
Roasted Chicken Breast	280	8	32
Salisbury Steak	360	9	45
Stuffed Pasta Shells	290	6	40
Sweet & Sour Chicken	340	7	54
Traditional Meatloaf	300	9	36
Mixed Grills:			
Chicken: w. Ginger Dipping Sce	450	9	59
w. Barbeque Dipping Sce	390	9	46
w. Honey BBQ Dipping Sce	390	9	46
w. Roasted Garlic Dipping Sce	420	9	49
w. Roasted Red Pepper	390	10	39
Steak: w. Teriyaki Dipping Sce	450	10	62
w. Zesty Dipping Sce	340	10	37
Medleys: Beef Teriyaki	310	7	39
Chicken Breast w. Veg. & Pasta	230	5	29
Chicken Carbonara	310	7	39
Chicken Fettuccine Alfredo	280	7	28
Country Glazed Chicken	230	5	29
Mandarin Chicken	280	3.5	43
Oriental Style Chicken	240	5	28
Rigatoni w. Broccoli & Chicken	280	7	34
Roast Turkey Breast	230	6	25
Sesame Chicken	260	6	34

Hot Pockets

	C	F	Cb
Per Pocket (1/2 Pkg)			
Barbecue Sauce w. Beef	340	12	47
Cheeseburger	340	12	46
Chicken Melt	360	18	39
Four Cheese Pizza, 1 pce	380	17	45
Ham & Cheese	320	14	37
Italian Style Meat Trio	390	21	39
Pepperoni & Sausage Pizza	350	18	39
Pepperoni Pizza	360	17	41
Philly Steak & Cheese, 1 pce	280	7	42
Toaster Pizza Pepperoni	200	10	21
Turkey & Ham w. Cheese	330	14	41
Croissant: 5 Cheese Pizza	400	23	36
Meatballs & Mozzarella	330	18	32

Jaclyn's

	C	F	Cb
Not Even 1 Gram Fat Pizza:			
1 slice, 4 oz	200	1	34

José Olé

	C	F	Cb
Mexi Minis: *Per Serving*			
Beef & Cheese, 4 pce, 3 oz	200	10	23
Beef & Chse Mini Taco, 4 pce, 3oz	200	10	23
Beef Steak Fajita Bowl, 12 oz	330	11	37
Cheese Mini Burrito, 3 pce, 3 oz	200	8	27
Chicken & Cheese, 4 pce, 3 oz	140	4.5	20
Chicken & Cheese Rolled Tacos	270	10	33
Chicken Monterey, 1 pc, 5 oz	320	7	47
Grill. Chick. Quesadilla,3 pce,3.4 oz	220	8	27
Shredded Beef Taquitos, 3 pce, 3 oz	160	5	24
Chimichanga: Chicken, 5 oz pce	330	12	45
Shredded Beef, 1 pce, 5 oz	400	19	43
Wraps: Steak Fajita, 1 pce, 4 oz	340	10	46
Chicken Fajita,1 pce, 5.3 oz	330	10	46
Steak & Cheese,1 pce, 5.3 oz	340	12	42
Chicken & Cheese,1 pce, 5.3 oz	330	11	40

Kid Cuisine

	C	F	Cb
Cheese Pizza	410	10	70
Chicken Nuggets	500	24	54
Fried Chicken	600	38	41
Fun Nuggets	390	18	46
Macaroni & Cheese	380	13	54
Parachuting Pork Ribettes, 7.55 oz	380	15	43
Pepperoni Pizza	610	22	88
Taco Roll-Up, 7.35 oz	360	13	50

Frozen Entrees & Meals (Cont)

Kroger Fish Portions

Per 2 Pieces, 4 oz	C	F	Cb
Batter Dipt, 2 pces, 4 oz	260	14	22
Crispy Crunchy, 2 pces, 4 oz	270	18	18

Lean Cuisine

Bowls: Entrée

	C	F	Cb
Chicken Fried Rice	420	7	67
Chicken Teriyaki	330	2.5	59
Creamy Chicken & Vegetables	390	7	57
Grilled Chicken Caesar	290	7	36
Teriyaki Steak	370	7	56
Three Cheese Stuffed Rigatoni	300	8	44

Everyday Favorites: Per Serving

	C	F	Cb
Angel Hair Pasta	240	4	43
Cheese Cannelloni	250	6	30
Cheese Ravioli	260	7	38
Chicken Chow Mein w. Rice	240	3.5	37
Chicken Enchilada Suiza w. Rice	280	5	48
Chicken Fettucini	270	6	33
Fettucini Alfredo	280	7	40
Grilled Chicken w. Penne Pasta	250	5	29
Lasagna w. Meat Sauce	300	8	41
Macaroni & Cheese	290	7	42
Roasted Potatoes w. Broccoli	240	5	37
Rst Chkn w. Lem. Pepper Fettuc.	250	7	32
Santa Fe Style Rice & Beans	300	5	54
Spaghetti w. Meat Sauce	300	5	51
Swedish Meatballs w. Pasta	290	7	35

Cafe Classics: Per Serving

	C	F	Cb
Baked Chicken	240	4.5	33
Baked Fish, 9 oz	290	6	40
Beef Portabello, 9 oz	220	7	24
Chse Ravioli w. Chunky Tom. Sce	260	7	38
Chicken Breast in Wine Sauce	210	5	24
Chicken Carbonara	260	8	29
Chicken in Peanut Sauce	260	6	32
Chicken Parmesan	270	5	37
Chicken Piccata	270	7	40
Chicken & Vegetables	250	5	33
Chicken w. Basil Cream Sauce	290	7	37
Fiesta Grilled Chicken	270	6	34
Glazed Chicken w. Veg. Rice	230	5	25
Herb Roasted Chicken	200	3.5	24
Honey Roasted Pork, 9.5 oz	240	5	31
MeatLoaf w. Whipped Potatoes	260	7	28
Roasted Garlic Chicken	230	5	29

Lean Cuisine (Cont)

Cafe Classics (Cont): Per Serving

	C	F	Cb
Salisbury Steak	290	9	26
Shrimp & Angel Hair Pasta, 10 oz	280	5	44
Sweet & Sour Chicken	320	3	57
Teriyaki Chicken	320	3.5	51
Thai Style Chicken	270	5	39

Skillet Sensations:

	C	F	Cb
Beef Teriyaki & Rice, 12 oz	290	4	50
Chicken Alfredo	320	7	42
Chicken Teriyaki, Rice, & Veg.	300	4	49
Chicken Oriental, 12 oz	290	5	40
Chicken Primavera	310	4.5	49
Garlic Chicken	350	6	54
Herb Chicken & Rst. Potatoes	270	4.5	38
3 Cheese Chicken	340	8	45

Dinnertime Selections: Per Serving

	C	F	Cb
Chicken Fettuccine w. Broccoli	410	8	55
Grilled Chicken w. Penne Pasta	360	7	47
Grilled Chicken Tuscan	290	6	43
Jumbo Rigatoni	360	8	56
Roasted Chicken	370	5	57
Roasted Chicken w. Mushrooms	370	5	57
Salisbury Steak Dinner	360	9	42

Lean Pockets

	C	F	Cb
BBQ Sauce w. Beef	290	7	48
Cheeseburger	290	7	45
Chicken Fajita	260	7	38
Chicken Parmigiana	290	7	44
Ham & Cheddar, 1 pce	280	7	40
Meatballs & Mozzarella	280	7	44
Pepperoni Pizza	290	7	42
Philly Steak & Cheese, 1 pce	280	7	42
Turkey/Broccoli/Cheese	270	7	39

Lightlife

Vegetarian Meals: Per Serving

	C	F	Cb
Meatless 'Lightburgers', 2.5 oz	120	2.5	12
Smart Deli Slices, 3 slices, 1½ oz	50	0	2
Smart Dogs, 1 link, 1½ oz	45	0	1
Tofu Pups, 1 link, 1½ oz	60	2.5	2
Wonderdogs, 1½ oz	55	1	1

Frozen Entrees & Meals (Cont)

Linda McCartney C F Cb

Vegetarian Frozen Entrees

	C	F	Cb
Macaroni & Cheese	470	22	50
South Western Style Rice & Beans	340	12	46
Veg. Burrito w. Spanish Rice	450	18	51
Vegetable Lasagna	350	13	42

Louis Kemp

Crab Delights,

	C	F	Cb
Surimi, 1/2 cup, 2.5 oz	80	0	10

Marie Callender's

Meals & Dinners

	C	F	Cb
Beef Stew w. Corn Bread	430	9	69
Beef Stroganoff	410	14	39
Breaded Fish w. Mac & Cheese	400	16	36
Cheesy Chicken w. Rice	470	20	39
Cheesy Rice Chick. Broccoli, 12 oz	390	13	44
Chicken Carbonara	520	19	57
Chicken Cordon Bleu, 1 dinner	490	23	38
Chicken Fried Beef Steak	640	41	46
Chicken Parmigiana, 1 dinner	680	34	63
Chicken & Potato Casserole	400	19	39
Chicken Teriyaki	420	35	72
Chili/Cornbread	480	21	49
Chunky Chicken & Noodle, 1 meal	650	36	54
Country Fried Chick. & Gvy,1 din.	660	34	63
Country Fried Pork Chop, 1 dinner	620	36	50
Grilled Chicken Breast w. Pasta	570	21	64
Ham Steak w. Macar. & Chse, 1 din.	410	13	43
Lasagna Bake	470	15	52
Lasagna w. Meat Sauce, 1 cup	270	12	25
Mac & Cheese	340	13	39
Meatloaf & Gravy w. Mashed Pot.	510	30	34
Roast Beef w. Mashed Potato	370	18	27
Stuffed Pasta Medley	470	19	53
Swedish Meatballs	560	25	56
Sweet & Sour Chicken, 1 dinner	520	16	73
Turkey w. Gravy/dress., 1 dinner	390	16	33
Turkey Medallions w. Pasta	630	32	58

Pot Pies: Per Pie

	C	F	Cb
Beef	510	32	40
Chicken, 1 pie, 9.5 oz	630	38	53
Chicken & Broccoli, 1 cup	630	45	41
Chicken Au Gratin, 1 cup	560	37	41
Turkey, 1 cup	500	31	40

Michelina's C F Cb

Per Serving

	C	F	Cb
Black Bean & Chili w. Rice, 8 oz	300	4	58
Chicken a la King	280	8	39
Chili-Mac, 8 oz	290	4	38
Fettucine Alfredo	390	16	45
Four Cheese Lasagna, 8 oz	290	7	42
Lasagna Pollo	280	9	33
Lasagna Primavera	270	10	34
Lasagna w. Meat Sce, 8 oz	240	7	29
Linguini w. Clams & Sauce	290	3	52
Macaroni Cheese	430	16	50
Meatloaf, Gravy, Mashed Potato	340	23	20
Noodles Stroganoff w. Beef, 8 oz	340	14	38
Noodles w. Chicken, 8 oz	300	10	40
Penne Pasta w. Mushroom Sce	280	8	41
Penne Pollo	290	8	39
Pepper Steak & Rice	260	4.5	34
Rigatoni Pomodoro Italiano	220	2.5	40
Risotto Parmigiana	460	21	50
Salisbury Steak	330	21	21
Shells & Cheese w. Jalapeno	360	12	45
Spaghetti & Meatballs	300	8	43
Spaghetti Marinara, 8 oz	250	2.5	44
Spaghetti w. Tomato Basil Sce	250	3	46
Standard Mac & Cheese	340	13	21
Standard Wheels & Cheese	360	13	43
Swedish Meatball Egg Noodles	360	13	45
Yu Sing: Chicken Fried Rice	360	8	58
Chicken Lo Mein	220	3.5	34
Roasted Garlic Chicken	220	3.5	34
Sweet & Sour Chicken w. Rice	340	4	67
Teriyaki Beef	240	2	51

NOTICE THIS IS AN EQUAL OPPORTUNITY KITCHEN

Frozen Entrees & Meals (Cont)

Mrs Paul's

	C	F	Cb
Battered: Fish Sticks, 6	240	11	13
Fish Portions, 2	280	17	22
Batter Dipped: Fish Sticks, 2	330	17	28
Crispy Crunchy: Fish Sticks, 5	200	14	20
Fish Fillets, 2	250	13	11
Breaded Fish Portions, 2	240	12	20
Crunchy Batter: Fish Fillets, 2	280	13	23
Flounder Fillets, 2	260	14	24
Haddock Fillets, 2	250	12	25
Healthy Treasures:			
Fish Sticks, breaded, 4 sticks	140	6	14
Fish Cakes, 2 cakes, 4 oz	190	7	24
Light Seafood Entrees: Fish Dijon	200	5	17
Fish Florentine	220	8	10
Fish Mornay	230	10	12

Nancy's

Quiche: Florentine, 1 quiche	440	26	35
Lorraine; Monterey, 1 quiche, aver.	480	29	34

Natural Touch (Vegetarian)

Per Serving

Breakfast Pattie, 1	80	3	4
Corn Dogs, 1	170	6	22
Hard Rock Cafe Burg., 1 pattie, 3 oz	220	15	2
Lentil Rice Loaf, 1" slice, 3 oz	160	7	16
Nine Bean Loaf, 1" slice, 3 oz	160	8	13
Okara Pattie, 1 pattie, 21/4 oz	120	5	6
Roasted Herb Chik'n, 1 fillet	110	2.5	9
Spicy Black Bean Burger, 1 pattie	110	1	15
Tex Mex Burger, 1 pattie (67g)	120	1.5	17
Thai Burger, 1 pattie (67g)	100	3.5	7
Vegan Burger, 1 pattie, 23/4 oz	70	0	6
Veggie Medley, 1 pattie (64g)	120	4	11
Vegetarian Chili, 1 cup, 8 oz	170	1	21

Old El Paso

Burrito: Bean & Cheese	300	9	44
Beef & Bean	320	10	47
Pizza, all types	250	9	30
Chimichanga, all types	350	18	38

Ore-Ida

	C	F	Cb
Bagel Bites: Per 4 Pieces, 3 oz			
Cheese & Pepperoni	200	7	26
Chse, Sausage & Pepperoni	200	6	27
Blasts: 3 Cheese, 6 pce, 3 oz	200	4.5	25
Chse, Saus. & Pepperoni, 6 pce, 3 oz	200	5	25
Pepperoni & Cheese, 6 pce, 3 oz	220	7	25
Deep Dish Minis: Per 2 Pieces			
Pepperoni & Cheese, 3.5 oz	280	12	26
Chse, Saus & Pepperoni, 3.6 oz	260	10	27
Lil' Calzones: Per 3 Pieces, 2.8 oz			
Saus., Pepperoni & Chse, 2.8 oz	200	6	22
Tater Dogs: 4 pce, 2.8 oz	240	15	16

Ortega

Beef Taco Filling, 1/3 cup, 2 oz	100	6	4
Beef Enchilada, 9.3 oz pkt	430	21	45
Cheese Enchilada, 93/4 oz pkt	390	17	47
Chicken Enchilada, 91/2 oz pkt	380	16	46
Fiesta Dips: 11 oz Pkg, 1/4 cup Serving			
4 Layer Dip	80	3.5	8
Nacho Beef	60	7	4
Nacho Chicken	80	5	4
Salsa & Beef	50	2	4
Skillet Fajitas: Steak, 1/2 c., 2 oz	35	1	3
Chicken, 3/4 cup, 21/2 oz	45	1	4
Nachos Ckn Supreme, 1/2 pkt, 11 oz	380	11	49
Bowls: Chicken Santa Fe, 1 bowl	420	9	63
Pepper Jack Grilled Chicken, 1 bowl	480	16	60
Cheddar Rice & Grilled Chkn, 1 bowl	450	14	59

Pita

Broccoli & Chse Pie, 1/4 pie, 5 oz	380	25	31
Cheese & Spinach Pie, 1/4 pie, 5 oz	370	23	32

Poppers

Cheese Sticks Mozzarella, (1) 1 oz	90	4.5	8
Stuffed Jalapenos Cr. Chse (5) 5 oz	370	23	34

PopStickers

Chinese Dumplings: w. Vege. Filling			
13 Dumplings, 8 oz	330	45	61
w. Vege. & Chicken Filling			
13 Dumplings, 8 oz	320	5	51

Frozen Entrees & Meals (Cont)

Puck's

C F Cb

Per Meal

	C	F	Cb
Breaded Chick. Parmagiana, 12 oz	540	21	58
Chick. & Spinach Pasta Wrap	460	11	68
Chicken Bolognese & Spaghetti	480	22	48
Chicken Pappardelle	460	18	47
Eggplant Parmesan	370	28	14
4 Cheese Lasagna; Meat Lasagna	490	22	51
4 Cheese Macaroni	610	33	51
Italian Sausage Pasta Wrap	700	29	67
Meat Lasagne, 12 oz	490	22	51
Meatloaf in Wine Sauce	560	32	36
Mushroom & Spinach Ravioli	260	18	54
Mushroom Lasagna/Tortellini	440	17	53
Penne Pasta w. Beef & Vege	410	18	38
Radiatore Pasta Primavera	310	10	41
Spicy Chicken Lasagna	470	21	45

Rosina

	C	F	Cb
Turkey Meatballs, 3 balls, 3 oz	170	9	7
Italian Saus. Bites, 4 bites, 2 oz	180	15	1
Swedish Meatballs, 6 balls, 3 oz	260	19	5

Safeway Select

Gourmet Club Meals: *Per Serving*

	C	F	Cb
Bacon Wrapped Sirloin Tip Fillets	350	27	0
Beef Meatloaf	180	9	9
Beef Sirloin Tip Fillets:			
w. Black Pepper Glaze	210	8	5
w. Teriyaki Glaze	250	9	3
Beef Tamales w. Sauce	240	12	22
Beer Battered Cod Fillets	160	7	13
Boneless Pork Shoulder Ribs	180	7	9
Cheese & Broccoli Potatoes	260	10	34
Cheese Enchiladas w. Mole Sauce	200	11	22
Chicken Breasts	230	12	13
Chicken Enchiladas	180	12	13
Chicken Fried Steak w. Gravy	330	12	27
Chicken Nuggets	210	12	10
Chicken Stew w. Dumplings	400	15	38
Chicken Strips	230	13	11
Chile Belleno w. Polenta, Cheese	510	27	46
Chili Pot Roast	160	5	8
Deluxe Beef Shepherd's Pie	360	20	17
Deluxe Chicken Pot Pie	480	28	36
Extra Lean Steakhouse Beef Patties	130	5	1
Fillet of Sole	190	10	18

Safeway Select (Cont)

C F Cb

Gourmet Club Meals (Cont):

	C	F	Cb
Gorditas	410	21	35
Italian Six Cheese Lasagna	310	12	34
Italian Style Penne Pasta	190	4.5	30
Jumbo Chicken Wings: BBQ Style	200	14	6
Hot Buffalo Style	160	10	1
Low Fat Chicken Fillets, average	130	2	6
Low Fat Turkey Lasagna	300	3	48
Macaroni & Cheese	350	18	30
Meat Lasagna	290	11	30
Mexican Style Lasagna	390	22	26
Mozzarella & Bacon Beef Stk Patties	300	25	0
Peppercorn Glazed Beef Kabobs	120	1	4
Pork Carnitas, Rice & Salsa	470	20	53
Pot Roast & Vegetables	210	6	15
Roasted Garlic Mashed Potatoes	190	10	22
Salisbury Steak w. Gravy	380	26	9
Seasoned Boneless Beef Strips	120	2.5	1
Southwestern Quesadilla	280	15	21
Southwestern Wraps	260	12	26
Stuffed Baked Potatoes, 1 potato	280	11	35
St Louis Style Pork Spareribs	370	23	17
Tamale Bake	400	23	32
Three Cheese & Bacon			
Stuffed Baked Potatoes	210	11	22
Vegetable Lasagna, 1 lasagna	310	17	27
Vegetable Quesadilla	330	15	33
w. Lemon Butter	120	2.5	5
w. Teriyaki Glaze	250	9	3

Stir Fry:

	C	F	Cb
Chicken & Vegetables	180	1.5	26
Chicken Fajita	130	2	14
Shrimp & Vegetable	140	0	24
Teriyaki Beef	190	3	28
Beef & Broccoli	260	14	19
Chicken & Pork Potstickers	330	10	54
Ginger Beef	310	17	22
Orange Chicken	390	17	35
Pepper Beef	270	16	16
Pork Fried Rice	330	17	32
Sesame Pork	410	21	28
Shrimp Fried Rice	300	13	33
Sweet & Sour Pork	250	3.5	42
Szechuan Chicken	250	11	28
Vegetable Potstickers	250	10	36

Frozen Entrees & Meals (Cont)

SeaPak | C | F | Cb
	C	F	Cb
Crunchy Clam Strips, 1 pkt, 5 oz	410	2.5	41
Popcorn Fish, 7 pces, 3 oz	240	11	23
Popcorn Shrimp, 15 pces, 3 oz	210	12	18

Seeds of Change
Per 11 oz Bowl
	C	F	Cb
Bowtie Primavera	380	12	51
Creamy Spinach Lasagna	370	16	36
Macaroni & Cheese	420	16	52
Mushroom Wild Pilaf	350	16	40
Penne Marinara	290	7	44
Seven Grain Pilaf	390	14	52
Spicy Peanut Noodles	370	12	53
Teriyaki Stir-Fried Rice	340	8	56

Skyline Chili
	C	F	Cb
Original Chili, 1 cup 8 1/2 oz	310	20	5
Chili & Beans, 1 cup 8 1/2 oz	350	1	63
Chili & Spaghetti, 1 cup 8 1/2 oz	340	13	37
Coney Calzones, 1 piece, 5 oz	340	17	33

SoyBoy (Vegetarian)
	C	F	Cb
Breakfast Links, 1 link, 1 oz	65	2.5	6
5-Grain Tempeh	135	6	9
Not Dogs, 1 link, 1.5 oz	95	3	10
Ravioli Rosa/Verde, 1 cup, 3.5 oz	180	3	29
Okra Courage Burgers, 1	130	5	8
Soy Tempeh, 3 oz	150	6	9
Tofu Ravioli, 1 cup, 3.5 oz	180	3	31

Stouffer's
Entrees: Per Meal
	C	F	Cb
Beef, Roast Potato & Peppers	300	6	44
Cheesy Spaghetti Bake	460	21	47
Chicken a la King	370	11	47
Chicken Pie, 10 oz	730	44	61
Creamed Chipped Beef	160	11	6
Fettucini Alfredo	520	28	51
Fish Fillet w. Mac. Cheese, 9 oz	410	16	44
Five Cheese Lasagna	340	11	39
Lasagna w. Meat Sauce, 10 1/2 oz	370	14	35
Macaroni & Beef w. Tomatoes	350	12	41
Macaroni & Chse, w. Broccoli	350	15	38
Macaroni & Cheese, 1 cup, 8 oz	330	16	32
Maxaroni, Macaroni & Cheese	390	17	44

Stouffer's (Cont) | C | F | Cb
Entrees (Cont): Per Meal
	C	F	Cb
Roasted Garlic Chicken	290	8	39
Spaghetti w. Meat Sauce	440	15	56
Spaghetti w. Meatballs	390	13	49
Stuffed Pepper, 10 oz	240	12	24
Swedish Meatballs w. Pasta	520	25	48
Tomato Sce & Italian Sausage	420	19	43
Tuna Noodle Casserole	360	16	36
Turkey Tetrazzini	400	19	36
Veg. & Chicken Pasta Bake	410	17	40
Yankee Pot Roast	320	9	40

Homestyle: Beef Pot Roast
	C	F	Cb
Beef Pot Roast	270	12	25
Baked Chicken in Gravy/Potato	260	11	18
Beef Stroganoff	350	15	37
Breaded Boneless Pork Cutlet	370	20	34
Fried Chicken & Mashed Potato	350	17	34
Meatloaf w. Whipped Potatoes	580	32	38
Roast Chicken w. Mushrooms	380	17	31
Roast Chicken w. Stuffing Bake	510	29	37
Roast Pork w. Sw.Pots, Stuff.	400	18	46
Salisbury Steak in Gravy/Onions	550	27	49
Veal Parmigiana	530	17	66

Family Style Recipes: Per Serving
	C	F	Cb
Chick. & Broc. Pasta Bake, 1/5 pkg	340	17	28
Chick. Cordon Bleu Pasta, 1/4	360	15	35
Grandma's Chick. & Veg. Rice Bake	360	15	36
Lasagna w. Meat Sce, 1/12 pkg	330	14	28
Macaroni & Cheese, 1 cup	370	18	37
Meatloaf in Gravy, 1 loaf, 5.5 oz	222	13	10

Hearty Portion: Fr. Chkn Brst, 15 1/8 oz | 520 | 16 | 66 |
| Pork w. Roast Potatoes, 15 3/8 oz | 570 | 15 | 75 |

Side Dishes: Corn Souffle
	C	F	Cb
Corn Souffle	170	7	21
Cheddar Potato Bake, 1/2 cup	250	15	21
Harvest Apples	210	4	43
Spinach Souffle	130	8	10
Welsh Rarebit	120	8	6
Whipped Potato & Gravy	320	19	31

Pot Pies: Chicken, 10 oz
	C	F	Cb
Chicken, 10 oz	730	44	61
Turkey, 10 oz	590	34	53

Skillet Sensations: Per 1/2 Pkg
	C	F	Cb
Broccoli & Beef	300	5	46
Chicken & Dumplings	280	8	33
Chicken Alfredo	470	16	52
Grilled Chicken & Vegetable	400	15	42
Homestyle Beef	370	15	37
Homestyle Chicken	370	9	43
Teriyaki Chicken	270	2.5	40

Swanson   C F Cb

	C	F	Cb
Pot Pie: Per Serving			
Flaky Crust Chicken Pot Pie	380	21	38
Flaky Crust Turkey Pot Pie	370	20	36
Standard Meal			
Boneless White Meat Fr. Chicken	450	18	50
Chicken Teriyaki *(Original)*	430	7	71
Chicken Teriyaki *(Standard)*	340	7	49
Classic Fried Chicken, $11^1/2$ oz	640	36	41
Fish 'N Chips	470	22	52
Grilled Glazed Turkey Medallions	380	11	45
Grilled White Meat Chick.w.Penne	310	11	31
Mexican Style Fiesta, 13.25 oz	470	16	63
Salisbury Steak	470	19	33
Turkey Brst. w. Stuffing & Gravy	420	15	39
Hungry Man Dinners: Mexican	690	27	87
Boneless Pork Rib	840	39	99
Boneless White Meat Fried Chick.	640	24	72
Buffalo Chicken Strips	870	28	106
Classic Fried Chicken, $16^1/2$ oz	790	40	75
Meatloaf	560	25	52
Mexican Style Fiesta	710	29	87
Salisbury Steak	470	19	33
Turkey Breast	630	20	82

TGI Friday's

	C	F	Cb
Chicken Quesadilla Rolls	250	11	26
Honey BBQ Wings	180	10	7
Mozzarella Sticks & Sce, 1 Serve	120	6	15
Potato Skins, 3 pc, 2.8 oz	210	11	19
South West. Egg Rolls, 1 pce 3 oz	190	9	20

Tyson

	C	F	Cb
Buffalo Style Chkn Strips (2), 3 oz	190	9	17

Uncle Ben's   C F Cb

	C	F	Cb
Breakfast Bowls: Per Bowl			
Egg, Cheese & Salsa, 7.5 oz	310	21	16
French Toast & Sausage, 6 oz	420	22	45
Pancakes: Apple Cinnamon, 6 oz	330	8	59
Peach & Pecan, 6 oz	300	7	54
Sausage, Egg & Biscuit, 7.5 oz	350	20	31
Mini Bowls (8 oz): Beef Taco Olé	350	15	42
Cheesy Mac & Cheese	330	12	39
Pepperoni Pizzeria	330	15	34
Noodle Bowls: Honey Ging. Chkn	430	5	69
Spicy Peanut Chicken	400	11	53
Spicy Thai Style Chicken	370	7	57
Pasta Bowls: Per 12 oz			
Chicken Fettuccini Alfredo	350	7	47
Garden Vegetable Lasagna	320	7	44
Parmesan Shrimp Penne	380	7	58
3 Cheese Ravioli	380	7	61
4 Cheese Lasagna	330	7	41
Rice Bowls: Per 12 oz, 340g			
Chicken Fried Rice	400	6	67
Chicken & Vegetable	360	4.5	56
Spicy Beef & Broccoli	370	4.5	62
Sweet & Sour Chicken	360	3	65
Teriyaki Chicken	380	3.5	66
Teriyaki Stir Fry Veg	360	3	74
Turkey, Wild Rice & Cranberries	360	4	61

Van De Kamp's

	C	F	Cb
Fish Sticks, Breaded, 6 stix, 4 oz	290	17	23
Battered Fillets, 2.6 oz fillet	180	11	12
Crispy Fish Fillets, 1 pce, 2.6 oz	160	8	15
Crisp & Healthy: Breaded, 1 fillet, 1.8 oz	85	1.5	12
Grilled: Italian Herb, 1, 4 oz	130	6	2
Breaded Butterfly Shrimp, 7, 4 oz	300	14	32
Lemon Pepper, 1, 3.6 oz	130	6	0
Salmon, Creamy Dill, 1	90	2.5	1
Tuna, Barbecue, 1, 1.8 oz	100	0.5	5
Tuna, Sesame Teriyaki, 1	110	1.5	4

Wampler Foods

	C	F	Cb
Turkey Burger, Seasoned (1) 4 oz	230	12	0

White Castle

	C	F	Cb
Cheese Burger, Microwaveable, 1 pkg, 3.7 oz	310	17	23

Frozen Meals • Frozen Pizzas

Weight Watchers   C   F   Cb

	C	F	Cb
Main Street Bistro Selections: Per Meal			
Basil Chicken, 9 oz	270	6	34
Fajita Chicken Supreme, 9.25 oz	280	7	33
Fire-Grilled Chick. & Vegies, 10 oz	280	5	40
Golden Baked Garlic Chick., 10 oz	280	6	40
Peppercorn Beef Fillet	230	8	24
Rst. Chicken w. Sour Crm, Chives	190	3.5	23
Slow Roast Turkey Breast, 10 oz	220	7	20
Smart Ones: Per Meal			
Chicken Enchiladas Suiza, 9 oz	280	8	38
Chicken Oriental	230	4.5	34
Chicken Stir Fry Bowl	300	6	45
Fettucini Alfredo w. Broc., 9.25 oz	270	6	39
Fiesta Chicken, 8.5 oz	210	2	35
Grilled Salisbury Steak	260	6	25
Lasagna Florentine, 10.5 oz	290	8	36
Lemon Herb Chicken Piccata	250	5	36
Mac. & Chse; Lasagna Bolognese	240	2.5	45
Ravioli Florentine, 8.5 oz	220	2	43
Santa Fe Style Rice & Beans, 10 oz	300	8	49
Teriyaki Chicken & Veg Bowl	280	3	48
Southwestern Style Chicken Bowl	230	2.5	35
Spaghetti Marinara, 9 oz	280	7	46
Spicy Penne Mediterranean	260	6	40
Spicy Szechuan Veg. & Chicken	230	5	34
Swedish Meatballs, 9 oz	280	7	34
Smartwiches: Ham & Cheddar	260	7	36
Average other varieties	270	7	38

Worthington (Vegetarian)

	C	F	Cb
Meatless: Bolono, 3 sl., 2 oz (57g)	80	3.5	2
Chicken Roll, 2 sl., 2 oz (57g)	90	4.5	2
Chicken, Diced, 1/4 cup, 2 oz	60	0	3
Salami, 3 sl., 2 oz (57g)	130	8	2
Smoked Beef, 6 slices, 2 oz	130	7	7
Smoked Turkey, 3 sl., 2 oz (57g)	140	9	5
Wham Veg. Roll, 1 3/8" sl., 2 oz	110	6	3
ChikStiks, 1 piece, 1 1/2 oz	110	7	3
Crispy Chic Patties, 1 pattie	170	9	15
Fillets, 2 pieces, 3 oz	180	10	8
FriPats, 1 pattie	130	6	4
Golden Croquettes, 4 pieces	210	10	14
Leanies, 1 link	100	7	2
Prosage Links, 2 links	60	2.5	2
Prosage Patties, 1 pattie, 38g	80	3	3
Stripples, 2 strips, 1/2 oz	60	4.5	2
Tuno (Tuna Substitute), 1/2 c., 2 oz	80	6	2

Frozen Pizzas   C   F   Cb

	C	F	Cb
Amy's: Per 1/3 Pizza			
Cheese; Spinach; Pesto	300	12	38
Roasted Vegetable, 4 oz	270	8	43
Soy Cheese; Veggie Combo, aver.	280	10	37
Mushroom & Olive	250	9	37
Bake to Rise			
Four Cheese, 1/6	330	13	39
Pepperoni, 1/6	350	15	39
Special Deluxe, 1/6	360	15	40
California Pizza Kitchen			
Large: Five Cheese, 1/6, 4.5 oz	350	15	35
Thai Chicken, 1/6, 4.5 oz	310	11	38
Small: BBQ Chicken, 1/3	280	9	33
Garlic Chicken, 1/3	290	12	30
Five Cheese & Tomato, 1/3	320	15	29
Portobello Mixed Mushr., 1/2	350	12	45
Rosemary Chicken Potato, 1/3	290	11	35
Thai Chicken, 1/3	290	10	33
Saus., Pepperoni & Mushr., 1/3	290	13	30
Celeste			
Pizza For One: Cheese, 1 pizza	390	19	42
Deluxe	440	23	42
Original Four Cheese	430	21	40
Pepperoni	420	23	39
Sausage & Pepperoni; Suprema	500	28	44
Zesty Chicken Supreme	360	16	40
Connie's Pizza			
Super, 1/6 pizza, 4.5 oz	260	14	22
Thin Crust, Sausage, 1/5	290	15	24
Di Giorno			
Rising Crust (Large): Per 1/6 Pizza			
Four Cheese	320	11	40
Sausage & Pepperoni	360	16	40
Spicy Chicken Supreme	320	10	40
Spinach, Mushroom & Garlic	300	9	41
Rising Crust (Small): Per 1/3 Pizza			
Four Cheese	270	9	34
Pepperoni	310	14	35
Sausage & Pepperoni	320	14	35
Spicy Chicken Supreme	280	9	35
Spinach, Mushroom & Garlic	260	8	36
Supreme	330	14	35
Deep Dish: Four Cheese, 1/8	320	11	40
Supreme, 1/8	310	17	25

Frozen Pizzas (Cont)

Di Giorno (Cont)	C	F	Cb
Cheese Stuffed Crust: Chse, 1/6	340	14	35
Pepperoni, 1/6	390	20	35
Sausage & Pepperoni, 1/6	360	16	39
Half & Half (Supreme/Pepperoni):			
Supreme, 1/6 pizza, 5.8 oz	410	20	41
Pepperoni, 1/6, 5.4 oz	400	19	40

Ellio's (McCain)	C	F	Cb
Cheese, 1 slice	160	5	22

Freschetta	C	F	Cb
Bakes & Rises (Large):			
4 Cheese, 1/5 pizza	390	16	46
Pepperoni, 1/6 pizza	360	17	38
Supreme, 1/6 pizza	370	17	39
Sauces Stuffed Crust:			
4 Cheese, 1/5 pizza	320	11	41
Sausage & Pepperoni, 1/5	350	15	41
Supreme, 1/5 pizza	360	15	42
Small Pizzas: Pepperoni, 1/2	440	20	47
Southwest Chkn Supreme, 1/2	350	12	47

Healthy Choice: *French Bread Pizza*	C	F	Cb
Solos: Cheese; Pepperoni, 6 oz	360	5	57
Supreme, 6.35 oz	360	5	58
Vegetable, 6 oz	320	5	50

Home Run Inn	C	F	Cb
Large: Cheese, 1/8 pizza	290	15	27
Sausage, 1/8 pizza	310	16	27
Small: Cheese, 1/6 pizza	260	13	26
Sausage, 1/6 pizza	280	14	26

Jack's (Kraft)	C	F	Cb
Original: Cheese, 1/3 pizza	330	13	38
Sausage/Pepperoni, 1/4 pizza	310	16	29

Jewel: Cheese, 1/3 pizza	310	11	40
Pepperoni, 1/4 pizza	290	13	32
Supreme, 1/4 pizza	320	15	32

Lean Cuisine: *French Bread Pizza*	C	F	Cb
Cheese, 6 oz	340	8	46
Deluxe, 6 1/8 oz	330	9	44
Pepperoni, 5 1/4 oz	300	7	44

Mr. P's Pizza	C	F	Cb
Cheese Pizza, 6.5 oz	410	11	58
Combination (Saus./Pepp.), 1	460	17	58

Mystic	C	F	Cb
Cheese, 1/3 pizza	360	15	36
House Special, 1/3 pizza	375	17	36
Pepperoni, 1/3 pizza	380	18	36

Old Italian	C	F	Cb
Microwaveable Little Pizza: Per 1 Pizza			
Pepperoni (1) 4.2 oz	350	16	41
Party (1) 4.2 oz	340	15	40

Puck (Wolfgang)	C	F	Cb
Large: 4 Cheese & Pesto, 1/4	440	23	38
Barbecue Style Chicken, 1/5	310	13	30
Italian Sausage & Pepperoni, 1/4	410	20	36
Small: BBQ Chicken, 1/2	330	13	32
Primavera Vegetable, 1/2	300	13	30
Spicy Grilled Chicken, 1/2	380	18	35
Thai Style Chicken, 1/2	390	18	36

Ralphs	C	F	Cb
Large (Self-Rising Crust):			
Four Cheese, 1/6 pizza	330	10	48
Pepperoni, 1/6	390	15	49
Supreme, 1/6	390	15	49
Small: Cheese, 1	440	11	62
Combination, 1	520	20	61
Pepperoni, 1	510	19	62

Red Baron	C	F	Cb
Bacon Scramble, 1 pizza	400	22	33
Classic (Large): 4 Cheese, 1/4	420	23	36
Pepperoni, 1/4 pizza	440	26	36
Sausage & Pepperoni, 1/5	360	21	29
Supreme, Special Deluxe, 1/5	350	20	30
Bake To Rise: 4 Cheese, 1/6	330	13	39
Pepperoni, Special Deluxe, 1/6	360	15	40
Deep Dish Pan Style:			
4 Cheese, 1/3 pizza	370	17	39
Supreme, 1/3 pizza	410	21	40
Deep Dish Singles: Cheese, 1	430	21	41
Pepperoni, 1	460	25	41
Supreme, 1	470	27	40
Deep Dish Mini Pizzas:			
Cheese, 4 pizzas	380	15	44
Pepperoni, 4 pizzas	400	20	41
Sausage & Pepperoni, 4 pizzas	420	20	41
Supreme, 4 pizzas	430	23	43

	C	F	Cb
Reggio's			
Family Size:			
Cheese, 1/6 pizza	320	12	38
Sausage, 1/6 pizza	330	12	38
Dinner Size: Cheese, 1/4 pizza	330	12	41
Pepperoni & Sausage, 1/4	400	18	41
Sausage, 1/4	380	16	41
Stop & Shop			
Single Serving: Cheese, 1	390	19	42
9 Slices: Cheese, 2 slices	350	10	49
Stouffer's *French Bread Pizzas*			
Cheese, 1 piece (1/2 pkg)	370	16	43
Deluxe, 1 piece	420	19	50
Extra Cheese, 1 piece	400	16	49
Pepperoni, 1 piece	410	20	47
Sausage, 1 piece	420	21	49
Three Meat, 1 piece	460	22	50
White Cheese/Garlic/Herbs, 1 pce	460	23	45
The Old City Cafe			
Mushroom Pizza, 1/4, 92g	165	3	28
Pizza De Deluxe, 1/4, 103g	195	3	29
Tombstone			
Original (Large): 4 Meats, 1/5	320	16	30
Classic Sauce, 1/5 pizza	300	15	30
Deluxe, 1/5	300	14	31
Extra Cheese, 1/4	340	15	37
Sausage & Mushroom, 1/5	300	14	30
Cheese Stuffed: Pepperoni, 1/6	380	20	33
Light (Large): Veggie, 1/5	230	6	31
Mexican Style (Large):			
Sausage, 1/4 pizza	380	18	38
Cheese Quesadilla, 1/3 pizza	360	17	37
Chicken Fajita, 1/4	300	14	29
Nacho Grande, 1/4	380	19	37
Pepperoni, 1/4	400	20	37
Original (Small 9"):			
Original, 1/3 pizza	280	13	29
Extra Cheese, 1/2	370	15	42
Classic Sausage, 1/3	270	13	28
Oven Rising: Pepperoni, 1/6	330	15	35
Thin Crust:			
3 Cheese, 1/4 pizza	350	20	27
Italian, 1/4 pizza	380	24	27
Pepperoni, 1/4 pizza	400	25	27

	C	F	Cb
Tony's			
Original: Cheese, 1/3 pizza	390	22	33
Sausage, 1/3 pizza	440	27	34
Supreme, 1/3 pizza	420	22	39
Thin Crust: Cheese, 1/3 pizza	290	12	31
Sausage, 1/3 pizza	330	16	32
Supreme, 1/3 pizza	340	17	33
Super Rise: 4 Cheese, 1/4 pizza	340	13	40
Sausage, 1/4 pizza	380	18	41
Totino's			
Crisp Crust Party Pizza: Per 1/2 Pizza			
Cheese	320	14	34
Pepperoni	380	21	35
Supreme	380	20	35
Verdi (Safeway Select)			
Self-Rising Crust (Large):			
Meat Magnifico, 1/6 pizza	370	15	41
Primo Pepperoni, 1/6	370	15	42
Quatro Formaggio, 1/6	300	9	41
Supremo Classico, 1/8	280	12	32
Self-Rising Crust (Small):			
Rstd Mushr. & Garlic, 1/3 pizza	230	7	33
Primo Pepperoni, 1/3	300	13	32
Roasted Vegetable Speciale, 1/3	240	7	33
Supremo Classico, 1/3 pizza	300	13	33
Weight Watchers (Smart Ones)			
Per Whole Pizza			
BBQ-Style Chicken Pizza, 218g	400	5	69
Four Cheese Pizza, 198g	400	9	58
Pepperoni Pizza, 212g	400	7	65
Veggie Ultimate Pizza, 186g	400	7	65

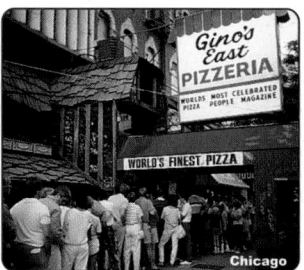

Chicago

Canned & Packaged Meals

Banquet

	C	F	Cb
Homestyle Bake: *Prepared, Per Serving*			
Creamy Turkey & Stuffing	260	12	29
Cheesy Ham & Hashbrowns	240	11	31
Country Chkn, Potato, Biscuit	380	13	55
Italian Pasta w. M'balls, Garlic Br.	370	16	46

B & M

	C	F	Cb
Baked Beans: *Per 1/2 Cup (41/2 oz)*			
Bacon & Onion w. Brown Sugar	190	2	36
Baked Beans w. Pork	180	2	33
Barbeque; Vegetarian	170	1	33
w. Natural Honey; Red Kidney	170	2	30
Yellow Eye Baked Beans	180	3	30

Betty Crocker

	C	F	Cb
Chicken Helper: *Per 1 Cup Prepared*			
Chicken & Herb Rice	260	7	26
Homestyle Chkn & Biscuit	440	11	53
Homestyle Chkn Dumplings	290	10	27
Southwestern Chicken	240	5	29
Average other flavors	300	9	28
Hamburger Helper: *Per Cup, Prepared*			
4-Cheese Lasagna; Stroganoff	330	14	31
Bacon Cheeseburger; 3-Cheese	380	17	35
Beef Pasta; Beef Stew, average	260	10	25
Cheddar & Broccoli	350	15	33
Cheddar Cheese Melt	310	12	31
Cheeseburger Macaroni	360	15	33
Cheesy Enchilada	380	16	40
Cheesy Hashbrowns; Chili; Pizza	290	10	31
Double Cheese Pizza	330	13	35
Lasagna; Ravioli; Sthwestern Beef	290	10	32
Nacho	350	16	30
Philly Cheesesteak	330	17	25
Potato Buds: Plain, 1/3 cup mix	80	0	18
As prepared, 1/2 cup	160	8	19
Suddenly Salad: *Per 3/4 Cup, Prepared*			
Classic	250	8	38
Ranch & Bacon	330	20	30
Roasted Garlic & Parmesan	260	11	33
Tuna Helper: *Prepared as Directed, Per Cup*			
Cheesy Pasta	310	14	32
Creamy Pasta	300	13	33
Tuna Melt; Creamy Broccoli	310	12	34

Campbell's: *Per 1/2 Cup, 41/2 oz*

	C	F	Cb
Barbecue; Old Fashioned Beans	170	2.5	29
Brown Sugar & Bacon Beans	170	3	29
Chili Beans	130	3	21
New England Beans	180	3	32
Pork & Beans in Tomato Sauce	130	2	24
Supper Bakes: *Per 1/6 Box, Prepared*			
Lemon Chick. w. Herb Rice	340	7	43
Herb Chick. w. Rice	330	7	40
Garlic Chicken w. Pasta	370	7	44
Savory Pork Chops	380	18	31

Cedarlane (Vegetarian)

	C	F	Cb
Bruschetta, Pesto, Mozz., Tom., (1)	100	5	10
Burrito, Beans, Rice, Chse., (1) 6 oz	260	1	48
Eggplant Parmesan, 1/2 pkg, 5 oz	190	8	16
Enchilada: Garden Veg., (1) 4.8 oz	140	3	20
Three-Layer Pie, 1/2 pkg, 5.5 oz	215	7	27
Focaccia: Tomato & Basil, 1/3 loaf	275	9	33
Mediterranean Stuff., 1/3 loaf	296	10	37
Lasagne: Cheese, 1/2 ctn, 5 oz	190	6	22
Garden Vege., 1/2 ctn, 5 oz	180	3	26
Pizza, Mini Bistro, (3) 4 oz	280	15	27
Rice Bowl: Terriyaki Veggie, 10 oz	460	6	86
Szechuan Veggie, 10 oz pkg	440	6	80
Wrap: Veggie "Ham" & Chse, 6 oz	350	10	36

Chef Boyardee

	C	F	Cb
Beefaroni, all types, 1 cup	260	9	35
Microwave Cup Meals: *Per Bowl*			
Beef Ravioli	190	3.5	28
Beef Ravioli & Meatballs	240	9	32
Lasagna; Pasta w. Chick. & Veg.	220	6	34
Spaghetti & Meatballs	210	7	28
Homestyle 15 oz Can: *Per Cup, 9 oz*			
Cannelloni	240	6	36
Cheese Tortellini in Tom. Sce	280	3	56
Chicken Alfredo w. Pasta	250	12	24
Rigatoni	250	10	31
Rotini in Tomato Sce	260	7	40
Mini Bites, *14.75 oz Can, Per Cup*			
Mini Beef Ravioli w. Meatballs	300	13	36
Mini Pasta Shells w. Meatballs	270	12	36
Mini Spaghetti w. Meatballs	280	13	31
Cheesy Burger Macaroni	220	6	32
Pepperoni Pizza Roli	320	11	46
Chef Jr: Micro Ravioli, 1 cup	220	5	36
Dinosaurs w. M'Balls in Tom.Sce	290	11	39
Other varieties, 1 cup, 9 oz	200	0.5	43

Canned & Packaged Meals (Cont)

Chef Boyardee (Cont)
Jumbo (14.75 oz Can): Per Cup

	C	F	Cb
99% Fat Free: Beef Ravioli	190	1.5	37
Cheese Ravioli	240	2.5	45
Lasagna	270	10	36
Spaghetti w. Jumbo Meatballs	280	13	30
Overstuffed Ital.Sausage Ravioli	280	4	50

Dennison's Chili: Per 1 Cup Serving (15 oz Can)
Chili Con Carne With Beans:

	C	F	Cb
Original; Hot, 1 cup	350	15	36
Chunky; Hot & Chunky	320	12	32
Micro Cup, 7.5 oz bowl	290	13	26
99% Fat Free: Beef Chili w. Beans	220	2	27
Turkey Chili w. Beans	210	3	29
Vegetarian w. Beans	180	1	35
Mild Green w. Beans	370	17	32
No Bean Chili Con Carne	330	18	21

Dinty Moore (Hormel Foods)

	C	F	Cb
1¹/₂ lb Can: Beef Stew, 1 cup	230	14	16
7¹/₂ oz Can: Beef Stew	190	10	15
Noodles & Chicken	200	9	21

American Classics: Per 10 oz Microwave Bowl

	C	F	Cb
Beef Pot Roast	200	3	19
Micro Cup: Beef Stew, 1 cup	160	7	16
Corned Beef Hash, 1 cup	350	22	19
Chilli con Carne, 1 bowl	290	13	26
Mac & Cheese	190	6	28
Chicken & Noodles	270	8	28
Chkn Brst/Rst Beef & Gravy w. Pot.	240	5	24
Hearty Lasagna	340	16	28
Salisbury Steak w. Potato	300	13	24
Turkey & Dressing w. Gravy	290	8	32

Don Miguel XLNT

	C	F	Cb
Flautas: Garlic Chicken, (2) 4 oz	250	5	40
Shredded Beef, (2) 4 oz	230	4.5	39
Tamales: Beef, (1) 3 oz	200	12	17
Chimichangas: Beef, (1) 4.8 oz	260	9	35
Chicken, (1) 4.8 oz	280	9	36

Dr. McDougall's: Per Cup

	C	F	Cb
Pasta w. Beans, Mediterranean	180	1	29
Pinto Beans & Rice, Sthwestern	190	2	38
Ramen Noodles; Chicken; Beef	140	1	39
Rice & Pasta Pilaf	210	1	36

Edamame (Vegetarian)
Soy Bean Rice Bowl: Per Bowl, 12 oz

	C	F	Cb
Kung Pao Vegetable	450	8	75
Szechuan Vegetable	410	4	77
Teriyaki Vegetable	460	4.5	86
Vegetable Fried Rice	450	8	78

Eden: Per ¹/₂ Cup, 4¹/₂ oz

	C	F	Cb
Baked Beans w. Sorghum, Mustard	150	0	27
Black Soy Beans	90	1.5	9
Chili Beans w. Jalapeno & Peppers	130	0	21
Ginger Blacks w. Ginger, Lemon	120	0	21
Lentils w. Onion, Bay Leaf	90	0	13

Fantastic: Per Packet

	C	F	Cb
Cup Meals: Cajun Rice & Beans	230	3	46
Bombay Curry Rice & Beans	250	1.5	52
Cha-Cha Chili	220	1	37
Chili Ole, average	260	2.5	48
Ready, Set, Pasta!, average	240	4	41
Spanish Rice & Beans	210	1.5	49
Spicy Jamaican	250	1.5	52
Tex Mex Rice & Pinto Beans	240	2.5	48
Vegetarian Chili	160	1	27
Couscous: Black Bean Salsa	240	1.5	46
Creole Vegetable	220	1.5	41
Nacho Cheddar	120	2	21
Sweet Corn	180	1	36
Noodles, average	140	1	27

Franco-American: Per Cup

	C	F	Cb
Spaghetti in Tom. Sce w. Cheese	210	2	41
Spaghetti O's: w. Tom. Sce & Cheese			
A to Z's	180	1	36
Garfield	210	3	39
Where's Waldo	200	2.5	38
Meatballs in Tomato Sce: A to Z's	260	9	33
Knights & Castles	270	10	33

Garden Gourmet

	C	F	Cb
Char-grilled Burgers, 2.6 oz	100	4	2
Vegetarian Drumsticks, 1.76 oz pce	90	4	10
Vegetarian Schnitzel, 3 oz schnitzel	100	4	5

Green Giant: Per Cup, 4.5 oz

	C	F	Cb
Pork & Beans w. Tomato Sce	240	2	46
Spicy Chilli Beans	220	2	40

Health Valley (Vegetarian)

	C	F	Cb
Fat-Free Beans & Chili:			
Chili Burrito/Enchilada, 1/2 cup	80	0	15
Chili in a Cup, all types, 3/4 cup	120	1	21
Chili, Fajito flavored, 1/2 cup	80	0	15
Honey Baked Beans, 1/2 cup	110	0	25
Mild/Spicy Vegetarian Chili:			
all flavors, 1/2 cup	80	0	15

Hormel: Per Cup

	C	F	Cb
Kid's Kitchen: Beans 'N Wieners	310	13	37
Beefy Macaroni	190	6	23
Cheezy Mac 'N Cheese	260	11	30
Cheezy Mac 'N Franks	300	16	26
Mini Beef Ravioli	240	7	34
Spaghetti & Mini Meatballs	230	9	26
Spaghetti Rings & Franks	240	9	32
Noodle Rings & Chicken	150	5	16
Spaghetti Rings w. Meatballs	230	7	35
Microwave Cup: Chili w. Beans	220	6	27
Chili no Beans	190	8	15
Lasagna w. Meat Sauce	210	6	29
Scalloped Potatoes & Ham	240	14	20
Spaghetti w. Meat Sce	220	7	31
Chili, 15 oz Can: Per Cup			
With Beans: Reg./Hot/Chunky	270	7	34
Homestyle Chili	330	19	24
Turkey (99% Fat Free)	200	3	26
Vegetarian (99% Fat Free)	200	1	38
Chunky No Beans	210	6	22
Hot/Chilli No Beans	210	9	17
No Beans, 1 cup	210	9	17
Tamales (15 oz Can): 2 Tamales	140	7	15
Natural Touch: Thai Burger (1) 2.4 oz	100	3.5	7
Breakfast Patty (1) 2.4 oz	80	3	4

Hy Top: Per Serving

	C	F	Cb
Deluxe Shells & Ched. Chse Dinner	410	16	51
Refried Beans, 1/2 Cup	150	2.5	24
Cans: Per 1 Cup			
Spagh. Rings & Tom. Meatballs	410	16	51
Spagh. Rings in Tomato Sce	190	0.5	40
Spaghetti in Tom. Sce & Chse	180	0	39
1 1/2lb Can: Beef Stew, 247g	190	7	18
15oz Can: Corned Beef Hash	430	28	28
Chili w. Beans, 270g	510	32	34

Hungry Jack Potatoes

	C	F	Cb
Casseroles: 1/2 cup, average	150	5	24
Idaho Mashed: 1/2 cup, aver.	155	5	21
Inst. Potato Flakes: 1/3 cup	80	0	18
Pot. Pancake Mix, 2 T., Made Up	90	1.5	16

Ken & Robert's: Veggie Burger

	C	F	Cb
Ken & Robert's: Veggie Burger	130	1	26
Veggie Pockets, average, 4.5 oz	250	8	39

Kraft Pasta Dinners: Per Cup, Prepared

	C	F	Cb
Deluxe: Four Cheese	320	10	44
Sharp Cheddar	270	4	38
Macaroni & Cheese:	320	10	44
Light	290	4.5	48
Light (Only 1 T. fat + skim milk)	290	6	47
Child's/Cartoon Pack	410	19	47
Easy Mac, 1 pouch	250	7	38
Velveeta: All varieties	360	13	46
Oven Classic Chicken Bake: 1/6 Pkt, Prepared			
Au Gratin; Traditional Roast	340	11	33
Herb & Garlic	320	8	34
Homestyle BBQ	360	6	43
Honey Mustard	380	10	43
Lemon	370	7	48
Roasted Garlic	310	10	28

Lipton Packet Meals
Per Cup, Prepared

	C	F	Cb
Rice & Sauce: Spanish	270	7.5	47
Cheddar Broccoli; Chicken	280	9	46
If no fat used in prep'n, deduct 55 Cals and 6g Fat			
Noodles & Sauce: Butter/& Herb	310	14	42
Chicken Flavor; Chick. Broccoli	300	11	42
If no fat used in prep'n, deduct 55 Cals and 6g Fat			
Pasta & Sauce: Creamy Garlic	350	13	47
Crmy Mushr./Tom.; Zesty Ched.	320	11	43
Mild Ched. Chse; Rst Garlic Chick.	290	10	40
Roasted Garlic Olive Oil w. Tom.	270	8.5	42
Other varieties, average	290	9	40
If no fat used in prep'n, deduct 55 Cals and 6g Fat			
Recipe Secrets: Golden Onion	50	1	9
Onion	20	0	4
Onion & Mushroom; Savory Herb	30	0.5	6
Vegetable	30	0	9
Sizzle & Stir: 1/6 Pkt, Prepared			
3 Cheese Alfredo Chkn & Penne	410	15	29
Savory Herbed Chicken & Pasta	340	9	28
Spanish Chkn; Teriyaki Stir Fry	360	9.5	34
Side Dishes: Per 1/3 Cup Mix (26g)			
Mash.Pot. w.Beef/Chick. Gravy	100	2	18

Canned & Packaged Meals (Cont)

Loma Linda (Vegetarian)	C	F	Cb
Big Franks: 1 link, 1.8 oz	110	7	2
Lowfat, 1 link, 1.8 oz	80	3	3
Chicken Supreme Mix, 1/3 cup mix	90	1	6
Chik Nuggets, 5 pieces, 3 oz	240	16	13
Dinner Cuts, 2 sl., 1.4 oz (41g)	90	1.5	3
Fried Chik'n/Gravy, 2 pcs, 3 oz	160	10	4
Gravy Quik, 1 Tbsp mix (1/4 pkt)	20	0	4
Linkettes, (1), 1 1/4 oz	70	4.5	1
Little Links, 2 links, 1.6 oz	90	6	2
Nuteena, 3/8" slice, 2 oz	160	13	6
Ocean Platter, 1/3 c. dry mix, 1 oz	90	1	8
Patty Mix, 1/3 cup dry mix, 1 oz	90	1	7
RediBurger, 5/8" slice, 2 oz	120	2.5	7
Sandwich Spread, 1/4 cup, 2 oz	80	4.5	7
Savory Din. Loaf, 1/3 cup, dry mix	90	1.5	7
Soyagen, 1/4 c. (1 oz) dry (make 1 c.)	130	6	12
Swiss Stake, 1 piece, 3 1/4 oz	120	6	8
Tender Bits, 6 pieces, 3 oz	110	4.5	7
Tender Rounds, 6 pieces, 2 3/4 oz	120	5	5
Vege Burger, 1/4 cup, 2 oz	70	1.5	2
Vita Burger Chunks, 1/4 cup, 3/4 oz	70	1	6
Vita Burger Granules, 3 T., 3/4 oz	70	1	6

Lunch Basket: *Per Serving*			
Microwave: Dumplings 'n Chicken	140	5	21
Hearty Beef Stew	170	9	17
Lasagna w. Meat Sauce	160	3	29
Pasta 'n Chick. w. Veg	150	5	22

Manischewitz			
Taco Dinner	290	12	38
Vegetarian Chili, 3/4 cup	145	1.5	31

Maruchan: *Per Pkt*			
Instant Noodles: all flavors, aver.	280	12	37
Instant Wonton, all flavors	200	12	19
Oriental Noodle, all flavors	290	12	38
Ramen flavors, 1/2 pkt, 1 1/2 oz	180	7	26
Wonton flavors, 1/3 pkt	90	5	9

Midland Harvest			
Fat Free & Lowfat Dry Mix:			
Taco Filling & Dip, 2.7 oz	50	0	7
Chili Fixin's, 8 oz	160	1	24
Sloppy Joe Fixin's, 3.6 oz	70	0	11
Burger Loaf Dry Mix: Per 3.2 oz	120	4	8
Frozen Patties: Sausage, 2 oz	80	4	4
Other varieties, 3.2 oz	120	4	8

Morningstar Farms (Vegetarian)	C	F	Cb
Better'n Burger, 1 pattie, 3 oz	80	0	8
Better'n Eggs, 1/4 cup, 2 oz	20	0	0
Breakfast Links, 2 links, 1 1/2 oz	80	3	3
Breakfast Patties:			
Frozen (1), 1 1/4 oz	80	3	3
Refrigerator Pack (1), 1 oz	60	2.5	3
Breakfast Strips, 2 strips	60	4.5	2
Buffalo Wings, 5 nuggets, 3 oz	200	9	16
Burger-Style Recipe Crumbles, 2/3 c.	80	2.5	4
Chik Nuggets, 4 nuggets	160	4	17
Chik Patties, 1 pattie	150	6	16
Corn Dog (Meat Free): 1 link	150	4	22
Mini, 4 pieces, 2.7 oz	170	4.5	21
Garden Vege Patties (1), 2 1/2 oz	100	2.5	9
Restaurant, 1 pattie, 3 1/2 oz	150	3.5	13
Grillers, 1 pattie, 2 1/4 oz	140	6	5
Grillers, Prime (1) 2 1/2 oz	170	9	5
Ground Meatless, 1/2 cup, 2 oz	60	0	4
Hard Rock Café Veggie Burger, 1	170	8	18
Harvest Burgers (1), 3.2 oz	140	4.5	8
Mushroom & Pepper Burger, 1	120	4	9
Oven Rstd Veggie Burger, froz., (1)	120	3	9
Quarter Prime Patties (1), 2 3/4 oz	140	2	6
Saus. Recipe Crumbles, 2/3 c., 2 oz	90	3	5
Scramblers, 1/4 cup, 2 oz	35	0	2
Spicy Black Bean Burger, 1 pattie	110	1	16
Veggie Dog, 1 link, 2 oz	80	0.5	6
Breakfast Sandwiches:			
Muffin/Scramblers/Pattie/Cheese	280	3	35
Muffin/Scramblers/Pattie	240	2.5	32
Stuffed S'wich, all types, average	290	8	42
Burger Kits (Dry):			
Garden Vegie Burger Kit, 1/4 pkg	80	0	6
Sth.West.Veggie Burger, 1/4 pkg	90	0	9

Natural Touch (Vegetarian)			
Canned & Dry Products			
Brown Gravy Mix, 1 Tbsp, (makes 1/4 cup)	20	0	4
Kaffree Roma, 1 rounded tsp, 2g	10	0	2
Mushroom Gravy Mix, 1 Tbsp, (makes 1 cup)	15	0	3
Roasted Soy Butter, 2 Tbsp, 1.1 oz	170	11	10
Tuno, 1/3 cup, drained, 2 oz	60	2	2
Vegetarian Chili, 1 cup, 8 oz	170	1	21
Continued Next Page			

Canned & Packaged Meals (Cont)

Near East	C	F	Cb
Prepared as Directed, Per Cup			
Couscous: Original Plain	230	2	46
Chicken & Herbs	270	6	51
Toasted Pine Nut	230	6	40
Creamy Parmesan	280	7	48
Roasted Garlic; Broccoli	220	4	41
Roasted Pecan & Garlic	240	9	37
Rice Pilaf	190	0.5	42

New Menu (Vitasoy) Vegetarian			
VegiBurgers, 3 oz	110	1	12
VegiDogs, 1 link, 1.5 oz	45	0	1
Tofumate (Season. Mixes): 1/4 pkt	25	0	4

Nile Spice: *Per Cup*			
Couscous: Lentil Curry	200	1.5	36
Minestrone	180	1.5	34
Parmesan	200	3	34

Nissan			
Cup Noodles, all types, average	300	14	38

Old El Paso: *Per Serving*			
One Skillet Mexican (Prepared):			
Rice Burrito, (1)	190	4	35
Salsa; Taco, average, (2)	460	16	56
Dinner Kits (Prep'd): Soft Taco	390	19	33
Burrito (1)	270	12	27
Hard & Soft Taco (2)	360	17	32
Shells, Taco Sce, Seasoning (2)	310	18	19
Fajita (2)	330	10	35
Taco Dinner (2)	300	17	19
Side Dishes: *Per Serving*			
Canned: Chili with Beans, 1 cup	240	11	19
Spanish Rice, 1 cup	140	1	30
Tamales in Chili Gravy (1)	320	19	31
Boxed: Chsy Mexican Rice 1/3 pkt	250	2	55
Spanish Rice, 1/3 pkt	280	4.5	55
Refried Beans: Reg., Black, 1/2 c.	100	0.5	17
w. Green Chilies, 1/2 cup	100	0.5	17
w. Cheese, 1/2 cup	130	3.5	18
w. Sausage, 1/2 cup	200	13	14
Fat Free varieties, 1/2 cup	100	0	18
Mexe/Pinto Beans, 1/2 cup	110	0.5	19
Black/Garbanzo Beans, 1/2 cup	100	1	17

Pasta-Roni: *Per Cup, Prepared*			
Angel Hair Pasta Primavera	330	16	39
Broccoli	340	15	41
Broccoli Au Gratin	280	10	41

Pasta-Roni (Cont):	C	F	Cb
Per Cup, Prepared			
Butter & Garlic	260	8	40
Chicken; Shells & White Cheddar	310	13	41
Chicken & Broccoli; Parmesano	370	16	49
Chicken & Garlic (Lowfat)	210	3	39
Creamy Garlic	420	25	41
Fettucini Alfredo, Reduced Fat	310	8	50
Garlic & Olive Oil w. Vermicelli	360	16	48
Homestyle Chicken	230	6	39
White Cheddar & Broccoli	400	19	48

Progresso: Beef Ravioli, 1 c., 9 oz	260	5	45
Cheese Ravioli, 1 cup, 9 oz	220	2	43
Italian Style Zucchini, 1/2 c., 4.2 oz	50	2	7

Pritikin: Vegetarian Chili, 1 cup	160	1	27

Ramen Noodles: *Per Serving*			
Beef/Chicken Flavor, 3 oz	190	8	27
Baked Noodle: 1/2 Block, 11/2 oz	140	1	30
Noodles: Fat Fried Shrimp, 11/2 oz	170	6	26
Other Flavors, 11/2 oz	160	6	26
Fried Cup: Beef, 1 packet, 2.2 oz	290	11	41
Lowfat: Average, 2 oz	215	1.5	45

Rice-A-Roni: *Per Cup, Prepared*			
Beef; Herb & Butter	310	9	52
Broccoli Au Gratin	370	17	47
1/3 Less Salt	320	11	50
Chicken	310	9	52
1/3 Less Salt	280	5	53
Lowfat	210	3	41
Chicken & Broccoli	230	6	41
Chicken & Garlic; Chkn Teriyaki	260	9	41
Chicken & Mushroom	360	14	52
Fried Rice	320	11	51
Long Grain & Wild Rice	240	6	43
Red Beans & Rice	290	7	51
Rice Pilaf; Risotto	310	9	51
Savory Chicken Vegetable	210	3	41
Spanish Rice	270	8	46
White Cheddar & Herbs	340	13	48
(Reduced Fat Recipe: If only 1 Tbsp fat is used			
instead of 2 Tbsp, deduct 35 calories and 4g fat.)			

Skyline Chili ~ Cincinatti's Famous			
Chili w. Beans, 1 cup, 81/2 oz	300	17	33
Original Chili, 1 cup, 81/2 oz	320	22	14
Chili & Spaghetti, 1 cup, 81/2 oz	320	15	25
Dip (in tub), 2 Tbsp., 1 oz	60	5	1

Canned & Packaged Meals (Cont)

Stagg Chili	C	F	Cb
(15 oz Can): Per 1 Cup (8.7 oz)			
Chili w. Beans: Classic/Dynamite	330	17	28
Country/Laredo	320	16	29
Fiesta Grille	240	9	25
Rancho House Chicken	290	9	32
Rio Blanco Chicken	250	12	19
No Beans: Steakhouse/Double	330	21	16
99% Fat Free: Veg. Gdn/4 Bean	200	1	37
Turkey Ranchers/Silvarado Beef	240	3	31

Sweet Sue	C	F	Cb
Chicken & Dumpling, 1 cup	240	7	31
Canned Whole Chicken:			
w/out giblets, 2 oz	80	5	0

Taco Bell: *Per 1/2 Cup*	C	F	Cb
Home Originals: Refried Beans	140	2.5	22
Fat Free Beans w. Green Chilles	120	0	23

Trader Joe's	C	F	Cb
Quiche: Broccoli & Cheddar, 6 oz	490	33	33
Mexicaine, 6 oz	510	36	29
Spinach & Mushroom, 6 oz	470	30	32

Tuna Helper ~ *See Betty Crocker, Page 72*

White Wave (Vegetarian)	C	F	Cb
Tempeh: Five Grain, 1/3 pkg	140	4	15
Original, 1/3 block, 2.7 oz	150	6	10
Sea Veggie, 1/3 block, 2.7 oz	120	3	11
Wild/Soy Rice, 1/3 block, 2.7 oz	140	5	13
Seitan: Chicken w. Broth, 5 oz	130	0	12
Traditional, 4 oz	140	0	4
Tofu: Baked: All flavors, 2 oz	120	6	3
Organic: Soft/Firm, 1/5 pkg, 3.2 oz	90	6	1
Fat-Reduced, 1/5 pkg, 3.2 oz	90	4	4
Extra Firm, 1/4 pkg, 3 oz	80	5	1
Soy Milks & Yogurts: See Pages 25, 28			

Wolf	C	F	Cb
Chili w. Beans: 227g Can	300	16	27
15 oz Can, 1 cup, 254g	330	18	30
Chili No Beans: 227g Can	390	27	18
15 oz Can, 1 cup, 248g	420	30	20
Chunky Beef w. Beans:			
15 oz Can, 1 cup, 254g	300	15	28
No Beans, 1 cup, 246g	330	22	18

Worthington (Vegetarian)	C	F	Cb
Canned & Dry Products			
Chic-Ketts, 2 slices (3/8"), 2 oz	120	7	2
Chili, 1 cup, 8 oz	290	15	21
Low Fat Chili, 1 cup, 8 oz	170	1	21
Choplets, 2 slices, 3 1/4 oz	90	2	3
Corned Beef, 4 slices, 2 oz	140	9	5
Country Stew, 1 cup, 8 1/2 oz	210	9	20
Diced Chik, 1/4 cup, 2oz	40	0	1
Dinner Roast, 3/4" slice, 3 oz	180	12	5
FriChik, 2 pieces, 3 oz	120	8	1
Low Fat FriChik, 2 pcs, 3 oz	80	3	2
Multigrain Cutlets, 2 sl., 3 1/4 oz	100	2	5
Numete, 3/8" slices, 2 oz	130	10	5
Prime Stakes, 1 piece, 3 1/4 oz	120	7	4
Prosage Roll, 5/8" slice, 2 oz	140	10	2
Protose, 3/8" slice, 2 oz	130	7	5
Savory Slices, 3 slices, 3 oz	150	8	7
Saucettes, 1 link, 1.3 oz	90	6	1
Sliced Chik, 3 slices, 3.2 oz	80	0.5	2
Smoked Beef, 6 slices, 2 oz	120	6	6
Smoked Turkey, 3 slices, 2 oz	140	10	3
Super-Links, 1 link, 1 1/2 oz	110	8	2
Tuno, 1/2 cup (drained), 2 oz	80	6	2
Turkee Slices, 3 slices, 3.3 oz	180	12	5
Vegetable Skallops, 1/2 cup, 3 oz	90	1.5	3
Vegetable Steaks, 2 slices, 2 1/2 oz	80	1.5	3
Vegetarian Burger, 1/4 c., 2 oz	60	2	2
Vegetarian Cutlets, 1 slice, 2.2 oz	70	1	3
Veja Links, 1 link, 1.1 oz	40	1.5	3
Wham, 2 slices, 1 1/2 oz	80	5	1
Continued Next Page			

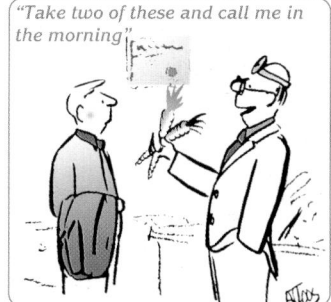

"Take two of these and call me in the morning"

Meals (Cont) ◆ Soy & Tofu

Yves Veggie Cuisine (Vegetarian)	C	F	Cb
Breakfast: Brkfast Links, (2) 1.8 oz	60	0	3
Breakfast Patties, (1) 2 oz	70	2	4
Canadian Veg. Bacon, 3 sl, 2 oz	80	0.5	1
Burgers: Veggie Burger, (1) 3 oz	120	2	9
Garden Vegetable Patties, (1) 3 oz	90	0	11
Blk Bean & Mushroom, (1) 3 oz	100	0	13
Veggie Chick 'N Burger, (1) 3 oz	120	3	6
Dogs: Good Dog, (1) 52g	80	2	2
Hot & Spicy Veggie Chili (1) 52g	70	1	3
Veggie Dog, (1) 46g	60	0	1
Jumbo Veggie Dog, (1) 76g	100	1.5	3
Tofu Dog, (1) 38g	45	0.5	2
Veggie Ground Round:			
1/3 cup, 1.93 oz (55g)	60	0	4
Veggie Meatballs, (1) 75g	120	3	28
Slices: Bologna, 2 oz (62g)	80	1	4
Pizza Pepperoni, 1.7 oz (48g)	70	0	4
Veggie Ham, 2 oz (62g)	80	0	6
Veggie Turkey, 2 oz (62g)	90	2	4
Veggie Entrees: Per 300g (10.5 oz) Tray			
Country Stew	170	0	24
Chili; Macaroni; Penne, average	230	2	38
Lasagne	300	3	51

Soybean Products

	C	F	Cb
Cheeses (Soy): See Page 40			
Miso, 1/2 cup, 5 oz	280	8	39
Cold Mountain: Red, 1 T., 0.5 oz	25	1	3
Mellow White, 1 Tbsp, 0.5 oz	35	0.5	6
Natto, 1/2 cup, 3 oz	190	10	13
Tempeh, 1 piece, 3 oz	170	6	14
Fried, 3 oz	250	14	14
SoyBoy, White Wave: See Page 67, 77			
Soybean Protein (TVP), 1 oz	90	0	7
Soy Beans: See Page 144			
Soy Drinks: See Page 25			

Tofu

	C	F	Cb
Azumaya Tofu:			
Soft (Silken), 3 oz	45	2	4
Firm, 3 oz	60	2.5	3
Extra Firm, 3 oz	75	3.5	10
Age (Tofu Puff), 1/2 oz	40	1.5	2
Nama-Age (Fried Tofu), 3 oz	130	5	8
Calco: Tasty Tofu, 3 oz	50	3	2
Hinoichu Tofu:			
Soft, 3 oz, 1" slice	45	2.5	5
Reg. (Japanese), 3 oz, 1" slice	60	3	6
Firm (Chinese), 3 oz, 1" slice	60	3	6
Extra Firm, 3 oz	90	5	10
Mori-Nu Tofu (Silken):			
Soft, 4 oz	60	3	3
Firm, 4 oz	70	3	3
Extra Firm, 4 oz	70	3	3
Nasoya Tofu: Soft, 3 oz	60	3	2
Silken, 3 oz	50	2	2
Firm, 3 oz	80	4	2
Extra Firm, 3 oz	90	5	1
Chinese 5 Spice Tofu, 3 oz	80	4	2
Pulmuone Tofu: Soft, 3 oz	45	2	5.5
Silken, 3 oz	45	2	5.5
Firm, 3 oz	55	2.5	6
SoyBoy: Firm Organic, 3 oz	100	5	2
X-Firm Organic, 3 oz	120	6	2
X-Firm LowFu, 3 oz	90	2	6
TofuLin, 2 oz	100	5	4
Baked, Seasoned, Smoked, 2 oz	100	5	3
Carribean Tofu, 2 oz	100	5	3
Tree of Life: Firm Raw, 3 oz	100	5	2
Reduced Fat, 3 oz	90	4	4
Tofu Stir Fried, 4 oz	120	8	3

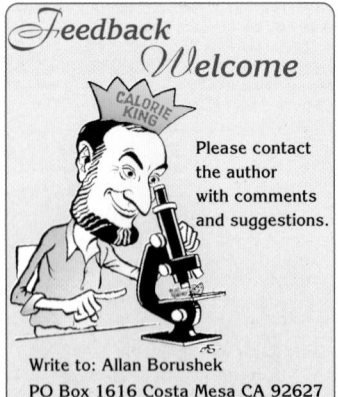

Feedback Welcome

CALORIE KING

Please contact the author with comments and suggestions.

Write to: Allan Borushek
PO Box 1616 Costa Mesa CA 92627
email: allan@calorieking.com

Soups

Homemade & Restaurant

Restaurant & Take-Out Per 8 fl.oz	C	F	Cb
Bean Medley	200	3	34
Beef Consomme	30	0	2
Borscht (w. Cream)	130	8	14
Bouillabaisse	400	15	10
Chicken & Corn	290	14	20
Chicken & Wild Rice	80	4	9
Chicken Consomme	50	0	2
Chicken Curry	180	8	18
Chicken Jambalaya	160	7	8
Chicken Noodle	80	2	12
w. Chicken	160	4	12
Chicken Soup	80	2	6
Chili with Beans	250	12	25
Clam Chowder	240	15	17
Corn & Crab	120	3	18
Corn Chowder	150	8	16
Cream of Broccoli	200	12	20
Cream of Potato	220	12	25
Cream of Mushroom	290	21	20
Creamy Pumpkin	210	10	26
Fish Chowder	220	15	6
French Onion	420	15	25
Gazpacho	60	0	13
Lentil Soup	250	9	28
Lobster Bisque	320	15	10
Matzo Ball (w.1 large ball)	180	7	24
Minestrone	140	2	14
Mulligatawny	300	15	8
Pea & Ham	240	10	25
Potato & Bacon	170	7	19
Shark Fin Soup	220	6	4
Spicy Shrimp Soup, 1 bowl	160	7	10
Split Pea Soup	150	6	18
Vegetable (Fat Free)	75	0	18
Vegetable Beef	80	2	10
Vichyssoise	200	9	15
Watercress	90	4	13

● Ethnic & Restaurant Section: Pages 169 - 174
● Fast Foods/Restaurant Section: Pages 175-250
(Arby's, Au Bon Pain, Boston Market, Dunkin' Donuts, Denny's, Schlotzsky's, Sizzler, Souplantation, Sweet Tomatoes)

Homemade Soups: Calculate calories, fat and carbohydrates from ingredients.

Bouillon Cubes & Powders

Bouillon Cubes: Average all types	C	F	Cb
Regular, 1 cube	8	0	1
Low Sodium (LiteLine)	12	0	1
Powders: Average, 1 tsp	8	0	1
Herb-Ox: Instant Broth & Seasoning, Beef, 1 envelope	10	0	2
Chicken; Vegetarian	10	0	2
Herbs, Spices: 1 tsp	5	0	1
Soup Oyster Crackers 40 small/20 large, 1/2 oz	60	2	8

Amy's

Per 1 Cup (1/2 Can)			
Black Bean Vegetable	110	1	22
Cream of Mushroom, 3/4 cup	120	9	10
Cream of Tomato, 1 cup	100	2	17
Lentil	130	4	19
No Chicken Noodle	90	3	12
Organic Vegetable Broth	35	0	8
Split Pea	100	0	19
Vegetable Barley	50	1	10

Bean Cuisine

Made as Directed: Per 1 Cup Serving			
13 Bean Bouillabaisse	240	0	18
Florentine/Country Bean; Barcelona	210	1.5	29
Basque Beans; Italian Market Bean	195	1.5	30

Betty Crocker

Bowl Appetit!: Per 2.7 oz Serving			
3-Cheese Rotini	370	12	52
Cheddar Broccoli Rice	300	8	52
Herb Chicken Veg. Rice	260	4	50
Homestyle Chkn Flavor & Pasta	260	6	42
Pasta Alfredo	360	11	51
Tomato Parmesan Penne	350	8	57

Birds Eye

Hearty Spoonfuls Soup Bowls (Frozen)			
Cheesy Cream of Broccoli	230	10	25
Chicken Noodle	140	1.5	19
Chicken, Rice & Vegetables	160	2	26
Italian Minestrone	240	4	37

Soups (Cont)

Campbell's C F Cb

Red & White Label
Per 1 Cup Prepared (from 1/2 Cup Condensed)

	C	F	Cb
Bean & Bacon	180	5	25
Beef Broth	15	0	1
Broccoli Cheese	110	7	9
Californian Veg.; Chicken Gumbo	60	1	10
Cheddar Cheese	130	8	11
Chicken Alphabet	80	2	11
Chicken Broth	30	2	1
Chicken Noodle/w. Stars	70	2	9
Chicken Vegetable	80	2	12
Chicken w. White & Wild Rice	60	1.5	10
Clam Chowder Manhattan	60	0.5	12
Clam Chowder New England	100	2.5	13
Cream of Asparagus; Celery	110	7	9
Cream of Broccoli; Shrimp	100	6	9
Cream of Mushroom	110	7	9
Cream of Mushroom w. Rstd Garlic	70	2.5	10
Cream of Potato	90	3	14
Curly Noodle	80	2	12
Double Noodle in Chicken Broth	100	2.5	15
French Onion	70	2.5	10
Golden Mushroom	80	3	10
Goldfish Pasta Chicken	70	2.5	8
Goldfish Pasta Tomato	110	5	25
Mega Noodle	70	1.5	10
Minestrone	100	2	16
Split Pea w. Ham; Green Pea	180	3.5	28
Tomato	80	0	18
Tomato Bisque	130	3	24
Tomato Noodle	120	1	25
Tomato Rice (Old Fashioned)	120	2	23
Vegetable	90	1	16
Vegetable & Beef; Turkey Noodle	80	2	10

Simply Home: Per 1 Cup Serving

	C	F	Cb
Chicken & Pasta; Chicken Noodle	90	1	14
Chicken w. Rice	100	1	19
Country Vegetable	110	0.5	23
Minestrone	140	1	27

Soup At Hand: Per 10 3/4 oz Ctn

	C	F	Cb
Blended Vege. Medley	110	2	21
Classic Tomato	120	0	26
Cream of Broccoli	160	9	17
Creamy Chicken	170	9	17

Soup & Recipe Mixes (Dry): Per 1 Tbsp

	C	F	Cb
Chicken Noodle/w. Broth	30	0.5	5
Onion	20	0	5

Campbell's (Cont) C F Cb

Chunky (Red Can):
19 oz Can: Per 1/2 Can Serving

	C	F	Cb
Baked Potato w. Cheddar, Bacon	180	8	23
Beef Rib Rst. w. Potato	110	1	17
Beef w. White & Wild Rice	140	1.5	23
Cheese Tortellini	110	2	18
Chicken & Dumplings	190	10	16
Chicken Broccoli Cheese	200	12	14
Chicken Corn Chowder	250	15	18
Classic Chicken Noodle	130	3	16
Grilled Chicken Veg. & Pasta	110	2	17
Grilled Sirloin Steak & Vegies	120	2	20
Hearty Bean & Ham	180	3	30
Hearty Chicken & Vegetable	90	2	12
Herb Rst. Chicken w. Pots. Garlic	110	2	17
Honey Rst. Ham w. Potatoes	130	2	20
New England Clam Chowder	300	18	26
Pepper Steak	140	3	17
Potato Ham Chowder	220	14	16
Salisbury Steak w. Mushr. Onion	150	4.5	18
Savory Chicken & Rice	140	3	18
Sirloin Burger	180	7	20
Slow Rst. Beef w. Mushrooms	110	2	17
Split Pea & Ham	180	3.5	27
Steak & Potato	130	2	18
Vegetable	160	4	15

10 1/2 oz Can: All flavors, 1 cup

	C	F	Cb
	120	3	20

Select: Per 1 Cup (approx. 1/2 Can)

	C	F	Cb
Beef w. Roasted Barley	130	1.5	21
Beef w. Portabello Mushrooms	120	3	14
Chicken & Pasta w. Garlic	110	2	17
Chicken Rice/Vegetables	100	1.5	18
Chicken w. Long Grain Rice	110	0.5	19
Creamy Potato w. Garlic	180	9	21
Fiesta Vegetable	120	0.5	24
Grilled Chicken w. Tomato & Veg.	100	1.5	17
Honey Rst Chkn w. Golden Potato	110	1	17
Herbed Chick. w. Rst. Veges	90	0.5	14
Italian Style Wedding	120	2.5	16
Minestrone	120	2.5	21
New England Clam Chowder	190	13	14
Fat Free	110	3	17
Roast Chicken w. Rotini & Penne	110	2	17
Rosemary Chicken w. Rst. Veg.	110	0.5	18
Tomato Garden	100	0.5	22
Vegetable	110	1	21
Vegetable Beef	120	3	15

Cup-A-Ramen

	C	F	Cb
Beef; Cajun Chicken, 1 cup	310	16	36
Chicken ; Shrimp, 1 cup	320	17	36

Dr McDougall's

Per Container Cup (Mix)

Minestrone & Pasta	180	1	31
Ramen Noodles, all flavours	150	0.5	29
Split Pea w. Barley	200	2	36
Tamale Pie w. Baked Chips	200	1.5	39
Tortilla Soup w. Baked Chips	190	1.5	37

Fantastic Cup Soups

Per Container Cup (Mix): Split Pea 190

		1	35
Cha Cha Chili	250	2	44
Corn & Potato Chowder	170	2	34
Creamy Soups: Average	150	2.5	27
Jumpin' Black Bean	210	1	39
Vegetable Barley	150	0.5	29

Big Soup Noodle Bowls: Per 1 Cup, 1/2 Pkg

Hot & Sour	140	2.5	25
Miso w. Tofu	110	1	21
Sesame Miso	100	1	19

Goodman's

Soup Mixes (Prepared): Per 1 Cup

Alphabet Vegetable	45	0	9
Noodle Soup	45	0.5	9
Onion Soup	30	1	5

Hain

Canned: Per 1 Cup

All Natural: Black Bean	90	0	18
Chicken Broth	25	2	1
Chicken Noodle	150	3	24
Mushroom Barley	130	1.5	26
Vegetable Broth	25	0	6
Wild Rice	80	1.5	15

Enjoy nutritious soup as part of a meal or as a snack. Soup is an excellent filler - especially to beat the 4.30pm snack syndrome. Choose low fat varieties.

Health Valley

	C	F	Cb
Per 1 Cup			
Bean Vegetable, 1 cup	140	0	32
Beef Broth	20	0	0
Carotene varieties, average, 1 cup	70	0	17
Chicken Broth, 1 cup	45	1.5	0
Chicken Noodle/Rice	130	2	20
Country Corn & Vege; Super Brocc.	70	0	17
Garden/Tomato Vegetable	80	0	17
Italian Minestrone	90	0	21
Lentil & Carrots	90	0	25
Mushroom Broth	10	0	2
Real Minestrone; Italian Plus	80	0	20
Rotini & Vegetables	100	0	20
Split Pea & Carrots	110	0	17
Pasta Soups: Pasta Fagioli, 1 cup	120	0	25
Other varieties, 1 cup	110	0	23
Organic: Black Bean; Split Pea	110	0	25
Mushroom Barley; Potato Leek	60	0	15
Lentil; Tomato; Minestrone, 1 c.	90	0	20
Vegetable, 1 cup	80	0	18
Dry Soups: 1/3 cup, average	120	0	24

Healthy Choice

Per 1 Cup

Bean & Pasta	100	1.5	18
Chicken & Dumplings	140	3	19
Chicken & Roast Garlic	130	2	21
Chicken Corn Chowder	150	2.5	29
Chicken Noodle	120	2.5	18
Chicken w. Rice	100	2	16
Classic Italian Bean & Pasta	100	1.5	17
Creamy Tomato	100	1.5	21
Garden Vegetable	120	0.5	27
New England Clam Chowder	120	1	22
Old Fashioned Chick. Noodle	120	0.5	27
Roasted Italian Style Chicken	130	2	17
Split Pea & Ham	170	2	28
Vegetable Clam	80	0.5	17
Zesty Gumbo	100	2	15

Hormel

Microwave Cup Hearty Soup: 1 Cup, 7 1/2 oz

Chicken w. Vegetable & Rice	110	2	17
Beef Vegetable	90	1	15
Beef & Ham	190	4	29
Chicken Noodle	110	2.5	13

Soups (Cont)

Imagine	C	F	Cb
Per Cup			
Organic Creamy: Broccoli	70	1.5	10
Butternut Squash	120	2	23
Portobello Mushroom	80	3	10
Potato Leek	90	2.5	14
Sweet Corn	100	3	15
Tomato	90	1.5	17
Vegetable Broth	30	0.5	5
Free Range Chicken Broth	20	0.5	2

Juanita's			
Per Cup			
Menudo Blanco/mas Picoso	170	7	12
Menudo Sin Maíz	170	9	1
Pozole	170	5	22

Knorr's Soup			
Taste Breaks: Per 1.6 oz Cup			
Beef Vegetable	150	2	27
Chicken Noodle/Vegetable	120	2	21
Corn Chowder	140	3	26
Hearty Lentil	200	1	38
Navy Bean	130	0.5	25
Potato Leek	130	2.5	22
Red Bean Chili	170	1	32
Split Pea	150	0.5	29
Tomato Penne	170	2	34
Noodle Cups: Per 2.1 oz Cup			
Fettucine Alfredo	230	4	41
3-Cheese Macaroni	230	3.5	41

Lipton			
Cup-a-Soup: Per Envelope			
Broccoli & Cheese	70	3	9
Cream of Chicken	70	2	12
Creamy Chicken Vegetable	80	4.5	10
Chicken Noodle	50	1	8
Recipe Secrets Mixes:			
Per Serving			
Beefy Onion	25	0.5	5
Chicken Noodle	80	2	11
Onion	20	0	4
Onion Mushroom	30	0.5	5
Savory Herb w. Garlic; Vegetable	30	0	7

Manischewitz	C	F	Cb
Condensed:			
Per 1/3 Cup (Unprepared): Chicken	15	0.5	2
Chicken w. 3 Matzo Balls	80	4	9
Four Bean	70	1	13
Lentil	140	2	24
Minestrone	90	1.5	16
Per 8 fl.oz Serving (Prepared)			
Borscht w. Beets	90	0	21
Borscht Low Calorie	25	0	6
Instant Cup (Mrs Manischewitz): Per Cup			
Black Bean	200	1	37
Chicken Noodle	140	2	26
Chicken Rice	130	1	28
Hearty Lentil	140	1	26
Minestrone	210	1.5	39
Potato Leek	100	1	39
Now Ready-To-Serve:			
Chkn Penne, 1 cup	100	1.5	14
Zesty Chicken Noodle, 1 cup	100	1.5	16

Miso Cup			
Original, 1 cup	30	1	3
Golden Seaweed, 1 cup	30	1	3
Organic: Traditional, 1 pkg	35	1	4
Reduced Sodium, 1 pkg	25	1	3

Nile Spice			
Per Cup			
Black Bean	170	1.5	36
Cheddar Broccoli	130	3	20
Chicken Flavored Vegetable	110	1.5	21
Country Mushroom	140	2.5	26
Lentil	180	1.5	31
Minestrone	140	1	30
Red Beans & Rice	170	1	36
Split Pea	200	1	35
Couscous: Parmesan	200	3	34
Other varieties, average	190	2	36

Pacific Foods			
Heat & Serve: Per Cup (8 fl.oz)			
All Natural Chicken Broth	15	0	2
French Onion	35	0	6
Organic Vegetable Broth	0	0	0
Creamy: 3-Potato	120	3	19
Corn Chowder	130	3	19
Tomato	100	2	16

Soups (Cont)

Progresso — C F Cb

Per 1 Cup Serving

	C	F	Cb
Beef Barley	130	4	13
Chickarina	130	5	12
Chicken with Wild Rice	100	1.5	15
Chicken Barley	110	1.5	16
Chicken Broth	20	1.5	1
Chicken Noodle	90	2	9
Chicken Rice w. Vegetable	90	2	13
Creamy Mushroom	180	14	12
Escarole in Chicken Broth	25	1	3
French Onion	50	1.5	9
Green Split Pea	170	3	25
Grilled Chicken Italiano	110	2.5	14
Grilled Steak w. Veg. Penne	120	3.5	13
Hearty Black Bean	170	1.5	30
Hearty Chicken & Rotini	90	1.5	12
Hearty Penne in Chicken Broth	80	1	14
Home Style Chicken w. Veges	90	1.5	11
Lentil	140	2	22
Macaroni & Bean	160	4	23
Manhattan Clam Chowder	110	2	11
Minestrone	120	2	21
New England Clam Chowder	190	10	21
Potato w.Broccoli & Cheese	160	6	21
Roasted Chicken Garden Herb	70	1.5	9
Roasted Chicken Italiano	80	1.5	10
Southwestern Style Corn Chowder	200	7	29
Split Pea w. Ham	150	4	20
Steak & Baked Potato	130	2.5	18
Steak & Mushrooms/Vegetables	100	2	12
Tomato; Tomato Basil	100	2	19
Tomato Vegetable Italiano	90	2	15
Tomato Rotini	140	5	30
Tortellini in Chicken Broth	70	2	10
Turkey Noodle	90	1.5	11
Turkey Rice w. Vegetable	110	1	18
Vegetable	90	1	17

99% Fat Free: Per 1 Cup Serving

	C	F	Cb
Beef Barley	130	2	20
Chicken Noodle	90	1.5	13
Lentil; Minestrone	130	1.5	20
New England Clam Chowder	110	1.5	18
White Cheddar Potato	100	1.5	20

Pritikin — C F Cb

Per Cup

	C	F	Cb
Black Bean w. Rice	200	1	37
Chicken Flavored Vegetable	160	1	27
Chicken Pasta	80	0	15
Fat Free Chicken Broth	10	0	0.5
Hearty Vegetable	90	0.5	16
Minestrone	130	0.5	25
Potato Broccoli	110	0	22
Split Pea	180	0.5	32
Vegetarian Vegetable	100	0	21

Puck

Canned: Per 1 Cup

	C	F	Cb
Chicken & Egg Noodles	150	5	16
Chicken & Vegetables	140	5	17
Chicken Parmesan	200	12	15
Chicken Pot Pie	220	13	16
Chicken w. Broccoli	180	10	14
Chick. w Rst. Pots & Garlic	180	8	16
Chicken w. Sweetcorn	200	10	20
Country Tomato w. Basil	140	6	20
Creamy Chicken	210	12	15
Hearty Lentil & Vegetable	180	2.5	31
Hearty Vegetable Beef	140	6	13
Hearty Winter Vegetable	140	6	21
New England Clam Chowder	240	13	18
Old Fashioned Beef Barley	140	5	16
Old World Minestrone	180	7	24
Roast Chicken w. Wild Rice	150	5	18
Spicy 7 Bean w. Italian Sausage	230	11	27
Steak & Potato	150	6	17
Thick Country Vegetable	170	7	23
Turkey & Noodle	140	6	11

Ralph's

	C	F	Cb
Chicken Broth, 1 cup	30	1	3
Fat Free/Reduced Salt, 1 cup	20	0	2

Rokeach

15 oz Can (Ready to Serve): Per Serving

	C	F	Cb
Barley & Mushroom	110	1	23
Chicken Consomme	50	4	0
Cream of Mushroom	120	7	13
Minestrone	170	1	32
Potato	100	1	20
Seven Bean	130	1	24
Split Pea & Egg Barley	190	1.5	35
Vegetable	110	1.5	22

83

Soups (Cont)

San-J	C	F	Cb
Mild Miso, 1 container	45	1.5	5
Dark Miso, 1 container	40	1.5	3

Shari Ann's	C	F	Cb
Per Cup			
Chicken Broth	20	1.5	1
Chicken Rice	90	2.5	12
Chicken Vegetable	90	2.5	15
Cream of Tomato	80	0	17
Great Plains Split Pea	150	0	26
Indian Black Bean & Rice	150	1	30
Italian White Bean	170	1	32
Organic Minestrone	120	2.5	20
Potato & Cheddar	100	2.5	15
Spicy French Green Lentil	130	0	22
Spicy Mexican Bean	210	1	38
Tomato & Roasted Garlic	50	0	12
Vegetable Broth	15	1	1
Vegetarian French Onion	60	0	9

Shelton's	C	F	Cb
Per Cup			
Canned: Chicken Broth	35	2.5	0
Black Bean & Chicken	170	4	22
Chicken Noodle	120	3	17
Chicken Tortilla	110	1.5	16
Vegetable Chicken	150	2	28
Ready-To-Eat: Chkn Noodle	120	3	14
Chicken Consomme	35	0	7
Mushroom Barley	110	2	17

Streit's	C	F	Cb
Cupa Soup: Per Serving			
Chicken Noodle; Mushr. & Barley	70	0.5	11
Garden Vegetable	70	0.5	13
Mild Chili; Split Pea	60	0	14
Tomato Couscous	80	0.5	18

Swanson	C	F	Cb
Per Cup			
Canned: Beef Broth	20	1	1
Chicken Broth	30	2	1
100% Fat Free	15	0	1
Vegetable Broth	20	1	3

Tabatchnick	C	F	Cb
Frozen: Per Serving (1 bag, 7 1/2 oz)			
Barley Mushroom	70	0	13
Cream of Spinach	90	4	11
Old Fashioned Potato	70	0	16
Pea	180	2	31
Vegetable	110	1	20
Yankee Bean	160	2	27

Uncle Ben's	C	F	Cb
Hearty Soup Mix: Per Serving (1/3 pkg)			
Black/Bean & Rice	150	1.5	28
Broccoli Cheese & Rice	110	2	19
Southwest Vegetable	90	1	19
White Bean & Pasta	100	1.5	18

Walnut Acres	C	F	Cb
Per Cup (250g)			
Autumn Harvest	100	2	19
Classic Minestrone	100	0	22
Country Corn Chowder	150	3	28
Cuban Black Bean	150	1	30
Four Bean Chili	140	1.5	28
Ginger Carrot	100	1	22
Mediterranean Lentil	130	0	26
Savory Tomato	120	2	23

Weight Watchers	C	F	Cb
Chicken Noodle, 10 1/2 oz	150	2	25
Chicken & Rice, 10 1/2 oz	110	1.5	17
Minestrone, 10 1/2 oz	130	2	23
Vegetable, 10 1/2 oz	130	1	27
Instant Beef/Chicken Broth, 1 pkg	10	0	2

Westbrae	C	F	Cb
Canned: Per Cup (240g)			
Alabama Black Bean Gumbo	140	0	26
Great Plains Savory Bean	120	0	23
Hearty Milano Minestrone	120	0	24
Louisiana Bean Stew	130	0	25
Mediterranean Lentil	140	0	24
New York Unchicken Noodle	60	1	10
Old World Split Pea	150	0	28
Santa Fe Vegetable	160	0	31
Spicy Southwest Vegetable	130	0	25

Herbs & Spices •Condiments

Herbs & Spices

Per 1 Teaspoon: Average all types	C	F	Cb
Average all types	5	0	1
Allspice, ground	5	0	1
Chili Powder	8	0	1
Cinnamon, ground	6	0	1
Curry Powder	6	0	1
Garlic Powder	9	0	2
Nutmeg, ground	12	0	1
Onion Powder	7	0	2
Parsley, dried	4	0	1
Pepper, black/red/white, aver.	6	0	1
Saffron	2	0	0
Tumeric, ground	8	0	1
Seeds: Fenugreek	12	1	2
Mustard, Poppyseed	15	1	1
Other types, average	7	0	1
Parsley Patch, Sesame, 1 tsp	16	1	1
Salt-free blends, average	10	0	2
All-purpose, 1 tsp	6	0	1

Seasonings & Flavorings

	C	F	Cb
Accent Flavor Enhancer, 1 tsp	10	0	0
Angostura Bitters, 1 tsp	12	0	3
Bacon Bits, average, 1 Tbsp	30	1	2
Bacon Chips (*Durkee*), 1 Tbsp	45	1	2
Best O'Butter, 1 tsp	10	<1	1
Bragg Liquid Aminos, 1 tsp	5	0	0
Butter Buds, 1 tsp	8	<1	2
Garlic Bread Sprinkle, 1 tsp	8	<1	1
Garlic Salt, 1 tsp	2	0	0
Italian Seasoning, 1 tsp	4	0	1
Lemon Pepper Season., 1 tsp	7	0	1
Meat Tenderizer, aver., 1 tsp	7	0	1
Molly McButter, 1 tsp	5	1	1
Mrs Dash Blends, 1 tsp	0	0	2
Perc Salt-free Seasoning, 1 tsp	8	0	2
Salad Sprinkles (*Lawry's*), 1 tsp	16	<1	2
Salad Supreme (*McCormick*), 1 tsp	10	<1	2
Salt: Regular, Sea Salt, Lite Salt	0	0	0
Seasoning Mixes, aver., 1/4 pkg	70	1	9
Taco Seasoning, 1/4 pkg	30	<1	4
Old El Paso: Chili Season. Mix, 1 T.	15	0.5	3
Cheesy Taco Season. Mix, 1 Tbsp	15	0.5	3
Taco/Burrito Seasoning Mix, 2 tsp	15	0	4
Enchilada Seasoning Mix, 2 tsp	10	0	2
Fajita Seasoning Mix, 1 tsp	10	0	3
Vegit Seasoning Mix, 1 tsp	5	0	1

Condiments, Sauces

Average of Brands & Homemade

	C	F	Cb
Apple Sauce: (Also see Page 143)			
Sweetened, 1/4 cup, 2 1/4 oz	45	0	11
Unsweetened, 1/4 cup, 2 oz	27	0	12
Bac O's (*Betty Crocker*), 1 tsp, 1/2 oz	60	3	4
Barbecue: Average, 1 Tbsp	25	0	6
Bearnaise Sce, 1/4 cup, 2 1/2 oz	190	19	5
Catsup (Ketchup): Reg., 1 Tbsp	15	0	4
Cheese, h/made, 1/4 cup, 2 1/2 oz	150	10	12
Chili Sauce: *Heinz,* 1 Tbsp	15	0	4
Del Monte, 1 Tbsp	20	0	5
Wolf Hot Dog, 1 Tbsp	15	1	2
Cocktail Sce: 1/4 cup	110	0	15
Cranberry, all types, 1/4 c., 2 1/2 oz	110	0	27
Escoffier Sauces, 1 Tbsp	20	0	4
Honey Mustard (*French's*): 1 tsp	5	0	1
Horseradish: 1 tsp	2	0	0
Sauce: *Sauceworks,* 1 tsp	20	2	0
Ketchup: Regular, 1 Tbsp	16	0	4
Heinz Lite, 1 Tbsp	8	0	2
Heinz Kick'rs, 1 Tbsp	20	0	4
Mushroom Sauce, 1/2 cup, 2 oz	50	2	5
Mustard, average, 1 tsp	0	0	0
Pesto, 1/4 cup, 2 oz	35	3	2
Pizza Sauce, cnd., 1/4 cup, 2 oz	25	0	5
Seafood Cocktail Sce, 1/4 cup	60	0	14
Soy Sauce, all types, av., 1 Tbsp	10	0	1
Sour Cream Sce, 1/2 cup	250	15	22
Spaghetti Sce: Average, 4 1/2 oz	135	6	19
Steak Sauce: *Heinz/A.1.,* 1 Tbsp	15	0	3
Lea & Perrins, 1 Tbsp	25	0	6
Str'berry Puree Sce: Unsweet., 2 T.	9	0	2
Sweet & Sour Sauce:			
Contadina, 2 Tbsp	40	1	8
Kikkoman Lite Soy, 2 Tbsp	10	0	1
La Choy, 2 Tbsp, 34g	60	0	14
Tabasco Sauce, 1 Tbsp	2	0	0
Taco Sauce: average, 2 Tbsp	10	0	2
Tartar Sauce: *Heinz,* 2 Tbsp, 30g	140	14	4
America's Choice, 2 Tbsp, 27g	160	17	1
Hellman's: Regular, 2 Tbsp, 30g	80	7	3
Lowfat, 2 Tbsp, 30g	40	1.5	4
Teriyaki Sauce: *Kikkoman,* 1 Tbsp	15	0	2
Vinegar: White or wine, 1 fl.oz.	4	0	1
White Sauce, 1/2 cup, 5 oz	130	7	12
Worcestershire Sauce, 1 Tbsp	5	0	1

Pickles • Gravy

Pickles & Relish

Average All Brands

	C	F	Cb
Bread & Butter Pickles, 4 sl.,1 oz	20	0	5
Chutney, 2 Tbsp, 1¼ oz	40	0	12
Dill Pickle:			
Slices, 4 slices, 1 oz	3	0	0.5
1 large, (3¾" x 1¼" diam.), 2¼ oz	12	0	3
Extra lrg (4" x 1¾" diam.), 5 oz	30	0	6
Halves: Small, 1 oz	3	0	0.5
Large, 2½ oz	8	0	2
Sweet, small, ½ oz	22	0	6
Gherkins, sweet, 1 med., 1 oz	15	0	7
Green Chilies, chopped, 2 Tbsp	5	0	1
Horseradish, 1 Tbsp	10	0	2
Jalapenos, pickled, 2 whole	5	0	1
Jalapeno Relish, 1 Tbsp, ½ oz	5	0	1
Mustard, aver. all brands, 1 tsp	5	0	0.5
Peppers: Hot/Mild, 1 oz	8	0	2
Pickled: Beets, ½ cup, 4 oz	75	0	19
Onions, 1 medium, ¾ oz	10	0	2
Cocktail Onion, 1 onion	2	0	0
Red Cabbage, ½ cup, 3 oz	60	0	13
Pickles:			
Sweet, 2 Tbsp, 1 oz	35	0	0
Large (3" x 3/4 diam.), 1¼ oz	40	0	10
Pickle in a Pouch, 1 large	12	0	3
Relishes: Sandwich Spread, 1 tsp	20	1	5
Cranberry-Orange, 1 Tbsp	30	0	7
Hot Dog (*Heinz*), 1 Tbsp	17	0	28
Sweet Pickle, 1 Tbsp	20	0	5
Sauerkraut, ½ cup, 3½ oz	25	0	5
Sweet Cauliflower	35	0	8

Salsa

Average all types:

	C	F	Cb
Regular, no oil, 2 Tbsp	15	0	3.5
w. Oil, homemade, 2 Tbsp	40	3	8
Chef's Kitchen, 2 Tbsp	10	0	2
Del Monte, all flavors, 2 Tbsp	10	0	2
Kaukauma, 2 Tbsp	15	0	3
Wild Oats, 2 Tbsp, 1 oz	10	0	2

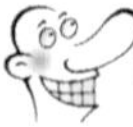

"Be sure to stay healthy, You can kill yourself later!"
(Yiddish Proverb)

Gravy

	C	F	Cb
Homemade Gravy:			
Thin, little fat, 2 Tbsp, 1 oz	20	1	3
Thick, 2 Tbsp, 1¼ oz	50	2	9
¼ cup, 2½ oz	100	4	18
Franco-American (Canned)			
Au Jus Gravy, ¼ cup, 2 oz	10	0	2
Beef/Mushrm; Turkey Gravy, 2 oz	25	1.5	3
Chicken Gravy, ¼ cup, 2 oz	40	3	3
Golden Pork Gravy, 2 oz	45	4	3
98% Fat Free, 2 oz	25	0	4
Franco-American (In Jars)			
99% Fat Free, ¼ cup, 2 oz	25	0.5	4
Pillsbury (Gravy Mixes)			
Brown; Homestyle, ¼ cup, 2 oz	15	0	3
Chicken, as prep., ¼ cup, 2 oz	20	0	4

Gravy-In-Jars-Homestyle

	C	F	Cb
Boston Market, all types, ¼ c., 2 oz	25	1	3
Heinz, reg., all types, ¼ c., 2 oz	25	1	3
Fat Free Rst. Turkey, ¼ c., 2 oz	10	0	2
Vons, all types, ¼ c., 2 oz	20	0.5	4

Tomato Products

	C	F	Cb
Whole/Chopped/Crushed/Diced			
1 cup, 8½ oz	50	0	10
In Aspic, ½ cup	50	0	12
w. Green Chili, 1 cup, 8½ oz	45	<1	11
Stewed, ½ cup	40	2.5	9
Wedges in Tom Juice, 1 cup	70	0.5	15
Salsa, average, 1 Tbsp	15	0	3.5
Tomato Ketchup:			
Regular, 1 Tbsp	16	0	4
Green (*Heinz*), 1 Tbsp	20	0	5
Tomato Paste, 2 Tbsp	25	0	5
Regular, 6 oz, ¾ cup	150	0	34
Tomato Puree, ½ cup	50	0	10
Tomato Sauce:			
Regular, ½ cup	40	0	9
Spanish Style, ½ cup	40	0	9
w. Mushrooms, ½ cup	40	0	9
w. Onions, ½ cup	50	0	11
Tomato Seasoning, 3 tsp	20	0	4
Sundried Tomatoes:			
Natural, 5-6 pces, 0.4 oz	22	0	5
In Oil, drained, 6 pces, ½ oz	60	4	5

Brands	C	F	Cb
Amy's: Per 1/2 Cup			
Family Marinara	50	1	8
Garlic Mushroom	120	7	10
Puttanesca	45	2	6
Tomato Basil	80	3	11
Barilla: Per 1/2 Cup			
Marinara; Sweet Peppers & Garlic	90	3	11
Roasted Garlic & Onion	90	3.5	11
Tomato & Basil	80	2.5	12
Bertoli/Five Brothers: Per 1/2 Cup			
Alfredo w. Mushrooms	160	12	6
Creamy Alfredo	220	20	6
Grilled Summer Vegetable	80	5	12
Imported Romano & Garlic	90	4	10
Marinara w. Burgundy Wine	80	3	13
Mushroom & Garlic	90	3	13
Olive Oil & Garlic	90	4	9
Olive w. Sundried Tomato	100	4	13
Oven Roasted Garlic & Onion	70	1.5	10
Roasted Red Pepper	80	3	13
Tomato Basil	80	2	10
Bookbinders: Per 1/2 Cup			
White Clam Sauce	300	30	4
Bullseye: BBQ, 1 Tbsp	25	0	6
Classico: Per 1/2 Cup			
Alfredo	220	20	6
Italian Sausage w. Pepper & Onions	70	3	80
Mushroom & Olive	50	1	10
Portobello Mushroom	60	1	11
Roasted Garlic Alfredo	220	20	6
Roasted Peppers & Onions/Garlic	60	2	9
Spicy Red Pepper	60	2.5	6
Spicy Tomato & Pesto	90	5	8
Sun Dried Tomato; 4 Cheese	80	4	8
Sun Dried Tomato Alfredo	220	18	8
Sweet Basil Marinara	70	2	11
Tomato & Basil	50	1	9

Brands (Cont)	C	F	Cb
Contadina			
Pasta Sauces: Per 1/2 Cup			
Alfredo Sauce	360	32	10
Lite	160	10	10
Garden Vegetable Sauce	40	0	9
Marinara Sauce	80	4	9
Mushroom Alfredo	200	14	12
Mushroom Marinara Sauce	70	2.5	11
Pesto w. Basil, Red. Fat	460	26	22
Pesto w. Sundried Tomato	380	30	20
Roasted Garlic Marinara	60	2	10
Pizza Squeeze Sce, 1/4 cup	35	1.5	6
Del Monte			
Pasta Sauces: Per 1/2 Cup			
Chunky Sce, average all varieties	60	1.5	11
D'Italia Pasta: Four Cheese	60	2	8
Other varieties	50	1.5	8
Spaghetti Sauce: Traditional	60	0.5	15
Garlic & Onion	60	1.5	11
w. Mushroom/Meat	70	1.5	14
Sloppy Joe Sauce, 1/4 cup, 67g	50	0	11
Dominick's: Per 1/2 Cup			
All Natural: Garl. & Onion; Marinara	80	4	10
Mushr. & Olive; Tomato & Basil	80	1	8
Italian Classics: Four Cheese	80	2.5	12
Portabella Mushroom	60	2	9
Puttanesca	70	3	8
Spicy Roasted Garlic	70	2	10
Sun Ripened Tomatoes	80	4	8
Tomato Basil	50	1	8
Estee			
Barbecue Sauce, 1 Tbsp	18	<1	3
Spaghetti Sauce, 1/4 cup, 4 oz	60	2	13
Steak Sauce, 1 Tbsp	14	<1	3
Enrico's			
Tomato Basil, 3.5 oz (100g)	65	2	10
Traditional Italian Style, 3.5 oz	55	0.5	11
Mushroom Onion, 1/2 cup (125g)	70	1	12
Other varieties, 1/2 cup (125g)	70	2	12
Emiril's: Per 1/2 Cup (123g)			
Puttanesca	80	5	9
Roasted Red Pepper	60	3	7
Vodka Sauce	130	8	13

Sauces ~ Pasta, Cooking

	C	F	Cb
Frank Sinatra: Per 1/4 Cup			
Alfredo; Pesto	160	14	4
French's Grill & Glaze			
Honey Mustard, 2 Tbsp	90	1	18
Teriyaki, 2 Tbsp	60	0	13
Garden Valley: Per 1/2 Cup			
Chunky Vege. Primavera	35	0.5	12
Four Cheese	35	1	8
Millina's Finest; Roasted Garlic	50	0	12
Sundried Tomato; Tomato Mushr.	50	0	11
Sweet Tomato Basil	60	0	13
Green Giant			
Sloppy Joe S'wich Sce, 1/4 c., 2.5 oz	50	0	11
Sloppy Joe Sauce & Meat	200	11	11
Hagerty Foods: Per 4 oz			
Artichoke	100	6	11
Asparagus Garlic	95	7	9
Healthy Choice: Per 1/2 Cup			
Four Cheese Creamy Alfredo	45	3	3
Garlic Lovers	45	0	10
Marinara w. Burgundy Wine	50	0.5	11
Mushroom Alfredo	45	3	3
Roasted Garlic & Romano	60	1	11
Sundried Tomato & Herb	60	0.5	12
Traditional Pasta Sauce	50	0	11
Super Chunky: Vege Primavera	45	0	9
Tomato, Mushroom Garlic	45	0	10
Heinz: Per 1 Tbsp (Approx. 1/2 oz)			
Barbecue Sauces, all flavors	35	0	9
Chili Sauce, 1 Tbsp	15	0	4
Horseradish Sauce	70	7	13
Mustard: Pourable/Mild, 1 Tbsp	8	<1	1
Spicy Brown	13	1	6
Seafood Cocktail Sauce	20	0	10
Steak Sauce 57	15	0	4
Tartar Sauce, 1 Tbsp	70	7	2
Tomato Ketchup	16	0	26
Worcestershire Sauce, 1 Tbsp	8	0	11
Sloppy Joe Sauce, 1/2 cup, 125g	70	0.5	14
Hunt's			
BBQ Sauce: Original, 36g, 2 Tbsp	50	0	13
Hickory & Brown Sugar, 38g, 2 T.	70	0	18
Manwich Sloppy Joe Sce, 1/4 c., 64g	30	0	6

	C	F	Cb
Hy Top: Per 1/2 Cup, 125g			
Spaghetti Sauce, all flavors	90	4	11
KC Masterpiece: Per 1 Tbsp			
Marinades: Garlic & Herb	30	1.5	4
Honey & Teriyaki	35	0.5	7
Original BBQ	40	1.5	7
Knorr (Sauce Mix)			
Made As Directed: Per 1/4 Cup, 2 oz			
Au Jus	8	0.2	1
Bearnaise	170	17	5
Classic Brown Gravy	25	1	3
Demi-Glace	30	1	4
Hollandaise	170	18	5
Hunter; Lyonnaise	25	0.3	4
Mushroom Sauce	60	3	5
Napoli Sauce	100	3	17
Pepper Sauce	20	1	3
Knudsen: Potato Toppings, 2 T	50	4.5	2
Kraft			
Sauceworks: Cocktail, 2 Tbsp	30	0.3	6
Horseradish, 1 tsp	20	1.5	0
Sweet 'n Sour, 1 Tbsp	30	0	7
Tartar: 1 Tbsp	50	5	2
Lemon & Herb, 1 Tbsp	75	8	0
Nonfat Tartar, 1 Tbsp	12	0	5
Barbecue Sauces: Average, 2 T.	50	0.5	9
Other Sauces: Mustard, 1 Tbsp	10	0	0
Horseradish: Reg./Cream Style, 1 T.	10	0	0
Sandwich Spread & Burger, 1 Tbsp	50	4	3
Sweet 'n Sour, 1 Tbsp	40	0.5	9
Las Palmas			
Red Chile Sauce, 1/4 cup, 2 oz	15	0.5	2
Enchilada Sauces: Green Chile	25	1.5	3
Hot/Original, 1/4 cup, 2 oz	15	0.5	3
Salsa: Mexicana. Mild, 2 Tbsp, 1 oz	5	0	1
Mexicana Hot/Medium, 2 Tbsp	10	0	2
Lawry's 30 Minute Marinade: Per 1 Tbsp			
Carriban Jerk; Teriyaki	25	0	6
Hawaiian; Dijon & Honey	20	0	3.5
Mediterranean; Lemon Pepper	10	0	2
Mesquite	5	0	1
Thai Ginger; Herb & Garlic	10	0	2
Libby's			
Sloppy Joe Sauce, 1/3 cup, 78g	45	0	10

Brands (Cont)

	C	F	Cb
McCormick Sauce Mixes			
Grillmates: Marinade, aver., 2 tsp	15	0	2
Sauce Blend Seasoning Mixes:			
Lemon Herb Chicken, 1 Tbsp	30	0	5
Chicken Fried Rice, 1 Tbsp	35	0	6
Stir Fry Chicken, 1 Tbsp	20	0	4
Chicken Teriyaki, 1¹/3 Tbsp	40	1	5
Mr Yoshida's			
Original Gourmet, 2 Tbsp, 30ml	90	0	20
Hawaiian Sweet & Sour, 2 Tbsp	35	0	9
Muir Glen: Per ¹/2 Cup (125g)			
Organic Pasta Sauce:			
Mushr. Marinara; Portobello Mushr.	50	0	11
Other varieties, average	50	1	11
Newman's Own: Per ¹/2 Cup			
Bombolina (Tomato & Basil)	100	5	15
Roasted Garlic & Peppers	70	2.5	11
Other flavors	60	2	9
Old El Paso			
Salsa: Thick 'n Chunky, 2 T., 1 oz	10	0	2
Homestyle; Green Chili; Verde			
2 Tbsp, 1 oz	10	0	2
Taco Sce, all varieties, 2 Tbsp, 1 oz	10	0	2
Enchilada Sce, all types, ¹/4 c., 2 oz	20	1	3
Grilling Sauces, all types, 2 Tbsp	60	0	14
Tom. & Gr. Chiles/Jalapenos,¹/4 c., 2 oz	10	0	2
Pace: Per 2Tbsp (1 oz)			
Piccente Sauce	10	0	2
Chunky Salsa, avg all types	10	0	2
Salsa Con Queso	45	3	4
Prego: Per ¹/2 Cup			
Extra Chunky: Garden Comb.	90	2	16
Garlic Supreme	120	3	23
Mushroom & Green Pepper	120	4.5	18
Mushroom Supreme	120	4.5	21
Pasta Bake: Per ¹/8 Jar			
Italian Sausage	90	3.5	12
3-Cheese Marinara	100	4.5	11
Hearty Meat Sauce	120	6	12
Tomato, Garlic & Basil	80	3.5	11
Mushroom w. Garlic & Onion	90	3	13

	C	F	Cb
Prego (Cont): Per ¹/2 Cup			
Regular: Diced Onion & Garlic	110	3	19
Flavored w. Meat	140	6	21
Fresh Mushroom; Traditional	150	5	23
Hamburger	120	4	17
Italian Sausage & Garlic	120	5	16
Mini Meatball	140	5	19
Mushroom & Garlic	110	2	20
Mushroom/Tomato Parmesan	120	3.5	19
Pepperoni	120	4.5	18
Roast Red Pepper/Herb & Garlic	110	3.5	17
Roast Garlic Parmesan	120	1.5	23
Savory Chicken	130	5	17
Three Cheese	100	2	18
Tomato, Onion & Garlic	110	3.5	19
Zesty Mushroom	120	4	20
Premier Japan(Organic)			
Garlic Tamari, 1 Tbsp	10	0	2
Ginger Tamari, 1 Tbsp	10	0	2
Thai Soynut, 1 Tbsp	25	2	2
Wasabi Tamari, 1 Tbsp	10	0	2
Ragu: Per ¹/2 Cup			
Meat Flavored Sauce	80	4	7
Traditional	70	3	8
Cheese Creations:			
Double Cheddar	200	18	6
Mushroom Green Pepper	110	3	16
Roasted Garlic Parmesan	240	22	6
Chunky Garden Style:			
Gard. Combo; Mushr. Gr. Pepper	100	3	16
Other varieties, average	110	3	18
Rich & Meaty: Classic Italian Style	150	10	9
Mama's Meat Sauce	130	8	8
Sausage, Peppers & Onions	160	11	9
Robusto!: Six Cheese	80	3	9
Italian Sausage & Cheese	100	4.5	11
Sauteed Onion & Mushr./Garlic	90	4	11
Tomato, Olive Oil, Garlic	90	4.5	9
Pizza Sauce: ¹/4 cup	30	1	4
Pizza Quick, average, ¹/4 cup	40	1.5	6
Rainforest Organic			
Ginger Curry, 1 Tbsp	15	1.5	1
Mango; Papaya Pepper, 1 Tbsp	5	0	1
Tamarind Spice, 1 Tbsp	5	0	1

Sauces ✦ Mayonnaise

Brands (Cont)

	C	F	Cb
Rinaldi: *Per 1/2 Cup*			
3-Cheese	90	2	15
Original; Meat/Mushroom	90	4	11
Tomato & Basil	80	2.5	11
Tomato, Garlic, Onion	80	2	
W: *Per 1 Tbsp*			
Mesquite Marinated Cooking	10	0	3
Teriyaki: Light; Marinade	25	0	5
Seeds of Change: *Per 1/2 Cup*			
Average all varieties	50	0.5	9
Sutter Home: *Per 1/2 Cup*			
Italian Style Pasta Sauce	80	2	12
Sicilian Style; Spicy Mediterranean	80	2	12
Marinara Pasta Sauce	70	2	11
Taj: *Per 1/2 Cup*			
Bombay Curry Simmer Sauce	90	5	10
Calcutta Masala Simmer Sauce	100	5	13
Kashmir Tandoori Marinade Sce	50	3	5
Seasoning Mixes: *Per 2 tsp*			
Meat Loaf; Sloppy Joe's	30	0	4
Beef Stew	15	0	3
Chili	40	1	6
Chicken/Taco Seasoning	25	0	4
Spaghetti Sauce: Italian Style, 1 T.	25	0	5
The Wizard's (Organic)			
Hot Nutz, 1 Tbsp	30	2	2
Hot Stuff, 1 Teaspoon	0	0	0
Vegetarian Worcestershire, 1 Tbsp	10	0	2
Troy's Sauces (Organic)			
Ginger Sauce, 1 Tbsp	5	0	1
Peanut Sauce, 1 Tbsp	30	2	1
Timpone's: *Per 1/2 Cup*			
Spaghetti Sauce: Classic	50	2.5	8
Family Recipe	80	3	7
Mom's	70	3.5	8
Tomaso's: *Per 1/2 Cup*			
Basil & Fresh Garlic; Spicy Eggplant	60	3	7
Black Olive Fresh Basil	40	2	5
Extra Garlic	55	2	8
Fresh Mushroom & Artichoke	50	2	7
Sugo Rosa	105	7.5	8

Brands (Cont)

	C	F	Cb
Tree of Life: *Per 1/2 Cup*			
Pasta Sauce Plus: All varieties	45	0	9
Organic: Classic Tomato	40	0	8
Average other varieties	30	0	7
Walnut Acres: *Per 1/2 Cup (125g)*			
Organic Pasta Sauce, average	50	1	9
Wild Oats: *Per 2 Tbsp, 1 oz*			
Wasabi; Seafood Marinade & Grill.	30	3	4
Korean Sesame Marinade & Grill.	30	0	8

Quick Guide

Mayonnaise

	C	F	Cb
Regular			
Average All Brands, 1 Tbsp	100	11	0
(Bestfoods, Kraft), 1 Tbsp	100	11	0
1/2 cup, 4 oz	800	88	0
Light/Reduced Fat			
Kraft; Best Foods, 1 Tbsp	50	5	1
1/2 cup, 4 oz	400	40	8
Hain, 1 Tbsp	60	6	2
Hellman's; Estee, 1 Tbsp	50	5	1
Smart Balance, 1 Tbsp	50	5	2
Smart Beat, 1 Tbsp	40	4	1
Weight Watchers, 1 Tbsp	25	2	1
Wild Oats, 1 Tbsp	35	3	1
Fat Free			
Kraft; Weight Watchers, 1 Tbsp	10	0	3
1/2 cup, 4 oz	80	0	16

Mayonnaise Type Dressing

	C	F	Cb
BAMA Dressing, 1 Tbsp, 0.5 oz	50	4	3
Gour Mayo (French's), 1 Tbsp, 0.5 oz	50	5	1
Miracle Whip Salad Dressing:			
Regular, 1 Tbsp, 0.5 oz	70	7	2
Light, 1 Tbsp, 0.5 oz	40	3	3
Free, 1 Tbsp, 0.5 oz	15	0	3
Nayonaise (Nasoya)			
(Tofu Base/Dairy Free/Eggless)			
Regular, 1 Tbsp, 0.5 oz	35	3	1
Fat-Free, 1 Tbsp, 0.5 oz	10	0	2

*It's only fattening
if you swallow it!*
(Virginia Graham)

Quick Guide **C F Cb**

Salad Dressings

Average All Brands
Per 2 Tbsp (Approx 1 fl.oz)

	C	F	Cb
Blue Cheese: Regular	150	16	2
Light/Reduced Fat	80	8	1
Caesar: Regular	140	14	2
Light/Reduced Fat	50	5	0.5
French: Regular	130	11	5
Light/Reduced Fat	50	3	4
Fat/Oil-Free	40	0	4
Italian: Regular	130	11	3
Light/Reduced Fat	70	7	2
Fat/Oil-Free	10	0	2
Ranch: Regular	180	18	3
Light/Reduced Fat	90	8	3
Fat-Free	50	0	2
Russian: Regular	130	10	3
Light/Reduced Fat	50	5	2
Fat-Free	30	0	3
Thousand Island: Regular	130	12	5
Light/Reduced Fat	50	4	3
Fat-Free	35	0	3

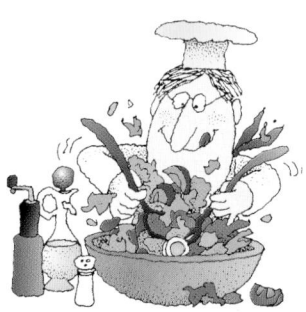

Enjoy a healthy salad
but don't drown it
in high-fat salad dressings.

Brands ~ Salad Dressings

Per 2 Tbsp (Approx 1 fl.oz)

	C	F	Cb
Annie's Naturals			
Caesar	120	11	1
Cowgirl Ranch	120	11	3
French	90	9	3
Gardenstyle (vinegar free)	120	12	3
Goddess	90	8	3
Organic: Buttermilk	70	7	1
Green Garlic	90	9	2
No Fat Yogurt	20	0	3
Red Wine & Olive Oil	160	17	1
Thousand Island	90	7	5
Tuscany Italian	80	7	5
Vinaigrette: Balsamic	100	10	3
Basil & Garlic	130	14	0.5
Black Olives & Truffle	110	12	1
Cilantro & Lime	100	10	2
Low Fat: Honey Mustard	45	2	6
Gingerly	40	2	4
Raspery	35	1.5	5
Roasted Red Pepper	70	6	3
Sea Veggie & Sesame	110	11	1
Shiitake & Sesame	120	13	1
Yellow Pepper & Tomato	70	7	2
Bernstein's			
Balsamic Italian	110	11	2
Cheese: Garlic Italian; Fantastico	110	11	2
Creamy Caesar	120	13	1
Fat Free Cheese & Garlic Italian	10	0	2
Italian	110	12	1
Olive Oil Vinaigrette	90	9	3
Red Wine & Garlic Italian	110	11	2
Restaurant Recipe Italian	130	13	1
Light Fantastic: Cheese Fantastico	25	1.5	3
Roasted Galic Balsamic	45	3.5	3
Bob's Famous			
Blue Cheese	140	15	1
Ranch Country	150	15	1
Roquefort	140	14	1
Tartar Sauce	170	16	2
Thousand Island	140	14	1
Brianna's			
Blush Vintage	100	6	12

Salad Dressings (Cont)

Per 2 Tbsp (Approx 1 fl.oz) | C | F | Cb

Cardini's

	C	F	Cb
Caesar, 2 Tbsp	160	17	1
Fat-Free Caesar	40	0	9
Light Caesar	80	7	5
Extra Virgin Olive Oil Italian	120	13	1
Honey Mustard	140	13	5
Kalamata Olive w. Romano Cheese	120	13	2
Lemon Herb	120	13	1
Parmesan Ranch	150	15	2
Poppyseed w. Shallots	160	14	8
Vintage White Wine	110	12	1
Zesty Garlic	120	13	2

Girards: *Per 2 Tbsp*

	C	F	Cb
Balsamic Basil	90	9	3
Caesar	150	16	1
Lite	80	7	2
Champagne	150	16	2
Lite Champagne	60	5	2
Greek Feta Vinaigrette	110	11	1
Honey Dijon Peppercorn	120	13	7
Olde Venice Italian	120	13	2
Oriental Chicken Salad	120	11	6
Original French	120	13	0
Raspberry	90	10	5
Romano Cheese	130	13	2
Shiitake Chardonnay	100	9	4
Spinach Salad	80	2	14
Fat Free: Caesar	40	0	9
Raspberry Vinaigrette	40	0	9

Good Seasons (Mix)
Prepared, 2 T. (Approx 1 oz)

	C	F	Cb
Blue Cheese, Cheese Garlic	145	16	2
Cheese Italian, Garlic & Herbs	145	16	2
Classic Dill, 1 pkg	28	0	5
Italian; Mild Italian; Zesty Italian	145	16	2
Italian Lite; Lite Cheese Italian	55	6	2
Ranch	115	12	2

Hidden Valley
Regular Range:

	C	F	Cb
Caesar w. Garlic	120	11	4
Cole Slaw	150	15	5
French w. Honey & Bacon	150	12	10
Original Ranch: w. Bacon	140	14	1
w. Garlic	130	13	2
w. Sundried Tomato	140	14	2

Per 2 Tbsp (Approx 1 fl.oz) | C | F | Cb

Hidden Valley (Cont)

	C	F	Cb
Light Range: B.L.T. Ranch	90	7	5
Original Ranch	80	7	3
Original Ranch w. Sour Cream	80	7	4
Fat Free:	30	0	6
French Honey & Bacon	50	0	11
Original Ranch	30	0	6

Knott's Berry Farm

	C	F	Cb
Honey Dijon, 2 Tbsp	130	13	4
Honey Poppyseed	120	9	10
Oriental Chicken Salad	130	11	5
Parmesan & Peppercorn	160	17	1
Roasted Garlic Caesar	140	14	3
Sun Dried Tomato	100	10	3
Low Fat: Raspberry	50	2	8
Tropical Fruit	45	1	9

Kraft
Regular Dressings: Per 2 Tbsp

	C	F	Cb
3 Cheese Ranch	170	18	1
Buttermilk Ranch	150	16	2
Caesar w. Bacon	150	15	1
Catalina	90	6	8
Classic Caesar	110	11	0.5
Coleslaw	150	12	8
Cucumber Ranch	140	15	2
Creamy Italian	110	11	3
French	120	12	4
Ranch w. Bacon	150	16	1
Roka Brand Blue Cheese	90	7	5
Thousand Island	110	10	5
Thousand Island w. Bacon	100	8	6
Zesty Italian	110	11	2
Kraft Free (Fat Free): Italian	10	0	2
Blue Cheese, Catalina, French	50	0	12
Caesar Italian	25	0	4
Classic Caesar; Ranch	50	0	11
Thousand Island; Sr Cream & Onion	45	0	11
Light Done Right!: Classic Caesar	70	6	3
Catalina	60	2	11
Ranch	70	4.5	7
Roka Blue Cheese	70	6	3
Thousand Island	70	4	7
3 Cheese Ranch	80	7	2
Special Collection: Caesar Italian	100	10	2
Balsamic Vinaigrette	90	8	4

Per 2 Tbsp (Approx 1 fl.oz)	C	F	Cb
Kraft(Cont)			
Classic Italian Vinaigrette	50	4	4
Sun Dried Tomato	60	5	4
Sweet Honey Catalina	130	11	8
Seven Seas: Viva Italian	90	9	2
Red Wine Vinaigrette	90	9	2
Litehouse: Caesar	140	14	1
Chunky Bleu Cheese	150	16	1
Coleslaw	90	7	7
Honey Mustard	130	14	3
Jalapeno Ranch	120	12	1
Lite Bleu Cheese	70	6	2
Ranch; Thousand Island	120	13	3
Maple Grove			
Fat Free: Caesar, 2 Tbsp	30	0	6
Honey Dijon	45	0	10
Marie's: 1000 Island	190	20	2
Blue Cheese	170	18	0
Caesar	150	13	8
Poppy Seed	190	20	2
Ranch (8 fl.oz ctn), 2 Tbsp	160	16	4
(15.5 fl.oz ctn), 2 Tbsp	170	19	1
Light: Blue Cheese	70	7	2
Ranch	70	7	2
Nasoya			
Vegi-Dressing *(Tofu Base/Dairy Free):*			
Thousand Island	60	4	6
Other flavors	60	5	3
(Nayonaise - See Mayonnaise)			
Newman's Own			
Balsamic Vinaigrette, 2 Tbsp	90	9	3
Caesar; Olive Oil & Vinegar	150	16	1
Creamy Caesar	170	18	1
Family Recipe Italian	120	13	1
Parmesan & Roasted Garlic	110	11	2
Parmesan Italiano	140	14	2
Ranch	180	18	2
Two Thousand Island	140	14	4
Pritikin: Honey Dijon	45	0	11
Dijon Balsamic; Zesty Italian	30	0	6
Honey French Style	40	0	10
Raspberry	35	0	11

Per 2 Tbsp (Approx 1 fl.oz)	C	F	Cb
San-J: Tamari Peanut	60	2	9
Tamari Sesame	45	2	5
Tamari Vinaigrette	45	3	4
Fat Free: Tamari Mustard	25	0	5
S & W			
Light: Italian	35	0	8
Red/White Wine; Raspberry Blush	40	0	10
Seeds of Change			
Balsamic/Greek Feta Vinaigrette	60	5	4
Italian Herb Vinaigrette	50	4	4
Spike Splashes!			
Original, 2 Tbsp	100	11	1
Salt Free	100	10	2
Fat Free	10	0	2
Spectrum			
Fat Free: Creamy Dill	25	0	4
Creamy Garlic	20	0	4
Sweet Onion & Garlic; Tstd Sesame	15	0	3
Lowfat: Blue Cheese Style	35	2	3
Creamy Roasted Pepper	45	2	5
Honey Dijon	35	2	4
Mango Madness	50	2	7
Southwestern Caesar	40	2	3
Zesty Italian	30	2	1
Subway Select			
Premium Collection: Caesar	170	16	1
Lite Blue Cheese; Lite Ranch	80	7	1
1000 Island	130	13	4
Jalapeno Ranch	100	10	1
The Spice Hunter: *Mix, As Prepared, Per 2 Tbsp*			
Caesar Salad, 2 Tbsp	150	13	1
Chinese Salad	140	12	2
Garlic & Herb	140	13	2
T. Marzetti's			
Regular: Balsamic Vinaigrette	100	9	4
Buttermilk	180	19	1
Creamy Caesar	150	17	0
Caesar Lite	70	6	2
Italian	100	10	3
Original Slaw	170	16	6
Ranch	160	17	2

Salad Dressings (Cont)

Per 2 Tbsp (Approx 1 fl.oz)	C	F	Cb
T. Marzetti's (Cont)			
Red Wine Vinegar & Oil	130	14	2
Roasted Garlic	150	15	2
Roasted Garlic Vinaigrette	130	10	8
Sesame Oriental	110	9	8
Sour Cream Blue Cheese	170	16	0
Sun Dried Tomato Vinaigrette	130	11	6
Vinaigrette Blue Cheese	120	11	4
Wild Berry Vinaigrette	100	9	4
Light: Buttermilk Ranch	80	8	2
Chunky Blue Cheese	90	5	5
Original Slaw	100	7	10
Tree of Life			
House Dressing: Cafe Venice	120	12	2
Maison Caesar	70	6	1
Shanghai Palace	80	7	3
Lowfat Free: Blue Cheese	15	1	2
Fat Free: Honey French	35	0	8
Italian Garlic	20	0	4
Oriental Ginger	15	0	3
Walden Farms			
Fat Free, Calorie Free Range			
Average All Types, 2 Tbsp	0	0	0
Weight Watchers			
Salad Celebrations Dressings			
Fat Free: Caesar (Single), 0.75 oz	5	0	1
Caesar, 2 Tbsp	10	0	1
Creamy Italian (8 oz), 2 Tbsp	30	0	7
French Style, 2 Tbsp	40	0	9
Honey Dijon, 2 Tbsp	45	0	11
Italian (8 oz), 2 Tbsp	10	0	2
Ranch Style, 2 Tbsp	35	0	7
Ranch (Single), 0.75 oz	25	0	6
Wild Oats			
Caesar Style	120	12	1
CreamyPeppercorn	100	10	1
Honey Toasted Sesame Ginger	100	10	3
Italian Balsamic Vinaigrette	80	7	5
Ranch	120	11	3
Thousand Isle	90	7	5
Williams Foods			
"Finally American"	160	15	5

Per 2 Tbsp (Approx 1 fl.oz)	C	F	Cb
Wishbone			
Regular: Chunky Blue Cheese	170	17	2
Caesar: Classic	110	10	2
Creamy Caesar	180	18	1
French: Deluxe French	120	11	5
Sweet 'N Spicy	140	12	6
Italian: Regular	80	8	3
House Italian	110	10	3
Robusto Italian	90	8	4
Ranch: Original	160	17	1
w. Garlic	150	15	2
w. Spring Onion	140	14	2
Russian: Regular	110	6	15
Thousand Island	130	12	7
Vinaigrette: Red Wine; Balsamic	60	5	3
Fat Free: Chunky Blue Cheese	35	0	7
Italian	15	0	2
Ranch	40	0	9
Dressing & Marinades: Per 2 Tbsp			
Asian Sesame	45	2	4
Balsamic Olive Oil & Herbs	35	2.5	4
Lemon Garlic & Herb	45	2.5	5
Tangy Honey Mustard	70	3.5	9
Just 2 Good!: Classic/Creamy Caesar	45	2	6
Classic/Creamy Caesar	40	2	5
Country Italian	30	2	3
Italian	35	2	5
Parmesan Peppercorn Ranch	45	2	6
Ranch	40	2	5
Thousand Island	60	2	9

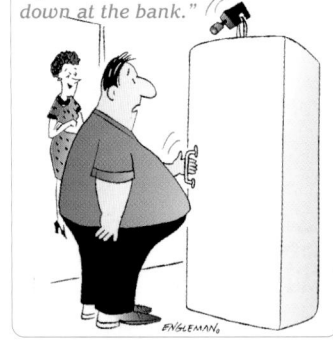

"I got the idea while down at the bank."

ENGLEMAN

Breakfast Cereals

Quick Guide   C F Cb
Cooked Cereals

	C	F	Cb
Buckwheat Groats, roasted:			
Dry, 1/2 cup, 3 oz	280	2	60
Cooked, 1 cup, 7 oz	180	1	39
Bulgar: Dry, 1/2 cup, 2 1/2 oz	240	1	53
Cooked, 1 cup, 6 1/2 oz	150	<1	34
Corn/Hominy Grits:			
Dry, 1/4 cup, 1.4 oz	145	<1	33
3 Tbsp, 1 oz	110	<1	25
Cooked, 3/4 cup, 6 1/2 oz	110	<1	25
Instant, 1 pkt, 0.8 oz	80	<1	18
w. Imitation Bacon Bits, 1 oz	100	<1	22
Cream of Rice, ckd, 3/4 c, 6 oz	90	0	20
Cream of Wheat:			
Regular, ckd, 3/4 cup, 6 oz	180	1	37
Quick, ckd, 3/4 cup, 6 oz	95	<1	20
Instant, ckd, 3/4 cup, 6 oz	110	1	23
Farina: Cooked, 3/4 cup, 6 oz	85	0	18
Millet, dry, 1/4 cup, 1 oz	100	1	20
Oat Bran: Raw, 1/3 cup, 1 oz	75	2	14
Cooked, 1/2 cup	45	<1	8
Oatmeal: Dry, 1/3 cup, 1 oz	110	0	19
Regular, ckd, 3/4 cup, 6 oz	110	2	19
1 cup, 8 oz	145	3	25
Instant: Regular, aver., 1 oz	100	2	18
Flavored, average	150	2	32
Quaker: *See Brands*			
Wheat Hearts, 1 oz dry, 3/4 c. ckd	110	1	21

Brans, Wheatgerm, Add-Ons

	C	F	Cb
Bran: Wheat, unprocessed,			
1 Tbsp, 3g	10	0	3
Rice Bran, raw, 1 Tbsp, 5g	16	1	2.5
1/3 cup, 1 oz	90	6	14
Oat Bran, 1 Tbsp, 5g	15	<1	3
1/3 cup, 1 oz	75	2	15
Wheat Germ, 1 Tbsp, 1/4 oz	25	1	3.5
1/4 cup, 1 oz	105	3	15
Fruit: Dried, average, 1 oz	80	0	21
Banana, 1/2 medium	50	0	23
Prunes in Syrup, 5, 3 oz	90	0	24
Honey: 1 Tbsp, 3/4 oz	65	0	17
Lecithin Granules, 1 Tbsp, 10g	50	5	1
Nuts: Almonds, 6 (1/4 oz)	40	4	5
Bee Pollen Granules, 1 T., 8g	25	1	2
Psyllium Husks, 1 Tbsp, 5g	10	0	1

Quick Guide   C F Cb
Cold Cereals
Average All Brands

	C	F	Cb
Bran Flakes, 3/4 cup, 1 oz	90	<1	21
Corn Flakes, 1 cup, 1 oz	110	<1	24
Granola, 1/4 cup, 1 oz	130	4	21
Oat Bran Cereal, 1/3 cup, 1 oz	110	1	22
Puffed Rice, 1 cup, 1/2 oz	55	0	12
Puffed Wheat, 1 cup, 1/2 oz	55	<1	12
Raisin Bran, 1/2 cup, 1 oz	85	<1	20
Rice Crisps, 1 cup, 1 oz	110	1	25
Shredded Wheat, 1 bisc., 3/4 oz	80	<1	18
Sugar-frosted Flakes, 3/4 c, 1 oz	110	<1	26
Wheat Flakes, 1 cup, 1 oz	105	<1	23

Ready-To-Eat Cereal

	C	F	Cb
Arrowhead: Amaranth, 1 c., 1.2 oz	130	1	23
Bran Flakes, 1 cup, 1 oz	90	1	18
Corn Flakes, 1 cup, 1.2 oz	130	0	30
Kamut Flakes, 1 cup, 1.1 oz	110	1	25
Maple Buckwheat Flake, 1 c., 1.5 oz	160	1	35
Multi Grain Flakes, 1 cup, 1.2 oz	140	1.5	29
Nature O's, 1 cup, 1.1 oz	130	2	24
Oat Bran Flakes, 1 cup, 1.2 oz	140	2.5	24
Perfect Harvest, 1 cup, 1.2 oz	140	2	25
Puffed Corn/Rice, aver., 1 c., 0.8 oz	60	0.5	12
Puffed Kamut, 1 cup, 0.6 oz	50	0	11
Puffed Millet/Wheat, 1 cup, 0.5 oz	60	0.5	12
Raisin Bran, 1 cup, 2 oz	190	1.5	40
Rice Flakes, 1 cup, 1.7 oz	80	1	19
Shredded Wheat, 1 cup, 2 oz	200	1	44
Spelt Flakes, 1 cup, 1.1 oz	100	0.5	23
Sweetened Nature O's, 1 c., 1.5 oz	160	2.5	31
Wild Wheat Flakes, 1 cup, 1.5 oz	160	0.5	37

Barbara's Bakery

	C	F	Cb
Breakfast O's, 1 cup	120	2	22
Brown Rice Crisps, 1 cup, 1 oz	120	1	25
Cinnamon Puffins, 3/4 cup, 1 oz	100	1	26
Corn Flakes, all types,1 cup, 1 oz	110	0	26
Crispy Wheats, 3/4 cup, 1 oz	110	0.5	25
Fruity Punch, 1 cup, 1 oz	110	0.5	26
Grain Shop, 2/3 cup, 1 oz	90	1	24
Shredded Oats, 1 1/4 cup, 2 oz	220	2.5	46
Shredded Spoonfuls, 3/4 cup	120	1.5	23
Soy Essence, 3/4 cup, 1 oz	100	0.5	25
Shredded Wheat, 2 bisc., 1.4 oz	140	1	31
Stars, Cocoa/Honey Crunch, 1 c., 1oz	110	0.5	26
Toasted O's, average, 3/4 cup	120	2	24

Breakfast Cereals (Cont)

Ready-To-Eat (Cont)

	C	F	Cb
Betty Crocker			
Scooby Doo! 25g	80	0	21
Breadshop			
Cranberry Crunch Muesli, 1 cup	200	3	44
Granola: Triple Berry Cr., 2/3 cup	220	7	36
Mocha Almond Crunch, 1/2 cup	210	7	34
Pralines in Cream, 1/2 cup	210	7	34
Vermont Maple, 1/2 cup	210	7	34
Super Natural, 1/2 cup	220	9	31
Straw. Blueb. Rasp., 1/2 cup	220	7.5	32
Kamut 'n Honey, 1 cup, 1 oz	120	3	22
Puffs 'n Honey, 3/4 cup, 1 oz	120	3	21
Sierra Crunch Muesli, 3/4 cup	190	3	38
Cap'n Crunch: All types, 3/4 cup	110	2	22
Cascadian Farms			
Honey Nut O's, 1 cup, 1 oz	120	1.5	24
Multi-Grain Squares, 3/4 c., 1 oz	110	0.5	25
Oats & Honey Granola, 2/3 c., 2 oz	230	6	42
Wheat Crunch, 3/4 cup, 1 oz	110	0.5	25
Chex: Corn, 1¼ cup, 1 oz	110	0	26
Wheat, 3/4 cup, 1.8 oz	190	1	41
Country Inn			
Green Gables Inn, 1/2 cup, 1.8 oz	210	7	36
Greyfield Inn, 3/4 cup, 1.8 oz	210	.5	39
Inn at Ormsby Hill, 1 cup, 2.1 oz	220	2.5	48
Dr McDougall's			
Oatmeal & Wheat, 1 cup, 2.4 oz	220	2	57
Oatmeal & 4 Grains,1 cup, 2.3 oz	210	1.5	52
Dominick's: Corn Flakes, 1¼ cup	120	0	24
Crispy Corn & Rice, 1¼ cup, 1 oz	120	0	26
Crispy Rice, 1¼ cup, 1 oz	130	0	28
Frosted Flakes, 3/4 cup, 1 oz	120	0	28
Fruit Rings, 3/4 cup, 1 oz	100	1	23
Tasteeos, 1¼ cup, 1 oz	120	2	24
Erewhon: Crisp Brn Rice, 1 oz	110	1	24
Aztec; Raisin Bran; Super O's, 1 oz	100	0	24
Fruit 'n Wheat, 1 oz	100	1	21
Wheat Flakes, 1 oz	100	0	24
Estee: Corn Flakes, 1 oz pkg	90	0	24
Raisin Bran, 1 oz pkg	90	1	21
Familia: "C.M.D.", 2/3 cup	230	7	38
Muesli, 1 cup, 2.1 oz	210	3	45
No Added Sugar, 1/2 cup	200	3	41
Swiss Crunch, 2/3 cup	250	11	33

	C	F	Cb
Glenny's			
Maple Frosted Corn, 1 oz	110	0	20
Oat/Rice Mini Puffs, 1 oz	110	0	21
General Mills			
Basic 4, 1/2 cup, 1 oz	100	1.5	21
Cheerios: Regular, 1 cup, 1 oz	110	2	22
Apple Cinnamon, 3/4 c., 1 oz	120	2	25
Frosted; Team, 1 cup, 1 oz	120	1	25
Honey Nut, 1 cup, 1 oz	120	1.5	24
Multi-Grain, 1 cup, 1 oz	110	1	24
Chex: Corn, 1 cup, 1 oz	110	0	26
Honey Nut, 3/4 cup, 1 oz	120	0.5	26
Morning Mix, 1 pouch, 1.15 oz	130	3.5	24
Multi-Bran, 1 cup, 2 oz	200	1.5	49
Rice, 1 cup, 1 oz	120	0	27
Wheat, 1 cup, 2 oz	180	1	41
Cinnamon Tst Crunch, 3/4 c., 1 oz	130	3.5	24
Cocoa Puffs: 1 cup, 1 oz	120	1	27
Milk & Cereal Bar, 1 bar, 1.4 oz	160	4	26
Cookie Crisp; Count Choc, 1 c., 1 oz	120	1	26
Fiber One, 1/2 cup, 1 oz	60	1	24
French Toast Crunch, 3/4 c., 1 oz	120	1.5	26
Frosted Mini Chex, 1 cup, 1 oz	110	0	27
Golden Grahams, 3/4 cup, 1 oz	120	1	26
Honey Nut Clusters, 1 cup, 2 oz	210	2	47
Kix: 1⅓ cup, 1 oz	120	0.5	26
Berry Berry, 3/4 cup, 1 oz	120	1.5	26
Lucky Charms, 1 cup, 1 oz	120	1	25
Oatmeal Crisp Almond, 1 c., 2 oz	220	5	41
Raisin Nut Bran, 3/4 cup, 2 oz	200	4	41
Reese's P'nut Butter Puffs, 3/4 cup	130	3	24
Total Corn Flakes, 1⅓ cup, 1 oz	110	0	26
Total Raisin Bran, 1 cup, 2 oz	180	1	43
Total Whole Grain, 3/4 cup, 1 oz	110	1	24
Trix, 1 cup, 1 oz	120	1.5	26
Wheaties: 1 cup, 1 oz	110	1	24
Energy Crunch, 1 cup, 1.95 oz	210	3	42
Hansen's Natural			
Per 1/2 Cup, 2 oz			
Orange & Chocolate Cereal	230	9	35
Stawb. & Yogurt Cereal	230	9	34
Toasted Nut Crunch Cereal	230	6	39
Tropical Cluster Cereal	210	5	36
Healthy Choice			
M/grain Raisin & Almond,			
3/4 cup, 1 oz	100	1	22
Flakes, 1 cup, 1.1 oz	100	0	26

Ready-To-Eat (Cont)

Health Valley	C	F	Cb
98% Fat Free Granola, 2/3 cup	180	1	43
Amaranth Flakes, 3/4 cup	100	0	24
Bran Cereal (w. Fruit), 3/4 cup	160	0	40
Corn Bran Flakes, 3/4 cup	100	0	24
Fiber 7 Flakes (100% Orig.), 3/4 c.	100	0	24
Golden Flax, 1/4 cup	190	3	38
Granola O's, all types, 3/4 cup	120	0	26
Healthy Crunches & Flakes, 3/4 c.	130	0	31
Healthy Fiber Flakes, 3/4 cup	100	0	23
Hot Cups: Apple; 10 Grain, 1 pkt	220	2.5	42
Maple; Banana, 1 pkt	240	2.5	46
Oat Bran Flakes, all types, 3/4 c.	105	0	26
Oat Bran/10 Bran O's, 3/4 cup	100	0	23
Orig. Soy Flakes 1 1/4 cup, 1.9 oz	190	1.5	35
Puffed: Honey Sweetened, 1 cup	110	0	24
Raisin Soy Flakes, 1 cup, 2 oz	190	1	39
Real Oat Bran, 1/2 cup	200	3	34

Heartland			
Granola, Lowfat, 1/2 cup, 2 oz	210	3	40
Original; Raisin, 1/2 cup, 2 1/4 oz	300	11	41

Kashi			
Breakfast Pilaf, 1/2 c., ckd, 5 oz	170	3	30
Cinna-Raisin Crunch, 1 c., 1.76 oz	150	1.5	39
GoLEAN Crunch!, 1 cup, 1.8 oz	190	3	36
Good Friends, 1 cup, 1 oz	90	1	24
Cinna-Raisin Crunch, 1 c., 1.75 oz	150	1.5	39
Heart to Heart, 3/4 cup, 1.2 oz	110	1.5	25
Honey Puffed Kashi, 1 cup, 1 oz	120	1	25
Kashi GoLEAN, 3/4 cup, 1.4 oz	120	1	28
Kashi Medley, 1/2 cup, 1 oz	100	1	20
Kashi Pillows, 3/4 cup, 1 oz	200	1	45
Organic Promise: Cranberry, 1 oz	110	1	26
Strawberry Fields, 1 cup, 1.1 oz	120	0	28
Puffed Kashi, 1 cup, 0.9 oz	70	0.5	13

Kellogg's			
Apple Jacks, 1 c., 1 oz	120	0	30
All-Bran: 1/2 cup, 1 oz	80	1	24
Bran Buds, 1/3 cup, 1 oz	80	0.5	16
with Extra Fiber, 1/2 cup, 1 oz	50	1	20
Apple Cinn. Rice Krispies, 3/4 c.	110	0	26
Apple Cinn. Squares, 3/4 c., 2 oz	180	1	44
Apple Raisin Crisp, 1/2 cup, 1 oz	90	0	23
Buzz Blasts,, 1 cup, 1 oz	120	2	24
Cinn. M'mallow Scooby-Doo, 1/2 cup	140	4	25
Cinn. Mini Buns, 3/4 cup	120	0.5	27

Kellogg's (Cont)	C	F	Cb
Complete Oatbran Flakes, 3/4 cup	110	0.5	23
Wheatbran Flakes, 3/4 cup	90	0.5	23
Cocoa Krispies, 3/4 cup	120	1	27
Common Sense O/Bran, 3/4 cup	110	1	23
Corn Flakes: 1 cup, 1 oz	110	0	24
Honey Crunch, 3/4 cup, 1 oz	120	1	26
Corn Pops, 1 cup, 1 oz	120	0	28
Cracklin' Oat Bran, 3/4 cup, 2 oz	190	7	35
Crispix: 1 cup, 1 oz	110	0	25
Cinnamon Crunch, 3/4 cup 1.1 oz	120	1	26
Double Dip Crunch, 3 3/4 cup	110	0	26
Froot Loops: 1 cup	120	1	28
Other types, 1 oz	120	1	28
Frosted: Flakes, 3/4 cup, 1 oz	120	0	28
Mini-Wheats, 3/4 cup, 1.8 oz	180	1	42
Bite Size, 1 cup, 1 oz	200	1	48
Fruity Marshmallow Krispies, 3/4 c.	110	0	25
Healthy Choice: Müeslix, 2/3 c, 2 oz	200	3	41
Lowfat Granola, 1 cup, 2.2 oz	220	3	48
Hunny B's, 1 cup, 1 oz	110	1	25
Just Right, 1 cup, 2 oz	210	2	48
Low Fat Granola: 1/2 cup, 2 oz	190	3	39
w. Raisins, 2/3 cup, 2 oz	220	3	47
Mickey's Magix, 1 cup, 1 oz	110	0.5	25
Mini Wheats:			
Raisin Squares, 3/4 cup, 1.8 oz	180	1	42
Strawberry Squares, 3/4 c., 1.8 oz	170	1	40
Frosted, 3/4 cup, 1.8 oz	180	1	41
Frosted Bite Size, 1 cup, 2 oz	200	1	48
Müeslix: Apple & Almond, 3/4 c.	200	5	39
Raisin & Almond, 2/3 cup	200	3	40
Nut & Honey Crunch, 1 1/4 c., 2 oz	220	2.5	46
Nutri-Grain: Almond, 1 1/4 c., 2 oz	180	3	38
Golden Wheat, 3/4 cup, 1 oz	100	1	23
Minis, 1 pouch, 1.55 oz	160	3	32
Cereal Bars, 1 bar, 1.3 oz	140	3	27
Twists, 1 bar, 1.3 oz	140	3	27
Yogurt Bar, 1 bar, 1.3 oz	140	3	27
Pokèmon, 1 cup, 1 oz	110	0.5	25
Pop Tarts: Spider-Man	200	5	37
Fruit/Frosted, aver. all flavors	200	5	37
Low Fat, all flavors	190	3	39
Pastry Swirls, 2.2 oz	260	11	37
Snak Stix, 1 pastry, 1.8 oz	200	5	37
Product 19, 1 cup, 1 oz	100	0	25
Raisin Bran, 1 cup, 2 oz	190	1.5	45
Raisin Bran Crunch, 1 cup, 1.9 oz	190	1	44

Breakfast Cereals (Cont)

Kellogg's (Cont)

	C	F	Cb
Rice Krispies: 1 1/4 cup	120	0	29
Treats, 3/4 cup	120	1.5	26
Bars, Original, 1 bar	90	2	18
Caramel/Peanut Butter, (1)	110	4	19
Double Choc Chunk, (1)	100	4.5	15
Scotcheroos, (1)	120	5	18
Smacks, 3/4 cup, 1 oz	100	0	24
Smart Start: Soy Protein, 1 cup	200	1.5	40
Original, 1 cup, 1.8 oz	180	0.5	43
Special K, 1 cup, 1.1 oz	110	0	23
Special K Red Berries, 1 cup, 1 oz	150	0	33
Special K Plus, 1 cup	210	2	47
Cereal Bars, 1 bar	90	1.5	18
Wheat Chex, 1 cup	170	1	38

McCann's Instant Irish Oatmeal

	C	F	Cb
Apple & Cinnamon, 1.23 oz (35g)	130	1.5	26
Maple & Brown Sugar, 1.5 oz (43g)	160	2	32
Original, 1 oz pkg (28g)	100	2	18

Mother's®

	C	F	Cb
Bumpers: Cocoa, 1 cup, 1.2 oz	120	0.5	29
Peanut Butter, 1 cup, 1.2 oz	130	2.5	26
Cinnamon Oat Crunch, 1 c., 2.1 oz	230	3	48
Groovy Grahams, 3/4 c., 1 oz	100	1	24
Honey Round-ups, 3/4 cup, 1 oz	110	0.5	24
Toasted Oat Bran, 3/4 cup, 1.1 oz	120	1.5	24
Toasted WheatGerm, 2 Tbsp, 1/2 oz	50	1	6

Nature's Path:

	C	F	Cb
Corn Flakes, 3/4 c.	115	0.5	26
Granola: Ginger Zing, 2/3 c.	270	11	37
SoyPlus/Hemp/Raspb., 1/2 cup	140	4	22
Heritage, all varieties, 3/4 c., 1 oz	115	0	24
Heritage Muesli, 1/2 cup, 2 oz	215	3	41
Honey'd Raisin Bran, 3/4 cup, 1 oz	110	0	25
Multigrain, 2/3 cup, 1 oz	110	0.5	24

New Morning

	C	F	Cb
Cornfetti, 3/4 cup	110	1	24
Cocomotion, 3/4 cup	100	5	22
Fruit-e-O's, 1 cup	120	1.5	25
Kamatios, 1 cup	120	1	25
Cocoa Crispy Rice, 1 cup, 2.1 oz	210	1.5	45
Corn/Honey Frost. Flakes, 1 c., 1 oz	120	1	25
Otios: Cocoa, 1 cup, 1.76 oz	170	1.5	21
Apple Cinnamon, 1 cup, 1 oz	90	1.5	21
Honey Almond, 1 cup, 1 oz	100	1	22
Original, 1 cup, 1 oz	120	1	21
Raisin Bran, 1 cup, 30g	90	0.5	22
Ultimate Oat Bran Flakes, 1 c., 28g	110	1	21

Post

	C	F	Cb
100% Bran, 1/3 cup, 1 oz	100	0.5	24
Alpha Bits, 1 cup	110	1	24
Banana Nut Crunch, 1/2 cup	240	6	44
Blueberry Morning, 1 cup	220	3	43
Bran Flakes, 3/4 cup, 1 oz	100	0.5	24
Cocoa Pebbles, 7/8 cup	115	1	25
Cranberry Almond Crunch, 1 cup	220	3	44
Fruit & Fibre, 1 cup, 2 oz	210	3	41
Fruity Pebbles, 1 1/4 cup	130	1.5	27
Golden Crisp, 1/2 cup	110	0	25
Grape Nut O's, 1 cup, 1.1 oz	120	0	28
Grape Nuts Flakes, 1/2 cup	110	1	24
Grape Nuts, 1/2 cup	210	1	47
Grape Nuts Raisin, 1/2 cup, 2 oz	200	1	47
Great Grains, 2/3 cup, 1.8 oz	200	6	38
Honey Bunches of Oats, 3/4 cup	120	2	26
Honeycomb, 1 cup	90	0.5	20
Marshmallow Alpha-Bits, 1 cup	130	1.5	27
Oreo O's, average, 3/4 cup	110	2.5	21
Raisin Bran, 2/3 cup, 1.4 oz	120	1	32
Shredded Wheat: Frosted, 1 cup	190	1	44
'N Bran, 1/2 cup	200	1	47
Honey Nut, 1 cup, 1.8 oz	200	1.5	43
Toasties Corn Flakes, 1 cup	90	0	20
Waffle Crisp, 1 cup	130	3	24

Quaker

	C	F	Cb
Breakfast/Cereal Bars: each	130	3	26
Ready to Eat: Oat Bran, 1 1/4 cup	210	3	41
100% Natural Granola: 1/2 cup	220	9	31
Lowfat, 2/3 cup	210	3	44
w. Raisins, 1/2 cup	230	9	34
Brown Sugar Bliss, 1cup, 1.7 oz	190	2.5	39
Cap'n Crunch: Regular, 3/4 c., 1 oz	110	2	23
Choco-Donuts, 3/4 cup, 0.9 oz	100	1	23
Honey Graham Oh's: 3/4 cup	110	2	23
Crunch Berries, 3/4 cup, 1 oz	110	2	23
Peanut Butter Crunch, 1 oz	110	3	21
Crunchy Corn Bran, 1 cup, 1 oz	90	1	23
Honey Nut Heaven, 1 cup, 1.7 oz	190	3.5	38
Life, all types, 3/4 cup	120	1.5	26
Oatmeal Squares, 1 cup, 1.8 oz	230	3	48
Puffed Rice, 1 cup, 1/2 oz	50	0	11
Puffed Wheat, 1 cup, 1/2 oz	55	0	13
Shredded Wheat, 3 biscuits	220	1.5	50
Unprocessed Bran, 1/3 cup	30	0	11

Breakfast Cereals ✦ Grains & Flours

Quaker (Cont)	C	F	Cb
Bagged: Cocoa Blasts, 1 cup	130	1	29
Apple Zaps; Fruitany O's, 1 cup	120	1	27
Frosted Flakers, 3/4 cup	120	0	28
Frosted/Honey Nut Oats, 1 cup	110	1	24
Frosted Oats/ Sweet Crunch, 1 cup	110	1.5	23
Rice Crisps, 1 cup	110	0	26
Fruitancy Oh's, 1 cup	120	1	27
Honey Crisp Corn Flakes, 3/4 cup	110	0	27
Honey Dipps, 1 1/4 cup	130	1.5	28
Grits: Regular, all types, 1 pkg	130	0.5	31
Instant: All types, 1 pkg	100	1	22
Quick'n Hearty (Microwave Oatmeal): Per Pkt			
Regular, 1 oz	110	2	19
Apple Spice; Cinn. Dble Raisin	170	2	35
Br. Sugar Cinnamon; Honey Bran	150	2	30
Instant Quaker Oatmeal: Per Pkt			
Oatmeal: Regular, 1 oz	100	2	19
Baked Apple; Banana Brd, 1.4 oz	150	2	31
Cinn. Roll; Fr. Vanilla, 1 1/2 oz	160	3	33
Fruit & Cream, 1 1/4 oz	140	2.5	27
Honey Nut, 1 1/2 oz	170	3.5	31
Maple/Br.Sug; Rais./Spice	160	2	33
Raisin Cinnamon Swirl, 1 1/4 oz	170	2	36
Dinosaur Eggs, 1.76 oz pkt	200	4	38
Kid's Choice, 1 pkt, aver., 1 1/2 oz	160	2.5	32
Nutrition for Women, 1 pkt	170	2	33
Quaker/Hot: Multigrain, 1/2 cup	130	1.5	29
Oat Bran, 1/2 cup	150	3	25
Whole Wheat Hot Nat. 1/2 cup	130	1	30
Oats: Quick/ Old Fash., Steel, 1/2 c.	150	3	27
Ralston: Bran Flakes, 3/4 c., 1 oz	110	1	24
Chex Multi Bran, 1 1/4 cup, 2 oz	220	2	46
Cocoa Crispy Rice, 1 c., 1 3/4 oz	200	1	45
Cookie Crisp, 1 cup, 1 oz	120	2	25
Frosted Flakes, 3/4 cup, 1 oz	120	0	28
Hot Ralston, 1/2 cup, 1.5 oz	150	1	31
Muesli: All types, avg.1 cup, 2 oz	200	3	41
Raisin Bran, 3/4 cup, 2 oz	190	1	41
Sun Flakes, 3/4 cup	110	1	33
Tasteeos, 1 1/4 cup, 1 oz	130	3	22
Stone-Buhr: Bran, 1/4 c., 0.5 oz	65	0	14
7 Grain, 1/3 cup, 1 1/2 oz	140	2	31
Weetabix: 2 biscuits, 1.23 oz (35g)	120	1	28
Wild Oats: CornFlakes, 3/4 c., 1 oz	100	0	24
Honey Frosted Flakes, 1 c., 1 oz	100	0	24
Oat Bran O's, 1 cup, 1 oz	120	1.5	25

Grains & Flours	C	F	Cb
Per 1/2 Cup (8 level Tbsp)			
Amaranth, 1/2 cup, 3 1/2 oz	350	6	60
Arrowroot, 1/2 cup, 2 1/4 oz	230	0	57
Barley: Regular, 1/2 cup, 3 1/4 oz	325	2	56
Pearled, raw, 3 1/2 oz	350	1	78
Flakes, 1/2 cup, 1 1/2 oz	150	0.5	33
Buckwheat: Regular, 1/2 c., 3 oz	290	3	61
Groats, roasted, dry, 3 oz	285	2	60
Roasted, cooked, 3 1/2 oz	90	0.5	19
Flour, whole-groat	200	2	42
Bulgur: Dry, 1/2 cup, 2 1/2 oz	240	1	54
Cooked, 1/2 cup, 3 1/4 oz	75	0.5	17
Carob Flour, 1/2 cup, 1.8 oz	95	0.5	25
Corn Kernels (blue/yellow), 3 oz	300	4	66
Corn Bran, 1/2 cup, 1.4 oz	85	5	32
Corn Flour/Masa, 2 oz	210	2	44
Corn Grits: Dry, 1/2 cup, 2 3/4 oz	290	1	62
Cooked, 1/2 cup, 4 1/4 oz	75	0.5	16
Corn Germ, toasted	245	2	21
Cornmeal: Average All Types			
3 Tbsp, 1 oz	100	0.5	22
1/2 cup, 2.2 oz	220	2	46
Mixes: same as above	220	2	46
Cornstarch: 1 Tbsp, 8g	30	0	7
1/2 cup, 2 1/4 oz	230	0	57
Couscous: Dry, 3 1/4 oz	345	0	72
Cooked, 4 oz	60	0	12
Farina: Dry, 3 oz	325	0	70
Cooked, 4.1 oz	60	0	13
Flax Seeds, 2 oz	280	12	22
Flour ~ See 'Wheat flour' Next page			
Garbanzo (Chick Pea), 1/2 c., 2 oz	200	3	35
Kuzu Root Starch, 1 Tbsp, 10g	35	0	8
Matzo Meal, 1/2 cup	260	1	55
Millet: Raw, 1/2 cup, 3 1/2 oz	375	4	76
Cooked, 1/2 cup, 4 1/4 oz	145	1	29
Oat Bran: Raw, 1/2 cup, 1.7 oz	115	2	31
Cooked, 1/2 cup, 4 oz	115	1	33
Oats, rolled/oatmeal:			
Dry/Groats, 1/2 cup, 1.5 oz	155	3	28
Cooked, 1/2 cup, 4.2 oz	75	1	13
Polenta: See Cornmeal			
Made Up, 1/2 cup, 5 oz	220	2	24
Potato flour, 1/2 cup, 3.2 oz	315	0	72
Psyllium Husks, 1 Tbsp (5g)	10	0	2
Quinoa, 1/2 cup, 3 oz	320	5	53
Rice: See Next Page			

Grains & Flours (Cont)✦ Rice

Grains & Flours (Cont)

Per 1/2 Cup (8 level Tbsp)

	C	F	Cb
Rice Bran, 1/3 cup, 1 oz	90	6	14
Rice Flour, 1/2 cup, 2 3/4 oz	290	2	63
Rice Polish, 1/2 cup	220	7	39
Rye Flour: Dark, 1 cup, 4 1/2 oz	415	3.5	88
Medium, 1 cup, 3 1/2 oz	360	2	79
Light, 1 cup, 3 1/2 oz	375	1.5	82
Rye Grain: 1/2 cup, 3 oz	280	2	59
Flakes, 1/2 cup, 1 1/2 oz	150	0.5	32
Semolina, 1/2 cup, 3 oz	305	1	61
Sorghum, 1/2 cup, 3.4 oz	325	3	72
Soybean Flakes, 1/2 cup, 1 1/2 oz	190	8	14
Soy Bean Flour:			
Defatted, 1 cup, 3 1/2 oz	330	1	34
Low-Fat, 1 cup, 3 oz	325	6	30
Full-Fat, 1 cup, 3 oz	370	18	27
Soy Meal, defatted, 1 cup, 4.3 oz	410	3	44
Tapioca, pearl, Dry: 1/2 c., 2. 7 oz	260	0	67
3 Tbsp, 1 oz	100	0	26
Teff (Seed) Flour, 2 oz	200	0.5	41
Tortilla Flour Mix, 1/2 cup, 2 oz	225	12	31
Triticale: 1/2 cup, 3.4 oz	325	2	70
Flour, whole-grain, 1/2 cup	220	1	47
Wheat: Average, 1 cup, 5 1/2 oz	320	2	68
Wheat Bran, unproc., 1/2 c., 1 oz	65	1	20
Wheat Flakes, 1/2 cup, 1 1/2 oz	160	0.5	32
Wheat Germ: 1/4 cup, 1 oz	105	3	15
Toasted, 1/4 cup, 1 oz	108	3	14
Wheat Flour:			
White, All Purpose/Self-Rising,			
1 level Tbsp, 0.6 oz	55	0	12
1/2 cup, 2.1 oz	225	0.5	47
1 cup, 4.4 oz	450	1	95
Whole Wheat, 1 cup, 4.2 oz	410	2	87

Also See Arrowhead Mills Cereals: Page 95

Eat it Today. . .
Wear it Tomorrow!

Brown Rice

	C	F	Cb
Average Short or Long Grain			
Raw/Dry: 1/2 cup, 3 1/2 oz	350	2.5	72
1 cup, 7 oz	700	5	144
Cooked: Hot, 1/2 cup, 3 1/2 oz	110	0.5	23
1 cup, 7 oz	220	1.5	46
Cold, 1/2 cup, 2 1/2 oz	90	0.5	19

White Rice

	C	F	Cb
Raw: Short/Med. Grain, 1 c., 7 oz	720	1	156
Long Grain, 1 cup, 6 1/2 oz	670	1	144
Glutinous, 1 cup, 6 1/2 oz	680	1	150
Cooked (Boiled/Steamed):			
Short/Medium Grain:			
Hot, 1/2 cup, 3 1/4 oz	120	0	27
1 cup, 6 1/2 oz	240	0.5	54
Cold, 1/2 cup, 2 3/4 oz	90	0	20
Long Grain: Hot, 1/2 c., 2 3/4 oz	100	0	22
1 cup, 5 1/2 oz	200	0.5	44
Cold, 1/2 cup, 2 1/2 oz	80	0	17
Glutinous/Sticky, ckd 1 c., 6 oz	170	0.5	36
Parboiled, ckd, hot, 1/2 c., 3 oz	90	0	20
Precook./Instant: Dry,1/2 c., 3 1/2 oz	370	0	80
Cooked, Hot, 1/2 cup, 3 oz	90	0	20
Wild Rice: Raw, 1 cup, 5 1/2 oz	570	13	120
Cooked, hot, 1 cup, 5 3/4 oz	165	0.5	35

Rice Dishes

	C	F	Cb
Chinese Fried Rice: 1/2 c., 2 1/2 oz	160	5	21
1 cup, 5 oz	320	13	42
2 cups, 10 oz	640	26	84
Mexican Rice: 1 cup	500	12	90
Taco Bell, 1 serving	190	9	23
Taco John's, 1 serving	250	5	44
Taco Time, 1 serving	160	2	30
Rice-A-Roni: See Page 76			
Rice Pilaf: Restaurant, 1 cup	270	7.5	43
Boston Market, 2/3 cup	180	5	32
Denny's, 1 serving	85	1	17
Rice w. Raisins/Pinenuts 1 cup	400	11	70
Risotto, 1 cup	420	18	65
Saffron Rice, 1 cup	370	12	66
Spanish Rice: 1 cup	390	9	72
El Pollo Loco, 1 serving	130	3	24
Sticky Thai Rice, plain, 1 cup	170	0.5	36
Sushi Rice, 1 Tbsp	25	0	6

- Macaroni includes all shapes and sizes; (e.g. spaghetti, fettuccini, shells, tubes, ziti, twists, sheets, cannelloni, manicotti, elbows).
- All regular macaroni products have the same cals/fat/carb. on a weight basis.
- 1oz Dry = approx. 2 1/2 -3 oz cooked.

Dry Spaghetti/Macaroni

	C	F	Cb
1 oz quantity	105	0.5	21
1lb box/pkg., 16 oz	1680	7	336
Elbows, 1 cup, 3 3/4 oz	395	2	77
Shells, small, 1 cup, 3 1/4 oz	340	2	66
Spirals, 1 cup, 3 oz	315	2	61

Cooked Spaghetti/Macaroni

	C	F	Cb
Plain, All Types (no added fat):			
Firm/Al Dente (8-10 mins.), 1 oz	42	0.5	8.5
Medium (11-13mins.), 1 oz	37	0.5	7.5
Tender (14-20mins.), 1 oz	32	0.5	7
(Longer cooking increases water absorbed)			
Spaghetti, 1/2 cup, 2 1/2 oz	90	0.5	18
Medium serving, 1 cup, 5 oz	185	1	37
Large (restaurant), 2 c., 10 oz	370	2	74
Elbows/Spirals, 1 cup, 5 oz	185	1	38
Small Shells, 1 cup, 4 oz	150	0.5	31
Protein-fortified: Dry, 1 oz	107	0.5	21
Cooked, 1 cup, 5 oz	230	0.5	44
Spinach/Vegetable: Dry, 1 oz	105	0.5	21
Cooked, 1 cup, 5 oz	180	0.5	37
Whole-wheat: Dry, 1 oz	100	0.5	21
Cooked, 1 cup, 5 oz	175	0.5	37

Fresh Pasta (Refrigerated)

	C	F	Cb
Plain/Spinach/Tomato, average:			
As purchased, 4 oz	325	2.5	64
Cooked, 1 cup, 5 oz	190	1	38
Home-made, without egg:			
Cooked, 1 cup, 5 oz	175	1	35
Buitoni			
Angel Hair, 1 1/4 cup, 3 oz	230	2.5	43
Fettuccine/Linguini: 1 1/4 cup, 3 oz	240	2.5	45
Spinach, 1 1/4 cup, 3 oz	260	4	43
Ravioli: Beef, 1 1/4 cup, 3.6 oz	330	9	46

Buitoni (Cont):	C	F	Cb
Ravioli: Chk., Herb Parm., 1 1/4 c., 3.6oz	310	9	44
Dblestuff. Mozz. Herb, 1 1/2 c., 4 oz	360	12	44
Four Cheese, 1 cup, 3 oz	290	9	38
Light, 1 cup, 3 oz	230	4	37
Garden Vegetable, 1 cup, 3 oz	250	5	39
Mini Beef, 1 cup, 3.5 oz	270	5	44
Rst Chick. & Garlic, 1 1/4 c., 4.5 oz	330	11	45
Tortellini: Chse & Rst Garlic 1 c., 3 oz	270	8	38
Chkn & Prosciutto, 1 c., 3.6 oz	360	13	45
Herb Chicken, 3/4 cup, 3 oz	260	7	40
Mozzarella & Herb, 1 cup, 3.6 oz	320	9	45
Mushroom & Chse, 1 c., 3.6 oz	290	6	46
Sundried Tomato, 1 cup, 3.6 oz	320	10	46
Sweet Italian Saus., 1 c., 3.6 oz	320	8	49
Three Cheese, 3/4 cup, 3 oz	250	6	39

Noodles

	C	F	Cb
Plain/Egg: Dry, 1 oz	108	1	20
1 cup, 1 1/3 oz	145	1.5	28
Cooked, 1 oz	38	0.5	7
1/2 cup, 2 3/4 oz	105	1	20
1 cup, 5 1/2 oz	210	2	40
Stir-Fried: 1 cup, 5 1/2 oz	270	9	40
2 cup serving, 11 oz	540	18	80
Yolk Free (Cooked): *Per Cup*			
'No Yolks' *(Foulds)*	210	2	40
Passover Gold *(Manischewitz)*	200	0	42
Chinese: Cellophane/Rice, dry, 1 oz	100	0	25
Chow Mein/hard, dry, 1 oz	150	5	17
Ramen Noodles: *See Page 76*			
Japanese: Soba, dry, 1 oz	95	0.5	21
cooked, 1 cup, 4 oz	110	0.5	24
Somen, dry, 1 oz	100	0.5	22
cooked, 1 cup, 6 oz	225	0.5	49
Japanese Style Pan Fried:			
Maruchan's Yaki-Sobu, 1 c., 5.6 oz	260	3	50
Udon *(Chikara),* aver., 7.5 oz pkt	250	1	52
Stir Fry/Yakisoba, 1 serve, 3.5 oz	220	2	44

Egg Roll Skins/Won Ton

	C	F	Cb
Egg Roll Skins:			
(Golden Dragon) 1 pce, 1 oz	80	0	18
(Wung Hung) 4 skins, 4 oz	300	0	64
Won Ton Wrappers:			
(Dynasty) 10 wrappers, 2.1 oz	170	1	36
Egg Roll/Spring Roll Wrapper:			
(Dynasty) 3 wrappers, 2.1 oz	170	1	36

Bread

Note: All breads have similar calories on a weight basis. However, volume may vary. For example, 1 oz of bread may equal 1 slice regular bread or 2 slices of a lighter bread. It is best to weigh bread used and calculate on 1 oz bread = 70 calories.

Quick Guide

Bread

	C	**F**	**Cb**
Average All Varieties:			
Thin slice (1/4") 1 oz	70	1	13
Extra thin slice 3/4 oz	55	<1	10
Light thin slice, 0.6 oz	40	<1	7.5
Toasting slice, 1.2 oz	85	1	16
Thick slice (3/8"), 1.5 oz	105	1.5	20
Large thick (1/2"), 2 oz	140	2	26
1-lb Loaf, 16 oz	1120	6	208

Toast has same calories as bread used.

1 thin slice + 1 tsp of fat	105	5	13
1 thick slice (3/8") +2 tsp fat	175	10	20

Breads

	C	**F**	**Cb**
Batard (8 oz), 1/4, 2 oz slice	140	0.5	28
Boule, 1/2" thick, 2 oz slice	130	0	29
Bran style/Dark, 1 oz slice	70	1	14
Buttermilk, average, 1 oz slice	80	2	13
Caraway Rye, 1 oz slice	70	0	15
Challah, 1 oz slice	85	2	14
Corn Bread, aver., 1 pce., 3 oz	180	7	36
Cracked Wheat Sourdough, 1 1/2 oz slice	130	0.5	27
Croutons, 2 Tbsp	35	1	6
Date & Nut, 1 oz slice	90	1	14
'Enriched' Breads, aver., 1 oz sl.	75	1	18
11-Grain, 1 oz slice	90	0.5	17
5-Grain Honey Wheat, 1 1/2 oz	110	1	23
Foccacia: Plain, 2 oz portion	150	4	23
Cheese & Garlic; Pesto, 2 oz	170	8	21
Tomato & Olive, 2 oz	120	2	20
French Stick/Baguette, 1 oz slice	70	1	15
French Toast, 1 slice, 2 1/4 oz	160	7	18
Sticks (Aunt Jemima), 1 pce, 1 oz	75	3	12
Garlic Bread, 1 pce. w. fat, 1 oz	125	6	14
Garlic Toast, (Pepp.Farm), 1.4 oz sl.	160	10	15
Italian Bread, 1 oz slice	75	1	15
Light Bread, aver., 0.8 oz slice	40	<1	7.5
1 oz slice	70	1	14
Melba Toast, 2 pces	25	0	6
MultiGrain, 1 slice, 1 oz	75	1	14
Fat Free, 1 oz	70	0	15
Nut/Health Nut, 1 oz slice	85	2	15

Breads (Cont)

	C	**F**	**Cb**
Oatmeal/Oatbran Bread, 1 oz sl.	70	1	13
Party Breads (Pepp. Farm): Rye, 1 sl.	15	<1	3
Dijon; Pumpernickel, 1 sl.	18	<1	3.5
Pita Bread, aver. all types, 2 oz	150	2	30
Mini/Pocket, 1 oz	75	1	15
Poppyseed (Vienna), 0.8 oz sl.	55	1	10
Pumpernickel, 1 oz slice	75	1	15
Cocktail size, 0.4 oz	30	<1	6
Raisin Bread, 1 oz slice	80	1	14
Raisin Walnut, 2 oz slice	160	3.5	29
Roman Meal, 1 oz slice	70	1	14
Country Potato & Oat, 1 1/2 oz	110	1.5	20
Rye: Average, 1 thin slice, 1 oz	75	1	13
1 thick slice, 2 oz	150	2	25
Cocktail size, 0.4 oz	25	<1	4
Sandwich Bread, 1 oz slice	70	1	13
Sandwich Pockets: Reg., 2 oz	150	1	30
Sourdough, 1 oz slice	70	1	12
Sprouted 7-Grain, 1.5 oz slice	110	1.5	18
Squaw, (33g) 1.1 oz slice	85	0.5	13
Turkish/Middle Eastern, 1 oz sl.	80	1.5	16

Bread Rolls & Buns

	C	**F**	**Cb**
Brown 'n Serve, average, 1 oz	80	2	15
Dinner Rolls: 1 small, 1 oz	85	2	15
1 medium (3" diam),1 1/2 oz	130	3	23
English Muffins, aver., 2 oz	140	2	27
Frankfurter/Hot Dog: 1 1/4 oz	100	2	19
1 1/2 oz size	120	2	23
French: 1 medium, 1.3 oz	110	1	24
1 large, 3 oz	240	2	52
Hamburger: Regular, 1 1/2 oz	120	2	23
Large, 3 oz	240	4	46
Hoagie/Submarine, 4 3/4 oz	400	8	77
Kaiser Roll, 2 oz size	170	3	18
Onion Roll, 2 oz size	170	2	20
Parker House Roll, 0.7 oz size	65	1	12
Party Roll, 0.6 oz	55	1	10
Sandwich Roll, 1.6 oz size	120	2	23
Soft Pretzel Bun (J & J), 3 oz	235	3	50
Sourdough Roll, 1 1/2 oz	100	1	18
Sweet Rolls, 1 oz	100	2	20
w. Icing, average	160	6	20
Wheat Roll: Small, 1 oz	75	0.5	14
Medium, 1 1/2 oz	110	1	20

Bagels ✦ Tacos ✦ Rice Cakes

Quick Guide

Bagels

		C	**F**	**Cb**
Average All Brands				
Plain/Onion:				
1 mini/bagelette, 1 oz		80	<1	15
1 small bagel, 2 oz		160	1.5	30
1 medium bagel, 3 oz		240	2	45
1 large bagel, 4 oz		320	3	60
Bagel Chips (New York Style),				
4 slices, 3/4 oz		90	2	17
Pizza Bagel, 6 oz each		380	7	60
Bagel Bites (Ore-Ida), 4 pces		190	7	25
Bagel Crisps (Burns Ricker), 1 oz		150	9	28

Bagel Brands

	C	**F**	**Cb**
Amy's Kitchen, average, 31/2 oz	235	2	50
Awrey's, 2.7 oz each	190	0.5	42
Cosco Bakery: Plain, 4 oz	300	1	61
Everything, 4 oz	330	3.5	62
Lenders, all flavors, 3.6 oz	280	3	55
Oroweat: Oatmeal, 3.4 oz	270	4	49
Multi-Grain, 3.4 oz	260	1.5	51
Sara Lee: Mini, average, 1 oz	80	0	15
Toaster Size, all types, 2.2 oz	160	0.5	33
3.4 oz Size (95g): Egg	260	2	50
Other flavors, 3.4 oz	260	1	55
4 oz Size (113g):			
Apple Cinnamon	310	1.5	64
Banana Walnut	350	7	61
Chocolate Chip	320	3.5	61
Cranberry Orange	310	1.5	64
Honey & Oat	310	2	61
New York Style, 41/2 oz	330	1	69
Sun Dried Tomato Basil	300	1.5	61
The Works	330	3.5	62
Western: All flavors, aver., 3 oz	230	1	47
Bagels: See Einstein Bros Bagels, Page 199			
Bagel Sandwiches: See Page 168			

Bagel Spreads

		C	**F**	**Cb**
Cream Cheese: Plain, 1 oz		80	8	2
Reduced Fat, 1 oz		60	5	2
Flavors: Lox, 1 oz		75	6	1
Raisin Walnut, 1 oz		90	6	8
Strawberry, 1 oz		60	3	7
Sundried Tomato, 1 oz		80	7	2
Vegetable, 1 oz		60	6	1

Bread Products

	C	**F**	**Cb**
Bread Crumbs, dry:			
Plain or seasoned, 1 oz	110	1	20
1 rounded Tbsp, 10g	35	<1	6
1 cup, 31/2 oz	390	5	73
Corn Flake Crumbs, 1 oz	110	1	20
Graham Cracker Crumbs, 1 oz	115	1	21
Keebler, 1 cup, 41/4 oz	520	14	84
Bread Dough: Frozen, 1 slice	75	<1	14
Refrigerated, French, 1" slice	60	1	13
Wheat/White, 1" slice	80	2	14
Breadsticks: Boboli, 1.75 oz	130	2	22
Stella D'oro: Sesame, (1)	50	2	7
Plain/Onion/Wheat, 1 pce.	40	1	7
Keebler/Lance, 2 sticks	30	<1	6
Salt Sticks, plain, 1 oz	110	1	20
Croutons: Aver. all brands, 1 oz	100	3	17
2 Tbsp, 10g	35	1	6
Coating Mixes:			
Seasoned, average, 1 oz	110	3	20
Featherweight, 1.4 oz pkg	72	<1	17
Pretzels: See Snacks ~ Page 126			
Stuffing: Average, dry mix, 1 oz	110	1	10
Made-up, 1/2 cup, 4 oz	180	9	11

Croissants ~ *See Page 112, 168*

Rice Cakes

		C	**F**	**Cb**
Average All Types/Brands:				
Regular size, 1 cake, 9g		35	0	7.5
Hain, Mini, average, 3g each		12	<1	2
Lundberg, all types, 15g each		60	<1	14
Quaker: Large, all flavors, 13g each	50	0	11
Crispy Mini's, average, 15g		70	2	12

Taco Shells

	C	**F**	**Cb**
Regular size, all types, each	55	3	6
Super Size, each	90	4	11
Mini Size, 1 taco	25	1.5	2
Salad Shell, flour (Azteca), 1.4 oz	180	11	19
Tortilla (Soft Taco), each	85	2	15
Corn Tortilla: 6", 1.2 oz each	45	0.5	9
Flour Tortilla: each, 1.75 oz	160	3	28
Lowfat	110	1.5	22
Burritos, 1 tortilla, 2.3 oz	190	5	32
Lowfat	110	1.5	22
Tostada Shells, each	55	3	6

Crispbreads ✦ Crackers, Cookies

Crispbreads | C | F | Cb

Per Crispbread/Cracker

	C	F	Cb
Ak-Mak: Sesame, 5 crackers, 1 oz	35	0	7
Finn Crisp: Original, rye,1	35	0	7
Other types,1	19	0	3
Kavli Norwegian: Thin,1	17	0	3
Thick,1	20	0	3
Malsovit, Meal Wafers.1	75	4	7
New York Flatbread Crisps, 1	35	0	7
Ry-Krisp: Natural, 1 crispbread	20	0	3
Seasoned,1	30	0	5
Sesame,1	25	1	3
Ryvita: Dark/Light, 1 piece	26	0	4
WASA: Breakfast; Sesame	50	0	9
Extra Crisp; Light Rye	25	0	5
Hearty Rye	45	0	9
Organic Rye	25	0	7
Sourdough Flatbread, 3	50	0	11
Sourdough Rye	35	0	7

Matzos

Manischewitz

	C	F	Cb
American Matzos, 1 board, 1 oz	115	2	22
Passover Matzos, 1 board, 1.1 oz	130	0	27
Passover Egg Matzos, 1.1 oz	130	2	27
Egg 'n Onion Matzo, 1 oz	112	1	23
Thin Salted Tea Matzos, 0.9 oz	100	1	21
Unsalted; Whole Wheat, 1 oz	110	0	24
Dietetic Matzo Thins, 0.83 oz	90	0	19
Crackers: Miniatures, 1 cracker	9	0	20
Passover Egg Matzo, 1 cracker	11	0	20
Matzo Meal, 1 cup, 4³/4 oz	515	2	110
Matzo Farfel, 1 cup, 2.7 oz	180	0.5	60
Grape Matzo, 1 each	110	0	25

World's Biggest Cookie!

Paul "Cookie" James

Quick Guide — Crackers | C | F | Cb

Average All Brands: Per Cracker

	C	F	Cb
Cheese Crackers: Plain, 1" square	5	0	0.5
Small, octagonal	10	0	1
Round (2" diam.)	15	0	1.5
Sandwich (Peanut Butter)	35	1	4
Graham, 2¹/2" square,1 cracker	30	0.5	5
Melba Toast, plain, 1 piece	20	0	4
Oyster & Soup Crackers, ¹/4 oz	60	2	10
(40 small oysters/20 lge hexagons)			
Rice Crackers: 1 small	9	0	2
Rice Snax (*Amsnack*), ¹/2 oz	60	1	12
Saltines, 2 crackers	25	1	4.5
Snack-type, 1 round cracker	15	0	3
Soda, 1 cracker, ¹/2 oz	60	2	10
Water Cracker (*Carr's*), regular, 1	32	0	7
Small, 1 cracker	14	0	4
Wheat, thin, 1 cracker	9	0	1
Zweiback Toast, 1 piece	30	0	5

Quick Guide — Cookies | C | F | Cb

Average All Brands: Per Cookie

	C	F	Cb
Biscotti: Small, 0.5 oz	65	2.5	10
Regular, 1 oz	130	5	20
Chocolate Chip Cookies:			
Small/Thin 0.5 oz	55	3	7
Regular, 1 oz	110	6	15
Large, 2.5 oz (*Mrs Field's*)	280	14	40
Jumbo, 4 oz	450	22	64
Oatmeal/Oatmeal Raisin:			
Small/Thin 0.5 oz	50	1.5	8
Regular, 1 oz	95	3.5	15
Large, 2.5 oz (*Mrs Field's*)	240	9	39
Jumbo, 4 oz	380	14	62
Peanut Butter:			
Small/Thin 0.5 oz	60	3	7
Regular, 1 oz	125	6.5	14
Large, 2.5 oz (*Mrs Field's*)	310	16	34
Jumbo, 4 oz	500	25	54
Lowfat Cookies			
Choc Chip (Lowfat), 1 oz (1)	100	1	21
Oatmeal Raisin (Fat-free), 1 oz (1)	90	0	20
Peanut Butter (Lowfat), 1 oz (1)	105	2	14

Crackers ✦ Cookies (Cont)

Brands	C	F	Cb
Per Cookie/Cracker (Unless Indicated)			
Archway: Coconut Macaroon	100	6	12
Apple/Date-filled Oatmeal	100	3	16
Apricot/Strawb.-filled Oatmeal	100	3.5	16
Aunt Bea's Pound Cake Cookie	100	4	16
Chocolate Chip: Drop	100	3.5	15
Ice Box	120	6	15
N' Toffee	130	6	18
Fat-Free: Oatmeal Raisin (1)	110	0	25
Cinnamon Honey Heart (3)	110	0	25
Devil's Food Cookie (1)	70	0	16
Frosty Lemon/Orange	110	4.5	17
Fruit & Honey Bar	100	3.5	18
Ginger Snaps: Regular (5)	150	5	23
Reduced Fat (5)	140	3.5	25
Iced (5)	150	5	23
Lemon Snaps (5)	150	7	20
Molasses	100	3	18
Oatmeal: Regular; Raisin	110	3.5	17
Iced	120	5	19
Ol' Fashioned Peanut Butter	120	6	15
Old Fashioned Windmill	90	3.5	14
Peanut Butter Choc	150	7	17
Peanut Jumble	110	6	13
Pecan Icebox	120	6	15
Ruth's Golden Oatmeal	120	5	18
Sugar Cookies (1)	100	3	16
Austin: Sandwich Cookies	240	2	36
Big Munch Wafer Bar, each	200	2.5	24
Cheese/Toast/Wheat Crackers, w. filling			
All types, average	200	2.5	29
Reduced Fat	170	1.5	25
Smackers Crackers, all types	130	1	32
Zoo Animal Crackers, all types	125	1.5	20
Zoo Animal Pretzels	200	0	40
Barbara's Bakery: Fig Bars, aver.	60	1	15
Animal Cookies, each	16	0.6	2
Cheese Bites, all types, 26 crackers	120	1.5	24
Coconut Almond, 1 bar, 1 oz	120	4.5	20
Crisp Cookies, all types (1)	80	4	11
Espresso Bean; Lemon Yog., 1 bar	120	3.5	22
Fat Free: Mini, all types, each	18	0	4
Rite Lite Rounds, 5 crackers	55	0.5	12
Roasted Peanut, 1 bar, 1 oz	130	4.5	20
Snackimals, 1 cookie	15	0.5	2
Wafer Crisps (3)	60	1	12
Wheatines, all types, 1 large square	50	1.5	10

Brands	C	F	Cb
Burns & Ricker			
Biscotti, average all types, (1)	70	2.5	10
Carr's			
Crackers: Table Water (5)	70	1.5	13
Monterey: Hearty Wheat (3)	60	2	9
Savory/Sesame (3)	70	3	9
Entertainer; Whole Wheat (2)	80	3.5	11
Cocktail, Croissant Orig. Gold (22)	140	3	21
Cookies: Bisc. for Tea (2)	140	6	20
Milk Choc Bisc for Tea (2)	130	6	16
Choccines (3)	150	9	16
Ginger Lemon Cremes (3)	140	6	19
Hob Nobs (2)	140	6	19
Imperials: Milk Chocolate (2)	140	7	18
Dark Choc (2)	150	7	19
Petites Bijoux (4)	140	5	21
Dominick's: Pecan Shortbread	100	6	11
Grahams: Cinnamon (8)	140	5	22
Fudge (3)	140	7	19
Honey (8)	150	6	22
Lowfat (9)	120	1.5	25
Saltine Crackers (5)	60	2	10
Sugar Wafers (5)	140	7	25
Unsalted Tops (5)	70	2	10
Cookies: Choc Chip Chewy (1)	100	5	14
Choc Chip Reduced Fat (3)	150	6	23
Old Fashioned: Assort.; Oatmeal	80	2.5	11
Sandwich Cremes, Chocolate	70	2.5	11
Striped Shortbread (3)	160	4	21
Vanilla Wafers (6)	160	6	23
Dr Soy: Average (2)	85	2	5
Entenmann's: Orig. Choc Chip (3)	150	7	20
Chocolate Brownie (2)	150	2	21
No Fat, 2 cookies	100	0	24
Soft Baked: Choc Chip	100	5	13
Gourmet English Toffee	100	5	13
Milk Choc Chip	100	5	13
Oatmeal Raisin, Fat Free (2)	100	0	23
White Choc Macadamia Nut (1)	100	6	12
Estee			
Chocolate Chip; Fudge Cookies	40	2	5
Coconut Cookies, Oatmeal Raisin	35	1.5	5
Fig Bars, each	50	0.5	11
Sandwich Cookies	55	2	6
Shortbread; Vanilla; Lemon	35	1.5	5

Crackers ✦ Cookies (Cont)

Per Cookie/Cracker (Unless Indicated)

	C	F	Cb
Famous Amos			
Butter Shorties	80	4.5	10
Chocolate Chip Cookie (1)	37	1.5	5
4 cookies, 1 oz	150	7	20
Belgian Style (4)	150	7	20
Choc Chip & Pecans (4), 1 oz	150	8	19
Chocolate Chunk	80	4	10
Oatmeal Choc Chip & Walnut (4)	150	7	19
Oatmeal Raisin (4), 1 oz	140	5	21
Pecan Shorties (1)	90	5	10
Lowfat: Iced Lemon (7), 1.1 oz	130	1.5	25
Iced Gingersnaps (7), 1.1 oz	120	1.5	25
Frookie			
Cookies, average all types	45	2	7
Animal Frackers	10	0.3	1.5
Apple Cinnamon Oatbran	45	2	7
Fruitins: Apple; Fig	60	1	12
Large Frooks, all types	120	4	18
Grandma's			
Choc Chip; Nutty Fudge	190	9	25
Fudge Choc Chip; Oatmeal Raisin	170	7	26
Old Time Molasses	160	4	29
Peanut Butter varieties, aver.	190	9	23
Cookie Bits, average (9)	150	7	22
Sandwich: Fudge (3)	180	5	31
Fudge Vanilla (3)	120	4	21
Vanilla (3)	180	5	32
Peanut Butter (5)	210	10	28
Rich & Chewy, 1 pkt	270	12	39
Sugar Wafers (3)	160	7	23
Tiny Bites (12)	280	12	39
Hain			
98% Fat-Free, all types (11)	110	0	23
Cheese Bites (22)	120	1.5	23
Cookie Jar Bits (Rice Cakes):			
Average all flavors, 17 bits	60	0.5	12
Mini Rice Cakes: Plain (8)	60	0	13
Oyster Crackers, Fat-Free (36)	60	0	13
Veg/Rice/Sesame Crackers (11)	140	6	19
Health Valley			
Graham: Amaranth; Oat Bran	15	0	3
Original Amaranth/Oat Bran	20	0.5	4
Healthy Pizza, all flavors (6)	50	0	11
Lowfat, all flavors (6)	60	1.5	10
Original Rice Bran	18	0.5	3

	C	F	Cb
Health Valley (Cont)			
Whole Wheat, all flavors	10	0	2
Cookies (each): Raisin Oatmeal	35	0	8
Apricot Delight; Date Delight	35	0	8
Healthy Biscotti, all flavors	60	1.5	12
Healthy Choc./Chips, all flavors	35	0	8
Jumbo, all flavors	80	0	19
Raspberry Fruit Center	70	0	18
Tarts: All types, 1 tart	150	0	35
Hy-Top			
Assorted Cookies (5), 1 oz	120	4	19
Assorted Sandwich Creme, aver.	80	3	12
Chewy-a-riffic	90	3.5	12
Chip-a-riffic (3)	170	9	23
Chocolate Chip (5), 1 oz	110	5	16
Honey Cinnamon Grahams (2)	120	4	21
Oatmeal	80	3.5	11
Iced Oatmeal	70	3	11
Pecan-a-riffic	100	5	11
Sugar	80	3	12
Vanilla Wafers (8), 1 oz	130	5	21
Jewel			
Animal Crackers (9)	140	3.5	25
Chip-A-Riffic (3)	180	9	24
Choc/Vanilla Sandwich Creme (2)	130	5	20
Chocolate Chip: Regular (3)	170	9	23
Chewy (1)	90	3.5	12
Chunky (1)	80	4.5	10
Choc Chunk, 1½ oz	200	9	26
Chocolate Sandwich Creme (2)	120	5	19
Cinnamon Grahams (8)	140	5	22
Cookie Jar Assortment (3)	150	9	23
Duplex Sandwich Creme (2)	120	5	19
Fudge Creme Wafer (3)	150	8	18
Fudge Marshmallow	110	4	18
Oatmeal; Oatmeal Old Fashioned	80	3.5	11
Peanut Butter (2)	140	5	14
Peanut Butter Chip, 1½ oz	210	12	21
P'nut Butter Fudge Wafer (2)	140	8	14
Saltine Crackers; Unsalted Tops (5)	60	1.5	11
Striped Shortbread (3)	170	8	20
Sugar Wafers (3)	140	7	20
Unsalted Top Crackers (5)	70	2	10
White Choc Macadamia, 1½ oz	200	10	26

Per Cookie/Cracker (Unless Indicated)

	C	F	Cb
Joseph's Cookies			
Sugar-Free (Bite Size):			
Almond (4)	100	5	13
Chocolate Chip (4)	100	5	13
Lemon (4)	95	5	15
Coconut (2)	105	5	14
Oatmeal: Pecan Shortbread (2)	100	5	14
Peanut Butter (2)	95	5	13
Lite: Choc Pecan B-Fit (2)	100	1	20
Peanut Butter Choc Chip (2)	120	4	20
Other varieties, average (2)	100	3	18
Keebler			
Crackers: Sandwich, 1 pkt, 1.3 oz	190	10	23
Club: Orig.; 50% Red. Sodium (4)	70	3	9
33% Reduced Fat (5)	70	2	12
Grahams: Regular (8), 1 oz	130	3.5	23
Lowfat varieties (9), 1 oz	115	1.5	24
Rumbly (20)	140	5	22
Snackin' (21), 1 oz	120	3.5	22
Munch'ems, average (40), 1 oz	140	5	20
Snax Stix, average (20)	130	5	18
Toasted: Reduced Fat (5)	60	2	10
Regular varieties (5)	80	3.5	10
Town House: Regular (5)	80	4.5	9
Reduced Fat (6)	70	2	11
Wheatables: Reduced Fat (13)	130	4	21
Other varieties (12)	140	6	20
Cookies: Classic Collection (1)	80	3.5	12
Chips Deluxe: Soft & Chewy (1)	80	3.5	11
Peanut Butter Cup; Rainbow (1)	80	4.5	9
Chocolate Lovers; Coconut (1)	90	5	11
Crunchy Walnut; Chips Deluxe (1)	90	5	9
Mini's, all types (4)	150	8	19
Cookie Stix (5)	140	6	20
Country Style Oatmeal w. Rais. (2)	140	6	18
E.L. Fudge Sandwich (2)	120	6	17
Mini Butter S'wich (7)	130	6	21
Double stuffed (2)	170	9	23
Fudge Shoppe: S'mores (3)	160	8	22
Deluxe Grahams, Reg. (3)	140	7	19
Double Fudge 'n Caramel (2)	140	7	20
Fudge Sticks (3)	150	8	20
Fudge Stripes (3)	160	8	21
Mini, 1 pkg (3)	270	13	38
Reduced Fat (3)	140	5	21
Mini's (4); Grasshopper (4)	150	7	20
Mini Grahams (10)	160	8	22
Keebler (Cont)			
Ginger Snaps (5)	150	6	24
Golden Fruit (1)	80	2	16
Iced Animal, (6)	150	5	24
Krisp Kreem, (5)	140	7	19
Lemon Coolers (5)	140	5	23
Sandies: 25% Red. Fat (2)	80	3	11
Choc Chip Pecan (1)	80	5	9
Pecan Shortbread, 1 pkg	300	17	33
Soft Batch, 0.5 oz all types, each	80	3.5	10
Choc Chunk types, 1 oz	130	7	17
Homestyle Oatmeal Raisin, 1 oz	130	4.5	20
Vienna Fingers: Regular (2)	140	6	21
Reduced Fat (2)	130	4.5	22
Wafers: Golden Vanilla Wafers (8)	150	7	20
Reduced Fat (8)	130	3.5	25
Rainbow (artif. flavored) (8)	130	5	20
Sugar: Vanilla (4)	150	8	18
Peanut Butter (4)	160	9	18
Sugar Free: Vanilla Creme (3)	130	6	19
Kraft			
White Cheddar Chse Nips (27), 1 oz	150	7	19
Teddy Graham Bearwiches (1)	150	7	21
Lance: Big Town, 1 pkg	250	11	38
Chocolate Chip, each	130	6	18
Dunking Sticks, each	180	10	22
Fig Bar, each	180	3.5	34
Fat Free: Apple/Cranberry, ea.	160	0	38
Oatmeal, each	130	6	18
Creme, each	240	10	35
Apple Bar, each	190	6	32
Peanut Butter, each	140	8	14
Peanut Butter Creme Wafer, 1 pkg	230	12	26
Little Debbie			
Apple Flips	150	5	24
Chse Crackers w. P'nut Butter (4)	140	8	16
Fudge Brownies (1)	270	13	39
German Choc Cookie Rings	140	8	18
Ginger Cookies	90	3	15
Marshmallow Pies, each	160	6	27
Nutty Bar (2), 2 oz	310	18	32
Oatmeal Creme Pies	170	7	26
Toasty Crackers w. P'nut Butter (4)	140	7	16
Yo-Yo's	130	6	21
Peanut Clusters, each	190	11	23
Figaroos, each, 1.5 oz	150	3.5	31
Peanut Butter & Jelly Sandwich	130	5	22

Crackers ✦ Cookies (Cont)

Per Cookie/Cracker (Unless Indicated)

	C	F	Cb
Lotte			
Chocolate (13), 1 oz	190	10	13
Koala Vanilla (13)	190	11	15
Koala Yummies (13), 1 oz	200	11	13
Peanut Butter (13)	190	10	11
Strawberry (13)	190	10	14
Lu Marie Lu			
Le Choclateur (3)	150	8	17
Le Petit Beurre (4)	150	4	25
Le Petit Ecolier (2)	130	6	17
Pim's: Orange; Raspberry (2)	90	3	17
Manischewitz			
Matzo Boards: See Page 104			
Biscotti: Toffee Crunch Macaroons	50	2.5	7
Choc. Chip Cappucino	70	2.5	10
Chocolate Macaroons, each	45	2	8
Matzo Cracker, Miniatures	9	0	2
Whole Wheat Crackers	9	0	2
M&M/Mars Co: *Per Bar*			
Cookie Bars, average, 1.2 oz	180	11	21
Mrs Fields' Cookies: *Per 1 Cookie, 2.5 oz*			
Butter; Butter Toffee	290	12	40
Chewy Fudge	300	14	40
Coconut Macadamia	280	13	39
Debra's Special; Milk Choc	280	12	39
Milk Choc w. Walnuts	320	17	37
Milk Choc Macadamia	320	18	38
Oatmeal Raisin	240	9	39
Peanut Butter	310	16	34
Pumpkin Harvest	270	14	31
Semi-Sweet Chocolate	280	14	40
with Pecans	300	16	37
with Walnuts	310	16	38
Triple Chocolate	300	14	41
White Chunk Macadamia	310	17	37
Nibblers: *Per 2 Cookies, 1 oz*			
Debra's Special	100	4.5	13
Milk Choc w/Walnuts	120	6	14
Milk Chocolate; Peanut Butter	110	6	15
White Chunk Macadamia	120	7	13
Nibblers (10 oz Ctn): *Per Cookies, 1.23 oz*			
Oatmeal Raisin w. Nuts	150	7	21
Milk Chocolate Chip	150	8	21
Semi Sweet Chocolate Chip	150	7	22
White Chunk Macadamia	160	8	21

Per Cookie/Cracker (Unless Indicated)

	C	F	Cb
Mother's			
ABC Cinnamon Grahams (1)	12	0.5	1.5
ABC Sugar Cookies (1)	12	0.5	1.5
Blasters (2)	120	6	17
Candy Chip (4)	150	7	21
Checkerboard Wafers	20	1	3
Chocolate Chip: Cookies	80	4	10
Cookies (bag) (1)	30	1	5
Cookie Parade Assortment, each	35	1.5	5
Chocolate Chip Parade	35	1.5	5
Angel Cookies	60	3	7
Circus Animal Cookies (1)	25	1	3
Cocodas Coconut	30	2	4
Coffee Creme S/wich (2)	180	7	26
Dinosaur Grrrahams (1)	65	1.5	12
Double Fudge	90	4.5	12
English Tea/Taffy Sandwich	90	3.5	13
Flaky Flix Fudge/Vanilla	70	3.5	8
Fudge Gauchos (2)	190	8	26
Gaucho Peanut Butter S'wich	95	5	11
Iced Raisin; Macaroon	80	4	9
Oatmeal Cookies: Regular	55	2.5	9
Butterscotch Chip	60	2.5	9
Iced; Chocolate Chip	65	2	11
Oatmeal Raisin Cookies	30	2	5
Oatmeal Walnut Choc. Chip	65	3	9
Peanut Butter	75	4.5	8
Striped Shortbread Cookies	55	2.5	7
Sugar Free: Shortbread (4)			
Choc & Lemon Sandwich			
Sugar Cookies	70	3	10
Sugared Lemon	75	4	9
Taffy	90	4	13
Murray® SugarFree Cookies			
Choc Chip/& Pecan (3)	160	9	19
Double Fudge (3)	140	6	23
Fudge-Dipped Wafer, Vanilla (4)	140	10	19
Lemon/Choc Cremes (3)	120	7	18
Lemon Crisp (4)	140	4.5	22
Peanut Butter (3)	150	7	18
Shortbread (8)	120	4.5	20
Vanilla Sugar Wafers (6)	160	9	21
Newman's Own			
Fig Newmans (2)	120	0	28
Snack Pack, 1.6 oz	140	0	33

Crackers ◆ Cookies (Cont)

Per Cookie/Cracker (Unless Indicated)

Nabisco

	C	F	Cb
Crackers: Cheese Nips (26), 1 oz	150	7	19
Air Crisps: Ritz, 1 oz (23)	140	5	22
Potato varieties, 1 oz (22)	120	3.5	21
Pretzel Original, 1 oz (23)	110	1	22
Wheat Thins, 1 oz (23)	130	4.5	21
Bacon Flavored Thins (7), 1/2 oz	80	4	9
Better Cheddars: Reg; Low Salt	7	0.3	1
Chicken in a Biskit (12), 1.1 oz	160	9	19
Garden Crisps (7), 1/2 oz	60	2	10
Honey Maid Graham, aver. (13)	120	2.5	24
Oysterettes (19), 1/2 oz	60	2.5	10
Ritz; Wheatsworth; Stoneground (1)	16	1	2
Mini Ritz (33), 1 oz	150	8	18
Ritz Bits S'wiches: Chse 1.5 oz pkt	230	14	23
Peanut Butter (4), 1 oz	160	8	18
Xtreme Cheese (13), 1 oz	160	10	16
Royal Lunch (1)	50	2	8
Sociables (7)	80	4	9
Swiss (7), 1/2 oz	70	3.5	10
Teddy Cheddy (23), 1 oz	150	6	19
Tid Bit, cheese (16), 1/2 oz	70	4	8
Triscuit Thin Crisps (14)	130	5	20
Triscuit Wafers: All types	20	1	1
Uneeda, Unsalted Tops	30	1	5
Vegetable Thins (7), 1/2 oz	80	4.5	9
Waverly (5)	70	3.5	10
Wheat/Oat Thins: (8), 1/2 oz	70	2	10
Big Wheat Thins (10)	140	6	20
Ranch (14)	150	7	19
Zings! 1 pkg, 1.8 oz	240	11	34
Cookies:			
Barnum's Animal Cracker	16	0.5	3
Biscos: Sugar Wafers	17	1	2
Waffle Cremes	35	2	4
Brown Edge Wafers	28	1	4
Bugs Bunny Graham Cookies	12	0.5	5
Café Creme: Vanilla Fudge (2)	200	10	27
Vanilla; Cappuccino (2)	160	8	22
Cameo Creme Sandwich	65	2.5	10
Choc Cherry Bar, 1 bar	130	2	26
Chocolate Chip Bite Size	10	0.3	2
Chocolate Chip Honey Grahams	5	0.1	1
Chocolate Snaps	17	0.5	3
Chocolate Wafers (Red. Fat)	14	0.2	3
Candy Blasts (1)	80	4	10

Per Cookie/Cracker (Unless Indicated)

Nabisco (Cont):

	C	F	Cb
Chips Ahoy!:			
Chocolate Chip (1)	80	4	10
Snack Pack (4), 1.4 oz	200	10	27
Chewy Chocolate Chip	85	4	12
Chunky Choc Chip; Cremewiches	80	4	10
Cookie Barz, 35g bar	180	10	23
Mini Chips Ahoy! (5)	150	7	20
Snack Pack, 1.5 oz (43g)	220	11	28
Peanut Butter (1)	80	4	9
Reduced Fat (1)	70	2.5	11
Famous Chocolate Wafers	28	1	5
Grahams	15	0.5	3
Honey Maid: Grahams, all types (2)	30	0.5	6
Low Fat Cinnamon Grahams (2)	28	0.4	6
Ideal Bars: Chocolate & Peanut	90	5	10
Lorna Doone Shortbread	35	1.5	4
Marshmallow Puffs; Mystic Mint	90	4	14
Marshmallow Twirls	140	6	20
Newtons: Fig (1)	110	2.5	22
Snack Pack, 2 pces, 2 oz	200	4	39
Fat-Free Fig (1)	90	0	22
Other Fruit Newtons (2)	90	0	22
Cobblers, Apple/Peach	70	0	17
Nilla Wafers: Original	15	0.5	3
Reduced Fat	15	0.3	3
Nutter Butter: Bites, each	15	0.6	2
P'nut Butter S'wich, 1.9 oz pkg	260	11	36
Oatmeal Crunch	15	0.5	3
Old Fash. Ginger Snaps	30	0.6	5
Oreo: Original, 3 cookies	160	7	23
Snack pkg, 2 oz	270	12	40
Cookie Barz, 1 bar	180	10	23
Reduced Fat, 3 cookies	130	3.5	25
Chocolate Creme, 2 cookies	150	7	20
Double Delight: Mint 'n Creme (2)	140	7	20
P'nut Butter & Choc Creme (2)	140	7	20
Double Stuf, 2 cookies	140	7	20
Fudge-Covered, 1 cookie	90	5	13
Mini Oreo: 9 pieces, 1 oz	140	6	21
Snack Pack, 1.5 oz (43g)	200	9	31
Pecanz	90	5	9
Pinwheels, Choc./Marshmallow	130	5	21
Teddy Cheddy Crackers (23), 1.1 oz	150	6	19
Teddy Grahams Snacks, all types	5	0.1	1

Crackers ◆ Cookies (Cont)

Per Cookie/Cracker (Unless Indicated)

Parmalat ~ Bed & Breakfast	C	F	Cb
Chocolate Chunk Pecan	130	8	14
Chunky Chocolate Chip	120	6	16
White Chocolate & Macadamia	130	7	15
Cranberry Raisin	110	5	17
Key Lime/Raspb. Fruit Center	140	6	22

Peak Freans: Trad. O'meal (2), 20g	90	3	15

Pepperidge Farm	C	F	Cb
American Collection: Sante Fe	120	4.5	18
Average other flavors	140	7	16
Biscotti: Figaro	110	4	14
Caruso; La Scala; Tosca	90	3	13
Chocolate Chunk Minis (4)	150	8	20
Fruit Cookies: Cherry Cobbler	70	2.5	11
Average other flavors	50	2	9
Dessert Bliss: Choc. Alm.; Mint Choc. (3)	160	8	22
Distinctive: Bordeaux; Pirouette	35	2	5
Brussels, 1 pkt, 0.7 oz	100	2	13
Brussels Mint; Milano (1)	65	3	7
Chantilly Raspberry (2)	120	6	23
Chessman; Toy Chest Butter	40	1.5	6
Double Choc. Milano	75	4	8
Geneva	55	3	6
Hazelnut Milano	65	3.5	8
Lido	90	4.5	11
Linzer Strawberry Filled	100	4	15
Milk Choc. Bordeaux	60	3	7
Milk Choc. Milano	170	9	21
Mint/Orange Milano	70	4	8
Goldfish: Plain, 55 pces, 30g	140	6	19
Flavor Blasted (51), 30g	150	8	17
Giant: Wheat (14)	140	5	21
Flavor Blasted, average (31)	145	7	19
Graham Snacks, average (38)	140	5	22
Nantucket: Choc Chunk Minis (4)	150	8	20
Double Choc Chunk (1)	140	7	18
Old Fashioned: Hazelnut	55	2.5	7
Brownie; Butterscotch Oatmeal	55	3	6
Chocolate Chip; Irish Oatmeal	45	2.5	6
Gingerman; Molasses Crisps	30	1	5
Lemon Nut Crunch	60	3	6
Oatmeal Raisin	55	2	8
Pecan Shortbread	70	4.5	7
Shortbread	70	3.5	8
Sugar	45	2	7
Sausalito, Choc Macadamia (4)	160	9	18

Pepperidge Farm (Cont)	C	F	Cb
Soft Baked: Caramel; Choc Chunk	130	6	13
Choc. Macadamia/Walnut	130	6	16
Oatmeal Raisin	110	4	17
Spritzers, all flavors (5)	140	7	21
Vanilla Raspberry Tart	60	1.5	12
Pirouline: 8 rolls, 1 oz	130	3.5	23
Salerno: Almond Windmill (2)	120	4.5	17
Bonnie Shortbread (4)	160	7	22
Butter Cookies: Original (6)	160	7	22
Reduced Fat (6)	150	5	22
Coconut Bar (4)	150	8	18
Creme Wafer Sugar-free (5)	190	13	18
Dinosaur Graham	70	2.5	11
Farm Animal Crackers (13)	140	5	22
Grahams: Cinnamon (2)	130	3.5	22
Chocolate (2)	130	3	24
Iced Oatmeal (2)	120	5	18
Mini Butter: Flavored (25)	150	6	20
Angel/Chocolate Creme (9)	140	6	20
Mini Dinosaur (15)	140	5	21
Mint Creme Patties (2)	130	7	16
Oyster Crackers: Regular (42)	60	1.5	11
Fat-Free (42)	60	0	12
Royal Crispy Stix (3)	150	8	18
Royal Stripes (3)	180	8	24
Saltine Crackers: Reg./Unsalted (5)	60	1.5	11
Fat-Free (5)	50	0	11
Santa's Favorites, aniseed (6)	150	5	22
Scooter Pie Choc Marshmallow	140	5	23
Sugar Wafers, assorted (5)	180	11	20
Vanilla Wafers (7)	130	5	21

Santa Fe Farms	C	F	Cb
Fat Free, average, 1 pkg	120	0	26
Sinful: Chocolate Chip (2)	150	7	19
All Butter Raisin & Oatmeal	130	6	20
Butter w. Soft Creme Raspberry (1)	70	3	12
Choc w. Vanilla Creme (2)	120	5	16

Snackwell's (Nabisco)	C	F	Cb
Choc Chip (3)	150	8	23
Coconut Creme (2)	110	4	19
Creme Sandwich, 1 pkg (4)	210	5	38
Double Choc Chip Bite Size (3)	130	4	22
Lemon Creme Sugar Free (3)	130	6	24
Mint Creme (2)	110	4	19
Oatmeal (1)	90	2.5	17
Peanut Butter Chip, 1 oz	120	4	20
Shortbread (3)	130	5	22

Cookies (Cont) · Refrigerated

	C	F	Cb
Snackwell's (Cont)			
Crackers: Cracked Pepper (5)	60	1.5	10
Wheat (5)	70	1.5	11
Stella D'Oro: Angel Wings	70	4.5	7
Almond Delight Chinese (1)	85	1	11
Angelica (1)	100	4	15
Anginetti (4)	140	4	23
Anisette Sponge (2)	90	1	19
Anisette Toast (3)	130	1	27
Banana Walnut Toast (1)	100	2	19
Blueberry Toast (1)	100	1	20
Breakfast Treats, Chocolate (1)	100	4	15
Biscotti (Hazelnut) (1)	100	3.5	15
Castelets, regular/chocolate (1)	70	3	9
Como Delight (1)	70	3.5	9
Fruit Delight Apple Cinnamon (1)	70	0	17
Golden Bars; Love Cookies (1)	110	4	16
Lady Stella Assortment (3)	130	5	19
Margherite, Reg./Low Sodium (1)	70	3	11
Swiss Fudge (1)	70	3	9
Sunshine: *Per Cracker, Unless Indicated*			
Cheez-It Crackers (1)	6	0.4	0.5
Big Cheez-It (1)	12	1	1
Cheez-It Cheddar Jack (26), 1 oz	160	10	16
Cheez-It Juniors (44), 1 oz	140	7	13
Heads & Tails, 1 pkt, 1.5 oz	210	9	28
Hi-Ho Crackers	17	0.5	2
Reduced Fat	14	0.5	2
Krispy: Regular	12	0.3	2
Oyster & Soup, 17 crackers	60	1.5	11
Reduced Fat	10	0	2
Party Mix: 1 pkt, 1.7 oz	230	9	32
Reduced Fat, ½ cup, 1 oz	130	3	21
Trader Joe's: Oatmeal Raisins (1)	250	11	37
Choc Chip Cookies (1)	270	13	36
Joe-Joe's Choc s/wich (1)	65	2.5	10
Weight Watchers: O'meal Rais. (2)	120	2	22
Apple Raisin Bars, each	70	2	14
Chocolate Chip (2)	140	5	22
Choc. S'wich Cookies (2)	140	3.5	23
Fruit Filled, 1 bar	70	0	16
Vanilla Sandwich Cookies (2)	140	3	25
Wild Oats: Ginger Snaps (5) 1 oz	130	5	20
Crunchy P'nut Butter (5) 1 oz	150	8	16
Oatmeal Raisin (5) 1 oz	130	5	20
Oat Choc Chip (5) 1 oz	130	5	20
Water Crackers (4) 0.5 oz	63	1.5	11

Thaw, Bake & Serve

	C	F	Cb
Big Country: Aver. all types (1)	100	4	15
Cookietree: *Per Cookie*			
Buttersugar; Cinn. Apple Oatmeal	120	5	17
Choc. varieties; Pecan/Macadam.	130	7	17
Cookie w. M&M's; Dble Fudge	120	6	17
Fat Free varieties, average	125	0	28
Peanut Butter/Chocolate	130	7	17
Raisin Oatmeal	110	3.5	18
Guiltless Indulgence (1.3 oz Cookie)			
Fat Free varieties, aver.	120	0	28
Lowfat Fudge/Choc., aver.	130	2	28
Grands!: *Per Biscuit*			
Blueberry; Golden Corn	210	9	28
Butter Tastin'; Buttermilk	200	10	24
Reduced Fat	190	7	27
Cinn. Raisin; Extra Fluffy; Wheat	200	8	28
Extra Rich	220	12	25
Flaky; Homestyle	200	10	25
Southern Style	200	10	24
Hungry Jack: Aver. all types (1)	100	4.5	14
Jewel: Buttermilk Biscuits (2)	100	1.5	20
Old Fashioned Biscuits (2)	100	1.5	20
Pillsbury Cookies: *Per 1 oz*			
Buttermilk; Country, each	50	1	3
M & Ms	130	6	17
Choc. Chip/Dbl Choc Chip Chunk	140	7	17
Choc. Chip. Reduced Fat	110	4	18
Chocolate Chip w. Walnuts	130	7	16
Holiday, all types (2), 1 oz	130	7	16
Oatmeal Choc. Chip; Reeses	125	6	16
Peanut Butter	120	6	16
SnackWells, Choc. Chip, Red. Fat	110	3	19
SnackWells, Chocolate Fudge	90	1.5	18
Sugar (2), 1 oz	130	5	20
Tender Layer Buttermilk	160	4.5	19
One Step Pan Cookies	130	6	19
Toll House (*Nestlé*)			
Choc Chip	140	6	20
Reduced Fat Choc Chip	130	3.5	23
Choc. Chip White; Chunk	150	6	22
Peanut Butter Choc Chip	150	7	20
Sugar	120	5	18

Cakes, Pastries, Croissants

Ready-to-Eat

	C	F	Cb
Angel Food: Plain, no oil, 2 oz	120	0	25
Plain with oil, 2 oz	160	1.5	25
w. Cream Frosting	230	7	37
Apple Fritters, 2 oz	360	22	38
Apple Pie: See Pies/Tarts Page 107			
Baklava, 1¹⁄₂" square, 1¹⁄₂ oz	110	6	13
Banana w. Butter Cream, 3 oz	300	13	40
Black Forest, 3 oz	230	10	34
Brownie, 3.5 oz	420	25	52
Bundt, 3 oz	300	17	35
Carrot Cake: Plain, 3 oz	230	8	41
w. Cream Cheese Frosting	380	21	42
Cheesecake: Small serving, 3 oz	260	18	24
Large serving, 5 oz	430	30	40
w. Lowfat Cheese/fruit, 3 oz	150	8	30
Cheesecake Factory: See Page 187			
Denny's Cheesecake, 1 slice	470	27	48
Cherry Cobbler, 5 oz	350	10	62
Chocolate Cake: Plain, 3 oz	220	11	40
w. Chocolate Frosting, 3 oz	320	15	42
& Cream Filling, 3¹⁄₂ oz	360	21	43
Cinnamon Crumb Cake, 4 oz	450	23	57
Cinnamon Roll, Large, 6 oz	630	27	87
Coffee Cake, 2¹⁄₂ oz	230	7	38
Cream Cheese Crumb, 4 oz	410	20	52
Cream Puff (custard fill), 4¹⁄₂ oz	300	18	26
Creme Horns, each	190	13	19
Croissants: See Next Column			
Cupcake: Plain, 1¹⁄₂ oz	140	6	25
w. Frosting	170	7	30
Danish Pastry: Small, 2 oz	220	10	25
Large, 4 oz	440	20	51
Date Nut Roll, ¹⁄₂" slice	80	2	12
Devil's Food, w. Frosting, 3 oz	460	25	55
Donut Holes, 1¹⁄₄" balls, 2 oz (5)	220	10	30
Donuts: See Page 108			
Eclair, Choc., Cust. fill, 3¹⁄₂ oz	240	14	23
Fig Bars, average, each	150	3	30
Fig Cake, ¹⁄₂ piece	110	2	21
Fruit Cake, Dark/Light, 1¹⁄₂ oz	165	7	26
Fudge Nut Brownie, each	340	13	56
Gingerbread: From mix, 3" sq.	200	6	37
Honey Bun, each	330	13	47
Key Lime Pie, 4.5 oz	440	22	54
Kolacky, Apricot/Rasp., ¹⁄₂ oz (1)	60	3.5	8

Ready-to-Eat (Cont)

	C	F	Cb
Lemon Cake, 2¹⁄₂ oz piece	220	9	40
Lemon Poppy Seed Creme, 3 oz	310	15	40
Mississippi Mud Pie, 4 oz	380	24	37
Mud Cake, 1 piece, 3¹⁄₂ oz	350	16	48
Orange Creme (Ring), 3 oz	300	15	40
Pineapple Upside Down, 2¹⁄₂ oz	230	9	37
Peach Melba, 3¹⁄₂ oz	300	8	52
Strawberry Creme, 3 oz	290	14	40
Strudel Bites, ³⁄₄ oz	85	4	12
Pecan Twirls, 1 piece	110	5	16
Pecan Pie, 3 oz	330	13	51
Pies & Tarts: See Page 109			
Pound Cake, 3 oz	420	27	42
Sponge: Plain, 2¹⁄₂ oz	190	3	36
w. Cream & Strawberry	325	8	38
w. Chocolate Icing	300	12	38
Raisin Bun, 1 bun, 2¹⁄₄ oz	180	2	37
Strudel, fruit, average, 3 oz	280	8	45
Sweet Roll, average, 1¹⁄₂ oz	155	7	24
Swiss Rolls, each	170	9	23
Tarts: See Page 109			
Tiramisu, 1 piece, 5 oz	400	29	30
Toaster Strudel, 2 oz	190	10	26
Turnovers, fruit, average, 3 oz	270	12	36

Croissants

Average All Brands

	C	F	Cb
Plain/All Butter:			
Petite, 1 oz	120	7	14
1 Medium, 1¹⁄₂ oz	180	10	21
1 Large, 2¹⁄₂ oz	300	18	35
Sweet: *Per Croissant, 3¹⁄₂ oz*			
Almond Croissant	420	25	39
Apple Croissant	250	10	30
Chocolate Croissant	400	24	36
Sandwiches: See Page 174			
Au Bon Pain: See Page 179			
Burger King: Croissan'wich, See Page 185			
Dunkin' Donuts: Plain	290	18	26
Almond	350	22	34
Chocolate	400	25	37
Sara Lee: All Butter, 1¹⁄₂ oz	180	9	19
All Butter Petite, 1 oz	120	6	13

Muffins, Sweet Rolls

Quick Guide   C F Cb
Muffins: Ready-to-Eat

Average All Types:

	C	F	Cb
Small, 1 oz	80	3	12
Medium, 2 oz	160	6	24
Large, 3 oz	240	9	36
Extra Large, 4 oz	320	12	48
Giant, 6 oz	480	18	60
Jumbo, 8 oz	640	24	96
English Muffin, 2 oz	150	2	29

Brands ~ Ready-To-Eat

	C	F	Cb
Awreys: Blueberry, 2.25 oz	210	9	29
Raisin Bran, 2.5 oz muffin	190	7	30
Carl's: Blueberry Muffin	340	14	49
Bran Muffin	370	13	61
Dunkin' Donuts: *See Page 197*			
Hostess: Mini, average, each	55	3	7
Blueberry; Raspberry, each, 4 oz	440	19	62
Jewel: English Muffin, 2 oz	130	1	25
McDonald's: Apple Bran, 4 oz	300	3	61
Oroweat: Cinnamon Rais., 2.4 oz	170	1	35
Extra Crisp; Sourdough, 2 oz	130	0.5	26
Health Nut, 2.3 oz	170	3	30
Otis Spunkmeyer: *Per Whole Muffin (4 oz)*			
Banana Nut, 4 oz	480	24	60
Cheese Streudel	440	20	60
Wild Blueberry	420	22	48
Our Daily Muffin: Each, 3 oz	120	0	31
Pepperidge Farm: Average	150	3	28
Ralphs: Banana, 4.5 oz muffin	470	21	62
Blueberry, 4.5 oz	410	16	60
Bran & Raisin, 5 oz	380	8	78
Sara Lee: Blueberry	220	11	27
Corn	260	14	30
Snackwell's: Blueberry, 1/6 pkt	120	0	28
Weight Watchers: *Per Muffin*			
Chocolate Chocolate Chip	190	2	39
English Muffin Sandwich	210	5	28
Fat Free, average, all flavors	165	0	39
Low Fat, average, all flavors	175	3	37

Muffin Mixes   C F Cb

Prepared: Per Muffin

	C	F	Cb
Betty Crocker: Apple Streusel	210	8	33
Banana Nut	170	6	27
Blueberry	160	6	25
Choc Chip; Cinn. Streusel	170	8	23
Wild Blueberry	170	5	28
Fat Free, all flavors	120	0	26
Duncan Hines: Blueberry, reg.	120	3	21
Bakery Style: Blueberry	190	6	32
Cinnamon Swirl	200	7	32
Cranberry Orange Nut	200	8	29
Pecan Crunch	220	11	27
Oat Bran Blueberry	110	4	17
Oatmeal & Apples/Walnuts	210	9	30
Pillsbury: Blueberry Lowfat	160	2	34
Cinnamon	160	4	27
Other varieties	180	5	30
Sweet Rewards: Fat Free	120	0	28

Sweet Rolls & Buns

Note: Weigh for actual weight as can be 10-50% higher than label weight.

	C	F	Cb
Cinnabon: Classic	730	24	114
Caramel Pecanbon, 1 serving	1100	56	141
Minibon, 1 serving	300	11	45
Entenmann's: Cinn. Bun, 2.15 oz	230	10	32
Reduced Fat, 2.15 oz	160	3	32
Cheese Swirl Buns, 3.4 oz	350	16	45
Cinnamon Swirl Buns, 1, 3 oz	310	14	42
Pecan Danish Ring, 1/6, 2 oz	250	15	25
Walnut Danish Ring, 1/8, 2 oz	240	15	25
Twists: Raspberry, 1/8, 2 oz	220	11	25
Nonfat, 1/8, 2 oz	140	0	32
Cinnamon Danish, 1/8, 2 oz	240	13	29
Lemon Danish, 1/8, 2 oz	210	11	27
Hostess: Honey Bun, Glazed, 2.7 oz	320	19	34
Actual weight up to 3.9 oz	460	27	49
Iced/Frosted, 3.5 oz	410	24	42
Little Debbie: Pecan Spinwheels, 1 oz	110	4	16
Mickey: Cinnamon Pastry, 4 oz	200	5.5	35
Cinnamon Nut, 2 1/2 oz	230	8	37
Raisin Cinnamon, 2 1/2 oz	200	4.5	35
Pillsbury: Cinnamon Roll, 1.5 oz	150	5	23
Reduced Fat, 1.5 oz	140	3.5	24
Svenhard's: Viking Size Cinn. Bun, 4 oz			
Actual weight up to 5.6 oz	650	35	79
Label data based on 4.8 oz	560	30	68

Donuts

Quick Guide

Donuts

Average All Brands

	C	F	Cb
Plain, 1³/4 oz	210	12	25
Sugared, 1³/4 oz	220	11	27
Glazed, 2 oz	250	12	34
Chocolate Iced, 2 oz	260	14	29

Brands

Buttercrumb

	C	F	Cb
Cinnamon, 1 cake, 1.6 oz	170	6	28

Dolly Madison Donuts

	C	F	Cb
Regular, 1³/4 oz	270	12	40
Gem varieties, 1/2 oz each	65	3	8
Powdered Mini, 1/2 oz each	60	3	8

Dunkin' Donuts: *See Fast-Foods, Page 197*

Dutch Mill: Plain, 1³/4 oz

	C	F	Cb
Plain, 1³/4 oz	210	12	25
Sugared, 1³/4 oz	220	11	27
Glazed, 2 oz	250	12	34
Double-Dipped Chocolate, 2 oz	280	17	31

Entenmann's Donuts

	C	F	Cb
Powdered, 1³/4 oz	230	14	25
Glazed Buttermilk, 2¹/4 oz	270	13	35
Light, 2 oz	190	7	31
Light Fantastic Fudge, 2 oz	210	9	40
Milk Chocolate Frosted, 2.4 oz	310	19	35
Dark Choc. Frosted, 2 oz	280	19	27

Hostess Donuts

	C	F	Cb
Cinnamon Sweet Roll, 2 oz	220	7	36
Regular: Plain, 1 oz	140	7	15
Chocolate Frosted, 1¹/2 oz	180	11	19
Pwd Sugar/Cinnamon, 1¹/2 oz	210	10	25
Old Fashioned; Glazed, 1¹/2oz	180	9	23
Blueberry, 1¹/2 oz	210	13	21
Hostess O's, Raspberry, 2 oz	230	10	34
Donettes: Regular, 1/2 oz	70	4	8
Chocolate, 0.6 oz	80	5	8
Crumb, 0.7 oz	80	3.5	10
Powdered, 1/2 oz	60	3	8

Jewel: Cinnamon Spiced, 2 oz

	C	F	Cb
Cinnamon Spiced, 2 oz	230	15	24

Krispy Kreme: *See Fast-Foods, Page 210*

Little Debbie Donuts

	C	F	Cb
Donut Sticks, 1.6 oz pkg	210	13	21
3 oz pkg	390	23	39

Brands (Cont)

Mickey

	C	F	Cb
Egg Fluff, 2, 1.65 oz	210	11	25
French Twirl, 2, 1.65 oz	240	16	21
Jumbo, aver. all types, 1, 1.5 oz	190	11	21
Mini, 2, 1 oz	130	8	15

Sara Lee Donuts

	C	F	Cb
Choc. Frosted Mini, 3/4 oz each	100	5.5	13
Powdered Mini, 1/2 oz each	85	4.5	9
Glazed, 1/2 oz each	110	5	14
Reduced Fat, 1/2 oz each	55	2.5	8

Tastykake Donuts

	C	F	Cb
Plain, 1¹/2 oz	190	10	22
Cinnamon, 1¹/2 oz	180	8	26
Frosted Rich, 2 oz	260	16	28
Glazed, Mini (6) 2¹/2 oz	270	12	38
Honey Wheat, 2 oz	210	8	32
Powdered Sugar, Mini (6) 2¹/2 oz	280	13	38

Van De Kamp's Donuts

	C	F	Cb
Old Fashioned: Plain	270	11	40
Chocolate, 2.4 oz	340	22	34
Powdered, 2 oz	240	11	35
Assorted, 2¹/4 oz	280	17	32
Mini Donuts: Chocolate, 4, 2 oz	290	17	32
Crumb, 4	220	8	35
Powdered, 4	250	13	33
Lowfat: Maple Buttermilk, 1	200	2	43
Chocolate Buttermilk, 1	200	2	43
Double Chocolate, 1	190	2.5	41
Powdered, 1	150	1.5	32

Zingers

	C	F	Cb
Devil's/Vanilla Food, 2 cakes	280	8	50

"Now cut that out!"

Pies & Tarts

Quick Guide   C F Cb

Pies ~ *Average All Brands*
1/8 of 9" Pie, 4 oz Serving

	C	F	Cb
Apple; Blueberry; Cherry	290	13	46
Boston Cream Pie	330	14	55
Chocolate Pie	300	18	35
Custard; Coconut Custard	250	13	27
Lemon Chiffon Pie	360	14	50
Lemon Meringue	270	11	42
Mince Pie	300	13	46
Pecan Pie	470	24	52
Pumpkin Pie	240	13	28
Strawberry Pie	230	9	37

Brands *Per Serving*

	C	F	Cb
Denny's: Apple Pie	470	24	64
Cherry Pie	630	25	100
Chocolate Peanut Butter	655	39	64
Chocolate Silk Pie	650	43	60
Dutch Apple Pie	440	19	55
Hershey's Choc Chunks N' Chips	600	36	58
Oreo® Cookies & Creme	650	40	67
Pumpkin Pie	235	7	38
Entenmann's			
Homestyle Apple, 1/6 pie, 4.3 oz	340	12	56
Hostess: Fruit; Cherry, 4.5 oz pie	470	22	65
Lemon, 4.5 oz pie	500	24	66
Long John Silver's: Per Serving			
Chocolate Crème Pie	280	17	29
Double Lemon Pie	350	18	41
Pineapple Crème Cheesecake	310	17	36
Marie Callender's			
Per 1/5 Pie: Apple	865	49	92
Blueberry	885	57	76
Boysenberry	860	57	82
Cherry	900	58	87
Banana Cream	630	28	67
Chocolate Cream	535	29	66
Coconut Cream	650	32	64
Per 1/4 Pie: Fresh Strawberry	615	28	89
Mince	885	59	97
Lemon Meringue	550	23	76
Pumpkin	615	28	80
Tastykake: Fruit, average	310	11	50
French Apple	360	12	61
Coconut Creme	390	20	47
Lemon Pie	300	13	44

Pastry & Pie Crusts   C F Cb

	C	F	Cb
Pie Crust: Baked, 9" diameter shell			
1 Pie Shell, 6 1/2 oz	900	60	79
2-crust shell, 11 1/4 oz	1500	93	137
Betty Crocker, 9", 1/8 shell	110	8	9
Boboli, thin Pizza Crust, 1/5, 2 oz	170	4	28
Hershey's Choc Crust, 1/8	110	5	14
Jewel, 1/8 of 9" crust	130	8	13
Keebler Graham Cracker, 1/8 of 9"	110	5	14
Reduced Fat, 1/8	90	3.5	14
Shortbread Crust, 1/8	110	5	14
Mrs Smith's Deep Dish, 9" (1/8)	110	7	11
Nabisco Oreo, 1/6 of 9" crust	140	7	18
Honey Maid Graham, 1/6, 1 oz	140	7	18
Nilla Pie Crust, 1/6, 1 oz	140	8	18
Pet-Ritz, all types, 1/8, 3/4 oz	90	5	10
Pillsbury (All Ready), 1/8 pie, 1 oz	120	7	13
Piecrust Sticks, 8 oz	960	64	90
Choux Pastry, raw, 1 oz	60	4	3
Filo Pastry: 4 sheets, 2 1/2 oz	210	2.5	40
Athens: 5 sheets, 2 oz	180	1	35
Mini Dough Shells, 2, 8g	45	2	1
Pepp. Farm, 2 sheets, 1 1/2oz	120	1	25
Flaky Pastry, 1 sheet, 6 oz	780	72	16
Puff (Pepp.Farm), 1/2 sheet, 4.5 oz	510	33	42
1/6 sheet, 1 1/2 oz	170	11	14
Bake & Fill Shell, 1.7 oz	190	13	16
Pizza Crust, 1/8 whole	90	1	16
Bisquick Baking Mix:			
Original, 1/3 cup, 1 1/2 oz	160	6	25
Reduced Fat, 1/3 cup, 1 1/2 oz	140	4	27

Pie Filling

	C	F	Cb
Canned: Average All Brands ~ Per 4 oz			
Apple, 4 oz	120	0	28
1 Can, 21 oz	600	0	145
Apricot, 4 oz	150	0	36
Blackberry, Blueberry, Cherry	120	0	28
Chocolate, Coconut, 4 oz	140	3	33
Lemon, 4 oz	200	2	47
Mincemeat, 4 oz	190	1	45
Peach, Strawberry	120	0	28
Pumpkin, 4 oz	170	0	40
Raisin, 4 oz	130	0	30
Raspberry, Black/Red, 4 oz	190	0	45
Strawberry, 4 oz	120	0	28

Cakes & Pastries - Packaged

Cakes & Pastries	C	F	Cb
Banquet: Crm Pies, aver., 1/3 pie	350	21	42
Cheesecake Factory: *See Page 187*			
Dolly Madison: Honey Bun, 3.75 oz	450	26	49
Cinn. Sweet Rolls (2), 4.25 oz	420	14	34
Dunkin' Stix, 3 stix, 4 oz	510	27	60
Eli's Frozen Cheesecakes: *Per 1/8 Pkg, 3 oz*			
Cookies N Creme; Choc. Caramel	320	23	11
Keylime; Original, average	320	22	26
Entenmann's			
All Butter Loaf, 1/6 loaf, 2 oz	210	9	30
Banana Cake, 1/8 cake, 2.5 oz	290	15	39
Brownie: Ultimate Fudge, 1	220	13	27
Light: Fudge, 1/10 strip, 1.4 oz	110	0	27
Lemon; Coffee, 1/8 strip, 1.9 oz	130	0	29
Buns/Twists: *See Page 115*			
Cheese-Topped Coffee, 1/8, 2 oz	200	9	26
Cheese-Filled Crumb Coffee, 2 oz	210	10	25
Chocolate Fudge, 1/6 cake, 3 oz	280	12	42
Chocolate Loaf, Light, 1/8, 2 oz	120	0	29
Creme-Filled: Choc Cupcakes, 1	160	0	39
Golden Cakes, 1 cake, 2.3 oz	280	15	34
Golden Loaf, (Light) 1/8, 1.7 oz	130	0	28
Louisiana Crunch, 1/9, 3 oz	330	14	48
Mocha Cake, 1/6 cake, 3 oz	340	17	45
New York Crumb Coffee, 1/10, 2 oz	250	12	33
Ultimate Crumb, 1/10, 2 oz	250	13	33
Grands!: Blueberry Biscuits, 2 oz	210	9	29
Cinnamon Rolls, 3.5 oz roll	300	7	54

Weigh packaged foods for actual weight. It can be up to 50% more than the label net weight (the minimum legal weight). Allow extra calories.

Hostess	C	F	Cb
Angel Food Cake, 1/8	160	1.5	33
Brownie Bites, each	57	3	7
Carrot Cake, 2 pcs, 3.5 oz	300	7	55
Coconut Cakes, Creme (1) 1 oz	130	7	16
Coconut Golden Cupcakes (1) 2 oz	200	7	33
Suzy Q's, 2 cakes, 2 oz	230	9	35
Twinkies, 1 pkg, 1.5 oz	150	5	25
Per Cake: Chocodiles	240	11	33
Chocolicious	190	7	30
Chocolate/Orange Cupcake, aver.	170	6	28
Crumb Coffee	130	5	19
Cup Cake, each	160	6	30
Dessert Cups, each	100	2	17
Ding Dongs	190	10	23
Ho Ho's, each	125	6	17
Honey Bun: Glazed, 2.7 oz	320	19	34
Actual weight up to 3.9 oz	460	27	49
Snoballs	180	5	31
Zingers: Chocolate, 1	200	7	33
Raspberry, 1	200	8	30
Vanilla, 1	210	7	36
Low Fat: Brownie	140	2.5	28
Cupcakes; Twinkies	135	1.5	28
Crumb Cakes	90	0.5	19
Jewel Bake Shop			
Choc Mini Cupcakes, 1 cake	100	12	30
Cinnamon Swirl Bread, 1 oz slice	160	2.5	30
Creme Horns, 1 horn	190	13	19
Elephant Ears, 2.5 oz	340	22	34
Fancy Jelly Roll, 1/6 roll, 2.7 oz	190	2.5	38
French Torpedo Roll, 2.7 oz	170	1	35
Gourmet Cinn. Rolls, 6 oz roll	640	29	88
Key Lime Meringue Pie, 1/6, 5 oz	340	12	55
Little Debbie			
Cakes: Coffee, 2, 2 oz	230	7	39
Choc Chip Snack, 2, 2.4 oz	290	14	42
Creme-filled Strawb. Cupcake ,1	200	9	29
Devil Cremes, 1.65 oz cake	190	8	29
Devil Squares, 2 cakes, 2.2 oz	270	13	37
Frosted Fudge , 1.5 oz cake	200	10	25
Swiss Cake Rolls, 2 cakes	260	12	39
Zebra Cakes, 2 cakes, 2.6 oz	330	16	45
Honey Buns, 1.75 oz bun	220	13	24
Manischewitz: Cheesecake, 3 oz	250	19	16
Marie Callender (Frozen)			
Cobbler, all types, 1/4 pie, 4.25 oz	390	19	45

Pepperidge Farm

	C	F	Cb
Cakes Supreme: *Per 3 oz Slice*			
Lemon Mousse	290	12	35
Chocolate Mousse	250	10	35
Boston Creme	260	9	32
Cream Cakes Supreme:			
Cream Cheese Carrot, 1/9, 3 oz	320	20	38
Pineap./Strawb. Crm., 2.7 oz slice	240	10	38
Old Fashioned Cakes: *Per 3 oz Slice*			
Butter Pound	290	13	39
Deluxe Carrot	310	16	39
Turnovers (Frozen): Apple, 3.2 oz	290	15	36
Raspberry, 3.2 oz	290	15	35
3-Layer Cakes: Coconut, 1/8, 2.5 oz	250	11	35
Golden, 1/8 cake, 2.5 oz	250	12	33
Fruit Squares: Apple/Blueb./Cherry	210	10	27

Rich's:

	C	F	Cb
Chocolate Eclairs (Frozen)	190	9	24

Sara Lee (Frozen)

	C	F	Cb
Cakes: *Per Serving*			
All Butter Pound, 1/6, 2.7 oz	320	16	38
Reduced Fat, 1/4, 2.7 oz	280	11	42
All Butter; Chocolate, 1/4, 2.7 oz	320	16	40
Banana Sundae, 1/10, 3 oz	270	14	32
Butter Streusel Coffee, 1/6, 2 oz	220	12	25
Choc Layer, 1/8, 3 oz slice	340	17	46
Dble Choc Layer, 1/8, 2.8 oz	260	13	33
Free & Light, 1/4, 2.7 oz	200	4	39
Golden Butter, 1/4, 2.7 oz	300	13	41
Pecan Coffee, 1/6, 2 oz	230	12	24
Red, White, Blueb. 1/10, 3 oz	210	8	31
Strawberry, 1/4, 2.7 oz	290	11	44
Dessert Cakes: Carrot, 1/6, 3.2 oz	320	17	39
Banana, 1/6, 2.3 oz	230	8	37
Layer Cakes: *Per 1/8 Whole*			
Strawberry Shortcake, 2.5 oz	180	7	27
Other flavors, average, 3 oz	260	13	32
Bars: 1 bar, 2.75 oz	190	14	14
Cheesecake: *Per Serving*			
Cherry/Strawberry, avg, 4.75 oz	340	12	53
Chocolate Chip, 4.3 oz	410	21	47
Peanut Butter Cup, 3.5 oz	380	22	3i4
New York Style Ch.cake: Classic, 1/6	500	30	50
Mixed Berry Swirl, 1/6	490	28	52
Choc Chip Cookie Crumble, 1/6	520	27	61
Classic Cheesecakes:			
Original Cream, 1/4 cake, 4.3 oz	340	18	38
Orig. Strawberry, 1/4 cake, 4.8 oz	330	12	49
French, 1/5, cake, 4.7 oz	410	25	41

Sara Lee (Cont)

	C	F	Cb
Cheesecake Singles: *Per Slice*			
Caramel Choc Pecan, 110g	400	25	37
Strawberry Drizzle, 113g	380	20	46
Bites: Carrot Cake Bites, 5 pces	370	25	32
Choc-Dipped Orig., 5 pces	480	33	40
Choc Praline Pecan, 5 pces	470	30	42
Toasted Almond, 5 pces	450	29	42
Triple Choc Fudge, 5 pces	170	8	24
Cream Pies (9"): *Per Serving*			
Choc. Silk; Coconut Crm, 1/5, 5 oz	500	32	49
Lemon Meringue, 1/6, 5 oz	350	11	59
Oven Fresh Pies (9"): *Per 4 1/2 oz (1/8 of Pie)*			
Apple; Cherry, average	340	16	46
Blueberry; Dutch Apple	355	15	53
Mince/Raspberry, average	380	19	48
Pecan	520	24	70
Pumpkin	260	11	37
Southern Sweet Potato	280	10	45
Deep Dish Pies: *Per 1/10 Pie (4.7 oz)*			
Cinnamon French Apple	360	15	48
Golden Peach	340	16	46
Orchard Apple	400	24	43
Individual Slices: *Per Slice*			
Apple/Cherry Pie, 4 oz	300	11	47
Carrot; Cookies N Cream, 3.5 oz	335	20	40
Lemon Icebox Pie, 3.5 oz	260	10	41
Southern Pecan Pie, 4 oz	470	23	62
Strawberry Swirl Ch'cake, 3.5 oz	300	17	31
Round Danish: Cheese, 1/6 whole	180	6	28
Butter Streusel/Pecan, 1/6	225	12	24
Raspberry, 1/6 whole	200	8	27
Deluxe Cinnamon Roll, 1/6 whole	320	15	41

TastyKake:

	C	F	Cb
Chocolate Jnr, 3.4 oz	320	12	52
Creme Filled Koffee Kakes, 3 oz	360	14	54
Koffee Kake Junior, 2 1/2 oz	250	8	40

Weight Watchers: *Per Serving*

	C	F	Cb
Brownie à la Mode	190	4	33
Chocolate Mousse	190	5	31
Chocolate Eclair	150	4	25
Choc. Chip Cookie Dough Sundae	190	4.5	35
Choc. Raspberry Royale	190	3	39
Double Fudge Brownie Parfait	190	2.5	39
Double Fudge Cake	190	4.5	36
French Style Cheesecake	170	4	28
Mississippi Mud Pie	160	5	24
New York Style Cheesecake	150	5	21
Strawberry Parfait Royale	180	2	35

Cakes & Dessert Mixes

Made As Directed	**C**	**F**	**Cb**
Betty Crocker			
Cakes (Super Moist): *Per 1/12 Cake (Prep'd)*			
Butter Recipe Yellow	260	11	36
Cherry Chip	300	13	41
Chocolate Chip	250	11	35
Creamy Swirls of Fudge, 1/9	210	8	32
Devil's Food	270	13	35
Other flavors, average	250	10	35
*Per 1/10 Cake (Prepared):*Carrot	320	15	42
Sour Cream	280	12	43
Light: White	210	3.5	43
Devil's Food; Yellow	230	4.5	43
If using No Cholesterol Recipe, deduct 40 cals and 4g fat.			
Angel Food Cakes: 1/12 mix	140	0	32
Brownie Mixes: *Per 1/20 Pkg (Prep'd)*			
Chocolate Chunk	180	9	25
Dark Chocolate	170	7	25
Fudge	170	7	24
Original Supreme	160	6	27
Peanut Butter; Walnut	180	9	24
Turtle (Caramel & Pecan)	170	8	23
Classic Dessert: Gold. Pound, 1/8	260	8	35
Boston Cream Pie, 1/10	200	4.5	38
Choc. Pudding Cake, 1/8	170	3.5	34
Date Bar, 1/12 mix, dry	160	7	23
Gingerbread Cake, 1/8	230	6	39
Lemon Chiffon, 1/16	140	3	26
Pineapple Upside Down, 1/6	400	14	64
Creamy Chilled: Banana Crm, 1/9	250	11	35
Chocolate French Silk, 1/8	270	11	39
Coconut Cream, 1/8	290	13	38
Cookies & Cream, 1/6	380	16	53
Sunkist Lemon Supreme, 1/9	320	13	52
Stir 'n Bake Mixes: *Per 1/6 Pkg*			
Carrot Cake w. Crm Chse Frosting	250	7	46
Chocolate Brownies	220	8	35
Coffee	200	6	36
Devil's Food Cake w. Choc. Frost.	240	8	42
3-Minute Snacking Cake: *Per 1/9 Pkg*			
Banana Walnut	180	6	31
Cinnamon Swirl	190	5	34
Golden Choc Chip	180	5	32
Supreme Dessert Bars: *Per Bar*			
Caramel Oatmeal; Choc. Chunk	180	9	24
Strawberry Swirl Cheesecake	180	19	20
Sunkist Lemon	140	4.5	24
Other varieties, average	170	8	24

Made As Directed	**C**	**F**	**Cb**
Aunt Jemima			
Coffee Cake, 1/8 cake, prep.	180	6	27
Duncan Hines			
Angel Food, 1/12 whole	140	0	30
Other flavors, average, 1/12	190	5	34
Cookies, all flavors, 1 cookie	65	3	8
Moist Deluxe Cake Mix:			
Average, 1/12 pkg, prepared	250	11	36
Lower Fat Recipe, 1/12 pkg, prep.	200	5	37
Estee			
Brownie, 1 pce, 2" x 2"	50	2	12
All cakes, 1/5 cake	200	4	38
Choc. Chip Cookie, 1 cookie	45	2.5	6
Jell-O-No Bake: *Prepared As Directed*			
Cheesecakes:			
Cherry/Strawberry, 1/9 pkg	300	13	42
Peanut Butter Cup, 1/8 pkg	360	23	38
Real/Homestyle, 1/6 pkg	360	17	42
Double Layer Lemon, 1/8 pkg	260	13	30
Manischewitz			
Apple Cake w. real apple, 1/6	260	10	43
Nancy's			
Petite Desserts, 1 tartlets, 0.6 oz	80	4.5	9.5
Pillsbury			
Moist Supreme: *Per 1/12 Cake (Prepared)*			
Angel Food	140	0	31
Devil's Food	270	14	33
French Vanilla; German Choc.	250	11	34
Funfetti	250	9	36
Other flavors, average 1/12	255	12	35
Streusel Coffee: 1/16 cake	260	11	37
Bundt: Hot Fudge, 1/12	350	20	39
Chocolate Caramel Nut, 1/16	290	18	28
Strawberry Cream Cheese, 1/16	300	17	34
Thick 'n Fudgy Deluxe Brownie (Mix Only):			
Chocolate Frosted, 1/16 pkg	150	4	27
Vanilla Frosted, 1/16 pkg	150	3.5	28
White Chunk, 1/16 pkg	120	4	21
w. Walnuts, 1/12 pkg	150	5	24
Double Choc, 1/16 pkg	120	2.5	23
Cheesecake Swirl, 1/18 pkg	110	3	19
Fudge, 1/20 pkg, mix	120	2.5	33

Frostings • Baking Ingredients

Cakes & Dessert Mixes (Cont)

Made As Directed

	C	F	Cb
Pillsbury (Cont)			
Deluxe Bar Mixes: *Per Serving*			
Apple Streusel	150	6	23
Chips Ahoy	150	5	25
Fudge Swirl Cookie	180	8	25
Lemon Cheesecake	190	10	22
Other flavors, average	175	7	26
Robin Hood: Yellow, 1/5 cake	280	13	37
Devil's Food, 1/5 cake	310	17	36
Sweet Rewards: Fat Free, 1/8	170	0	40
Reduced Fat, all flavors, 1/12	200	5	37
Brownie Mix: Supreme, 1 pce	150	4	27
Lowfat Fudge, 1/18 pkg	130	2.5	27
Snackwell's			
Brownie: Devil's Food, 1/12	150	2.5	28
Fudge, 1/12	150	2.5	29
Cakes: Devil's Food, 1/6 cake	200	4	38
White; Yellow, 1/6 cake	210	4.5	39
Cookies: Choc. Chip, 1/18, 1 oz	110	3	19
Chocolate Fudge, 1/18, 1 oz	90	1.5	18
Streusel Squares, 1.5 oz piece	150	3	31

Cake Frostings

	C	F	Cb
Betty Crocker			
Ready-to-Spread/Rich & Creamy:			
All flavors, 2 Tbsp	130	5	24
Whipped Deluxe, 2 Tbsp	100	5	15
Sweet Rewards: Red. Fat, 2 Tbsp	125	2	25
Frost. Mixes: C'nut Pecan, 2 T. prep	160	8	21
Duncan Hines: *Per 2 Tbsp, 1.2 oz*			
Creamy Homestyle, avg all flavors	140	5	23
Pillsbury: *Per 2 Tbsp (approx.1/12 Tub)*			
Caramel Pecan	150	8	19
Chocolate; Choc. Fudge/Mocha	140	6	21
Chocolate Cream Cheese	140	6	21
Chocolate Walnut	150	7	20
Coconut Pecan	160	10	17
Cream Cheese; Lemon	150	6	24
Dark Choc	130	6	20
All other flavors	150	6	23
Decorators, Choc., 1 Tbsp	70	2	11
Sweet Rewards			
Average all flavors, 1 Tbsp	120	2.5	24

Baking Ingredients

	C	F	Cb
Almond Paste:			
(Marzipan), 1 oz	125	7	12
Baking Powder: Regular, 1 tsp	3	0	0.5
Cream of Tartar, 1 tsp	2	0	0.5
Bisquick Baking Mix:			
Original, 1/3 cup, 11/2 oz	170	6	25
Reduced Fat, 1/3 cup, 11/2 oz	150	2.5	28
Butter/Margarine: 1/2 cup, 4 oz	820	91	0
Carob Flour, 1/2 cup	90	0.5	26
Chocolate Baking Bars: *Average All Brands*			
Unsweetened, 1 oz	150	15	8
Grated, 1 cup, 4 1/2 oz	680	68	36
Semi-sweet, 1 oz	160	8	18
Bitter-sweet/White Baking 1 oz	160	9	17
Chocolate Baking Chips: *Average All Brands*			
Milk Choc./Semi Sweet 1 oz	160	8	20
1/4 cup, 11/2 oz	240	12	30
1 cup, 6 oz	960	48	120
Cocoa Powder, Baking: *Nestle*, 1 T.	15	1	3
1/3 cup, 1 oz	80	4	12
Hershey's, 1 Tbsp	20	0.5	3
1/3 cup, 1 oz	115	3.5	21
Coconut, dried: Unsweet., 1 oz	190	18	7
Sweetened/flaked, 1 oz	135	9	14
1/2 cup, 1.3 oz	175	12	18
Toasted *(Baker's)*, 1 oz	170	13	17
Coconut Cream/Milk: *See Page 37*			
Cornstarch, 1 Tbsp	30	0	7
Flour: white: 1 Tbsp, 0.6 oz	55	0	12
1 cup, 4.4 oz	450	1	95
Whole Wheat, 1 cup, 4.2 oz	410	2	87
Flavor Extracts: *Average All Brands*			
Imitation, 1 tsp	15	0	3.5
Pure Extract, 1 tsp	20	0	4
Almond, Vanilla, 1 tsp	10	0	3
Fruit Pectin: Swtnd, 1 Tbsp, 1/2 oz	35	0	10
Unsweetened, 1 Tbsp	2	0	0.5
Gelatin, dry, 1/4 oz pkg	30	0	0
Lemon/Orange Peel, 1/4 cup	30	0	4
Rennin, 1 pkg (11g)	12	0	3
Sprinkles: All types, 1 Tbsp, 1/2 oz	70	3	10
Vinegar, aver. all types, 1 oz	4	0	1
Whey, sweet, dry, 1 oz	90	0.5	20
Yeast: Active, dry, 1/4 oz pkg	15	0	2
Fleischmann's, 0.6 oz pkg	15	0	2
Bakers, compressed, 1 oz	25	0	3
Brewers; Torula, 1 oz	80	0.5	11

Puddings, Desserts, Gelatin

Ready-To-Serve

	C	F	Cb
Instant Pudding, Reg., 1/2 cup	170	4	30
Reduced Calorie: *D-Zerta; Estee*	70	0	12
Jell-O, sugar-free, 1/2 cup	80	2	11
Royal, sugar-free, 1/2 cup	100	2	17
Del Monte Pudding Snacks	130	4	24
Fat Free Vanilla	90	0	20
Dr McDougall's Rice Pudd., 3 oz	310	1.5	69
Hershey's Portable Pud., 2.25 oz	100	3	16
Hunt's Snack Pack: Per 3.5 oz Cup			
Puddin' Cakes: Choc Brownie	180	7	27
German Choc Cake	160	3.5	30
Puddin Pie: Lemon Meringue	130	2.5	24
Apple; Choc Mud	170	7	26
Dessert Favorites: Dulche de Leche	140	5	23
Banana Cream Pie	140	6	20
Imagine Foods: **Natural Pudding (Cups)**			
Chocolate, 1/2 cup, 3.7 oz	160	3	34
Banana; B'scotch; Lemon, 1/2 pkg	140	3	30
Jell-O			
Pudding Snacks (6 Pack)			
Choc./Caramel, 4 oz (113g) each	150	4.5	27
Fat Free, 4 oz snack	100	0	23
Chocolate/Vanilla; Van. Swirls	160	5	27
Cheesecake Snacks, aver., 4 oz	150	4.5	25
Pudding Pops: Regular	80	2	12
Deluxe Chocolate covered	200	10	24
Creme Savers (1) 113g	130	3	25
Jewel: **Chef's Kitchen**			
Rice Pudding, 1/2 cup, 4.5 oz	230	8	35
Tapioca Pudding, 1/2 cup, 4.5 oz	170	8	35
Jolly Rancher: Reg., 3.5 oz cup	100	0	25
Sugar-free, all flav., 3.5 oz cup	10	0	2
Kozy Shack: Banana; Van., 4 oz	130	3	22
Lite, 4 oz	110	1	22
Rice Pudding, 4 oz cup	140	3	24
Creme Caramel Flan 1 cup, 4 oz	150	4	25
Choc./Tapioca Pudding, 4 oz	140	3	25
Manischewitz: Choc., 1/2 cup	110	0.5	26
Passover Gold Noodle, 1/2 cup	140	2	28
President's Choice			
Key Lime Pie (36oz) 1/8 pie, 4.5 oz	440	22	54
Mississippi Mud Pie (36oz) 1/9, 4 oz	380	24	37
Swiss Miss Pudding Snacks			
Swirls, Choc. Pudd. Snacks, 3 1/2 oz	150	5	23
Tapioca: 1 pudding cup, 3 1/2 oz	120	3.5	21
Fat Free varieties, 3 1/2 oz	90	0	20
Weight Watchers (Frozen)			
Chocolate Mousse, 2 3/4 oz	190	5	31

Homemade Puddings

	C	F	Cb
Apple Tapioca, 1/2 cup	150	0	32
Bread Pudding, 1/2 cup	250	8	40
Blancmange, 1/2 cup	140	5	19
Chocolate, 1/2 cup	190	6	30
Corn Pudding, 1/2 cup	135	4	21
Crème Brûlée, 1/2 cup	400	35	16
Plum Pudding, 2 oz	170	3	32
Rennin Dessert, 1/2 cup	115	4	16
Rice with Raisins, 1/2 cup	200	4	38
Sponge Pudding, 3 1/2 oz	340	16	45
Tapioca Cream, 1/2 cup	110	4	15
Trifle, 1/2 cup	180	7	26

Custards

	C	F	Cb
Custard Mix			
Jell-O (Americana) Golden Egg:			
Dry, 1/6 pkg	80	0	19
Prep. w. 2% milk, 1/2 cup	140	2.5	19
Jello Flan, w. 2% milk, 1/2 cup	140	2.5	20
Royal-Flan: Prep. w 2% milk, 1/2 c.	130	2.5	18
Homemade Custard			
Baked, plain, 1/2 cup, 4 1/2 oz	150	7	16
w. skim milk, artif. sweetened	70	3	4
Boiled, 1/2 cup	165	7	18

Meringues

	C	F	Cb
Meringue Swirl, 1/2 oz	50	0	8
Meringue Shell, 1 oz shell	100	0	16
(Add extra calories/fat/carbohydrate for fillings)			

Jell-O • Cups • Parfait

	C	F	Cb
Gelatin Mix: *Jell-O, Royal ~ Made Up*			
Regular, all flavors, 1/2 cup	80	0	18
Sugar Free/Low Cal., 1/2 cup	8	0	0
Gel Gelatin/Parfait: *Per 1/2 Cup*			
Ida Mae, 1/2 cup	60	2	10
Winky: Strawberry (109g)	110	1.5	22
Rainbow (130g)	100	0	24
Reser's, Dessert Parfait (110g)	100	2	19
Mrs Crockett's Kitchen, Str. Parfait	160	4	26
Gel Snack Cups, *Del Monte/Jell-O*	70	0	17
Jell-O Extreme Gel Snack (1)	60	0	14
Jolly Rancher Portable Gel Snacks,			
All types, 1 tube, 2.25 oz	60	0	15

Quick Guide

Pancakes

	C	F	Cb
Plain: *Average All Types*			
Small (3" diam.), 3/4 oz	50	2.5	6
Medium (4" diam.), 1 1/4 oz	80	3	11
Large (5" diam.), 2 1/2 oz	160	6	21
Add Extra for Syrups/Butter			
Pancake Syrup: Regular, 1 Tbsp	50	0	13
1/4 cup	200	0	52
Lite, 1 Tbsp	25	0	6
1/4 cup	100	0	24
Butter/Margarine: Regular, 1 T.	100	11	0
Whipped, 1 Tbsp	70	7.5	0

Restaurant Style Pancakes

	C	F	Cb
Denny's			
Hot Cakes, Plain, 3	490	7	95
w. Syrup & Butter	725	17	130
Original Grand Slam Breakfast	795	50	65
w. Syrup & Margarine	1030	60	101
Maple Flav. Syrup, 1 serving	145	0	36
Whipped Margarine, 1/2 oz	90	10	0
Hardees			
3 Pancakes (no fat)	280	2	56
w. Sausage Pattie	430	16	56
w. 2 Bacon Strips	350	10	56
IHOP (International House of Pancakes)			
Pancakes (Syrup/Butter extra):			
Buttermilk, 1 (2 oz)	110	3	17
Short Stack, 3	330	9	51
Full Stack, 5	550	15	85
Buckwheat, 1 (2 oz)	110	4	15
Country Griddle, 1 (2 oz)	120	3.5	19
Harvest Grain 'N Nut, (2 1/4 oz)	180	9	20
Crepes (Egg Pancakes), 1 (2 oz)	120	6	14
Waffles (Plain): Regular, 1 (3 oz)	310	15	37
Belgian: Regular, 1 (4 oz)	390	19	48
Crepe: Egg, 1 (2 oz)	120	6	14
McDonalds			
Hotcakes, Plain (3)	340	8	58
w. Marg. (2 pats) & Syrup (1)	600	17	104
Perkins			
Buttermilk, 3, plain	440	12	70
Harvest Grain: Short Stack, Plain, 3	270	2	56
w. lowcal Syrup	295	2	63
5-Stack w. Lowcal Syrup	475	3.5	93

Brands

	C	F	Cb
Aunt Jemima			
Frozen: Lowfat, 3	130	2	33
Original; Blueberry, 3	200	3	40
Pancake & Waffle Mix:			
Original, 1/3 cup, prepared	240	6.5	38
Complete, 1/3 cup	160	2.5	32
Mini Pancakes (13)	240	4	46
Thaw & Pour B'milk Pancake Batter:			
1/2 cup, 4 x 4" pancakes	260	3.5	51
Betty Crocker Pancake Mixes			
Complete Original, 3	200	3	40
Complete Buttermilk, 3	200	2.5	40
Bisquick (Shake 'N Pour)			
Pancake & Waffle Mixes:			
Average, all types, 3	200	3	38
Hungry Jack Pancakes			
Mixes: Per 1/3 Cup (prep.)			
Buttermilk: Complete, 1/3 cup	160	1.5	32
Original, w. 2% Milk, Oil, Egg	290	13	32
w. Skim Milk, Oil, Egg Whites	220	6	32
Extra Lights: Complete	150	2	30
Microwave: Buttermilk, 3	270	4.5	51
Original, 3 pancakes	270	4.5	51
Northern Pines: Complete Gourmet			
3 x 4" pancakes, 3.5 oz	380	7	71

Waffles

	C	F	Cb
Homemade: 7" waffle, 2 1/2 oz	245	13	26
From Mix: 7" waffle, 2 1/2 oz	205	8	28

Frozen Waffles

	C	F	Cb
Aunt Jemima: Blueberry, 1	95	3	15
Buttermilk, 1	100	3	17
Eggo *(Kelloggs):* Banana Bread, 1	95	3	6
Chocolate Chip, 1 waffle	100	3.5	16
Cinnamon Toast, 1 set	96	3	15
Homestyle, average, 1	95	3.5	15
Nut & Honey, 1	110	4.5	15
Nutri-Grain, 1	85	2.5	14
Special K (fat free), 1	60	0	13
Waf-fulls, all types, 1, 2 oz	160	5	26
GO-LEAN (Kashi): Average, 1	90	1.5	16
Hungry Jack: Blueberry, 1 waffle	105	4	17
Buttermilk; Homestyle, 1	95	3	16
Mini Funfetti, 1	65	2	11

Sugar, Syrup, Jam, Honey

Sugar

	C	F	Cb
White Sugar, granulated:			
1 level teaspoon, 4g	15	0	4
1 heaping teaspoon, 6g	25	0	6.5
1 cube, 1/2"	24	0	6.5
Single portion, 1 packet	25	0	6.5
1 Tablespoon, 12g	48	0	12
1 ounce, 1 oz	110	0	20
1 cup, 7 oz	770	0	203
1 pound	1760	0	464
Brown Sugar:			
1 Tbsp, 13g	50	0	13
1 ounce, 1 oz	109	0	28
1 cup, not packed, 5 oz	540	0	140
1 cup, packed, 7 3/4 oz	845	0	218
Powdered/Confectioners:			
Sifted, 1 cup, 3 1/2 oz	385	0	98
Unsifted, 1 cup, 4 1/4 oz	460	0	117
Other Sugars			
Glucose, 1 oz	110	0	27
Tablets (Dex 4), 1	15	0	4
Barley/Wheat/Rye Malt, 1 Tbsp, 3/4 oz	60	0	14
Cinnamon Sugar, 1 tsp	15	0	4
Dextrose, 1 oz	110	0	27
Fructose: 1 tsp	15	0	4
3 Tbsp, 1 oz	110	0	27
FruitSource: 1 oz (powder)	110	0	27
Sorbitol, 1 oz	110	0	27
Turbinado Sugar, 2 Tbsp, 1 oz	110	0	27
Unrefined Cane Sugar, 1 oz	110	0	27

Sugar Substitutes

	C	F	Cb
DiabetiSweet, 1 teaspoon (Carbohydrate as Sugar Alcohol)	9	0	4
Equal: Tablet/Liquid	0	0	0
Granulated, 1 pkg	4	0	1
NutraSweet Spoonful, 1 tsp	2	0	0.5
Nutra Taste, 1 pkt	0	0	0
Sprinkle Sweet, 1 tsp	2	0	0.5
Stevia, 1 pkt	0	0	0
Sugar Delight, 1 pkt	8	0	2
Sugar Like (Bateman's), 1 tsp	4	0	1
Sugar Twin: 1 pkt	3	0	0
Sugar Substitute, 1 tsp	2	0	0
Sweet 'N Low, 1 pkt	0	0	1
Sweet One, 1 pkt	0	0	0
Walgreens Wal-Sweet, 1 pkt	0	0	0
Weight Watchers Sweetener, 1 tsp	4	0	1

Honey, Jam, Preserves

Average All Brands	C	F	Cb
Honey: 1 tsp, 1/4 oz	22	0	5.5
1 Tbsp, 3/4 oz	65	0	17
1 ounce, 1 oz	86	0	23
1 cup, 12 oz	1030	0	269
Single Portion, 1/2 oz pkg	43	0	11
Jams/Jellies/Marmalade/Preserves			
Regular, 1 tsp, 1/4 oz	18	0	5
1 Tbsp, 3/4 oz	55	0	16
1 ounce	75	0	22
Single Portion, 1/2 oz pkg	38	0	11
Apple/Fruit Butters, 1 T., 0.6 oz	20	0	6
Fruit Spreads: Regular, 1 tsp	16	0	4
Low Sugar, 1 tsp	8	0	2
Low Cal. (Featherweight), 1 tsp	4	0	1
Jelly: Regular, average, 1 tsp	18	0	4.5
Imitation, Low Calorie, 1 tsp	4	0	1

Syrups, Molasses

Syrups: *Average All Types & Brands*
(Corn/Rice/Maple/Pancake/Sundae/Waffle)
Includes *Aunt Jemima, Cary's, Karo, Hershey's, Hungry Jack, Log Cabin, Mrs Butterworth's*

	C	F	Cb
Regular/Dark/Light Color:			
1 Tbsp, 1/2 fl.oz	55	0	14
1/4 cup (4 Tbsp)	220	0	55
Single Portion: 1 1/2 oz pkg	170	0	42
Lite: 1Tbsp	25	0	6
1/4 cup (4 Tbsp)	100	0	25
Sugar-Free: Cary's, 2 Tbsp, 1 oz	18	0	5
Cozy Cottage, 2 Tbsp, 1 oz	10	0	3
Molasses: Dark/Light: 1 T., 3/4 oz	55	0	14
1 cup, 11 1/2 oz	880	0	224
Blackstrap: 1 Tbsp, 3/4 oz	47	0	13
1 cup, 11 1/2 oz	750	0	208

Icecream Toppings

Average All Types & Brands (Hershey's, Kraft, Smuckers)	C	F	Cb
Butterscotch, Caramel, 2 Tbsp	140	1	30
Chocolate, Hot Fudge, 2 Tbsp	140	4	22
Fat Free (Hershey's), 2 Tbsp	100	0	23
Pineapple, Strawberry, 2 Tbsp	110	0	28
Smuckers: Guilt-Free, all flavors	100	0	24
Magic Shell, 2 Tbsp	210	15	18
Milky Way, 2 Tbsp	130	3.5	24
Lite Hot Fudge, 2 Tbsp	90	0	23

Quick Guide

Chocolate

Average All Brands

	C	**F**	**Cb**
Milk Chocolate, regular:			
Plain/Nuts/Fruit, average, 1 oz	150	10	13
1½ oz Bar	225	15	23
2 oz Bar	300	20	30
4 oz Block	600	40	60
8 oz Block	1200	80	120
1 Pound, 16 oz	2400	160	240
Dark/White Chocolate, 1 oz	150	10	16
Chocolate-coated:			
Almonds, 5-6, 1 oz	160	11	11
Clusters, nut, 2, 1 oz	160	11	15
Coffee Beans, 1.4 oz	180	10	23
Creme/Cordial Centers, 1 oz	120	4	21
Fudge, 1 oz	125	5	18
Macadamias, 2-3 pces., 1 oz	180	13	11
Mints, 1 med., 11g	45	1	9
Nougat & Caramel, 1 oz	120	4	21
Peanuts, 12 med., 1 oz	160	11	15
Raisins, 30 med., 1 oz	120	4	21
Cooking Chocolate:			
Sweet/Semi-sweet, 1 oz	160	8	18
Chips, ¼ cup, 2½ oz	210	12	24
Unsweetened, 1 oz	150	15	8
Carob: Plain, 1 oz	160	11	9

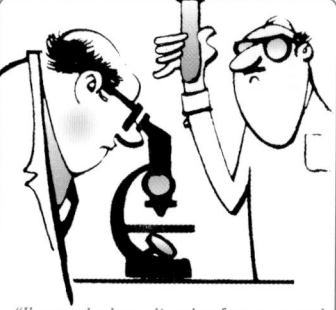

"I've worked on vitamins for years and I've discovered that the three most important elements necessary to life are breakfast, lunch and dinner."

Brands & Generic

Per Piece/Serving	**C**	**F**	**Cb**
Abba Zaba, 2 oz bar	250	5	48
Absolutely Almond, 2.5 oz bar	380	23	40
Aero Bar *(Nestlé)*, 1.45 oz bar	210	13	26
After Dinner Mints, 1 small	45	1	9
After Eight Mint, each	35	1.2	6
Air Head, 2 bars, 1 oz	120	1	30
Allen Wertz: Simply Sugar Free			
Coffee Time (decaf), 4	45	1.5	8
Coffee Toffee, 6	120	3	23
Other types, 4	120	2.5	24
Almond Joy, 1.76 oz bar	240	13	29
King Size, 2 pces, 1.6 oz	220	12	27
Snack, 1, 0.68 oz	90	5	11
Bites (18) 1.4 oz	230	14	23
Almond Roca, 1 pce	70	5	6
Almonds, sugar-coated, 7, 1 oz	130	5	20
Almond Clusters *(Trader Joe's)*,			
2 pce, 1.2 oz	210	14	5
Altoids *(C & B)*, each	3	0	1
Amazin' Fruit, 1 bag, 1.9 oz	180	0	41
Andes: Creme de Menthe; Cherry Jubilee			
Choc covered Patty, (3), 1½ oz	180	3	35
Thins, aver. all flav., (8), 1.4 oz	210	13	22
Anthon Berg: Cognac, each	180	8	25
After Dinner Sweet:			
Marzipan w. Madeira, 1.4 oz	175	7.5	26
Marcipan Brod	120	7	13
Asteroid *(Nestlé)*, 54g	260	10	40
Baby Ruth, King Size, 3.7 oz bar	480	24	66
2.1 oz bar	280	13	34
Fun size, each	100	4.5	17
Snack, 1 bar, ¾ oz	100	5	12
Baci *(Perugino)*, each	85	5	8
Bar, 1.58 oz	230	15	27
Bar None, 1.5 oz bar	240	14	23
Barley Sugar, 1 pce., 0.2 oz	23	0	6
Baskin31 Robbins, 3 pce, 0.5 oz	60	1	13
Big Hunt, 2 oz	230	3	47
Bit-O-Honey, 1.7 oz	200	3.5	41
Chews, 6 pces, 1.4 oz	170	3	34
Blow Pops, each	50	0	14
Bonus Bar, 2.1 oz bar	290	16	34
Boston Baked Beans, 30 pces, 1 oz	135	5	20
Brach's: Almond Supremes,11	220	15	18
Butterscotch Disks, 3, 0.6 oz	70	0	16
Choc Bridge Mix, 16, 1.4 oz	190	9	25

Candy, Chocolate (Cont)

Per Piece/Serving	C	F	Cb
Brach's (Cont):			
Circus Peanuts, each	25	0.6	3
Clusters, 3	220	14	19
Double Dip Choc Peanuts, 15	220	14	19
Golden Butter/Internation. Toffee	25	0.6	5
Lemon Drops, 4, 0.6 oz	50	0	13
Malted Milk Balls, 15	190	9	27
Milk Maid Caramel, 18	170	5	30
Orange Slices Hi-C, each	50	0	13
Breath Savers, all types, each	10	0	2
Brite Crackers, 1 bag, 1.5 oz	140	0	32
Brock: Candy Corn, (10) 0.7 oz	75	0	18
Gummy Bears; Sour Balls, each	26	0	6
Lemon Drops, each	20	0	5
Orange Slices, each	35	0	9
Spice Drops, each	12	0	3
Starlight Mints, each	20	0	5
Toffee, each	25	0.8	5
Bubble Gum: See 'Gum'			
Buncha Crunch, 1/2 cup, 1.4 oz	200	10	26
Burnt Peanuts, 40 pces, 40g	190	8	32
Butterfinger:			
Hug Size, 3.7 oz bar	480	18	75
2.1 oz bar	270	11	41
Fun size, each	100	3.5	15
Mini, each	20	1	7
Snack, 2, 1.3 oz	170	7	27
Butterfinger B.B's, 1.7 oz bag	220	9	34
Buttermints, 18 pces, 1 1/2 oz	160	0	40
Butterscotch: 5 pces	120	2.5	20
Buttons (Walgreens), 3, 18g	70	0	16
Chips, 1 oz	150	7	36
Discs (Sathers), 3, 0.6 oz	110	0	16
Candy Cane, Medium, 5", 1/2 oz	50	0	12
Candy Corn, 1 oz	110	0	24
4 oz pkt: 24 pces, 1 1/2 oz	150	0	37
Candy Jar Mix (Jewel), 3, 17g	70	0	17
Candy Necklaces, 20g each	80	0.5	20
Caramels:	30	1	6
Chocolate, each	25	0.3	6
Creams, 3 pces, 1 1/4 oz	130	3	23
2.75 oz pkt, 5 pces, 1 1/2 oz	160	3.5	30
Hershey's Classic Caramels:			
Soft 'n Chewy, 3 pces	80	2	15
Choc Creme Filled, 3 pces	80	3	13
Caramel Nips, each	30	1	6
Caramel Popcorn, 1 cup, 1 oz	120	1.5	26

Per Piece/Serving	C	F	Cb
Caramel Truffles (Godiva), 1 pce	110	6.5	11
Caramello (Hershey's) 1.6 oz bar	220	10	29
Snack, 0.66 oz	90	4	12
Cadbury, 1.6 oz bar	210	9	29
Kingsize, 2.7 oz bar	360	16	49
Certs: Breath Mints, 1 pce	6	0	2
Sugar-free, 1 piece	7	0	2
Charleston Chew, 1 bar, 53g	230	7	40
Cherry Sours (Sathers), 11, 1 1/2 oz	150	0	38
Chews, all types, 1 oz	110	1	25
Chocolate Mints (Hershey's), each	20	0.5	4
Chocolate Parfait Nips, each	30	1	5
Chuckles Jelly: each	35	0	9
Jujubes, each	10	0	3
Chunky Bar (Nestlé), 1.4 oz	210	11	24
Chupa Chups, 1 pce, 0.42 oz	50	0	11
Cinnamon Bears (Walgreens), 5	150	0	38
Cinn. Buttons (Walgreens), 3 pce	70	0	17
Cinnamon Drops (Sathers), 19 pce	150	0	36
Coconut Stacks, 4, 41g	190	6	33
Coffee Go Coffee/Cappuccino, ea.	18	0.4	4
Coffee Rio-Gold, each	15	0.5	1
Collard & Bowser: Eng. Toffee, 2	80	4	12
Corn Nuts, 1/3 cup, 1 oz	130	4	20
Cote d'Or: Bouchee, each	130	8	12
Chokotoff, each	210	9	30
Nougatti	150	8	19
Bar & Nuts,1.3 oz	220	18	12
Cotton Candy, 1 oz	70	0	17
Cough Drops: See Page 130			
Cracker Jack, 1.25 oz box	150	2.5	29
Crisped Rice: Almond, 1 bar	130	6	18
Choc Chip, 1 bar	115	4	18
Crispy Rice Snacks, 1 bar	70	2.5	10
Crows, 7 oz pkg	150	0	37
Crunch: 5 oz bar	725	38	90
King Munch, 2.75 oz bar	400	20	51
1.55 oz bar	230	12	29
Fun size, each	50	2.5	7
Snack (3), 1 1/2 oz	220	11	28
Pieces, 1/4 cup, 38g	190	10	25
White Bar, 1.4 oz bar	220	13	23
Crunch Berries Treats, 1.6 oz bar	190	4.5	36
Decadence (NuBar) Bar, 1.3 oz	140	2.5	30
Dots, 12 dots	150	0	37
Double Dip Stick, 1 stick	16	0.5	3

Per Piece/Serving	C	F	Cb
Dove: Dark/Milk, 1.3 oz bar	200	12	22
Bar, 6 oz	920	56	104
Miniatures, each	30	2	3
Drops Candy (9)	100	0	24
Dum Dum Pops *(Spangler)*, 1 pop	25	0	6
English Toffee, 1 pce	48	3	5
Eda's Sugar Free, all flav., 5, 1/2 oz	40	0	15
Estee Dietetic Candies:			
Caramels, all flavors, 1 pce	30	1	5
Chocolate, Dark/ Mint, 1/2 bar	200	14	23
Gummy Bears; Gum Drops, 1 pce	7	0	1.5
Hard Candies: Butterscotch, 2	25	0	6
Assorted Fruit Lollipops, 5	60	0	15
Peppermint, 3	30	0	7
Mint/Toffee, 5	60	0	15
Lollipop	30	0	8
Milk Chocolate, 1/2 bar, 4 oz	230	17	17
Peanut Butter Cups, 1 cup	40	3	3
Fructose Sweetened, 1 cup	40	2	3
Peanut Brittle, 1/3 box, 1.5 oz	240	9	28
5th Avenue: 2 oz bar	280	13	35
King Size bar	460	20	64
Snack Size, 0.58 oz	80	3.5	1
Fanny May: Single wrapped pces			
Mint Meltaway Patty, 1.5 oz	250	17	22
Pixie, 1.5 oz	215	12	24
Trinidad, 1.5 oz	205	11	24
Fast Break, 2 oz	270	13	34
Ferrero Rocher: each	75	5	6
3 pces, 1.3 oz	220	15	17
Fifty 50 Snack Bars:			
Peanut Butter, 2	200	14	16
Almond Choc., 7 pce, 1 1/2 oz	210	15	20
Crunch Choc., 1.1 oz	160	11	19
Fruit & Nut Choc., 7 pce, 1 1/2 oz	200	14	21
Milk Choc., 3 pce, 1/2 bar, 43g	210	14	25
Mini bars, 8 bars, 1 oz	140	9	16
Fluffy Stuff *(Harms)*, 0.6 oz bag	70	0	17
Fondant: Choc-coated, 1.2 oz	130	3	28
Mint, 1 oz	105	0	27
Franklin Crunch 'N Munch:			
all varieties, average, 1.25 oz	170	7	30
Fran's: Gold Bar, 1.75 oz	260	14	34
Gold Bites (Almonds), 1	130	7	17
Fruit Crystals *(Walgreens)*, 3 pces	70	0	17
Fruit Drops, each	6	0	1
Fruit Gems *(Sunkist)*, 3, 1.1 oz	105	0	26

Per Piece/Serving	C	F	Cb
Fruit Leathers, average, 0.5 oz	45	0	12
Fruit Pastilles, 1 roll, 1.4 oz	100	0	26
Fruit Rolls, 1 roll	80	0	20
Fruit Roll-Ups, 1/2 oz	50	0	12
Fruit Runts *(Walgreens)*, 1T., 1/4 pkt	60	0	14
Fruit Shapes *(Fruitfield)*, 1 oz (10)	100	0.5	9
Fruit Waves, 0.5 oz	50	0	12
Fudge: Chocolate/Vanilla, 1 oz	115	3	20
with Nuts, 1 oz	120	4	21
Choco. Marshmallow, 1 oz	120	5	18
w. Nuts, 1 oz	125	5.5	18
Peanut Butter, 1 oz	105	2	21
Ghirardelli: Milk/Dark Chocolate,			
1.25 oz bar	185	12	20
w. almonds, 1.5 oz bar	220	14	25
Choc Nuts & Chews, 1 pce	55	3.5	5
Godiva: Hearts, each	45	2	6
Almond Butter Dome, 1 pce	80	6	6
Bouchee au Chocolate, 1 pce	220	13	23
Cordial Assortment, each	60	2.5	9
Gold Ballotin, 1 pce	70	3.5	9
Milk/Dark/IvoryAssortment, each	75	4	8
Nut & Caramel, each	75	4	6
Truffle Amaretto, 1 pce	110	6.5	12
Golden Almond Bar, 1 bar	520	34	40
Golden 111 Bar, 1 bar	500	30	52
Go Lightly: Box Candies, 4	60	0	15
Bags: Assorted Taffy, 6	140	3	36
Vanilla Caramels, 5	150	6	31
Super Free Choc Crunch (7) 1 1/2 oz	180	13	23
Goobers Peanuts, 1 pkg, 1.4 oz	210	13	20
Good & Fruity, 1 box, 1.8 oz	140	1	35
Snack Size, 1 box, 17g	60	0	15
Good & Plenty, 1.8 oz box	160	0	40
Snack Size, 1 box, 17g	60	0	14
GooGoo Cluster, 1 bar, 1.75 oz	240	11	32

Rev. Dr Robert Schuller

*Inch by inch
Life's a cinch*

*You'll never win
If you don't begin!*

Candy, Chocolate (Cont)

Per Piece/Serving	C	F	Cb
GUM: *Per Piece*			
Bazooka, each	30	0	7
Beechies	6	0	2
Big League Chew	10	0	2
Bubble Gum Balls (*Hershey's*)	10	0	2
Bubble Yum	25	0	6
Sugarless	10	0	3
Candilicious	30	0	2
Carefree (Sugarless/Regular)	5	0	2
Chiclets	5	0	1
Clorets, stick	10	0	2
Dentyne	6	0	2
Estee, bubble/regular	5	0	2
Extra (*Wrigley's*),			
Sugar-Free Bubble Gum, 1	5	0	2
Freshen-Up	13	0	2
Hubba Bubba: Regular	23	0	6
Sugar-free, average	14	0	0.5
Ice Breakers, 1 stick	5	0	2
Sonic Boom Bubble Gum	15	0	3
Sticklets	7	0	2
Super Bubble	15	0	4
Trident: Slab	5	0	1
Soft Bubble Gum	9	0	1
Wrigley's, all flavors	10	0	2
Gum Drops: 1 small	15	0	3
1 large, 0.4 oz	40	0	7
6 oz pkt: 4 pces, 1.4 oz	130	0	31
Gummi Bears: 1 bear	17	0	4
8 bears, 1¹⁄₂ oz	140	0	32
Gummi Novelties (*Walgreens*), 6	150	0	22
Gummi Savers, each	12	0	3
Gummi Sweet Tarts, 1 bug, 1.5 oz	150	0	34
Gummi Watch, 1, 2 oz	105	0	24
Gummi Worms, each	25	0	5
Guylian: No Sugar Added			
Milk Chocolate, 8 squares, 1 oz	126	9	15
Dark Chocolate, 8 squares, 1 oz	117	9	14
Halvah (*Joyvah*):			
Plain/Marble, ¹⁄₂ bar, 2 oz	390	25	18
Choc.coated Sesame, ¹⁄₂ bar, 2 oz	380	23	20
Hard Candy: All flavors, 1 oz	110	0	28
1 regular piece	18	0	5
Heath: Original, 1.4 oz bar	210	12	24
Bites, 1.4 oz	210	12	25
Snack, 0.33 oz	50	3	6

Per Piece/Serving	C	F	Cb
Hershey's:			
Bar: 1.55 oz bar	240	14	25
King Size bar, 2.6 oz	410	25	38
w. Almonds, 1.45 oz	230	14	20
Cookies 'n' Creme, 1.55oz bar	230	12	26
Bites: Almond Joy (18)	230	14	23
Cookies 'n' Creme (7)	90	5	10
York (15), 39g	150	3	31
Milk Choc w. Almond (17)	220	14	20
Cookies 'N Mint: 1.55 oz bar	230	12	27
Snack, 0.6 oz	90	4.5	11
Crunchy Cookie Cups, 1.4 oz	210	12	23
Hugs: Regular (1), 4.5g	25	1.5	3
Regular (9), 40g	220	13	23
w. Almonds (9), 40g	230	13	22
Kisses: Milk Choc./Almond (1)	25	1.5	3
Milk Chocolate: 1.55 oz bar	230	13	25
Kingsize, 2.6 oz bar	400	23	42
7 oz bar, ¹⁄₅ bar	200	12	21
w. Almonds Snack, 0.6 oz	90	6	8
Miniatures, 5 pces, 1.5 oz	230	13	25
Nuggets: Snack, aver. all bars (1)	50	3	6
P'nut Butter Crispy Rice, (1)	230	13	25
Special Dark Choc., 1.45 oz	230	13	25
Sweet Escapes:			
1.4 oz bar, average	180	7	27
Snack, average all bars (1)	80	3.5	12
Whoppers, 10 pce	100	4	16
Honeycomb: Plain, 1 oz	115	0	27
Choc-coated, 1 oz	125	1	28
Hot Tamales: 1 box, 60g, 2.1 oz	220	0	55
Sathers, 19 pces, 1.4 oz	150	0	36
Ice Blue Mints (*Walgreens*), 3, 17g	70	0	17
Jawbreakers (*Sathers*), 3, 17g	70	0	17
Jellies, 3 medium, 1 oz	120	0	30
Jells Raspberry (*Joyva*), each	70	1	8
Jelly Beans: Small, 22 beans, 1 oz	100	0	24
Regular, 12 beans, 1 oz	100	0	24
1 bean	8	0	2
Jumbo, 1 bean	20	0	5
Jewel, 13 beans, 1.4 oz	140	0	36
Sathers/Walgreens, (17) 40g	150	0	37
Wonderbeans, 33 beans	100	0	24
Jelly Bellys: each	4	0	1
32 pces, 1.4 oz	150	0	37
1 tin, 2.5 oz	250	0	65
Jelly Rings (*Jewel*) (3) 1.5 oz	160	0	39

Candy, Chocolate (Cont)

Per Piece/Serving	C	F	Cb
Jolly Rancher: Candy (1)	40	0	9
Fruit Chews (6), 1.4 oz	150	1.5	33
Hard Candy (3), 18g	70	0	17
Jolly Jellies, 7 oz	120	0	30
Lollipops, 1 pce, 0.6 oz	60	0	16
Sugar Free, 4 pces, 0.5 oz	35	0	14
Junior Mints: 1.84 oz box	210	3.5	40
16 pces, 1.4 oz	160	2.5	34
Juicefuls: Red Raspb., (3), 0.6 oz	60	0	15
Assorted Fruits, 1 pce	20	0	5
Jujubes, all types (6), 1.4 oz	3	0	3
Juju Mix (Sathers), 11 pce, 1 1/2 oz	150	0	36
Juju Toys, 6 pce, 1.4 oz	150	0	37
Jujyfruits, 1 box, 0.2 oz	40	0	10
Kit Kat: 1.5 oz bar	220	11	27
2.6 oz bar	365	21	40
Big Kat, 1.94 oz	290	15	35
Bites (15), 1.4 oz	200	10	25
King Size, 3 oz bar	440	22	54
Multipack, each	80	4	10
Snack, 3 (2 pce bars), 1.65 oz	240	12	30
Wafer Bar, 2 pce, 0.56 oz	80	4	10
Krackel: 2.6 oz bar	390	21	45
Snack size, 0.3 oz	45	2.5	5
Kraft: Caramels, (5), 40g	160	3.5	30
Kudos: 1 oz bar, aver. all types	120	5	20
M&M's Milk Choc Minis, 0.8 oz	90	2.5	17
Snickers, 0.8 oz	100	3.5	16
Lance: Popscotch, 1.2 oz pkg	160	6	24
Chocolaty Peanut Bar, 2 oz bar	320	18	30
Peanut Bar, 1.8 oz pkg	260	14	24
Lemon Drops, 3, 1/2 oz	50	0	12
Sugar Free (Walgreens), 5, 1/2 oz	35	0	14
Lemonhead, 10, 1/2 oz	60	0	14
Licorice:			
Average all types, 1oz	100	0	25
Bites (Switzer), each	12	0	1
Chews (Panda), each	10	0	2
Tid Bits, each	5	0	1
Twists: Black/Red, aver. 1 pce	30	0	7
American Licorice Co.: Laces, 1	35	0	8
Stick, (1) 0.5 oz	45	0	11
Choco Sticks, (4) 1.4 oz	145	0	35
Red Bites, 1.4 oz	140	0	34
Super Red Ropes, 1 rope, 2 oz	200	0	46
Vines, 1 pce	70	0	17

Per Piece/Serving	C	F	Cb
Lifesavers: Large size, 1 candy	15	0	4
Regular, all flavors, 1 candy	9	0	2
1 Roll (14 candies), 1.14 oz	130	0	32
Creme Savers (1)	23	0.5	4
Sugar-free Delites: *Per Candy*			
Orchard Fruits; Summer Blend	5	0	2
Butter Toffee; European Collect.	9	0.5	3
Gummi Savers, 1.5 oz roll	140	0	32
Lollipops Fruit, 1 pce, 0.4 oz	45	0	11
Pepomint, 4 mints	60	0	15
Lik-m-aid (Nestlé), 1.7 oz	60	0	15
Lindt: Lindor, Balls, average	73	4	8
Dark Choc Truffles, each	70	6	4
Lollipops, each, 0.2 oz	20	0	5
Lollipops C Pops (Glenny's), each	35	0	8
Mamba, 9 pces, 1 1/2 oz	160	2	36
M&M's: Plain, 1.7 oz pkg	240	10	34
Milk Chocolate, 1 pce	4	0.2	0.5
20 pces, 0.6 oz	80	4	10
1/4 cup, 1.5 oz	210	9	30
Almond Choc., 1.3 oz pkg	200	11	21
1.5 oz pkg	230	13	25
Caramel, 1/4 cup, 1.5 oz	220	11	28
Crispy, 1.65 oz	220	9	34
King Size, 1/2 pkg, 1.6 oz	220	9	32
1.5 oz pkg	220	11	26
Minis, Mega Tube, 1.94oz tube	270	11	37
Peanut: 1.7 oz pkg	250	13	30
Fun Size, 0.7 oz pkg	110	5	13
Peanut Butter: 1.6 oz pkg	240	13	27
Fun Size, 0.7 oz pkg	110	6	12
Mars Bar: All varieties, 1.76 oz	240	13	31
Fun size, 1 bar	95	5	12
Marshmallows: Firm/Soft, 1 oz	90	0	23
Regular size, 6 pce, 33g	110	0	26
Mini-Marshmallow, 1/2 c., 30g	100	0	24
Choc-coat. Twists (Joyva), ea.	95	2	10
Kraft: Mini, 1/2 cup	80	0	21
Creme, 2 Tbsp	40	0	10
Jet-Puffed, 5 pces	90	0	23
Funmallows, each	25	0	6
Miniature, 1/2 cup	100	0	25
Teddy Bear, 1/2 cup	50	0	12
Marshmallow Egg, 1 egg	110	0	24
Marzipan: 1 oz	140	7	16
Mauna Loa: Choc., 2.5 oz bar	420	29	36
Choc. coated Macadamias, 9	230	17	19

Candy, Chocolate (Cont)

Per Piece/Serving	C	F	Cb
Mega Fruit Gummi, each	10	0	2
Mexican Hats, (9)	100	0	24
Mentos, each	10	0	2
Milkfulls (Storck): (6), 1.4 oz	170	3	35
Mike & Ike: 1 pkg, 2.1 oz	220	0	55
19 pce, 1.45 oz	150	0	36
Milk Choc. (Hershey's): 1.55 oz bar	240	14	25
Eggs, candy coated (4)	90	4	12
w. Almonds, 1.45 oz bar	230	14	20
Milk Choc. Crisp, 1.45 oz bar	205	11	22
Milk Duds, 1.85 oz pkg	240	9	37
Milk Shake Bar, 1.8 oz bar	220	7	37
Milky Way: Regular Bar, 2 oz	270	10	41
Fun size, 2 bars, 1.4 oz	180	7	28
King Size, 3.63 oz bar	480	18	72
Midnight, 1.76 oz bar	220	4.5	36
Miniatures, (5) 43g	190	7	30
Milky Way Lite, 1.57 oz	170	5	34
Miniatures, 1.4 oz pkg (5)	150	4.5	29
Midnight Bar, 1.75 oz	220	8	36
Mints: Uncoated, 1 oz	100	0	23
1 small mint (3/4" diam.)	7	0	2
1 large mint (1 1/2" diam.)	30	0	7
Mon Cheri (Ferrero), 4 pces, 45g	260	18	20
Mounds: 1.75 oz bar	240	13	29
Snack, 0.68 oz	90	5	11
Mr Goodbar:			
King Size, 2.6 oz bar	420	26	38
1.75 oz bar	270	16	27
Snack, 0.3 oz	45	3	4
Necco Candy Wafers (3) 57g	15	0	4
Neuhaus, average all types	80	5	7
Newman's Own: Pepp. Cups, 1 pkg	170	11	20
P'Nut B. Cups (Milk/Dark), 3, 1 pkg	180	12	17
Nibs, all types, 1 pouch, 0.5 oz	45	0	11
Nips (Pearson), all flavors, 2, 14g	60	2	10
Nite Bite (Glucose Bar)	100	3.5	15
Nothing But Nuts Butter Toffee			
3 Tbsp, 1 oz	200	15	9
Nougat, 2 pces, 1 oz	115	1	25
Chocolate Covered, 1 oz	120	4	20
Nougat Nut Cream, 3.5 oz	340	31	50
Now & Later (Nabisco), 1 pkg	270	2.5	63
Nutrageous Bar, 3.4 oz	520	30	52
Snack, 0.6 oz	90	5	9
Oh Henry! 1.8 oz bar	240	10	32

Per Piece/Serving	C	F	Cb
100 Grand, 1.5 oz bar	190	8	30
Orange (Lindt), 6 block, 40g	190	10	24
Orange Slices: (Jewel), 3, 41g	140	0	36
(Walgreens), 3, 43g	150	0	36
Pastel Mints (Walgreens), 33 pce	150	0	38
Patteez (Sweet n' Low), 1/2 ctn, 5	120	2.5	32
PayDay Bar, 1.85 oz bar	260	13	27
King Size, 3.4 oz	480	26	50
Snack, 0.7 oz	100	5	11
Peanut Bar, 1.6 oz bar	210	14	20
Peanut Butter Bars, 3 pces, 18g	80	1.5	15
Peanut Butter Cups: See Reese's; Newman's Own			
Peanut Brittle, 1 oz	130	5	20
Peanut Chews (Goldenberg's), ea.	60	3	21
Peanut Riesen (5), 41g	190	7	28
Peanuts, choc-covered, each	25	1.5	2
Pearson's Mint Patties, 5, 38g	150	2.5	31
Pecan Roll, 1/3 bar, 40g	200	10	26
Peppermints, 7 small, 0.5 oz	50	0	12
Hershey's, 3 pces	60	0	15
Peppermint Twists, 2, 13g	60	0	12
Pez, 1 roll	30	0	6
Planters: Choc. Peanuts (25) 7 oz	220	13	20
Orig. Peanut Bar, 1.6 oz	230	14	22
Popcorn: See Snacks Page 131			
Positively Pecan, 2.5 oz bar	390	24	38
Pralines: Small, 0.3 oz	38	2	5
1 large piece, 1.4 oz	180	10	24
Pretzels: Choc-covered,			
3 miniature, 1.15 oz	150	5.5	23
1 regular, 1 oz	130	4.5	20
Pretzel Flipz (Nestlé), 8, 1 oz	130	5	19
Raisinets, 1 pkg, 1.7 oz	210	8	33
Raspberry Cream, each	80	2.5	5
Red Hot Dollars, 7 pce	100	0	24
Reese's: Chocolate Bar, 2.8 oz	420	24	43
Candy (Multipack), each	95	5.5	9
Miniatures, each	40	2.5	4
Peanut Butter Bites (7)	90	6	9
Mini, 1 pce	42	2.5	5
Peanut Butter Cups 1.6 oz pkg	250	14	25
Kingsize, 2.8 oz	420	24	43
Mini, 1 pce, 0.27 oz	40	2.5	4
Peanut Butter Eggs (1), 0.6 oz	90	5	8
Reese's Pieces (25), 1.63 oz pkg	230	11	26
Snack Size, (2), 1.2 oz (34g)	190	11	19
ReeseSticks, Kingsize, (2), 1.5 oz	230	13	23

Per Piece/Serving

	C	F	Cb
Rice Crunchy Bars: 1 bar, 19g			
average all flavors	60	0	14
Rice Krispies Treats: 1.3 oz bar	150	3.5	29
Chocolate Chip, 1.3 oz bar	160	5	28
Riesen Choc. Chew, (5) 1.4 oz	180	7	29
Peanut & Milk Choc, (5)	190	7	28
Ritter Sport: Plain Choc, 50g	260	16	26
w. Hazelnuts, 1/2 pkg, 50g	290	19	24
Rocky Road, 1.8 oz bar	240	11	34
Robin Eggs: Large, 2 pces	70	2	13
Medium, 4 pces	90	3	15
Mini, 10 pces	70	2.5	13
Rolo, all types (3), 0.64 oz	80	2.5	13
Root Beer Barrels, 3, 0.5 oz	60	0	16
Russell Stover Candy: Creams (1)	60	2	10
Almond Delight, 2 oz	290	17	32
Caramel Bar, 46g	230	11	20
Jelly Cups (P/Nut Butter), 2, 34g	140	9	14
Mint Dream	160	8	19
Pecan Delight (Sugar Free), 2 oz	260	18	27
Pecan Delight, 2 oz bar	310	20	27
Pecan Roll, 50g	260	18	23
Salt Water Taffy (Sathers), 5, 43g	150	2.5	34
Seashells (Guylian) 1 shell	65	4	6
Sesame Crunch, 3 pces	80	4	7
Simply Lite, 1/2 ctn, 36 pieces	130	5	18
Simply Sugar Free: See Allen Wertz			
Sixlets (Hershey), 24 pces	90	3.5	15
Skittles: Sour, 1.8 oz bag	200	2	44
Orig./Trop./Wild Berry, 2.17 oz bag	240	2.5	54
Fun Size, 1 bag, 0.7 oz (20g)	80	1	18
King Size, 4 oz bag	450	45	132
Large bag (16 oz): 1/4 cup, 1.5 oz	170	1.5	37
Mint (Pepp./Sprmint), 1.6 oz pkg	180	2	40
Skor Toffee Bar, 1.4 oz	220	13	24
Smarties Candy Rolls, 1 roll	25	0	5
Snackwell's Raisin Dips, 5 oz	160	5	34
Snickers: 2.07 oz bar	280	14	35
3.7 oz bar	510	24	63
Cruncher, 2.54 oz	370	21	41
King Size, 1/2 oz, 1.2 oz	170	8	21
Munch Bar, 1.4 oz bar	230	15	17
Fun size, each	95	5	12
Miniatures, each	42	2.5	5
Creme Egg, each	170	10	19
Snack, 2, 40g	190	10	24
Sno Caps, 2.3 oz pkg	300	13	48

Per Piece/Serving

	C	F	Cb
Soft Chews (Maalox), 1 chew	20	0.5	4
Soft 'N Chewy Butter Toffee, ea.	32	0.5	7
Soft Drops (9)	100	0	24
Soft Hot Dollars (11)	90	0	23
Sonic Boom Pops (Walgreens), ea.	60	0	14
Sour Brite Crawlers, 13 pces	140	0	31
Sour Punch: All types, 2 oz	190	1	45
1 straw	20	0	5
Spearmint Leaves: (Jewel), 5, 40g	140	0	35
(Walgreens), 5, 1 1/2 oz	150	0	38
Spice Drops, 10 pces, 1 1/2 oz	130	0	33
Spree Candies: Original, 8 pces	60	0	14
Chewy Spree, 8 pces	50	0	12
Starburst: Candy Canes, 0.5 oz	70	0	18
Fruit Chews, each	20	0.4	4
2 oz pkg	240	4.5	48
Fruit Twist, each	35	0	8
Fruit Twist, 2 oz pkg	190	1	45
Jellybeans, 1.5 oz	150	0	38
Jellybean Egg, 2 oz	200	0	51
Tropical Fruit, 2.07 oz pack	240	4.5	48
Starlight Mints: 3 pces, 1/2 oz	60	0	16
Suckers (Walgreens), 1 sucker, 11g	45	0	11
Sugar Babies, 1.7 oz bag	190	2	43
Sweet 'N Low: Chews, each	14	0	3
Sugar-Free Hard Candy, each	8	0	2
Peanut Butter Wafer Bars (1)	52	3	7
Sweet Escapes: See Hershey's			
Sweet Success Bar, 1 bar	120	4	23
Sweet Tarts (Nestlé), 7, 1/2 oz	50	0	13
Symphony, 1.5 oz bar	240	15	22
Snack: Chocolate (1), 0.6 oz	100	6	10
w. Almds & Toffee (1), 0.5 oz	80	5	7
Taffy, 1 pce, 1/2 oz	55	0.5	12
3 Musketeers: 2.13 oz bar	260	8	46
Fun size, each	70	2	13
Miniatures, each	25	0.5	5
Snack, 2, 33g	140	4.5	26
Tang-a-Roos: 1 roll	24	0	6
Tarts (Walgreens), 4 pce, 15g	60	0	15
Tails (Walgreens), 8 pce, 15g	60	0	15
Tastetations (Hershey's): Pep'mint	20	0	8
Butterscotch; Caramel; Choc	20	0.5	4
Terry's Choc Orange, (5), 1.5 oz	230	12	27
Tic Tac, all varieties, each	1.5	0	0
Toblerone: 50g (1.76 oz) bar	270	15	32
1 bar, 100g, (3.5 oz)	540	30	63
1/3 bar, 33g	180	10	21

Candy, Chocolate (Cont)

Per Piece/Serving	C	F	Cb
Toffees: Regular, 1 oz	150	9	15
Tongue Torchers (Walgreens), 3	70	0	17
Tootsie Roll Midgies (Walgreens), 6	160	3	33
Tootsie Roll, 2.25 oz roll	260	4	54
Treasures (Nestlé): (4), 1.6 oz	240	16	26
Nestlé Crunch, 3	160	8.5	23
Butterfinger Pieces, 3	180	9	23
Creamy Caramel, 3	180	9	22
Peanut Butter Miniatures, 3	180	12	17
Trolli: Gumm Candy, av. 5 pc	120	0	29
Truffles: Regular, 1 pce, 0.4 oz	60	4	5
Large (Godiva), 0.75 oz	110	6.5	12
Extra Large (J.Schmidt), 1 1/2 oz	220	13	24
Turtles (Nestlé), each	85	4.5	10
Twists (Sugar Free): Licorice; Strawberry, 6 twists, 40g	140	0	32
Twix: Caramel 2 oz pkg	280	14	37
King Size, 3.35 oz pkg	480	24	64
Fun Size: 0.5 oz	80	4	10
2 oz pkg, 2 bars	280	14	37
Peanut Butter, 0.9 oz	140	8.5	14
Snack, 1 cookie, 0.5 oz	80	5	8
Twizzlers: Candy, aver., 1 pce, 8g	30	0	8
Pull 'n' Peel, Cherry (1), 1 oz	90	1	19
Velamints Sugar Free, 1 pce	10	0	2
Werther's: Original, 3 pce, 15g	60	1	13
Chocolates (5), 20g	110	6	13
Whatchamacallit Bar, 1.6 oz	230	11	28
Snack (1), 0.58 oz	80	3.5	10
Whitman's:			
Pecan Roll, 2 oz roll	300	20	26
Sampler, 3 pces, 1.4 oz	200	11	25
Assorted; Dark Chocolate, 1 pce	65	3	9
Snoopy Treats, 2 pces	190	10	24
Whoppers: 1.75 oz bag	230	9	37
Yogurt Candy: Plain, 1 oz	120	6	15
Coated Raisins, 1 oz	120	4	21
York Mints, 1.5 oz patty	145	5	34
Snack size, 0.5 oz	55	1	11
Peppermint Patties, 3	150	2.5	30
York Peppermint Pattie, 1.4 oz	160	3	32
Zachary Old Fash. Creme Drops, 3	170	3	36
Zagnut: 1.75 oz bar	230	10	31
Snack size (1), 0.5 oz	70	3	9
Zero Bar, 1 pce, 0.6 oz	70	2.5	12
Zingos, 3 pce, 2g	5	0	2

Carob Candy

Per Piece/Serving	C	F	Cb
Carob: Plain/Natural, 1 oz	160	11	9
Carob coated: Raisins, 1 oz	130	8	15
Almonds/Peanuts, 1 oz	150	10	14
Malt Balls, 1 oz	135	8	15
Caramels, 1 oz	110	4	18
Dates, 1 oz	125	5	20
Soybeans	145	9	16
Trail/Party Mix, 1 oz	140	9	15
Carob Chips, unsweetened, 1 oz	140	7	19
Carob Bars: Avg, Plain/Nut, 1 oz	160	11	13
Fruit & Nut, 1 oz	155	10	13
Mint/Orange, 1 oz	160	11	14
Carafection: Cashew Coconut Crunch, 1/2 Bar, (42g) 1.5 oz	250	14	5
Caroby Natural Touch, 3 oz	450	27	36

Cough Drops

	C	F	Cb
Beech Nut, 1 drop	10	0	2
Diabetic Tussin, 1 drop	0	0	0
Halls Defense Vit. C, 1 drop	15	0	4
Halls Fruit Breezers, 1 drop	14	0	4
Halls Menthol Drops, 1 drop	15	0	4
Sugar Free, 1 drop	6	0	4
Halls Plus, 1 drop	18	0	5
Helps Cough, all flavors, 1	14	0	3
Listerine Lozenge (Amer. Chicle)	9	0	2
Luden's Throat Drops, all flavors, 1	10	0	2
Sugar Free, 1 drop	0	0	0
Pine Bros, 1 cough drop	10	0	2
Ricola: Cough Drops, 1 drop	12	0	3
Sugar-Free Lemon Mint, 2 mints	0	0	1
Rite Aid, Menthol Cough, 1 drop	12	0	3
Robitussin: Regular, 1 drop	14	0	3
Honey Cough, 1 drop	40	0	10
Sugar Free Throat, 1 drop	10	0	2
Sunny Orange Vit. C, 1 drop	12	0	3
Rolaids/Sodium Free, 1	4	0	1
Sathers Peppermint Lozenges, 1	13	0	3
Squibb Cough/Throat Loz.'s, 1	16	0	4
Sucrets (Beecham) Lozenges, 1	10	0	2
Wintergreen Loz. (Walgreens), 1	13	0	3
Cough Suppresant Liquids: See Page 139			

Home-Popped Popcorn

	C	**F**	**Cb**
Popping Corn Kernels:			
2 Tbsp, 1 oz	100	1	22
(makes approx. 3½ cups)			
Air-popped (no oil), plain, 1 oz	100	0	22
1 cup (6g)	20	0	4
Oil-popped, plain, 1 oz	140	8	10
1 cup (11g)	55	3	4
Popcorn Oil, 1 Tbsp	120	14	0

Microwave Popcorn

Average All Brands (Popped)

Butter: Regular, 1 cup	35	2	4
Light, 1 cup	25	1	4
Act II Popcorn:			
Butter, 1 cup, 0.3 oz	35	2	4
4 cups, popped, 1 oz	140	8	16
Light Butter, 1 cup, 0.2 oz	25	1	4
5 cups, popped, 1 oz	125	4	20
Butter Lovers, 1 cup, 0.3 oz	45	3	4
3.5 cups, 1 oz	160	10	14
Butter Lovers (Reduced Fat), 1 c.	30	1.5	4.5
4.5 cups, 1 oz	130	6	20
American Fare (K-Mart):			
Butter, 1 cup, 0.3 oz	37	2.5	4
3.5 cups, 1 oz	130	9	14
Light Butter, 1 cup, 0.3 oz	28	1	5
3.5 cups, 1 oz	100	4	17
Healthy Choice			
Butter, 6 cups	100	2.5	22
Natural, 6 cups, 1 oz	100	2	22
Newman's Own: Butter, 1 oz	170	11	16
Light Butter Flavor, 3½ cups	110	3	20
Orville Redenbacher's: *Per 1 Cup Popped*			
Corn on the Cob, 1 cup, popped	35	2.5	3
Movie Theater Butter, 1 cup	30	2	3
4 cups, popped, 1 oz	120	8	12
Light Movie Theater Butter, 1 cup	20	1	2
4 cups, 1 oz	80	4	8
Double Feature Jumbo, 1 cup	30	2	3
Smart Pop!:			
94% Fat Free Butter, 1 cup	20	0.5	4
Butter Light, 1 cup	20	0.5	3
Sweet 'n Buttery, 1 cup	45	3.5	4
Butter, 1 cup	35	2	4

Bagged Popcorn

	C	**F**	**Cb**
Average All Brands (Ready-to-Eat)			
Regular: Plain, ½ oz pkg	80	5	7
1 oz pkg	160	10	14
4 oz pkg	640	40	56
Box (store/airport), 2 oz	320	20	28
Bag (9" high x 5" wide), 3 oz	480	30	42

Brands ~ Bagged Popcorn

Act II Popcorn:			
Butter Toffee: ¾ cup, 1 oz	110	1	27
w. Peanuts, ¾ cup, 1 oz	120	2.5	24
Supreme w. Pecans, Almonds, ¾ c.	130	5	22
Boston's: Fat Free, ⅔ cup, 1 oz	100	0	23
Lite, 2 cup, 1 oz	140	6	19
Gourmet Super Prem., 2 c., 1 oz	160	11	13
40% Less Fat, 2¾ cup, 1 oz	140	6	17
Cracker Jack: Original, ½ c., 1 oz	120	2	23
Fat Free varieties, ¾ cup, 1 oz	110	0	26
Crunch 'N Munch: ½ cup, 1 oz	140	5	22
Buttery Toffee, ⅔ cup, 1 oz	150	6	22
Caramel w. P'nuts, ⅔ c., 1.2 oz	140	3.5	25
Fiddle Faddle: Skippy ¾ c., 1 oz	130	3	23
Honey Nut, ½ cup, 1 oz	130	3.5	24
w. Real Planters Peanuts, ⅔ cup	130	3	24
Hixon's: Caramel Corn, 1 oz	125	4.5	20
Cheese Corn, 1 oz	160	11	15
Korn Krunch: *(Kornfections Treasures):*			
Almond Pecan (Sugar Free), 1 oz	150	8	19
Orville Redenbacher:			
Butter Toffee, ⅔ cup, 1.1 oz	140	4.5	24
Skippy P'nut Butter, ¾ c., 1 oz	130	3	23
Choc. Lovers Poppycock, ½ c., 1 oz	140	5	21
Heath Toffee Candy, ½ c., 1 oz	140	1.5	23
Pecan Delight: Poppycock, ½ c.	150	7	20
Pizza Hut: Cheese Pizza, 2 oz bag	360	26	26
Simmons (Fat Free): ¾ c., 1 oz	110	0	25
Weight Watchers: Butter, ⅔ cup	90	2.5	14
Wild Oats: All types, 2.5 cup, 1 oz	160	10	15

Movie Theater Popcorn

Small (7 cups): Plain	400	27	30
with Butter	580	47	30
Medium (16 cups): Plain	900	60	70
with Butter	1170	90	70
Large (20 cups): Plain	1150	76	90
with Butter	1500	116	90

Potato Chips, Pretzels, Tortilla Chips

Potato Chips/Crisps

	C	F	Cb
Average All Brands			
Regular:			
Plain or flavored, 1 chip	9	1	1
17 chips, 1 oz pkg	150	10	15
4 oz quantity	600	40	60
Pringles, 14 crisps, 1 oz	160	11	15
Large, 5.75 oz can	920	63	86
Snack Stack, 23g tub	140	9	12
Ruffles, 14 chips, 1 oz	160	10	14
Reduced Fat: *Pringles,* 1 oz	140	7	20
Crunch Tators, 1 oz	140	7	19
Kettle Fry *(Eagle),* 1 oz	150	8	16
Sun Chips, 1 oz	140	6	19
Lowfat/Baked varieties, 1 oz	110	1.5	23
Fat Free:			
Childer's/Louise's, 1oz	100	0	22
Pringles (Fat Free), 1 oz	70	0	15
Lay's Wow!, 20 chips, 1 oz	75	0	18
Ruffles Wow!, 17 chips, 1 oz	75	0	17
Cheddar Sour Crm, 15, 1 oz	75	0	16

Corn & Tortilla Chips

	C	F	Cb
Corn Chips:			
Average all types, 1 oz	160	10	15
8 oz bag	1280	80	120
Doritos: (12), 1 oz	150	7	20
Nachos; 4-Cheese, 1 oz	140	8	17
3D's Nacho Cheesier, 1 oz (32)	130	5	19
Fritos (Sabrositas), 1 oz	150	9	17
Pringles, Torengos (13) 1 oz	140	9	15
Tortilla Chips: Average, 1 oz	150	8	22
(1 oz = approx. 12 chips or 13 strips)			
Boston: Baked, 13 chips, 1 oz	110	1.5	23
Doritos: 18 chips, 1 oz	140	6	20
Light, 13 chips, 1 oz	130	5	20
Wow! Nacho Cheesier, 1 oz	90	0.5	16
Frito Lay, Baked, (15) 1 oz	120	3.5	21
Garden of Eatin', 1 oz	140	7	28
Keebler Suncheros Light, 1 oz	150	8	18
Kettle: Average, 1 oz	140	6	18
Padrino Reduced Fat, 1 oz	130	4	22
Torengos, 13 chips, 1 oz	140	9	15
Utz: Lowfat Baked, 8 chips, 1 oz	120	1.5	23
Wild Oats: 14 chips, 1 oz	150	7	18

Pretzels

	C	F	Cb
Average All Brands			
Hard Baked Pretzels:			
1 oz	110	2	22
Sticks, thin, 2 1/4" (9/oz), 1	12	0	3
Twists, thin, 1/4" thick, (5/oz), 1	25	0.2	5
Dutch (2 3/4" x 2 5/8") 1/2 oz, 1	55	1	11
Sourdough *(Shultz),* 3/4 oz, 1	80	0	17
Fat Free Pretzels:			
Snyders (1), 1 oz	100	0	22
Mini (20), 1 oz	110	0	25
Utz Wheels/Nuggets, 1 oz	100	0	22
Rold Gold: Sticks, 48, 1 oz	100	0	23
Sourdough Nuggets, 12, 1 oz	100	0	23
Sourdough Hards (1), 3/4 oz	80	0	17
Thins, 12, 1 oz	110	0	24
Twists, 16, 1 oz	110	1	22
Tiny Twists/Sticks, 18, 1 oz	100	0	23
Low Fat Pretzels:			
American Fare Mini Twists, 1oz	120	1	23
Frito Lay, Rold Gold:			
Butter Checkers 20 pcs., 1 oz	110	1.5	22
Braided Twists, (8) , 1 oz	110	1	23
Choc-coated: *(Nestlé),* 1 oz	130	6	20
White Fudge covered *(Nestlé),*			
1 oz, 7 pieces	140	6	19
Yogurt, *(Wild Oats)* 8 pcs., 1.4 oz	210	10	27
Soft Pretzels (Twists) average:			
Plain: Regular, 2.5 oz	190	0	41
King Size, 5 oz	390	0	83
Big Cheese, 5 oz	380	7	61
Peanut Butter filled *(Tr. Joe's)* 1 oz	160	7	18
Frito Lay Pretzels			
Flavor Twists, 23 pc. 1 oz,	160	10	16
Rold Gold Flavor Rush, 1/3 c. 1 oz	150	7	20
Braided Twists, 8 sticks, 1 oz	110	1	23
Auntie Anne's: See Fast-Foods Pg. 180			
Snyder's of Hanover Pretzels			
Logs (7) 1oz	120	1	21
Homestyle (15), 1 oz	120	1	24
Mini (20), 1 oz	110	0	25
Super Pretzel: Jalapeno, 5 oz	360	0	78
Bavarian Twist, 3 oz	210	3	41
Cinnamon Raisin w. Icing, 5 oz	420	4	76
Sweet Dough Twist, 3.7 oz	300	3	60

Snacks	C	F	Cb

Note: Actual weight of packaged snacks is usually 5-10% more than label Net Wt. For accuracy, weigh snack and allow extra calories for any extra weight.

Item	C	F	Cb
Bacon Cheese Crackers, 1 oz	140	6	14
Banana Chips, 1/4 cup, 1 oz	150	8	20
Beef Jerky: Average, 1 oz	70	1	3
Beef Sticks (Frito-Lay's) 0.3 oz	50	4	1
Bugles: Original, 1/3 cup, 1 oz	160	9	18
Baked Bugles, 1 1/3 cup, 1.1 oz	130	3.5	23
Cajun Jerky, 1 1/2 oz	150	6	6
Carrot Chips (Hain)	160	9	26
Cheddar Lites (Health Valley) 1 oz	120	3	21
Cheese Crackers, 1 oz	130	6	18
Cheese Filled (Frito-Lay's)	210	11	24
Cheese Curls, 1 1/4 cup, 1 oz	160	9	19
Reduced Fat (Utz), 1 oz	140	6	21
American Fare, 1 1/4 cup, 1 oz	140	5	22
Cheese Nips (Nabisco) (29) 1 oz	150	6	19
Cheese Puffs: Average, 1 oz	150	10	15
Lowfat, 1 oz	140	5	20
Health Valley, 1 1/2 cup	110	3	21
No Fries, 1 oz	110	0	23
Cheese Straws, 4 pieces	110	7	8
Cheese Twists, 23 twists, 1 oz	150	8	19
Cheetos: Regular all flavors, 1 oz	160	10	15
Light, cheese flavored, 1 oz	140	6	19
Cheez Balls, 45 balls, 1 oz	150	10	15
Reduced Fat, 45 balls, 0.73 oz	100	4.5	13
Cheez Bopps (Boston's), (28) 1 oz	130	6	17
Cheez Curls/Doodles, 1 oz	160	12	15
Cheez Mania (Planters), 35, 1 oz	160	10	15
Cheez It: White Cheddar, 1 pkt	210	11	26
Cheese Sandwiches, 1 pkt	220	13	21
100% Real Cheese, 1 pkt	220	12	23
Chex Mix: General Mills, 1.1 oz	150	10	15
Bold 'N Zesty (40% less fat), 1/2 c.	140	6	20
Chedder (50% less fat), 1/2 c.	130	5	20
Traditional (60% less fat), 2/3 c.	130	4	21
Churros (Mex. Pastry) 10", 1.2 oz	140	9	12
Cinna Chips (T.J. Cinn.) 3, 1 oz	110	4	19
Combos: (Oven Baked):			
Crackers, 1/3 cup, 1 oz	140	7	18
1 cup, 3 oz	420	21	54
Pretzels, 1/3 cup, 1 oz	130	4.5	19
1 cup, 3 oz	390	14	57
Cookies: See Pages 104-111			
Corn Chips: See Page 132			

Snacks (Cont)	C	F	Cb
Corn Crunchies/Spirals, 1 oz	160	10	15
Corn Crisps (Pringle), 1 oz	140	7	18
Corn Nuts, 1/3 cup, 1 oz	130	4	20
Corn Puffs (Health Valley) 2 c., 1 oz	120	1.5	25
(Pirate's Booty) 1 oz	130	5	18
Dunkaroos (1 tray, 1 oz	130	4.5	20
Flavor Twists (Fritos), 1 oz	160	10	16
French's Potato Sticks 3/4 c., 1 oz	180	12	16
Fruit Snack Cups: See Page 143			
Funyun's Onion flavor, 1 oz	140	7	18
Goldfish (Pepperidge Farm) 1 oz	140	7	18
Gold-N-Chees (Lance), 1 3/8 oz	180	7	25
Handi Snacks (Kraft), Bearwiches	150	7	21
Honey Mustard Onion Pieces			
(Snyder's) 1 pkg, 2 oz	280	13	35
Hot Peanuts (F.'o Lay), 1 3/4 oz pkg	310	25	10
Keebler: Wheatables Snack Mix,			
Toasted Honey, 1/2 cup, 1 oz	130	5	20
Peanut Butter Crunch, 1/2 c., 1 oz	160	7	20
Chse & P'nut Butter			
Sandwich Cookies, 1 pkg	250	12	30
Koolstuf: All flavors, 1 bar, 1.3 oz	130	3	27
Lance Sandwich: Bonnie, 1 pkg	160	7	23
Capt. Wafers: Choc-O-Mint, pkg	190	10	23
Sour Dough w. Cheddar, 1 pkg	240	15	23
Other varieties, average, 1 pkg	200	10	22
Lunchables: Fudge Brownie	250	9	42
'S'Mores	200	6	35
Munchos, 16 pieces, 1 oz	160	10	16
Nabisco: Chips Ahoy, 1.3 oz	150	7	20
Chips Ahoy! Cookie Barz, 35g	180	9	23
Nutter Butter Bites (10)	150	6	20
Oreo, 1.3 oz	160	7	24
Oreo Cookie Barz, 1 bar	180	9	23
S'Mores	200	6	35
Sportz, Cheese Nips (38), 1 oz	150	7	19
Sweet Crispers (18), 1 oz	135	3	25
Nibblers (Snyder's): Regular (13)	130	3	23
Sourdough Fat Free (16)	120	0	25
Onion Rings (Lance), 1 pkg	120	6	16
Oriental Mix (Rice Snacks), 1 oz	155	7.5	15
Rice Snacks (Wild Oats) 2/3 c. 1 oz	110	0	25
Oyster Crackers (Bradshaw's), 1 oz	140	5	14
Party Mix (Flavor Tree) 1/4 c., 1 oz	160	11	14
Pirate's Booty w. White Ched., 1 oz	130	5	18
Popcorn: See Page 131			

Snacks • Vending Machines

Snacks (Cont) | C | F | Cb

	C	F	Cb
Pork Skins/Rind: Baken-ets, 1 oz	160	10	0
Grande, 2/3 cup	80	5	0
Lance, 1 pkg	65	4	1
Potato Chips: See Pages 132			
Potato Puffs (Health Valley) 1 oz	110	3	21
Potato Skins (TGI Friday's) 1 oz	150	9	17
Potato Sticks (French's) 3/4 c., 1.1oz	180	12	16
Puffs: 1 2/3 cup, 1 oz	140	8	17
8 oz pkg	1120	64	136
Quakes Rice Snacks (Quaker)			
Apple Cinnamon (8) 16g	60	0	15
BBQ, Ranch, Sour Crm (10) 16g	70	2.5	12
Caramel Corn (7) 15g	60	0	13
Cheddar/Nacho Cheese (9) 15g	70	2.5	11
Chocolate (7) 15g	60	1	13
Ranch Puffs (No Fries) 1 oz	110	0	23
Rice Chips, Bar-B-Q/Onion, 1/2 oz	70	3	9
Santitas (Frito Lay) 1 oz	140	6	20
Sesame Sticks (Cityfarm) 1 oz	160	11	13
Snack Crackers (No Fries) 1 oz	110	0	24
Soy Nuts: Dry Roasted, 1 oz	130	6	9
Choc-coated, 12-15 pces, 1/2 oz	70	4	7
Spicers Wheat Snacks, 1 1/2 oz	150	7.5	18
Sport Jerky Ostrich,			
(Wild Oats) 1/2 oz	25	0	0
Sun Chips (Frito Lay) 1 oz pkg	140	6	19
TastyKake, Koffee Kake Jnr	250	8	40
Chocolate Jnr	320	12	50
Creme Filled Koffee Kakes	360	14	54
Toast/Cheese Crackers, 1 pkg	205	10	23
Tortilla Chips: See Pages 132			
Tostitos: Regular, average, 1 oz	140	8	18
Fat Free, 1 oz	90	0	20
Trail Mix (Nuts/Seeds/Dried Fruit):			
Regular, 3 Tbsp, 1 oz	130	8	13
Tropical, 3 Tbsp, 1 oz	120	5	19
w. Chocolate Chips, 1 oz	140	9	13
Turkey Jerky Teriyaki (Oberto)	80	0.5	0
Vegetable Snacks/Chips, 1 oz	130	4	24
Veggie Chips, 1 oz	130	5	18
Veggie Stix, 1 oz	140	7	15
Wahoos, 1 oz, 23 pces.	140	8	18
Weight Watchers: Chse Curls, 1/2 oz	70	2.5	10
Apple Chips, 3/4 oz pkg	70	0	18
Yogurt Raisins, 1 oz	130	6	20

Fruit Snacks | C | F | Cb

	C	F	Cb
Betty Crocker:			
String Things, 1 pouch, 0.75 oz	80	1	17
Lucky Charms Fruit Shapes,			
1 pouch, 0.9 oz (25g)	80	0	20
Squeezit, average, 1 bottle	100	0	25
Nabisco: Rugrats; Wacky Faces (1)	80	0	18
Blues Clues; Dora the Explorer (1)	60	0	14
Fruit Rolls, 1 roll, 0.74 oz	80	2	16
Sunkist: All flavors, 1 pch, 0.9 oz	80	0	21
Fruit Snack Cups: See Page 143			

Vending Machines

	C	F	Cb
Brownie, frosted	180	9	24
Cheese Balls, 1 oz	150	8	16
Choc Chip Cookies, 4	130	7	19
Choc Milk, 8 fl.oz	225	9	26
Coca Cola Classic, 12 fl.oz	140	0	35
Diet Coke, 12 fl.oz	1	0	0
Corn Chips, 1 oz	160	10	15
Danish Pastry, 2 oz	220	10	25
Donut, plain, 1 3/4 oz	210	12	25
Fruit Pie, 4 oz	290	13	46
Granola/Cereal Bars	130	3	26
Hershey's, 1.55 oz bar	240	14	25
Hot Fries, 1 oz	140	10	11
Kellogg's Rice Krispies Treat	120	1.5	26
Lance: Captain's Wafers, 1 pkg	230	12	26
Big Town, 1 pkg	250	11	38
M & M's: Plain, 1.7 oz	240	10	34
Peanuts, 1.7 oz	250	13	30
Milk: Whole, 8 fl.oz	150	8	12
Reduced Fat, 2%, 8 fl.oz	120	5	12
Milky Way, 2 oz	270	10	41
Onion Rings, 1 oz	120	6	16
Orange Juice, 8.75 fl.oz	120	0	28
Peanuts, roasted, 1 oz	165	14	6
Popcorn, plain, 1 oz	160	10	14
Pork Skins, 1 oz	160	10	0
Potato Chips, 1 oz	150	10	15
Reduced Fat, 1 oz	140	7	20
Pretzels, 1 oz	110	2	22
Raisins, 1/2oz pkg	40	0	9
Reece's Peanut Butter Cups, 1.8 oz	280	17	28
Snickers, 2.1 oz bar	280	14	35
Tortilla Chips, 1 oz	150	8	22

Granola, Sports & Diet Bars

Note: Actual weight of bars is usually 5-10% more than label Net Wt. Weigh bar and allow extra calories.

Per Bar

	C	F	Cb
All Goode: Organic, 1.66 oz bar	210	9	29
Amazin! P'nut; Cashew, 1.62 oz	210	11	29
Choc Peanut, 1.75 oz	200	9	29
Nutty Choc. Apricot, 1.75 oz	200	10	26
Amway Positrim Food Bars, 1 wrap	210	9	26
Arbonne Balanced Nutr., 1 bar	190	4.5	24
Atkins Advantage Bar, aver., 60g	240	13	11
Balance: Regular, aver., 1.76 oz	200	6	23
Outdoors, av. all types, 1.76 oz	200	6	21
Kid Sport: Double Choc, 1.76 oz	200	6	27
Creamy Peanut Butter, 1.76 oz	190	6	28
Balance + Bar, 50g (1.76 oz)	200	6	22
Snack, Honey, Peanut, 25g	100	3	11
Barbara's Bakery: Real Fruit	50	0	13
Cereal Bars, fruit filled	110	0	24
Granola Bars, average, 3/4 oz	80	2	15
Bariatrix: Nutra Bars, 47g	170	5	23
Proti Bars (15g Protein), 41g	130	5	14
Right Choice Bars, 40g	140	3	24
BioX Bio Protein: 81g	300	7	37
Body Smarts: Choc. P'nut Crunch	210	6	34
Yogurt Berry Crunch	200	5	35
Boost: Choc./Strawb. Crunch	190	6	30
Boulder Bar Endurance, 2.5 oz	220	4	43
Burn-IT: 50g bar	180	3	13
Cap'N Crunch, all types, 0.8 oz	90	2	17
Carbolite: Choc Almond, 1.75 oz	230	17	25
Choc Crisp Bar, 1.75 oz	250	17	27
Milk/Dairy Choc, avg, 1.75 oz	250	19	28
CarbRite Diet *(Doctor's),* 2 oz	180	3	25
Carb Solutions: *Per 2.1 oz Bar*			
Choc. Cappuccino Crisp	240	9	14
Choc. Toffee Hazelnut	250	10	14
Cr. Choc. Peanut Butter	240	10	14
Frosted Blueberry	230	8	15
Carnation Breakfast Bars, 35g (1.2 oz):			
Granola (Honey/Choc), average	130	2.5	26
Choc Chip/P.nut Butter, average	150	5	24
Champion Nutrition, Lemon Dream	180	3	25
Cheetah *(NutraFig),* 2.25 oz bar	210	2	43
Choice, all types, 1.23 oz bar	140	4.5	19
Clif Bar: *Per 2.4 oz (68g) Bar*			
Apr.; Cranb. Apple Cherry	220	2	44
Choc Almond Fudge	230	4.5	39
Carrot Cake; Choc Chip/Brownie	240	4	43
Cookies 'n Cream	230	3.5	39
Ginger Snap	230	3.5	42

Clif Bar (Cont): *Per 2.4 oz Bar*	C	F	Cb
The Ice Series	250	5	42
Luna, 48g bar	180	5	24
Mojo: Honey Rstd, 1.5 oz bar	200	6	26
Honey BBQ Alm.; Mix Nuts, 1.5 oz	200	7	25
Creamy Cinnamon Bar, 1.4 oz	180	8	14
Designer Whey Protein, 2.7 oz	260	6	7
Dr Soy: Protein Bar, Lemon, 1.76 oz	180	2.5	28
Chocolate/Peanut, 1.76 oz	185	4	27
EAS·HP: Muscle Drive, 2.82 oz	280	7	24
EAS: Results For Women, 1.94 oz bar			
Cranapple; Wildberry	200	6	28
Cookies & Cream	190	5	17
EcoBar, all flavors, 1 bar	170	5	30
Edgebar, 2 oz (57g) bar	220	2	42
Energia Bar, 2.25 oz	230	2	41
Ensure Choc Fudge Bar	130	3	20
Entenmann's: Multi-Grain, 1.3 oz	140	3	25
Extend Bar, 40g	160	3	30
Extreme Body, 3 oz bar	340	8	24
Extreme Ripped Force, 45g	160	4	33
Fi-Bar Nectar Granola Bars, 1 oz	100	0	22
Chewy & Nutty Bar, 1.2 oz	140	4.5	23
Fi-Pro-Tein *(R-Kane),* 1.2 oz bar	107	1	16
Figurines Diet Bar, aver., 1 bar	110	6	12
Fruitein Energy Bar, 1.3 oz	130	3	14
Gatorade Energy Bars, 2.3 oz	260	5	47
General Mills: *Milk 'n Cereal*			
Chex; Cheerios, Cocoa Puffs 1.4 oz	160	4	26
Cinnamon Toast Crunch, 1.6 oz	180	4	31
GeniSoy: Nature Grains, 2.3 oz	230	3	41
Peanut Butter Fudge	230	5	31
Soy Nutty, 1.76 oz	190	5	26
Glucerna, Nutr'l Bar, 38g	140	4	24
Grove Organic Energy Bars, 2 oz	250	10	30
Hain: Mini Munchies Rice	90	1.5	2
Hansen's: *Per 1.76 oz Bar*			
Crunch: Choc. Banana	180	2.5	37
Orchard Fruit	170	2.5	37
Yogurt Strawberry	190	3	38
Chocolate Brownies, average	190	5	24
Hardbody, 2.5 oz, 71g	280	7	41
Health Valley: Fruit/Granola Bars	140	0	34
Cereal: Strawberry Cobbler	130	2	27
Healthy Recipes *(Novartis)*	150	4	21
HeartBar, Orig., Cranberry, 50g	190	3	27
HMR Benefit Bar, 1.1 oz	160	5	22

Granola, Sports & Diet Bars (Cont)

Per Bar	C	F	Cb
IDN (*Nu Skin*): AppSignal, 2 wafers	25	0	5
Glycobar, 42g (1.48 oz)	170	5	28
ProGRAM-16 Bar, 65g (2.28 oz)	250	5	34
Iron-Tek: Vanilla Fudge, 2.73 oz	290	5	21
Triple Decker Protein, 2.3 oz	250	10	27
Jenny Craig: Meal Bars, 1.97 oz			
Milk Choc; Lemon Meringue	210	5	32
Choc Peanut; Yogurt Peanut	220	5	33
Oatmeal Raisin	210	3	35
Jewel Granola Bars: Cereal	140	3	27
Choc Chip/P'nut Butter	130	4.5	20
Lowfat varieties	110	2	22
Jolt Bar (*Nutra Tech*) 40g	140	3	24
Kashi Golean Bars: Avg, 78g	290	5	53
Kudos: *M&M's*	90	2.5	17
Snickers, 23g	100	3.5	16
Choc Chip/Fudge; P. Butter, 28g	125	5	20
Kraft: Philadelphia Cream Cheese, average of all bars, 1.5 oz	190	12	18
Krave (*Kellogg's*): P'nut Butter, 48g	200	7	29
Chocolate Delight, 48g	200	6	31
Lean Body, 76g	300	6	15
Metab-o-Lite (w. Ephedra) 1.23 oz	130	4	21
Met-Rx: "Big 100", avg, 100g	340	3	51
After FX: Choc Chip, 3 oz	300	9	13
Double/Peanut Fudge, 3 oz	250	8	13
Protein Plus, 3 oz	200	0	15
Source One: all types, 1 pkg	190	3	30
MightyBite Choc. Bar, 25g	100	4	11
MLO Bio Protein, 2.85 oz	300	7	39
Mountain Lift Energy Bar	220	4.5	34
Muscle Tech: 3 oz Bar	220	4.5	34
Meso-Tech Chunky Choc Chip	340	8	38
Nitro-Tech, average	290	8	6
Myoplex Plus Deluxe, 90g	340	7	43
Myoplex HP: Mocha, 2.3 oz	250	5	30
Lite, all flavors, 1.97 oz	190	4	27
Carb Sense, 2.47 oz,			
Choc Dipped Strawberry	250	6	23
Lo Carb, 2.47 oz	250	6	3
Natrol Prolab, 1.76 oz bar	190	6	12
Naturade, Total Soy, 2.1 oz	250	8	32
Nature Valley Granola: Average	180	6	27
Lowfat varieties	110	2	21
Nature's Best: Solid Protein, 2.75 oz			
Honey Almond; Cherry Vanilla	290	4	11
Chocolate Raspberry	290	4	11
Nature's Best (Cont):			
Blueberry Cheesecake	280	4	14
Choc. Peanut Butter; S'Mores	290	7	12
Chocolate Mint	290	7	12
Cookie Dough Chip; Dble Choc	290	4	10
Nature's Plus: Energy Bar, 1.45 oz	140	4.5	23
Chinese Herbal, 1.5 oz	150	4	20
Calcium Almond Blitz, 1.5 oz	150	2.5	29
Spiru-tein, all flavors, 1.4 oz	150	4	20
New You: Choc Chip, 1.65 oz	170	3.5	25
Lemon Crisp, 1.65 oz	170	3	26
Peanut Butter, 1.65 oz	185	5	25
NiteBite (Time-release Glucose Bar)			
Choc. Fudge; P'nut Butter, 25g	100	3.5	15
NuBar Decadence, 1.3 oz	140	2.5	30
Nutiva (Hemp, Sunflower), 40g	205	14	15
Nutra Blast, average, 47g	160	4	27
Nutri-Grain: Cereal/Twist bars	140	3	27
Low Fat Granola Bars, 21g	80	1.5	16
Fruit-full Squares, 49g bar	190	6	33
Nutrilite Positrim Food Bar, 50g	210	9	26
Odwalla, 2.2 oz	245	5	45
100% Bar, 50g	190	6	31
Perfect Rx Nutrition Bar, 100g	340	3	50
Planters: Peanut Bar, 1.6 oz	230	11	22
Pounds Off Bar: All flavors	220	4	35
Power Bar: Harvest, 2.3 oz	240	4	45
Dipped Harvest 2.3 oz	260	5	45
Performance, average all, 2.3 oz	230	2.5	45
Pria, 0.98 oz	110	3	17
Protein Plus, 2.75 oz	290	5	38
PR Bar Ironman, 49.6g	200	6	22
Precision, all flavors, 50g	200	7	18
Pro 42: 3.7 oz bar	270	6	8
Almond Rocky Trail	380	8	13
Chocolate Attack	350	7	11
PB Choc Chip	410	10	14
PB Collision	370	9	11
Promax: Dble Fudge Brownie, 75g	270	5	34
Other flavors, 75g	280	5	36
Prozone Nutrition Bar, 50g	195	6	18
Pure Protein Sports Bar: *Per 78g (2.75 oz) Bar*			
Chewy Choc Chip	285	5	16
Peanut Butter	280	7	9
Other varieties, average	270	4	15

Per Bar	C	F	Cb
Quaker Chewy Granola Bars:			
Choc Chip	120	4	21
Cookies 'n Cream	110	2	22
Peanut Butter	110	3.5	18
Peanut Butter & Choc Chunk	120	3.5	20
Other varities, average	120	3.5	22
Low Fat varieties, average	110	2	22
Quaker Fruit & Oatmeal Cereal Bars:			
Average all varieties, 37g bar	130	3	26
Bites: All varieties, 37g pouch	140	2.5	27
Restart: Peanut Butter, 1.25 oz	140	4	10
Strawb. Banana; Chocolate	130	2.5	21
Revival Soy Protein: 60g bars,			
Choc. Tempt.; M'mallow Crunch	220	3	30
Peanut Butter/Chocolate Pal	240	6	30
Rice Krispies Bar (Kellogg's), 28g	120	4	20
Coco Pops Bar, 22g	100	3.5	16
Treats Squares, 22g	90	2	18
Slim-Fast Bars: Per Bar			
Ultra Slim-Fast Snack Bars,			
Crispy Peanut Caramel	120	4	21
Peanut Butter Crunch	130	4	21
Rich Chewy Caramel	120	4	22
Meal On-The-Go Bars (56g),			
average all varieties	220	5	35
Breakfast & Lunch Bars (34g),			
Dutch Chocolate	140	5	20
Peanut Butter	150	6	19
Snacbar (Champion Nutr.), 1 bar	180	3	24
Snackwell's: Per Bar			
Cereal Bars	120	0	29
Hearty Fruit & Grain	130	3	26
Chewy Granola, Fudge-Dipped	130	3	26
SoBeBars (Market America): Per Bar			
Meal Replacement Bars, Choc	296	6	42
Peanut	300	7	44
Tropical	290	4.5	47
Wafers, 2	10	0	3
Source One (Met-Rx), 1 pkg, 62g	190	3	30
Spirutein Energy Bar, 1.4 oz	150	4	20
Energy: Cocoa, 65g (2.3 oz)	210	3	41
Steel Bar, 3 oz, 85g	330	6	52
Steel Pro, 85g	330	6	15
Sweet Rewards: Choc. Chip	110	2	23
Brownie; Fat Free	120	2	30
Sweet Success (Nestlé):			
Choc Bars	100	3.5	23
Snack Bars, 33g (1.2 oz)	120	4	23

Per Bar	C	F	Cb
Thermo Speed Bar, 85g	280	5	24
Think: Protein Bar, 2.3 oz	280	9	18
Think Thin! Lo Carb Diet,			
average all bars, 2.1 oz	240	10	18
Thunder Bar, all flavors	220	2	44
Tiger's Milk: 35g Bar	130	2.5	24
Peanut Butter varieties	150	6	19
Protein Rich	145	5	18
Tiger Sport, 65g	230	2	43
Twinlab: Ultra Fuel, 2¹/₂ oz	230	0	42
Protein Fuel, 3 oz	340	6	12
Soy Sensations, 1.76 oz	180	5	23
Hi Energy, 2 oz	230	7	25
Ironman Triathlon, 56.8g	230	7	25
Ultimate Lo Carb: Per 2.1 oz Bar			
Crunchy Peanut Butter	270	10	23
Other varieties, average	250	7	25
Ultimate Protein Bar:			
Choc./Dream; P'nut Butter, 78g	280	6	20
Berries 'N Yogurt, 40g (1.4 oz)	140	3	14
Chocolate Choc Dream, 40g	140	2.5	10
Universal Muscle, 56.7g	280	5	35
Usana: Nutribar, 41g	150	4	20
Fibergy Bar, 48g	180	2.5	37
Verve (Wholefoods Mkt), 2.4 oz	240	5	41
Viactive (Mead Johnson), 1.6 oz	180	4.5	29
Vita-Trim (Market America):			
Choc./Peanut Bar, 78g	320	6	44
White Lightning, 85g	320	5	27
Whole Foods: Everyday Bars, 1.76 oz			
Choc Fudge/Raspberry	172	4	17
Honey Peanut Yogurt	200	4.5	18
Worldwide Sport Nutrition: Per 2.75 oz Bar			
Pure Protein: Lemon Chiffon	270	5	27
Blueberry Cheesecake	270	6	27
Chewy Choc Chip	280	7	28
Choc Deluxe	240	4.5	27
Cinnamon Graham	270	6	26
Peanut Butter	280	7	26
Raspberry Vanilla	280	5	29
S'Mores	270	6	31
Vanilla Malted	280	5	24
White Choc. Mousse	270	6	25
Xetalean (Nature's Bounty), 40g	140	4.5	21
You Are What You Eat, 56g	220	5	39
Zone Force/Perfect, aver., 50g	195	6	21

Nuts

Per 1 oz Unless Indicated	C	F	Cb
Acorns, raw 1 oz	105	7	12
Almonds, Dried/Dry Roasted:			
Whole, 24-28 med., 1 oz	170	15	7
1/2 cup, 2 1/2 oz	420	37	17
Chopped, 1/2 cup, 2 1/4 oz	380	34	16
Sliced, 1/2 cup, 1 2/3 oz	280	25	12
Choc. coated (5-6), 1 oz	160	11	14
Oil Rstd *(Blue Diamond)*, 1 oz	175	17	3.5
Almond Meal (partially defatted)			
1 cup (not packed), 2 1/4 oz	260	11	11
Honey Roasted, 1 oz	170	13	8
Brazil Nuts, 8 medium, 1 oz	185	19	3.5
Cashews, Dry or Oil Roasted:			
14 large/18 med./26 small, 1 oz	165	14	10
1/2 cup, 2.4 oz	400	33	23
Honey Roasted, 1 oz	160	12	11
Chestnuts, aver. all: Dried, 1 oz	105	1	22
Raw/Fresh, 5-6 nuts, 1 oz	60	1	13
Canned, water chestnuts			
sliced/whole/drained, 1 oz	23	0	5
Coconut:			
Flesh (no shell), 1 oz	100	10	4
Raw: 1 pce. (2"x2"x1/2"), 1.6 oz	160	15	7
1/2 medium (4 1/2" diam.)	650	62	30
Dried (Desiccated):			
Unsweetened, 1 oz	187	18	17
Sweetened, shredded, 1 oz	140	9	13
Grated, 1/2 cup, 1.3 oz	185	12	18
Cream (can.), 1/2 c., 5.2 oz	285	26	12
Milk (canned), 1/2 c., 4 oz	225	24	3
Water (center liq.), 1/2 cup, 4 1/4 oz	23	0	4.5
Filberts or Hazelnuts:			
Shelled, 18-20 nuts	180	18	4.5
Chopped, 1/4 cup	180	18	4.5
Ground, 1/4 cup	120	12	3
Ginko Nuts, can., 14 med., 1 oz	32	0	6
Hickory, 30 small nuts	190	18	5
Macadamia Nuts, shelled:			
Raw, 7 med./14 small, 1 oz	200	21	4
1/2 cup, 2.3 oz	460	48	10
Oil roasted, 1 oz	205	22	3.5
1/2 cup, 2.4 oz	490	52	8
Choc. coated, 2-3 pces, 1 oz	180	13	15
Mixed Nuts: 18-22 nuts, 1 oz	175	13	7
Planters: Dry Roasted/Honey	170	15	7
Oil Roasted, all types	180	16	7
Sweet Roasts, 26 pces, 1 oz	160	12	10
Kettle: Choc Lover's Mix, 1 oz	130	17	16

Per 1 oz Unless Indicated	C	F	Cb
Nut Toppings:			
Chopped, 1 Tbsp, 1/4 oz	40	4	1.5
Peanuts:			
Raw/Dried: In shell, 1 oz	117	10	3
Shelled, 1 oz	160	14	4.5
Boiled, 1 oz, 1.1 oz	102	7	7
Roasted, 30 lge./60 sml., 1 oz	165	14	6
1 cup, 5.1 oz	840	71	31
Chopped, 3 Tbsp, 1 oz	165	14	6
Planters: Oil Roasted, 1 oz	170	15	5
Beer Nuts, 1 oz pkg	170	14	7
Choc-coated, 1/2 cup, 2 1/2 oz	380	25	36
Cocktail, oil roasted, 1 oz	170	14	6
Dry Roasted, 1 oz	160	14	6
Honey Roasted, 1 oz	150	11	10
Honey/Dry Roasted, 1 oz	160	13	7
Spanish Oil Roasted, 1 oz	170	14	5
Sweet 'n Crunchy, 1 oz	140	8	16
Pecans: Kernel halves, 1 oz	190	19	5
(20 Jumbo or 31 large halves)			
1 cup halves, 3.8 oz	720	73	20
Chopped, 1/2 cup, 2 oz	380	30	10
Oil Roasted, 1 oz	195	20	4.5
Honey Roasted, 1 oz	200	18	5
Pilinuts, dried, 1/4 cup, 1 oz	205	23	1
Pinenuts, dried, 1 Tbsp, 10g	50	5	1.5
Pistachios:			
Unshelled, 1/2 cup, 2 oz	165	14	7
Shelled, 1/4 c., 45 nuts, 1 oz	165	14	7
Lance, 1 1/8 oz package	180	14	8
Planters: Dry Roasted, 1oz	170	15	6
Fruit 'n Nut Mix, 1 oz	150	9	13
Nut Topping, 1 oz	180	16	6
Tavern Nuts, 1 oz	170	15	6
Trail Mix, 3 Tbsp, 1 oz	140	9	15
Sesame Nut Mix: *Planters,* 1 oz	160	12	8
Soy Nuts: Dry Roasted, 1 oz	130	6	9
1/2 cup, 3 oz	390	18	28
Dr Soy: Choc coated, 1 oz pkg	130	4.5	18
Honey Roasted, 1 oz pkg	140	6	21
Flavors, average, 1 oz	150	7	8
Walnuts:			
Black, 15-20 halves, 1 oz	175	16	3.5
Chopped, 1/4 cup	190	18	4
Ground, 1/4 cup	120	12	2.5
English/Persian:			
14 halves, 1 oz	185	18	5
Chopped, 1/4 cup	195	19	5

Seeds

	C	F	Cb
Alfalfa Seeds, sprout., 1/2 c., 1/2 oz	5	0	1
Caraway, Fennell, 1 tsp	10	0.5	1
Cottonseed Kernels, rst., 1 Tbsp	50	4	2
Flax Seeds, 3 Tbsp, 1 oz	150	10	11
Lotus Seeds, dried, 1/2 c., 1/2 oz	50	0.5	10
Poppy Seeds, 1 tsp	15	1	1
Pumpkin & Squash Seeds, whole:			
Roasted/Tamari, 1 oz	125	5.5	3
1/2 cup (32g)	140	6	3.5
Dried, 1 oz	155	13	5
Safflower Kernels, dried, 1 oz	150	11	10
Sesame Seeds: Dried, 1 Tbsp, 9g	50	4.5	2
Roasted/Toasted, 1 oz	160	14	7
Sunflower Kernels/Seed:			
Dry Roasted, 1 Tbsp, 8g	45	4	1.5
1/4 cup, 1 oz	160	14	6
Oil Roasted, 1/4 cup, 1 oz	180	17	6
Watermelon, dried, 1/4 cup, 1 oz	160	14	4.5

Quick Guide

Peanut Butter

	C	F	Cb
Average All Brands:			
1 tsp, 6g	35	3	1.5
1 Tbsp, 0.6 oz, (17g)	105	8.5	3.5
2 Tbsp, 1.2 oz, (34g)	210	17	7
1 oz Quantity (28g)	170	14	6
1/2 cup, 5 oz	850	70	30
Jif "Sensations" Berry Blend, 1 T.	100	8.5	5
Chocolate Silk, 1 Tbsp, 0.6 oz	95	7.5	7
Peanut Wonder, 1 Tbsp	50	2	5.5
Smucker's Honey Swtnd., 1 Tbsp	100	8	4
Goober Grape/Strawb., 1 Tbsp	90	5	4
Skippy, honeynut, 1 Tbsp, 16g	95	8	4

Other Nut & Seed Butters

	C	F	Cb
Almond Butter, 1 Tbsp, 1/2 oz	105	9	2.5
Almond Butter Honey Roasted	90	7	5.5
Beanut Butter, 1 Tbsp, 1/2 oz	88	5.5	7
Cashew Butter, 1 Tbsp	92	7	4.5
Cashew Peanut Date Butter	95	7	4
Hazelnut Butter, 1 Tbsp	100	10	2.5
Pecan Butter, 1 Tbsp	110	11	3.5
Pistachio Butter, 1 Tbsp	100	8.5	5
Sesame Butter/Tahini, 1 tsp	30	3	1
1 Tbsp, 1/2 oz	90	8.5	2
Sunflower Seed Butter, 1 Tbsp	95	8	4

Supplements

	C	F	Cb
Aloe Vera Juice, undil., 2 fl.oz	5	0	1
Barlean's Flax Oil, 3 capsules	27	3	0
Cod Liver Oil, 1 Tbsp	120	13	0
Evening Primrose Oil, capsules, 1	5	0.5	0
Fiber Supplements: Tabs, 1	1	0	0
Bios Life 2, 1 packet	10	0	2
Metamucil, 1 packet	5	0	0
Regular, 1 rounded Tbsp	34	0	8
Sugar-Free, 1 Tbsp	6	0	1
Fish Oil Capsules, average, 1	10	1	0
Flax Oil Capsules, 2	10	1	0
Garlic Tablets/Capsules, each	3	0	0
Lecithin Granules, 1 Tbsp, 10g	50	5	1
Protein; Powders, average, 1 oz	100	0.5	0
Tablets, 20 tabs, 1/2 oz	70	0.5	0
Seaweed: Dried, 1 oz	85	0.5	22
Soaked, drained, 1 oz	15	0.5	3
Spirulina, 1 tablet	2	0	0.5
Vitamins/Minerals: Tabs/Caps, 1	2	0	0
Vitamin E Capsules, each	5	0.5	0
Yeast: Tablets, 2 tabs	4	0	0.5
Flakes, 1 heaping Tbsp, 1/3 oz	30	0.5	4
Powder, 1 heaping Tbsp, 1/2 oz	50	0.5	6

Cough & Pharmaceutical

	C	F	Cb
Cough/Cold Syrups: *Per 1 Tbsp*			
Regular: w. sugar, 1 Tbsp	35	0	9
w. alcohol, 1 Tbsp	46	0	9
Sugar-Free *(Diabetic Tussin)*, 1 T.	0	0	0
Cough Drops/Lozenges: *See Page 130*			
Antacids: Average, 1 tablet	4	0	1
Liquid, 1 Tbsp	6	0	1
Sudafed Syrup, 1 tsp	14	0	3
Tylenol Liquid: Child, 1 tsp	17	0	4
Extra Strength, 1 tsp	11	0	3

Nut eaters are healthier and live longer say medical researchers. Nuts are a nutritious source of protein, vitamins, minerals and fiber. Their fat and fiber content can help to lower blood cholesterol, but watch the quantity if overweight.

Fresh Fruit

Weights As Purchased	C	F	Cb
Acerola, 1 cup, 20 pcs, 3$^{1}/_{2}$ oz	30	0	7.5
Apples: whole, average all varieties:			
1 small (4 per lb), 4 oz	70	0	17
1 medium (3 per lb), 5$^{1}/_{2}$ oz	90	0	23
1 large (2 per lb), 8 oz	135	0	34
I extra large, 11 oz	185	0	46
without skin, $^{1}/_{2}$ medium	35	0	9
Caramel Apple, 1 medium	170	0	42
Nut Coated, 1 medium	230	5	46
Apricots: 1 small (12 per lb)	17	0	4
1 medium (8 per lb), 2 oz	25	0	6
1 large (5-6 per lb), 3 oz	35	0	8
Avocado (w/out seed/skin):			
Average, $^{1}/_{2}$ medium, 3$^{1}/_{2}$ oz	160	15	6
1 salad slice, $^{1}/_{2}$ oz	25	2	1
Mashed/Puree, 2 Tbsp, 1 oz	50	4.5	2
$^{1}/_{4}$ cup, 2 oz	90	9	4
Californian, $^{1}/_{2}$ medium, 3 oz	160	14	8
Mashed/Puree, $^{1}/_{2}$ c., 4 oz	210	18	12
Florida, $^{1}/_{2}$ medium, 5$^{1}/_{2}$ oz	170	13	14
Mashed/Puree, $^{1}/_{2}$ c., 4 oz	125	10	9
$^{1}/_{2}$ cup cubed, 3 oz	105	8	8

Note: Avocados are nutritious and contain no cholesterol. Fat is mainly monounsaturated and benefits blood cholesterol. Excellent substitute for butter or margarine on bread or crackers.

	C	F	Cb
Banana: 1 small (4 lb), 4 oz	55	0	13
1 medium (3 per lb), 5 oz	80	0	20
1 large (2$^{1}/_{2}$ per lb), 7 oz	105	0	25
w/out skin, 1 medium, 3$^{1}/_{4}$ oz	80	0	20
$^{1}/_{2}$ cup, mashed, 4 oz	105	0	25
Berries: (Blueberries/Black/Boysenberries)			
$^{1}/_{2}$ cup, 2.5 oz	40	0	10
1 pint, 14 oz	220	1	56
Breadfruit, $^{1}/_{2}$ cup, 4 oz	115	0	28
Cantaloupe: Flesh/no skin, 1 oz	8	0	2
$^{1}/_{2}$ small, 20oz (w/skin/seeds)	125	1	30
$^{1}/_{2}$ medium, 28oz (w/skin/seeds)	175	1.5	42
1 slice, 2.5 oz (w/out skin)	20	0	5
1 cup pieces/balls, 5.5 oz	55	0	13
Carambola (Star Fruit), 1 med	50	0	4
Cassava, $^{1}/_{3}$ cup	120	0	27
Cherimoya (Custard Apple), 4 oz	110	1	27
Cherries: Sweet, 8 fruit, 2 oz	40	0	10
$^{1}/_{2}$ lb (30 cherries)	145	0	37
Sour, 8 fruit, 2 oz	25	0	6
$^{1}/_{2}$ lb (30 cherries)	100	0	23

Weights As Purchased	C	F	Cb
Coconut: Fresh, 1 piece, 1 oz	100	10	3
Shredded, fresh, $^{1}/_{2}$ cup	150	14	6
Sweetened, dried, $^{1}/_{2}$ cup	235	16	22
Crabapples, $^{1}/_{2}$ cup slices, 2 oz	40	0	9
Cranberries, $^{1}/_{2}$ cup, 2 oz	20	0	5
Currants: Per $^{1}/_{2}$ Cup			
European Black, raw, 2 oz	35	0	8
Red & White, raw, 2 oz	30	0	7
Custard Apple, raw, 4 oz	110	1	27
Dates ~ See Dried Fruits			
Durian, flesh, 4 oz	165	6	28
Elderberries, $^{1}/_{2}$ cup, 2$^{1}/_{2}$ oz	55	0	13
Feijoas, 1 medium, 2$^{1}/_{2}$ oz	35	0	7
Figs, green/black: 1 med., 2 oz	40	0	10
1 large, 3 oz	60	0	15
Fruit Salad, fresh, average,			
$^{1}/_{2}$ cup, 3$^{1}/_{2}$ oz	60	0	15
1 cup, 7 oz	120	0	30
Gooseberries, raw, $^{1}/_{2}$ c., 2$^{1}/_{2}$ oz	30	0	7
Grapefruit: Average all types,			
$^{1}/_{2}$ fruit, 10 oz (6 oz flesh)	55	0	13
1 cup sections w. juice, 8 oz	75	0	17
Grapes: Average, 1 cup, 5$^{1}/_{2}$ oz	100	0	24
1 small bunch, 4 oz	70	0	17
1 medium bunch, 7 oz	125	0	31
1 large bunch, 16 oz	285	0	71
Granadilla, flesh, 3$^{1}/_{2}$ oz	95	0	23
Groundcherries, $^{1}/_{2}$ cup, 2$^{1}/_{2}$ oz	35	0	8
Guava: 1 fruit, 4 oz	80	0	15
$^{1}/_{2}$ cup, 3 oz	40	0	9
Honeydew: 1 wedge (7"x 2" wide),			
8 oz (with skin)	50	0	12
1 cup cubes/balls, 6 oz	60	0	14
Honey Murcots, 1 only, 5 oz	45	0	11
Jaboticaba, flesh, 4 oz	75	2	15
Jackfruit, flesh, $^{1}/_{8}$ average, 4 oz	105	0	25
Jambos (Brazil Cherry), flesh, 4 oz	35	0	8
Java-Plum, 4 plums, $^{1}/_{2}$ cup	25	0	6
Jujube, flesh, 4 oz	65	0	16
Kiwifruit, 1 medium, 3 oz	45	0	11
1 large, 4 oz	60	0	15
Kumquats, 5 medium, 3$^{1}/_{2}$ oz	60	0	15
Kiwano, $^{1}/_{2}$ medium, 5 oz	35	0	8
Langsat, Duku, 1 medium, 2 oz	25	0	5
Lemon, 1 medium, 4 oz	20	0	5
1 wedge, 1 oz	5	0	1.5
Peel, 1 Tbsp	4	0	1

Weights As Purchased	C	F	Cb
Limes, 1 only, 2 oz	20	0	5
Loganberries, froz., 1/2 c., 2^1/2 oz	40	0	9
Longans, 5 fruit, 1/2 oz	10	0	2.5
Loquats, 4 fruit, 2^1/4 oz	25	0	6
Lychees, 4 fruit, 2^1/4 oz	25	0	6
Mamey Apple, 1 whole, 3 lb	430	4	100
1/4 fruit (1 cup flesh), 7 oz	100	1	23
Mandarin: 1 small, 3 oz	25	0	6
1 medium, 4 oz	35	0	8
1 large, 6 oz	55	0	11
Mango: flesh, 1/2 cup sl., 3 oz	48	0	11
1 whole, medium, 11 oz	140	0	34
Melon, avg, 1 cup, cubes/balls, 6 oz	60	0	14
Monstera Deliciosa (Taxonia),			
Edible part, 4 oz	50	0	11
Mulberries, 20 fruit, 1 oz	15	0	3
Nashi Fruit (Asian Pear), 1 med., 7 oz	85	0	21
Nectarines, 1 medium, 4 oz	50	0	12
1 large, 5^1/2 oz	70	0	17
Oheloberries, 1/2 cup, 2^1/2 oz	20	0	5
Olives (Pickled): Green, 1/2 oz lrg, 1^1/2 oz	45	5	0.5
Ripe, Grk. Style, 10 med., 1 oz	70	7	2
Ripe (Black), Californian:			
1 small/medium	5	0.5	0.3
1 large/extra large	6	0.5	0.5
1 jumbo	7	0.5	0.5
1 colossal	11	1	0.5
1 super colossal	13	1	1
Oranges: Average all varieties,			
1 small, 5 oz (with skin)	50	0	12
1 medium (3" diam.), 7 oz	70	0	17
1 large, 10 oz	100	0	24
Flesh only, 1 cup, 6 oz	80	0	19
Californian Valencia,			
1 medium (2^3/4" diam.), 6 oz	60	0	15
Californ. Navels (3" diam.), 7 oz	60	0	15
Sunkist Navel, 14 oz	130	0	32
Florida Orange, 1 medium, 7 oz	70	0	17
Peel, 1 Tbsp	0	0	0
Papaya: 1/2 cup, cubed, 2^1/2 oz	30	0	7
1 medium, 16 oz	120	0	28
Green (unripe), 1/2 cup, 3^1/2 oz	20	0	5
Passionfruit, 1 medium, 1^1/4 oz	20	0	4.5
PawPaw (see Papaya)			
Peaches: 1 med. (4 per lb), 4 oz	35	0	8
1 large, 6 oz	55	0	13
1 extra large, 10 oz	90	0	22

Weights As Purchased	C	F	Cb
Pears: Bartlett, 1 small, 4 oz	60	0	15
1 medium, 6 oz	90	0	22
1 large, 8 oz	120	0	30
1 cup slices, 5.8oz	100	0.5	25
Asian, 1 medium, 7 oz	85	0	21
Bosc, 6 oz	90	0	22
D'Anjou, 1 medium, 8 oz	120	0	30
Forelle, 1 medium, 7 oz	85	0	21
Red Pear, 5 oz	80	0	20
Seckel (Wash'ton), 2^1/4 oz	35	0	9
Pepino, 1/2 medium, 4 oz	20	0	4
Persimmons: Native, 1 oz	30	0	7
Japan. (2^1/2"d. x 2^1/2"h), 7 oz	120	0	30
Seedless (Maui), 1 md., 5 oz	100	0	25
Pineapple (no skin):			
1 thin slice, (1/2"), 2 oz	28	0	7
1 thick slice, (3/4"), 3 oz	40	0	10
1 cup, diced, 5^1/2 oz	75	0	19
1 medium, 1^1/2 lb (peeled)	525	0	130
Canned: *See Page 143*			
Pitanga, 3 fruit, 1 oz	6	0	1
Plaintains, 1/2 cup slices, 2^1/2 oz	90	0	22
Plums: Average all types,			
Mini/Damson, (1" diam.), 1/2 oz	8	0	2
Small (1^3/4" diam.), 2 oz	30	0	7
Medium (2^1/4" diam.), 3 oz	45	0	10
Large (2^1/2" diam.), 4 oz	65	0	15
Pomegranates, 1/2 fruit, 5 oz	55	0	13
Pummelo, flesh, 1/2 cup, 4 oz	35	0	8
Prickly Pears, 1 fruit, 5 oz	50	0	11
Quince, 1 medium, 3^1/2 oz	55	0	14
Rambutan (Rambotang),			
Red/Yellow, 1 medium, 2 oz	15	0	4
Raspberries, 1/2 cup, 2 oz	30	0	7
Rhubarb, raw, 1/2 cup, 2 oz	15	0	3
Sapodilla (Chico), 1 md., 7^1/2 oz	140	2	33
Sapotes, 1/2 cup, 5.5 oz	150	0	37
Soursop, 1 cup pulp, 8 oz	150	0	38
Strawberries: 1 cup, 5^1/2 oz	45	0	10
6 medium/3 large, 2 oz	15	0	3
1 pint, 12 oz	95	0	22
Chocolate Dipped, 2 medium	45	2.5	6
Sugar Apples, 1/2 cup pulp, 4 oz	120	0	30
Tamarillo, 1 medium, 3 oz	20	0	3
Tamarind: 1 fruit, 1/4 oz	5	0	1
Tangelo: 1 small, 4 oz	30	0	7
1 medium, 5 oz	40	0	9

Weights As Purchased	C	F	Cb
Tangelo: 1 large, 7 oz	55	0	12
Tangerine, 1 medium, 4 oz	50	0	12
Tangor, 1 medium, 4 oz	35	0	7
Tomatillos, (3) 3 oz	20	0	5
Tomato: Grape, 3 medium	8	0	2
Yellow Tear Drop, 4 med., 1 oz	8	0	2
Cherry, 1 medium, ³/4 oz	5	0	1
1 small, 3 oz	25	0	6
1 medium, 5 oz	35	0	8
1 medium slice	5	0	1
1 large, 7 oz	50	0.5	11
1 giant salad, 10 oz	70	1	16
Canned Tomatoes/Products: *See Page 86*			
Tree Tomato (Tamarillo), 3 oz	20	0	5
Ugli Fruit, Tangelo type, 5 oz	40	0	2
Watermelon: Flesh only/no skin, 1 oz	9	0	2
1 cup cubes or balls, 4¹/2 oz	50	0	12
1 thick (1") slice (¹/4 circle, 4¹/2"radius)			
9 oz w. skin / 5¹/2 oz no skin	50	0	12
1 thin (¹/2") slice (¹/4 circle)	25	0	6
1 thick (1") slice (¹/2 circle)			
18 oz w.skin	100	1	24
1 whole melon (15" long, 7¹/2"diam.)			
20 lb w.skin/10lb no skin	1450	19	324
Wax Jambu (Rose Apple), 2 oz	10	0	2

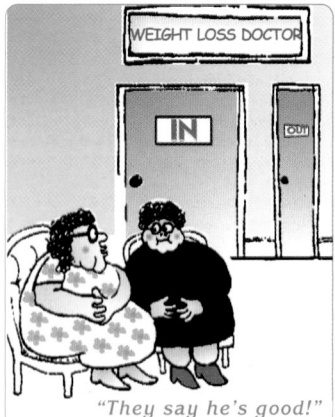

WEIGHT LOSS DOCTOR

IN — OUT

"They say he's good!"

Dried Fruit

	C	F	Cb
Apples, 5 rings, 1 oz	75	0	18
Apricots, 8 halves, 1 oz	65	0	15
Banana Chips, ¹/2 cup, 1¹/2 oz	160	5	18
Banana Flakes, 4 Tbsp, 1 oz	80	0	20
Cranberries, swtn. dr.,¹/3 c., 1.4 oz	130	0	33
Currants, ¹/4 cup, 1¹/4 oz	100	0	24
Dates: 5 medium dates, 1¹/2 oz	120	0	28
Large Calif., 3 dates, 2 oz	160	0	37
¹/2 cup, chopped, 3 oz	240	0	57
Figs, 3 medium figs, 2 oz	145	0	34
Longans; Lychees, 1 oz	80	0	19
Mango Slices, 4 strips, 1 oz	70	0	15
Mixed Fruit, 1 oz	70	0	16
Papaya Spears, 1 oz	75	0	17
Peaches, 2 halves, 1 oz	60	0	14
Pears, 3 halves, 2 oz	75	0	17
Pineapple, 1 oz	80	0	18
Prunes (dried Plums): w. pits, 1 oz	60	0	14
1 Medium (60/lb)	16	0	4
1 Large (50/lb)	22	0	5
1 Extra Large (40/lb)	27	0	6
Without pits, 4 med., 1 oz	70	0	17
Cooked: w. sugar, ¹/2 c, 5 oz	200	0	47
w/out sugar, ¹/2 c, 4¹/2 oz	125	0	30
Raisins: 2 Tbsp, 1 oz package	90	0	22
¹/2 cup, 2.8 oz	260	0	62
Sunsweet: Fruitlings, ¹/3 c., 1.5 oz	130	0	31
Plums (5) 1.4 oz	100	0	24

Candied Glacé Fruit

	C	F	Cb
Apricot, 1 medium, 1 oz	100	0	25
Cherry, 3 large, ¹/2 oz	50	0	12
Citron/Fruit Peel, 1 oz	90	0	21
Fig, 1 piece, 1 oz	90	0	21
Ginger, 1 oz	95	0	23
Pineapple, 1 slice, 1¹/4 oz	120	0	30

Fruit Leather/Rolls

	C	F	Cb
Average All Brands, 1 oz	100	0	24
Fruit By The Foot, 1 roll, ³/4 oz	80	0	17
Fruit Gushers, 1 pouch, 1 oz	90	1	20
Fruit Roll-Ups, 1 roll, ¹/2 oz	50	0	12
Stretch Island Leathers, 2 pces, 1 oz	90	0	21
Sunkist Fruit Roll, 1 roll	75	0	18

Other Fruit Confectionery/Snacks/Bars
~ *See Snacks/Granola Bars Page 133-137*

Canned Fruit & Snacks

Canned/Bottled Fruit

Solids & Liquids:
Per 1/2 Cup (Approx. 4 1/2 oz)

	C	F	Cb
Apples: sweetened	70	0	17
Apricots: In water/diet	35	0	9
In juice/lite	60	0	15
In syrup	105	0	27
Black/Blueberries: Heavy syrup	115	0	30
In light syrup	110	0	26
Cherries, pitted, in water	55	0	14
In light syrup	85	0	21
In heavy syrup	110	0	28
In extra heavy syrup	130	0	33
Maraschino, 5, 1 oz	50	0	12
Pie, 2/3 cup, 5 oz	60	0	14
Fruit Salad: In water/diet	35	0	9
In juice/Light	60	0	16
In heavy syrup	95	0	25
Gooseberries: Light syrup	90	0	23
Grapefruit: Juice pack	45	0	15
In light syrup	75	0	20
Lychees: Canned, 1/2 cup, 4.5 oz	105	0	26
Mixed Fruit: In water/diet	40	0	10
In fruit juices/light syrup	60	0	15
In heavy syrup	100	0	25
Peaches (halves/slices): In water/diet	30	0	8
In juice/light	50	0	14
In light syrup	70	0	19
drained, 1/2 peach	40	0	11
In heavy syrup	100	0	26
Pears: In water/diet	35	0	9
In juice/light	60	0	16
In heavy syrup	100	0	26
Pineapple: All types			
In own juice	70	0	17
In heavy syrup	90	0	22
Slices, drained, 2 slices			
In own juice, drained	30	0	7
In heavy syrup, drained	45	0	11
Plums: In water	50	0	14
In juice	75	0	20
In light syrup, 3 plums	85	0	21
In heavy syrup, 1/2 cup	160	0	41
3 plums	120	0	31
Prunes: In heavy syrup	120	0	32
4 prunes	70	0	18
In Liqueur, 1/2 cup, 125g	280	0	70
In Water, 1/2 cup	135	0	32
Raspberries, in heavy syrup	120	0	30

Solids & Liquids:
Per 1/2 Cup (Approx. 4 1/2 oz)

	C	F	Cb
Strawberries: In water	25	0	7
In heavy syrup	120	0	31
Tropical Fruit Salad: In light syrup	80	0	18
In heavy syrup	95	0	21

Fruit Snack Cups

	C	F	Cb
Mott's: Healthy Harvest, 4 oz cup	50	0	13
Blues Clues; Fruitsations, 4 oz c.	90	0	22
Del Monte Fruit Cups: Per 4 oz Cup			
Fruit Cocktail: In water/diet	40	0	11
In juice/light	55	0	15
In light syrup	80	0	21
In heavy syrup	95	0	25
Mandarin Orange cup	70	0	17
Mandarin Oranges: In water	40	0	10
In light syrup	80	0	20
Peach/Pear/Lite	50	0	13
Fruit Rageous cup	90	0	22
Fruit to Go, 4 oz cup	70	0	18
Pop Top Snack Cans:			
Fruit Cocktail, 8 1/2 oz can	190	0	47
Lite Sliced Peaches, 8 1/4 oz can	115	0	28
Dole Fruit Bowls			
4 oz Bowls: Peaches/Mandarin Or.	70	0	17
Mixed Fruit	80	0	19
Pineapple/Tropical Fruit	65	0	15
7 oz Bowls: Pineapple Chunks	90	0	23
Sliced Peaches	120	0	29
Tropical Fruit	100	0	25
Fruit 'n Gel Bowls 4.3 oz: Reg.	90	0	22
Reduced Sugar	50	0	13
Tree Top: Fruit Rocketz, 1 tube	45	0	11
Natural Apple, 1 Pkg., 4 oz	50	0	12
Vons: Mixed Fruit,			
In heavy syrup, 1 cup, 4.5 oz	90	0	22
In lite syrup, 1 cup, 4.5 oz	60	0	13

Apple & Fruit Sauces

	C	F	Cb
Apple Sauce:			
Regular/sweetened, 2 Tbsp, 1.1 oz	23	0	5
4 oz package cup	80	0	20
1/2 cup, 4.5 oz	90	0	22
Mott's Cinnamon, 1/2 cup, 4.5 oz	110	0	27
Cranberry Sce: Whole Berry, 1 T.	14	0	3
1/4 cup, 2 1/2 oz	110	0	27
Jellied Cranberry, 1/4 cup	110	0	27

Vegetables

Edible Portion ~ Raw Weight	C	F	Cb
Alfalfa Sprouts, 1/2 cup, 1/2 oz	5	0	1
Artichokes, Globe/French:			
1 medium, 4 1/2 oz	65	0	15
1 large, 8 oz	105	0	23
Artichoke Heart, 1/2 cup, 3 oz	40	0	10
Asparagus, raw/froz.: 4 med. spears	15	0	3
Cuts & tips, 1/2 cup, 3 oz	25	0	5
Bamboo Shoots, ckd, 1/2 c, 4 oz	15	0	3
Beans: Green/Snap, 1/2 c, 2 oz	20	0	4
Dried Beans, average all types:			
(Kidney, Brown, Haricot, Lima,			
Mung, Navy, Pinto, Red, White)			
Raw, 2 Tbsp, 1 oz	95	0.5	18
1 cup, 7 oz	665	3	126
Cooked, 1 oz	35	0	7
1/2 cup, 3 oz	105	0	21
Bean Sprouts, avg, 1/2 cup, 3 oz	25	0	3
Beets: Cooked, 1/2 c, slices, 3 oz	25	0	6
1 beet, 2" diam., 2 oz	17	0	4
Beet Greens, ckd, 1/2 c., 2 1/2 oz	20	0	4
Bell Pepper: *See Peppers*			
Bitter Melon/Gourd, 1 c. pces, 4 oz	22	0	5
Black Eyed Peas, ckd, 1/2 c., 2 oz	160	0	32
Bok Choy (Chinese Chard), 3 oz	13	0	3
Breadfruit, 1/4 small fruit	100	0	25
Broadbeans (Fava Beans):			
Green (in pod), raw: 4 pods			
(3 1/2 oz w. shell; 1.2 oz beans)	30	0	6
1 cup beans (no shell), 4 1/2 oz	110	1	22
Mature Seeds: Raw, 1 c., 5.3 oz	510	2	87
Cooked, 1/2 cup, 3 oz	95	0	17
Broccoli: Raw, 1/2 cup, 1 1/2 oz	12	0	3
1 spear (5 oz edible)	40	0	8
Cooked, 1/2 cup, 3 oz	25	0	5
BroccoSprouts, 1/2 cup, 1 oz	16	0	2
Brussel Sprouts, ckd, 1/2 c., 3 oz	35	0	8
Butterbeans, ckd, 1/2 cup, 3 oz	90	0	20
Cabbage: Avg, ckd, 1/2 c., 2 1/2 oz	15	0	2
Raw, shred., 1/2 cup, 1 1/4 oz	8	0	1
Carrot: Ckd, 1/2 cup sl., 2 1/4 oz	35	0	8
Raw, 1 medium (7 1/2"), 3 oz	33	0	8
Raw, 1 lb, (5-6 med)	175	0	44
4 sticks (4"), 1 1/2 oz	15	0	3
Shredded, 1/2 cup, 2 oz	25	0	6
Cauliflower: cooked:			
1 floret, 1/2 c. 1" pces, 3 oz	15	0	3
1/2 medium (15 oz raw)	100	0	20

Edible Portion ~ Raw Weight	C	F	Cb
Celeriac, 1/2 cup, raw, 2 3/4 oz	30	0	7
Celery: 1 stalk, 7 1/2", 1 1/2 oz	5	0	1
Diced, 1/2 cup, 2 1/4 oz	10	0	3
Chard (Swiss), 1/2 c., ckd, 3 oz	20	0	4
Chayote Squash, 4 1/2 oz	30	0	7
Chick Peas (Garbanzo Beans):			
Dry, 1 cup, 6 oz	550	10	92
Cooked, 1 cup, 6 oz	270	4	45
Chicory, Greens, 1/2 cup, 3 oz	20	0	4
Chicory/Witloof: *See Endive*			
Chili Peppers: *See Peppers*			
Chinese Long Bean, sliced, 1 c., 3.2 oz	45	0	8
Chives, chopped, 1 Tbsp	1	0	0
Choy Sum, 3 oz	13	0	3
Cilantro (Coriander), 1 Tbsp	1	0	0
Collards, ckd, 1/2 cup, 3 oz	15	0	4
Corn, yellow/white:			
Raw, kernels, 1/2 c., 2 3/4 oz	65	1	14
Ear (5"x 1 3/4"), 5 1/2 oz	80	1	17
Trimmed to 3 1/2" long	65	1	14
Cooked, kernels, 1/4 c., 1 1/2 oz	35	0.5	7
(Also see Frozen & Canned Corn Page 146-147)			
Courgette: *See Zucchini*			
Cress, Garden, 1/2 cup, 1 oz	10	0	2
Cucumber, 1 whole, 11 oz	40	0	12
1/2 cup slices, 2 oz	5	0	1
Daikon Radish, 3 oz	18	0	4
Dandelion Greens, 1/2 cup, 1 oz	15	0	3
Endamame: Shelled, 2/3 cup, 3 oz	120	5	9
in pods, 4 oz	60	3	5
Eggplant: 1/4 medium, 4 oz	35	0	8
1/2 cup, 1" pieces, 1 1/2 oz	10	0	2
1 slice, fried, 1 oz	75	4	10
Endive, Belgian/French:			
1 med. head (6"), 2 1/2 oz	12	0	3
Fava Beans: *See Broadbeans*			
Fennel, 2 oz	10	0	3
Gai Choy Cabbage, ckd, 1 cup	20	0	5
Gai Lan (Chinese Kale), 3 oz	35	0	7
Garlic, 1 clove	4	0	1
Ginger: 1/4 cup slices, 1 oz	20	0	4
Crystallized (sugared), 1 oz	95	0	20
Horseradish, 1 pod, 3/4 oz	4	0	1
Jerusalem Artichoke, 1/2 cup	60	0	14
Jicama, raw, 1/2 cup, 3 oz	25	0	5
Kale, 1/2 cup, 2 oz	20	0	4
Kohlrabi, 1/2 cup, cooked, 3 oz	25	0	6

Edible Portion ~ Raw Weight	C	F	Cb
Leek, cooked, 1 whole, 4 oz	40	0	9
Lentils, green/brown: Dry, 1 oz	95	0.5	16
Dry, 1 cup, 6 3/4 oz	650	2	109
Cooked, 1/2 cup, 3 1/2 oz	115	0.5	20
Lettuce, 1 c., chop./shred., 2 1/2 oz	10	0	2
Butterhead, 2 leaves, 1/2 oz	2	0	0.5
Cos/Romaine, 1/2., shred., 2 1/2 oz	4	0	1
Iceberg: 1 leaf, 3/4 oz	3	0	1
1 medium head, 15-16 oz	60	0	15
Lima Beans, baby, ckd,1/2 c., 3 oz	90	0	17
Lotus Root, 10 slices, ckd, 3 oz	60	0	15
Mung Bean Sprouts, 1/2 cup	15	0	3
Mushroom: Raw, 1/2 cup, 1 oz	10	0	2
Cooked, 1/2 cup, 2 1/2 oz	20	0	3
Mustard Greens, 1/2 cup, 1 oz	7	0	1
Okra, ckd., 1/2 cup, slices, 2 3/4 oz	25	0	6
Onions: Raw, 1 small, 2 oz	20	0	5
1 medium, 4 oz	40	0	9
1 large, 8 oz	80	0	19
1 jumbo, 16 oz	160	0	38
1/2 cup, chopped, 3 oz	30	0	7
Dehydrated flakes, 1/4 c, 1/2 oz	45	0	11
Rings, breaded/fried, 2 rings	80	5	9
Ore-Ida, 4 pces	220	11	27
Scallions, 2 oz	15	0	4
Spring, 1/4 cup, chopped, 1 oz	6	0	1
Parsley, chopped, 1/2 cup, 1 oz	10	0	2
Parsnips, 1 medium, 4 oz	80	0	20
Cooked, 1/2 cup slices, 2 3/4 oz	65	0	16
Peas: Green, 1/4 cup, 1 1/2 oz	35	0	6
raw, with pods, 1/2 lb	70	0	13
Snow Peas (8-9 pods), 1 oz	10	0	2
Split, dry, hulled, 1 oz	50	0	10
cooked, 1 cup, 7 oz	230	1	41
Peppers:			
Bell: 1 medium, 5 oz	25	0	6
1/2 cup, chopped, raw, 1 3/4 oz	12	0	3
1 ring (3" diam. x 1/4" thick)	2	0	0
Sweet, 1 medium, 5 oz	35	0	9
Chile: Green/Red, 1 1/2 oz	18	0	4
Habanero, 1 only, 8g	11	0	2
Pigeon Peas, cooked, 1/2 cup	85	1	16
Pimientos, 3 medium, 3 1/2 oz	25	0	5
Poi, 1/2 cup, 4.2 oz	135	0	33
Pumpkin, mashed, 1/2 cup, 4 oz	25	0	6
Purslane, cooked, 1/2 c., 2 oz	10	0	2

Edible Portion ~ Raw Weight	C	F	Cb
Potatoes: Raw (with skin):			
1 Baby, Gourmet, 2 oz	45	0	11
1 Small, 3 oz	65	0	15
1 Medium, 5 oz	110	0	26
1 Peeled, 4 oz	90	0	22
1 Large, 8 oz	180	0	44
1 Extra large (Russet), 12 oz	270	0	65
1 Jumbo (Russet), 16 oz	360	0	88
Baked (no fat); large, 10oz raw:			
Plain, with skin, 7 oz	220	0	51
without skin, 5 1/2 oz	145	0	34
With Toppings: + 2 tsp fat	290	8	51
+ Sour Cr./Chives, 2 Tbsp	270	6	53
+ Plain Yoghurt, 2 Tbsp	240	1	55
+ Grated Cheese, 1 oz	330	9	56
+ Cottage Cheese, 2 oz	280	2	56
Potatoes (Cont):			
Mashed w. milk and fat, 1/2 c.	110	4	14
Roasted (w. fat), 1 small	155	8	21
Garlic Potatoes, 4 oz	120	2	22
Hash Browns: w. Butt. Sce, 2 1/2 oz	125	6	10
Homemade, 1/2 cup, 2 1/2 oz	165	10	10
Potato Skins: (w. Cheese topping),			
1 whole (8 oz baking), 4 oz	240	13	22
French Fries: Small serve, 2 1/2 oz	220	12	14
Medium serve, 4 oz	350	20	22
Froz., uncooked, 18 fries, 4 oz	185	7	22
Oven-heated, 18 fries, 4 oz	185	7	22
Take-Out, 1 cup, 5 oz	440	25	28
McDonald's: Small, 2.4 oz	210	10	26
Medium, 5 oz	450	22	57
Supersize, 7 oz	610	29	77
Fried, 18 fries, 3 oz	275	15	16
Au Gratin, 1/2 cup, 4.3 oz	160	9	22
Pancakes, 1 only, 5 oz	90	5	9
Kugel, 5 oz	300	20	26
Puffs, fried, 4 puffs, 1 oz	65	3	37
Scalloped, 1/2 cup, 4 1/4 oz	105	4	13
Stuffed Baked Potatoes:			
See 1-Potato-2 ~ Fast-Food Section			
Ore-Ida Frozen Potatoes: See Page 147			
Potato Salad, 1/2 cup, 4 1/2 oz	180	10	14
Radish: aver., 10 only, 1 1/2 oz	10	0	2
Oriental, 1/2 c. slices, 1 1/2 oz	10	0	2
Rutabagas, ckd., 1/2 c. cubes, 3 oz	30	0	7
Salsify, ckd, 1/2 c. slices, 2 1/2 oz	45	0	11
Sauerkraut, 1/2 cup, 4 oz	25	0	5

Vegetables - Fresh or Frozen (Cont)

Edible Portion ~ Raw Weight

	C	F	Cb
Seaweed: Average, dried, 1 oz	50	0	13
Soaked, drained, 1 oz	15	0	4
Nori/Laver, dried, 6 sheets, 1/2 oz	35	0	5
Shallots, chopped, 1 Tbsp	7	0	1
Sorrel, raw, 1/2 cup, 4 oz	23	0.5	4
Soybeans: Mature, dry, 1 oz	110	5	9
Dry, 1/2 cup, 3 1/2 oz	385	18	22
Cooked, 1/2 cup, 3 oz	105	5	6
(Soy Products/Tofu/Tempeh: See Pages 78)			
Spinach, cooked, 1/2 cup, 3 oz	20	0	4
Creamed, 1/2 cup, 4 1/2 oz	140	12	8
Raw 1 cup, 1 oz	20	0	4
Squash: Summer, raw, 1/2 c., 2 1/4 oz	13	0	3
cooked, 1/2 cup slices, 3 oz	18	0	4
Winter, cooked,			
Acorn, 1/2 cup cubes, 3 1/2 oz	55	0	14
1/2 medium (10 oz raw wt.)	85	0	22
Butternut, 1/2 c. cubes, 3 1/2 oz	40	0	10
1/4 medium (9 oz raw wt.)	95	0	23
Spaghetti, 1/2 cup, 2 3/4 oz	23	0	5
Succotash, ckd, 1/2 cup, 3 1/3 oz	110	1	23
Sweetcorn: *See Corn*			
Sweet Potatoes: Cooked with Skin (no fat)			
1 medium, 4 oz	120	0	28
No skin, mashed, 1/2 c., 5 1/2 oz	170	0	40
Swedes, 1/2 cup, 3 oz	45	0	10
Swiss Chard, ckd chop., 1 cup, 6 oz	35	0	7
Taro, cooked, 1/2 cup, 2 oz	95	0	23
Tomatoes *(See Pg. 142):* 1 sm., 3 oz	20	0	5
1 medium, 5 oz	35	0	8
1 large, 7 oz	45	0	10
Cooked, 1/2 cup, 4 1/4 oz	30	0	7
Fried, 1 small, 3 oz	60	4	5
Tomatillo, 1 oz	7	0	1
Turnips: White, ckd, 1/2 cup, 3 oz	15	0	4
Greens, ckd, 1/2 cup, 2 1/2 oz	15	0	3
Water Chestnuts: 4 nuts	40	0	10
1/2 cup slices, 2 1/4 oz	65	0	15
Watercress, 10 sprigs, 1 oz	4	0	1
Yam: Cooked, 1/2 c., 2 1/2 oz	80	0	20
Baked, 1 medium (6") 8 oz	260	0	62
1 large (9") 12 oz	390	0	93
Yardlong Bean, 1 pod, 1/2 oz	7	0	1
Yucca Root, 2.5 oz	60	0	14
Zucchini: 1 medium, 10 oz	45	0	10
1/2 cup slices, cooked, 3 oz	13	0	3

Frozen Vegetables

Birds Eye

	C	F	Cb
Brocc./Carrots/W. Chestnuts, 1 cup	35	0	6
Broccoli/Corn/Red Peppers, 3/4 cup	50	0.5	11
Broccoli/Cauli./Carrots, 1 cup	30	0	5
Brussels Sprouts/Cauli./Carrots	35	0	5
Carrots/Corn/Green Beans, 2/3 cup	60	0.5	11
Cauliflower/Carrots/Pea Pods, 1 cup	30	0	5
Chopped Spinach, 1/3 cup	20	0	2
Baby: Corn Blend, 2/3 cup	60	0.5	11
Bean & Carrot Blend, 1 cup	30	0	5
Broccoli Blend, 1 cup	70	1.5	8
Baby (Cont): Broccoli Florets, 1 c.	25	0	4
Gold & White Corn, 2/3 cup	80	1	15
Pea Blend, 3/4 cup	40	0	7
Sweet Pea, 2/3 cup	70	0.5	12
Simply Grillin':			
Garden Herb, 1 cup, 4.3 oz	140	6	19
Potatoes & Onions, 1 c., 4.4 oz	180	7	25
Rstd Corn & Pot., 3/4 cup, 3.5 oz	140	5	19
Roasted Garlic, 3/4 cup, 3 1/2 oz	120	4.5	17
Pasta Secrets: Ranch, 1 c., 6.6 oz	300	15	29
Italian Pesto, 1 cup, 6.4 oz	240	9	32
Primavera, 1 c. 6.7 oz	230	10	26
Three Cheese, 1 cup, 6 oz	230	8	31
Zesty Garlic, 1 cup, 6 oz	240	10	31
Stir Fry: *Prepared (Includes Pasta)*			
Asparagus, 2 cup	90	0.5	16
Green Bean, 1 3/4 cup	100	0.5	19
Voila! Meals: *See Page 59*			

Green Giant

	C	F	Cb
Vegetables: Asparagus Cuts, 2/3 cup	25	0	4
Corn: Nibblers, 1 ear	70	0.5	14
Extra Sweet Niblets, 2/3 cup	70	1	13
S/Western & Rst Peppers, 3/4 c.	90	1	18
Green Bean Casserole, 2/3 cup	100	5	11
Honey Glazed Carrots, 1 cup	90	3.5	13
Le Sueur Baby Sw. Peas, 2/3 cup	60	0.5	11
Spinach, 1/2 cup	25	0	3
Veges In Cheese & Cream Sauce: *Prepared*			
Alfredo Vegetables, 3/4 cup	80	3	9
Broccoli & Cheese, 2/3 cup	70	2.5	9
Brocc., Cauliflower, Carrots, 2/3 c.	70	2.5	10
Cauliflower & Cheese Sce, 1/2 cup	60	2.5	8
Creamed Spinach, 1/2 cup	80	3	9
Cream Style Corn, 1/2 cup	110	1	23
Green Bean Casserole, 2/3 cup	90	5	9

Vegetables - Frozen, Canned or Bottled

Frozen Vegetables (Cont)

	C	F	Cb
Green Giant (Cont)			
Rice & Vegetables: Prepared			
Cheesy Rice & Brocc., 1 pkt, 10 oz	300	5	56
Oriental Rice, 1 pkt, 10 oz	340	12	52
Rice Medley, 1 pkt, 10 oz	280	4	52
Rice Pilaf, 1 pkt, 10 oz	230	3.5	44
White & Wild Rice, 1 pkt, 10 oz	280	6	51
French Fries: Country, 18 fries, 3 oz	120	4	19
Crispers 17 pces, 3 oz	210	12	23
Crispy Crunchies, 13 fries, 3 oz	160	8	20
Fast Food Fries, 35 fries, 3 oz	160	7	22
Ore-Ida (As Purchased):			
Pasta Accents: Per 1 Cup, Cooked			
Alfredo Broccoli	105	4	14
Crmy Cheddar w. Broc./Carrots	125	4	18
Garden Herb	115	3.5	16
Garlic Seas. w. Broc./Corn/Carrots	130	5	18
Primavera	140	4.5	19
Three Cheese	150	4.5	21
White Cheddar	135	4	18
Funky Fries: Cinna-Stiks (17) 3 oz	300	17	27
Cocoa Crispers, 17 pces, 3 oz	300	16	31
Crunchy Rings, 11 pces, 3 oz	230	11	26
Kool Blue, 17 pces, 3 oz	250	15	21
Golden Crinkles, 13 pces, 3 oz	120	3.5	19
Golden Fries, 17 pces, 3 oz	120	4	20
Golden Twirls, 17 pces, 3 oz	160	7	22
Oven Chips, 7 pces, 3 oz	160	7	22
Shoestrings, 40 pces, 3 oz	150	6	22
Steak Fries, 9 fries, 3 oz	110	3.3	19
Texas Crispers, 8 pces, 3 oz	140	6	20
Waffle Fries, 9 fries, 3 oz	150	7	21
Zesties, 12 pces, 3 oz	150	7	20
Hash Browns: Toaster, 2 patties	220	12	25
Potatoes O'Brien, 3/4 c., 2 oz	60	0	14
Onion Rings: Gourmet, 4 pces, 3 oz	210	10	28
Onion Ringers, 6 pces, 3.2 oz	220	12	25
Sweet Potatoes: 4 oz	80	0	18
Tater Tots: 9 pces, 3 oz	170	8	21
Mini, 19 pces, 3 oz	180	10	18
Onion 9 pces, 3 oz	150	7	21
Twiced Baked: Potatoes, 1, 5 oz	190	7	26
TGI Friday's			
Potato Skins, 3 pces, 3¹/2 oz	210	11	19
Wild Oats: Oven Fries, (18) 3 oz	130	4	24
Potato Poppers (Bites), (10) 3 oz	130	8	14

Canned/Bottled

	C	F	Cb
Solids & Liquid			
Artichoke Hearts: Plain, 1 oz (1)	30	0	8
Marinated, 1 oz	60	5	2
Asparagus, 1/2 cup, 4¹/2 oz	20	0	3
Bamboo Shoots, 1 cup, 4¹/2 oz	25	0	4
Bean Salad, 1/2 cup, 3 oz	90	0	23
Bean Sprouts, 2/3 cup	10	0	2
Beans: Green, 1/2 cup, 4¹/4 oz	20	0	4
Baked Beans, 1/2 cup, 4¹/2 oz	120	<1	18
Butter Beans, 1/2 cup, 4¹/2 oz	90	0	20
Italian, cut, 1/2 cup, 4¹/2 oz	30	0	7
Kidney Beans, 1/2 cup, 4¹/2 oz	105	<1	20
Lima Beans, 1/2 cup, 4¹/2 oz	80	0	15
Pinto Beans, 1/2 cup, 4¹/2 oz	100	<1	20
Beets: Sliced/Whole, 1/2 c., 4¹/2 oz	35	0	7
Crinkle/Pickled (Del Monte) 1/2 c.	80	0	20
Carrots: Sliced, 1/2 cup	35	0	8
Honey Glazed (Green Giant) 1/2 c.	45	3.5	13
Corn: Kernels, 1/2 cup, 4¹/2 oz	80	0.5	20
Drained Solids, 1/2 cup, 3oz	65	0.5	15
Creamed style, 1/2 cup, 4¹/2 oz	100	0.5	24
Garbanzo/Chick Peas, 3 oz	100	2	20
Green Chilies: diced, 2 Tbsp, 1 oz	5	0	1
Hearts of Palm, (1), 1.2 oz	9	0	2
Mushrooms: 1/2 cup, 2¹/2 oz	20	0	4
in Butter Sauce, 2 oz	30	1	3
Onions: Pickled, 1 med., 3/4 oz	10	0	2
Cocktail, 1 onion	2	0	0.5
Peas, 1/2 cup, 3 oz	60	0	11
Peppers: Hot Chilli, 1 only, 1 oz	8	0	2
Sweet, undrained, 2¹/2 oz	15	0	3
Jalapeno, w. liq., 1/2 c. chopped	17	0	3
Fried, drain, 2 Tbsp, 1 oz	60	5	3
Salsa, average all types, 2 Tbsp	15	0	3.5
Sauerkraut, undrained, 1/2 c., 4 oz	25	0	6
Spinach, 1/2 cup, 3¹/2 oz	25	0	3.5
Succotash: w. Cr. Style Corn,1/2 c.	100	1	23
w. whole kernels, undrained	80	1	17
Sweetcorn: See Corn			
Sweet Potato: 1/2 cup, 3¹/2 oz	105	0	24
Candied (Green Giant) 3/4 cup	240	7	41
Tomatoes, Sundr.: Natural, 5-6 pce	22	0	5
in Oil, drained, 6 pces, 1/2 oz	60	4	6
Tomato Products: See Page 86			
Vegetables, mixed, 1/2 cup, 4 oz	45	0	8
Yams: in Light Syrup, 1/2 cup, 4 oz	105	0	25
Candied, 1/2 cup, 5 oz	170	0	46
Zucchini in Tom. Sce., 1/2 c., 4 oz	30	0	8

Vegetables • Salads

Take-Out Salads & Vegetables

Avg. All Outlets: Per Serving

	C	F	Cb
Antipasto Salad, 1 cup	140	10	2
Bean Salad, 1/2 cup	110	4	17
Bulgur Salad, 1/2 cup	70	2	12
Caesar Salad, Classic, 1 cup	200	14	15
Side Salad, no dressing	25	0	6
Carrot Raisin: No dress., 1/2 cup	20	0	5
with dressing, 1/2 cup	65	5	5
Chef Salad: Regular, no dressing	620	37	8
w. 2oz 1000 Island	860	61	8
Chicken Salad Platter, 6 oz	200	8	12
Coleslaw: Traditional, 1/2 cup	150	8	18
w. low cal dressing	60	1	12
Corn, Mexican, 1/2 cup	240	12	33
Cucumber, non-oil dress, 1/2 cup	60	0	14
w. Oil dressing, 1/2 cup	140	12	8
Eggplant Salad, 1/2 cup	75	5	7
Fettucini w. veges, 1/2 cup	110	5	15
Garden Salad, no dressing	35	0	8
Greek Salad, 1 cup	120	10	7
Greek Vegetables, 1/2 cup	140	12	7
Lettuce, hearts, 1/4 head	20	0	4
Lobster Salad Platter, 6 oz	200	8	12
Macaroni Salad, 1/2 cup, 4 oz	180	13	13
Nicoise, 1 cup	450	32	18
Pasta Salad, 1/2 cup	160	8	16
Pineapple Coconut Slaw, 1/2 cup	150	10	14
Potato Salad: Dijon	140	7	17
w. Mayonnaise, 1/2 cup	170	10	17
Lowfat, 1/2 cup	110	1.5	21
Rice Salad, 1/2 cup	150	10	13
Saffron Rice, 1/2 cup	130	3	24
Spinach Salad	180	13	13
Tomato & Mozzarella, 1/2 cup	180	14	10
Tabouli, 1/2 cup	150	6	22
Three Bean Salad, 1/2 cup	80	5	9
Tortelini w. Basil Pesto, 1/2 cup	170	10	19
Waldorf w. Mayo, 1/2 cup	160	12	12

Signature Salads: Per 6 oz Serving
(Supplied to Deli's and Institutions)

	C	F	Cb
Antipasto Salad, 6 oz	510	50	4
Artichoke Salad, marinated	400	41	8
California Medley	120	7	15
Cheese Agnolotti	250	8	23
Chicken Salad	420	33	11
Crabmeat Flavored	450	38	20

Signature Salads (Cont)

	C	F	Cb
Egg Salad	300	23	14
Fresh Button Mushroom	190	16	6
Garden Olive	630	67	3
Ham Salad	400	32	14
Prima Pasta Salad	360	30	18
Seafood Pasta Del Mar	170	10	21
Seafood with Crab & Shrimp	420	34	20
Shrimp Salad	360	32	8
Tuna Salad	450	36	14

Fast-Food Restaurants: *See Page 175*

Fresh Salad Packs

Pre-Packaged (Supermarkets)

	C	F	Cb
Dole: Complete: Caesar, 3 1/2 oz	170	13	8
Oriental, 3 1/2 oz	120	6	13
Romano, 3 1/2 oz	150	12	9
Spinach Bacon, 3 1/2 oz	170	10	18
Sunflower Ranch, 3 1/2 oz	160	16	5
Special Blends (no added dressing):			
Aver. all varieties, 2 cups, 3 oz	15	0	3
Regular Salad Packs (no added dressing):			
Classic Coleslaw, 3 oz	25	0	5
Classic Iceberg, 3 oz	15	0	4
Zesty Italian, 7 oz	110	0	4
Fresh Express: *Per Package*			
Chicken Caesar, 1 pkg, 183g	240	16	13
Chick. Crmy. Ranch, 1pkg. 194g	230	14	15
Chicken Teriyaki 1pkg, 193g	250	15	17
Salad Kits: Per Serving, Prepared			
Caesar, 2 cups	160	14	7
Caesar w. Light Dressing, 2 cups	100	7	8
Caesar Supreme, 2 cups	150	12	7
Oriental, 1 1/2 cups	140	9	13
European, 2 1/2 cups	15	0	3
Ready Pac: Average all types	15	0	2

Salad Toppings

	C	F	Cb
Bacon Bits, average, 1 Tbsp	30	1.5	2
Chow Mein Noodles, dry, 1/2 cup	120	5	13
Croutons, 2 Tbsp, 10g	35	1	6
Olives, 5 medium	25	2	0
Potato Chips, 1 oz	150	10	15
Sunflower Seeds, 1 Tbsp, 8 g	45	4	1.5
Tortilla Chips, 1 oz	150	8	16

Quick Guide

Orange Juice C F Cb

Average ~ Fresh or Sweetened:

	C	F	Cb
1/2 Cup, 4 fl.oz	55	0	13
Small Glass, 6 fl.oz	82	0	20
Regular Glass, 8 fl.oz	110	0	26
8 3/4 fl.oz Box	120	0	28
10 fl.oz Bottle	140	0	32
11 1/2 fl.oz Can	160	0	36
16 fl.oz Bottle	220	0	52
20 fl.oz Bottle	280	0	72
64 fl.oz/1/2 Gallon	880	0	208

Juices ~ Generic

Average All Brands: Per 8 fl.oz Unless Indicated

	C	F	Cb
Aloe Vera Juice, unsweet., 2 oz	5	0	1
Apple Juice: 8 fl.oz	115	0	30
10 fl.oz Bottle	145	0	36
16 fl.oz	230	0	60
Carrot Juice: Fresh, 6 fl.oz	60	0	14
Sweetened, 6 fl.oz	75	0	17
Cranberry Juice, Cocktail/Blend	120	0	34
Fruit Blends, average, 8 fl.oz	120	0	31
Fruit Nectars, average, 8 fl.oz	140	0	35
Grape Juice, 8 fl.oz	160	0	40
Grapefruit Juice, 8 fl.oz	100	0	23
Lemon/Lime Juice: 1 Tbsp	4	0	1.5
1 cup, 8 fl.oz	60	0	21
Concentrate, 1 tsp	0	0	0
Noni Juice: Tahitian, 2 Tbsp, 1 fl.oz	10	0	2
Southern Cross Botanicals, 1 fl.oz	6	0	2
Tahiti Traders, 1 fl.oz	20	0	5
Orange Juice, 8 fl.oz	110	0	26
Passion Fruit Juice (Fresh):			
Purple, 1 cup, 8 fl.oz	125	0	34
Yellow, 1 cup, 8 fl.oz	150	0	36
Papaya/Peach Nectar, 8 fl.oz	140	0	35
Pear Nectar, 8 fl.oz	150	0	40
Pineapple Juice, 8 fl.oz	110	0	27
Prune Juice, 8 fl.oz	180	0	43
Strawb./Raspberry Juice, 8 fl.oz	100	0	23
Tangerine Juice, 8 fl.oz	100	0	25
Tomato Juice, 8 fl.oz	50	0	12
Vegetable Juice, 8 fl.oz	50	0	12
Wheat Grass Juice, 1 fl.oz 'Shot'	5	0	1
2 fl.oz 'Shot'	10	0	2

Quick Guide

Fruit Smoothies C F Cb

Average All Brands

	C	F	Cb
Fruit Only: 8 fl.oz cup	105	0	25
12 fl.oz	160	0	38
16 fl.oz	210	0	50
24 fl.oz	320	0.5	76
Fruit + Nonfat Milk/Soy:			
12 fl.oz	190	0.5	40
16 fl.oz	250	0.5	53
24 fl.oz	380	1	80
Fruit + Nonfat Frozen Yogurt/Sherbet:			
12 fl.oz	210	0.5	47
16 fl.oz	280	0.5	62
24 fl.oz	420	1	94

Juice Brands

Per 8 fl.oz Unless Indicated

	C	F	Cb
Apple & Eve: Naturally Cranberry	120	0	30
Cranberry/Raspberry Apple	120	0	30
Arizona: Grapeade, 8 fl.oz	120	0	29
Crazy Cocktail; Lemonade	110	0	27
Mucho Mango; Orangeade	105	0	27
Pina Colada	140	1	34
Bright & Early			
Orange Juice (Chilled/Frozen)	120	0	30
Grape Juice (Frozen)	140	0	33
Campbell's			
Tomato Juice, 8 fl.oz	50	0	10
10.5 fl.oz	60	0	12
V-8 100% Vegetable Jce, 8 fl.oz	50	0	10
V-8 Splash, all flavors, 8 fl.oz	110	0	27
Capri Sun: Avg all flavors, 6.75 oz	100	0	28
Chiquita: Frozen Concentrates, prepared:			
Average all varieties, 8 fl.oz	130	0	32
Del Monte			
Pineapple Juice: Fresh, 8 fl.oz	110	0	27
From Concentrate, 8 fl.oz	130	0	32
Prune Juice, 8 fl.oz	170	0	42
Tomato Juice: Fresh, 8 fl.oz	40	0	10
From Concentrate, 8 fl.oz	50	0	12
Snap-E-Tom Cocktail, 11.5 fl.oz can	70	0	15
Fruit Smoothie Blenders: Per 5.5 fl.oz			
Average all flavors	160	0	40

149

Fruit & Vegetable Drinks & Juices (Cont)

Per 8 fl.oz Unless Indicated   **C** **F** **Cb**

Dole
	C	F	Cb
100% Fruit Juice Blends:			
Average all varieties, 8 fl.oz	120	0	29
Fruit Drink Blends:			
Average, 8 fl.oz	130	0	31
Spicy Vegetable Blend, 12 fl.oz	80	0	16

Donald Duck
	C	F	Cb
100% Orange Jce (+Calcium), 8 fl.oz	120	0	29

Eden: Organic Apple, 8 fl.oz
	C	F	Cb
Eden: Organic Apple, 8 fl.oz	80	0	23

Five Alive: Citrus beverage, 8 fl.oz
	C	F	Cb
Five Alive: Citrus beverage, 8 fl.oz	120	0	30

Florida's Natural
	C	F	Cb
Orange Juice, 8 fl.oz	110	0	26
Grapefruit Juice, 8 fl.oz	100	0	24

Fresh Samantha
	C	F	Cb
Banana Strawberry	150	1	12
Carrot/Orange; The Big Bang	100	0	8
Grapefruit	90	0	7
Mango Mama/Tangerine	120	0	10
Raspberry Dream	120	1	10
Protein Blast	160	1	10
Desperately Seeking C	110	0	5

Fruit Whips: Per 8 fl.oz Bottle

Smoothies: Berry/Lemon/Orange/Tropical
	C	F	Cb
All flavors, 236ml (8 oz)	125	0	29

Fruitopia
	C	F	Cb
Apple Raspberry, 8 fl.oz	75	0	19
20 fl.oz Bottle	190	0	48
Other flavors, average, 8 fl.oz	115	0	29
20 fl.oz Bottle	290	0	72

Goya Nectar
	C	F	Cb
Apricot Nectar, 12 fl.oz can	130	0	31
Pear Nectar, 12 fl.oz can	240	0	59

Hansen's: Natural Juice Cocktail
	C	F	Cb
Regular, all flavors, 8 fl.oz	110	0	28
Low Calorie Peach Mango	10	0	4

Smoothies: *Per 11.5 fl.oz Can*
	C	F	Cb
Fruit flavors, regular	170	0	43
Lite: Cranberry; Raspberry	50	0	13
Energy Island Blast	170	0	42
Colada Blast	190	0	45
Power Berry Blast	170	0	42
Protein Banana Blast	210	2	46
Vita Citrus Blast	170	0	42

Per 8 fl.oz Unless Indicated   **C** **F** **Cb**

Hawaiian Punch
	C	F	Cb
Fruit Juicy, Red, 6 fl.oz	90	0	22
Box, 8.45 fl.oz	120	0	30

Hi-C
Orange Juice
	C	F	Cb
Chilled/Premium Choice, 8 fl.oz	110	0	30
10 fl.oz bottle	140	0	36
Calcium Rich, 8 fl.oz	120	0	33
Other Juices Drinks: Aver., 8 fl.oz	130	0	32
8.45 fl.oz box, average	135	0	33
11.5 fl.oz can	180	0	45

Hood
	C	F	Cb
Grapefruit Juice (Select)	100	0	23
Natural Blenders, average	130	0	32
Orange Juice: Select	120	0	30
Calcium Rich	120	0	30

Jamba Juice (California): See Page 206

Jera's Juice (Boston): Per 24 fl.oz
	C	F	Cb
Berry Blitz	440	2	105
Cape Codder	335	0.5	80
Citrus Burst	320	1.5	8
Flu Fighter	280	1	67
Mango Passion	290	0	68
Orange Bite	280	1.5	62
Razzle Dazzle	380	1	94
Soy Smoothie (7g protein)	320	3.5	68
Strawberry Smile	345	0.5	84
Triathlete (15g protein)	300	1.5	71
Whey-Out Protein (27g protein)	325	1.5	56

Jui2ce: All flavors, 8 fl.oz bottle
	C	F	Cb
Jui2ce: All flavors, 8 fl.oz bottle	95	0	23

Juicy Juice
	C	F	Cb
Apple Grape, 8.45 fl.oz box	120	0	10
Berry, 8.45 fl.oz box	130	0	30
Punch, 8.45 fl.oz box	140	0	32
Tropical, 8.45 fl.oz box	150	0	26

Kern's Nectars
	C	F	Cb
Pineapple Coconut Nectar, 6 fl.oz	140	0	26
11.5 fl.oz box	210	0	48
Other nectars, average, 6 fl.oz	110	0	27

Kool Aid
	C	F	Cb
Koolers, average, 8.45 fl.oz	140	0	37
Fruit Drinks, average, 8 fl.oz	100	0	25
Sugar Free, 8 fl.oz	5	0	0

Knott's: Sparkling Ciders, 325 ml
	C	F	Cb
Knott's: Sparkling Ciders, 325 ml	110	0	25

Fruit & Vegetable Drinks & Juices (Cont)

Per 8 fl.oz Unless Indicated	C	F	Cb
Knudsen: Per 8 fl.oz Bottle			
Fruit Juices: Apple	110	0	28
Apple Blends, all varieties	120	0	30
Black Cherry; Prune	180	0	43
Creamed Papaya	40	0	10
Grape; Pomegranate	150	0	37
Grapefruit	100	0	23
Guava Strawberry	110	0	27
Just Blueberry	100	0	24
Just Boysenberry	90	0	23
Just Cranberry; Tomato	60	0	14
Kiwi Strawberry	120	0	30
Natural Breakfast	110	0	27
Orange	100	0	23
Pear	120	0	30
Pineapple Coconut	130	0	32
Raspberry Peach	150	0	31
Razzleberry	130	0	33
Nectars: Coconut	140	5	26
Apricot; Peach	120	0	30
Other Nectars, average	130	0	36
Blends: Average all flavors	120	0	30
Citrus Juices:			
Rio Red Grapefruit	140	0	35
Lemonade (Natural)	120	0	30
Floats: Orange	140	0	33
Spritzers: Aver. all flavors, 12 oz	170	0	43
Lights, all flavors, 12 oz	110	0	28
TeaZers: All flavors, 12 oz	110	0	28
Very Veggie: 8 fl.oz	50	0	10
Simply Nutritious:			
Blackberry Hibiscus Mist	100	0	24
Ginseng Boost	110	0	27
Inner Strength	110	0	26
Lemon Ginger Echinacea	120	0	30
Mega C	130	0	31
Mega Green; Gingko Alert	120	0	30
Morning Blend; VitaJuice	120	0	30
Krasdale			
Cranberry Apple	170	0	42
Cranberry Juice Cocktail	130	0	32
Cranberry Raspberry	150	0	37
Libby's: Orange Juice, 8 fl.oz	105	0	25
Juicy Juice, average, 8 fl.oz	140	0	34
Nectars, 1 can, 11.5 fl.oz	220	0	52

Per 8 fl.oz Unless Indicated	C	F	Cb
Luzianne: Per 8 fl.oz Prepared			
Smoothies: Mixed Berry	90	0.5	19
Peach Mango	90	0	19
Strawberry Banana	80	0.5	18
Mauna La'i Hawaiian: 8 fl.oz	130	0	32
Mistic (Mega 24 fl.oz)			
Average All flavors, 8 fl.oz	120	0	30
24 fl.oz	360	0	90
Minute Maid			
Orange Juice, Premium, 8 fl.oz	110	0	27
Blends: Average all flavors, 8 fl.oz	120	0	30
Powders: Aver. all flavors, 8 fl.oz	120	0	30
Pink Lemonade, 8 fl.oz	110	0	28
Chilled Singles: Per 16 fl.oz Bottle			
Berry/Tropical Punch	240	0	60
Lemonade/ Orange Juice	220	0	55
Juices to Go: All flav., 10 fl.oz	160	0	40
Boxed Juices: Per 8.45 fl.oz			
Cherry Grape; Tropical Punch	130	0	32
Orange/Apple Juice; Berry; Fruit	120	0	31
Calcium Juices, 8 fl.oz	120	0	29
Mott's			
Apple Raspb., Fruit Punch, 10 fl.oz	145	0	36
Apple Cranb., Grape Apple, 10 fl.oz	180	0	42
Clamato Tomato Cocktail, 8 fl.oz	60	0	11
Fruitsations: all flavors, 4 oz	85	0	22
Grapefruit (from conc.), prep.	120	0	28
Juice Paks: All flavors, 8.45 fl.oz	120	0	30
Mini Motts, 4.23 oz	60	0	14
Orange Juice (from conc.)	130	0.5	30
Mountain Sun Organic: Per 8 fl.oz			
Black Cherry; Cranberry Zip	120	0	30
Lemonade; Wild Cranberry	110	0	27
Limeade	100	0	24
Plain Apple; Spiced Cider	120	0	30
Other flavors	130	0	32
Naked Juice: Per 8 fl.oz, 1/2 Bottle			
Apple Juice, 8 fl.oz	120	0	29
Banana Blueberry; Boysenberry	140	2	34
Banana Date	240	4	46
Berry Blast; Wise Guy	130	0	30
Carrot Beet/Celery/Spinach	100	0	21
Carrot-U-Copia	80	0	13
Chocolate Dream	190	2	38
Grapefruit Juice	110	0	23

Fruit & Vegetable Drinks & Juices (Cont)

Per 8 fl.oz Unless Indicated	C	F	Cb
Naked Juice: *Per 8 fl.oz, 1/2 Bottle*			
Carrot-O-Copia	80	0	13
Green Machine	140	0.5	35
Lemons Juiced	130	0	32
Mighty Mango; Orange Jce Nirvana	110	0	24
Orange Carrot Banana	120	0	27
Papaya Strawberry	100	0	24
Power-C	120	5	29
Protein Drink (6g protein)	170	1.5	33
Protein Zone (17g protein)	220	4	32
Raspberry Ale	140	0	35
Tangerine Scream	110	0	25
Turbo C	110	0	27
Well-Being	140	0	32
Zenergy	160	0	37
Zippitea	80	0	20
Soy Shakes: Choc (9g protein)	210	2	38
Vanilla (8g protein)	170	1	33
Nantucket Nectars			
100% Juices: Apple Raspberry	140	0	34
Grape Juice	160	0	39
Grapefruit Juice	100	0	24
Orange Passionfruit	120	0	29
Pineapple Orange Banana	140	0	35
Premium Orange Juice	120	0	29
Pressed Apple Juice	100	0	25
Ruby Red Grapefruit	100	0	25
The Original Peach	120	0	30
Juice Cocktails: Cranberry	140	0	34
California Melonberry	110	0	28
Cranberry Apple	140	0	34
Juice Cocktails (Cont): Guava	130	0	33
Diet Green Tea	5	0	1
Diet Iced Tea	5	0	1
Fruit Punch	130	0	32
Grapeade	130	0	33
Kiwi Berry	120	0	30
Orange Mango	130	0	32
Papaya	120	0	30
Pineapple Orange Guava	120	0	30
Watermelon Strawberry	120	0	30
Lemonades: Authentic/Pink	120	0	30
Super Nectars: Chai Green Tea	90	0	23
Gingko Mango	150	0	38
Green Angel	140	0	39
Protein Smoothie	120	1	38

Per 8 fl.oz Unless Indicated	C	F	Cb
Nantucket Nectars (Cont)			
Super Nectars (Cont):			
Red Guarana Tea	110	0	26
Strawberry Smoothie	120	0	30
Vital C	130	0	32
Vitamin Smoothie	110	0	27
Newman's Own			
Lemonade (Reg./Pink), 8 fl.oz	110	0	27
Ocean Spray: *Per 8 fl.oz*			
Apple Juice (from conc.)	110	0	28
Bl. Cherry; Crazy Kiwi; Mega Melon	130	0	33
Cranberry:			
Cranberry Grape	170	0	41
Cranberry Juice Cocktail	140	0	34
Light Style (Low Calorie)	40	0	10
Other Cranberry flavors, avg	150	0	35
Caribbean Colada; Cran-Mango	130	0	32
Cranicot; Cranapple; Cranblueberry	160	0	41
Crantastic Fruit Punch	150	0	37
Fruit/Holiday Punch; Tangerine	130	0	32
Grapefruit: 100% Juice	100	0	24
Other flavors, average	125	0	31
Lemonade flavors, average	130	0	32
Orange Juice (from concentrate)	120	0	31
Kiwi Strawb.; Summer Cooler	120	0	31
Ruby Red & Strawberry	140	0	34
Ruby Red & Mango/Tangerine	130	0	33
Cravin' Less Sugar: Grape	90	0	22
Kiwi Strawberry	70	0	17
Tropical; Cranberry Wildberry	80	0	19
Odwalla: *Per 8 fl.oz Unless Indicated*			
Carrot, Orange, Apple	100	0	23
C Monster, 16 fl. oz	300	0	72
Femme Vitale	130	0	29
Fruitshake Blackberry	160	0	40
Grapefruit Juice	90	0	34
Lemonade	90	0	24
Mango Tango	150	0	37
Mo Beta, 16 fl. oz	280	0	70
Orange Juice	120	0	34
Serious Energy	150	0	36
Strawberry Banana/Go Man Go	100	0	25
Super Protein, 16 fl.oz	400	0	40
Wellness (Echinacea)	150	1	33

Fruit & Vegetable Drinks & Juices (Cont)

Per 8 fl.oz Unless Indicated	C	F	Cb
Orange Julius: Per 16 fl.oz			
Orange	265	0	65
Pina Colada	300	0	75
Strawberry	340	0	85
Raspberry Cream Supreme	510	20	82
Tropical Cream Supreme	510	25	71
PS - Private Selection (Ralphs)			
Lemonade (Premium Juice), 8 fl.oz	110	0	29
Orange Juice, 8 fl.oz	110	0	27
Mango Nectar, 8 fl.oz	140	0	35
Realemon - Realime (Borden)			
Lemon/Lime Juice (from concentrate)			
1 teaspoon	0	0	0
2 Tbsp, 1 fl.oz	6	0	2
Santa Cruz			
Natural 100%: Aver. all varieties	120	0	30
Sparkling varieties, 8 fl.oz	150	0	33
S&W			
Apple Juice, 8 fl.oz	120	0	30
Orange Juice, 6 fl.oz can	90	0	22
Grapefruit Juice, unswt'd, 8 fl.oz	105	0	25
Tomato Juice, 8 fl.oz	30	0	7
Squeezit			
Average all flavors, 6.75 fl.oz	90	0	23
Snapple			
Cranberry Royal, 10 fl.oz	150	0	38
Fruit Drink Blends, 8 fl.oz	120	0	30
Grapeade; Orangeade 8 fl.oz	120	0	30
Orange Juice, 10 fl.oz	130	0	30
Whipped Snapple (Fruit Smoother):			
Aver. all flavors, 297ml bottle	160	0	40
Snap.E Tom			
Tom. & Chile Cocktail, 11.5 oz can	70	0	15
Sunny Delight			
Florida Citrus, 6 fl.oz	90	0	22
Calcium Rich, 6 fl.oz	150	0	37
Sunny Delight Lite, 6 fl.oz	20	0	5
Tropical Fruit Punch, 6 fl.oz	90	0	22
Sunsweet			
Prune Juice/w. Pulp, 6 fl.oz	180	0	43
Superfood: Juice, 8 fl.oz	140	1	32

Per 8 fl.oz Unless Indicated	C	F	Cb
Tampico: Citrus Punch, 1 cup	100	0	25
Mango/Trop. Frt. Punch, 1 cup	110	0	28
Tang			
Fruit Box (8.45 fl.oz): Aver. all flav.	140	0	34
Pouches, average all flavors (1)	100	0	26
Mix: Made up, 6 fl.oz			
Regular (2 Tbsp dry)	90	0	22
Sugar Free	7	0	0
Tree of Life: Black Cherry	180	0	43
Concord Grape	160	0	40
Cranberry Nectar	150	0	38
Other varieties, average	130	0	33
Tree Top: Per 6 fl.oz			
Apple Juice; Apple Citrus/Pear	120	0	30
Apple Cranberry/Grape	130	0	32
Fruit Juice Punch, 10 fl.oz	150	0	37
Grape/Grape Fruit Juice; Sparkling	120	0	30
Orange Juice	120	0	28
Tropicana			
Blends: Berry; P'apple, 8 fl.oz	130	0	32
Pure Premium: Orange Juice	110	0	26
Orange Juice + Fiber	120	0	30
Ruby Red	120	0	28
Season's Best: Orange Jce, 7 fl.oz	100	0	24
10 fl.oz bottle	130	0	33
11.5 fl.oz can	140	0	36
Grapefruit Juice, 8 fl.oz	160	0	40
Tropics: Average all flav., 8 fl.oz	110	0	26
Twister: Average, 8 fl.oz	120	0	32
10 fl.oz bottle	150	0	40
11.5 fl.oz can	160	0	40
Light: average, 8 fl.oz	35	0	10
10 fl.oz bottle	50	0	11
V8® Juices & Drinks			
V8 100% Vegetable Juice, 8 fl.oz	50	0	10
1 Can, 12 fl.oz	70	0	15
V-8 Splash, all flavors, 8 fl.oz	110	0	27
Diet V-8 Splash, all flavors, 8 fl.oz	10	0	3

Continued Next Page

> *Success is 1% Inspiration and 99% Perspiration.*

Fruit Juices (Cont) ◆ Nutritional Drinks

Per 8 fl.oz Unless Indicated **C** **F** **Cb**

Veryfine

	C	F	Cb
Apple Cranberry	130	0	33
Fruit Punch	140	0	36
Grape Juice (100%)	150	0	37
Grape Drink	110	0	28
Grapefruit Juice (100%)	90	0	20
Pink	120	0	30
Guava Straw.; Lemon Lime	120	0	30
Orange Juice (100%)	120	0	24
Orange Drink	140	0	35
Papaya Punch	120	0	30
Pineapple Orange	130	0	32

Welch's

	C	F	Cb
100% Grape Juice, 8 fl.oz	170	0	42
100% White Grape Juice, 8 fl.oz	160	0	39
Fruit Juice Cocktails: *Per 8 fl.oz*			
Grape; Strawberry Breeze	130	0	33
Country Pear; Wild Raspberry	145	0	35
Tomato Juice, 8 fl.oz	50	0	10

Whippy Snapple: Per 10 fl.oz

	C	F	Cb
Smoothies: Citrus	150	0	39
Pineapple Orange	100	0	41

Wild Oats

	C	F	Cb
Down to Earth, average 8 fl.oz	140	0	34
Beautiful Juices, average 8 fl.oz	120	0	27

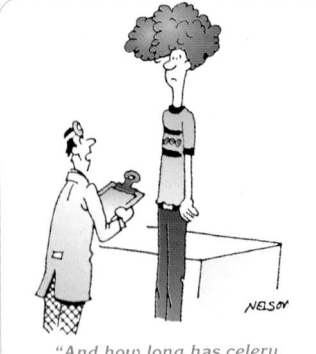

"And how long has celery been your basic diet."

Nutritional Shakes/Drinks

Per 8 fl.oz Unless Indicated **C** **F** **Cb**

	C	F	Cb
ABB: Carbo Force, 18 fl.oz	440	0	109
Diet Force, 22 fl.oz	5	0	0
Extreme Ripped Force, 22 fl.oz	100	0	24
Lean Protein, 18 fl.oz	110	0	2
Pure Pro Shake, made up, 12 fl.oz	160	0.5	4
Ripped Force, 18 fl.oz	100	0	23
Speed Stack, 18 fl.oz	5	0	1
AllSport, all flavors, 8 fl.oz	70	0	18
Amino Force, 22 fl.oz	390	0	75
Amway Positrim Drink Mix, 1 pkt	160	4	27
Fat Free Mix, 1 pkt, 65g	230	0	50
Arbonne Meal Shakes, 1 pkt, 46g	190	4.5	25
Arizona: Rx Energy, 16 fl.oz	240	0	60
Rx Power, 16 fl.oz	210	0	52
Rx Total Trim, 8 fl.oz	5	0	1
Total Sport; Ginseng, 16 fl.oz	130	0	16
Atkins Shake: Mix, 2 scps, 1.5 oz	170	8	1.5
Balanced: Diet, 11 fl.oz can	180	1	34
Choc Royale; Fr. Vanilla, 11 fl.oz	180	2	35
Strawb.; Vanilla, 11 fl.oz can	230	3	36
Kids Chocolate, 8 fl.oz can	160	3	30
Bariatrix Shakes, 1 serving	100	2	6
Proti-Max Meal, 67g	250	3	20
Bawls Guarana, 8 fl.oz	130	0	32
Biochem Ult. Protein, 2 scp, 2 oz	200	0	10
Blue Thunder, 22 fl.oz	310	0	43
Body Fuel (w. NutraSweet), 8 fl.oz	4	0	1
Body Works (Shasta), 12 fl.oz	90	0	22
Boost: Ready-To-Drink, 8 oz	240	4	41
Boost High Protein, 8 fl.oz	240	6	33
Boost Plus, 8 fl.oz can	360	14	45
Breeze Juice Drink, 8 fl.oz can	160	0	31
Bulk Force, 1 pint bottle	750	0	163
Carb Mate, bottle, 16 fl.oz	28	0	7
Carboplex (Nutra Life), 31g	120	0	30
Carnation Instant Breakfast			
Powder: 1 reg. envelope, 37g	130	1	28
No Sugar Added, 1 envel., 21g	70	1	12
Ready-To-Drink, avg,, 10 oz	220	3	37
CeraSport, 34g pkt (makes 16 fl.oz)	150	0	32
Champion Nutrition:			
Heavywt Gainer 900, 4 sc., 5.4 oz	630	10	101
Lean Gainer, 3 scoops, 2.7 oz	280	4	11
Super H. Wt Gainer, 4 scoops	900	29	108
Choice dm (Mead Johnson), 8 fl.oz	250	12	25

Nutritional Shakes & Drinks (Cont)

Per 8 fl.oz Unless Indicated	C	F	Cb
Cytomax, 8 fl.oz	65	0	13
Designer Whey, Prot. Blast, 16 fl.oz	170	1	1
Ensure: High Calcium, 8 oz can	225	6	31
Ensure Bal'd Bkfst, choc pouch	140	0.5	30
Ensure Fiber, 8 fl.oz can	250	6	42
Ensure Light, 8 fl.oz can	200	3	33
Ensure Plus, 8 fl.oz can	360	13	47
Ensure Regular, 8 fl.oz can	250	6	40
Glucernos, 8 fl.oz can	220	11	22
Powder, made up, 1/2 cup	250	9	34
Enterex Diabetic (w/fiber), 8 fl.oz			
(Carbohydrates as Maltodextrin)	237	9	27
Exceed (Weider): Powder, 2 Tbsp	70	0	17
Liquid, 12 fl.oz box	105	0	26
Fruit2O (Veryfine), 8/16/20 fl.oz	0	0	0
G-Up, 8.4 fl.oz can	220	0.5	55
Gatorade: Frost, 8 fl.oz	50	0	14
Energy Drink, 12 fl.oz	310	0	78
ThirstQuencher, 8 fl.oz	50	0	14
Nutrition Shake, 325ml can	370	6	62
Genisoy: Shake, 1 scoop, 35g	120	0	17
Protein Powder, 1 scoop, 29g	100	0	0
Go-Go: Sports, 8.4 fl.oz	90	0	24
Relax, 8.4 fl.oz	80	0	26
Immune, 8.4 fl.oz	90	0	24
HMR 500 Shakes, 1 pkt	100	0	16
HMR 120, 1 serving	120	1.5	16
Hansen's: Anti-Ox, 243ml can	110	0	31
Energy: Original, 246ml can	120	0	32
Endurance Formula, 246ml can	110	0	27
Power Formula, 246ml can	140	0	36
Energade: Stamina, 243ml can	110	0	31
Citrus/Orange, 243ml can	60	0	16
Slim Down, 246ml can	0	0	0
b. well; d. stress, 243ml can	110	0	31
Smoothies: Per 1.5 fl.oz Can			
Energy: Colade Blast	190	0	45
Island Blast	170	0	42
Power, Berry Blast	170	0	42
Protein, Banana Blast	210	2	46
Vita Smoothie, Citrus Blast	170	0	43
Health Source Soy, 2 scoops, 1 oz	100	1	4
Herbalife (Thermogetics F.1), 1 oz	100	1	14
Hydra Fuel (Tury Labs)	65	0	16
Hype Energy, all flavors, 12 fl.oz	90	0	22
IDN (Nu Skin): Aloe Fountain, 2 fl.oz	20	0	5
Amino Build, 3 scoops, 1 1/2 oz	160	1	12

Per 8 fl.oz Unless Indicated	C	F	Cb
IDN (Cont): Splash C w. Aloe, 1 sc.	80	0	20
Creatine Blast, 1 scoop, 1 1/2 oz pkt	130	0	32
Appeal: French Delight, 2 oz pkt	210	2	33
Swiss Truffle, 2 oz pkt	220	2.5	33
Appeal Lite HT	120	1.5	26
Sportalyte, 1/2 pkt (makes 8 fl.oz)	70	0	17
Isopure (Nature's Best), 20 fl.oz	160	0	0
Jevity (Abbott): w. Fiber, 8 oz can	250	8	37
Kashi GoLEAN Shakes: Van., 325ml	220	2.5	36
Chocolate, 325ml	230	3	32
Powdered, 1 pkt, 71g	250	1.5	30
Knudsen: Isotonic Sports, 8 fl.oz	60	0	15
ReCharge, all flavors	80	0	18
Simply Nutritious, 1/2 bot., 16 fl.oz	60	0	14
Kombucha: Vit. Enriched, 8 fl.oz	30	0	7
Wonder Drink, 8.5 fl.oz	65	0	16
Lipovitan: EB3, 8.2 fl.oz	110	0	29
Mass Recovery, 1 pint bottle	380	0	60
Max, made-up, 8 fl.oz	96	0	24
Met-Rx: Defense/Energy, 8.3 oz can	120	0	32
Energy, 8.3 fl.oz can	120	0	32
Protein Shake, 11 fl.oz can	200	3	19
Protein Plus, 15 fl.oz can	190	3.5	3
Met-Rx: Nutrition Drink Mix, 72g	260	2	22
RTD 40 Shake, 15 fl.oz can	240	3	15
Met-Rx ORS, Endura (Metagenics)	60	0	15
Metabolife Meal Shakes, 11 oz can	220	3	40
Metabolol: Endurance, 2 scps, 52g	200	5	24
Metabolol II, 2 scoops, 66g	260	3	40
Metaform: Lean Mass, 2 scoops	140	0	13
Protein Powder, 76g pkt	270	2	21
Proton, 45g pkt (1.6 oz)	170	1	15
Myoplex: Shake, 11 fl.oz	200	4.5	24
Powder, 1 pkt, 2.7 oz	280	2	24
Lite Powder, 1 pkt, 2 oz	190	1.5	20
Nature's Best: Isopure			
Zero Carb, 2 scoops, 2.1 oz	200	0	0
Low Carb, 2 scoops, 2.3 oz	210	0	3
Perfect Whey, 2 scoops, 0.7 oz	90	1.5	1
Nitro Speed, all flavors, 18 fl.oz	110	0	7
Nutrament (Mead Johnson): 12 fl.oz	360	10	52
Optifast 800: Powder, 1 serving	160	3	20
Ready-To-Drink, Chocolate	160	3	20
Pedialyte (Abbott)	25	0	6
Power Dream (Imagine Foods):			
Java Jolt, 11 fl.oz	240	4.5	42
Mango Passion, 11 fl.oz	320	4.5	65
Chai, 11 fl.oz	200	3	35

Nutritional Shakes & Drinks (Cont)

Per 8 fl.oz Unless Indicated

	C	F	Cb
Powerade: Regular, 8 fl.oz	70	0	19
20 fl.oz bottle	175	0	48
Light, 8 fl.oz	25	0	7
20 fl.oz bottle	65	0	17
PowerBar Power Gel: Chocolate	120	1.5	28
Other flavors, 41g pack	110	0	28
Pro-formance, all flavors	100	0	25
ProBalance, 8.45 fl.oz	300	10	39
Pro-Cal 100 (R-Kane), 1 pkt	105	2	7
Pure Pro, 22 fl.oz bottle	180	0	2
Recharge (Knudsen), all flavors	80	0	18
Red Bull Energy Drink, 8.3 fl.oz	113	0	28
Red Devil: Energy Drink, 12 fl.oz	120	0	31
Red Tiger Energy Drink, 8.2 fl.oz	115	0	28
Relode Gel, 0.75 oz pkt	80	0	20
Resource (Novartis): Plus, 8 fl.oz	360	11	52
Standard 8 fl.oz pak	250	6	40
Diabetic, 8 fl.oz pak	250	11	23
Fruit Beverage, 8 fl.oz pak	180	0	36
Yogurt Flav'd Beverage, 8 fl.oz	250	4	45
Revenge Pro (Champ. Nutr.), 1 oz	100	2	1
Sport, 25g scoop	90	0	23
Revival Soy: Plain,1 oz pkt.	110	1.5	2
Vanilla w/Fructose, 2 oz pkt.	220	2	31
Unsweetened/Aspartame, 35g	120	2	6
Rite Aid: Nutritional Suppl. 8 oz	250	6	40
Rite Aid Plus, 8 oz	360	11	50
Sav-on Nut'l: 8 fl.oz can	360	13	47
Light, 8 fl.oz can	200	3	33
Scan Diet (Soy-base), 1 scoop	160	3	21
Slim-Fast: Ready-To-Drink (cans),			
Shakes, all flavors, 325ml	220	3	40
Juices, all flavors, 340ml	220	1	46
Powder Mix: 1 scoop, 1 oz	100	1	20
w. 8 oz fat-free milk	190	1	32
Slim-Fast Soy Protein:			
Café Mocha, 2 scoop, 1/3 cup	170	1.5	26
Ultra Slim-Fast Mixes: Regular flav., average			
1 scoop, 1/3 cup, 33g	120	1	25
w. 8 oz fat free milk	200	1.5	36
Choc Delite w. Soy Protein,			
2 scoops, 1/2 cup, 48g	170	2	25
w. Fruit Juice Mix,			
1 scoop, 1/4 cup, 31g	100	1	17
w. 8 oz fruit juice	220	1	42
Snapple Sport, all flavors	80	0	20
SoBe: Energy/Power, 8 fl.oz	120	0	32
Juice Elixers, 8 fl.oz	90	0	24
Liz Blizz; Lizard Lightning	130	0	33
Adrenaline Rush, 8.3 oz can	140	0	37
SoBe Lean, all flavors, 8 fl.oz	5	0	1
SoBeShakes (Market America), 1 pkt	210	2	26

	C	F	Cb
Solaray Soytein (Protein Energy Meal),			
Natural, 1 heaping scoop, 24g	70	0.5	5
Flavors, avg, 1 hpg scoop, 32g	115	1	13
Spiru-Tein: 8 fl.oz can	220	5	23
Powder, 1 scoop, 34 g	100	0	11
Sustacal: Liquid, 8 fl.oz can	240	6	33
Basic, 8 fl.oz can	250	9	34
Sustacal Plus, 8 fl.oz	360	14	45
Powder, 2 oz + water	200	1	36
Sweet Success (Nestlé):			
Healthy Shake, 10 fl.oz can	200	3	37
Fruit Flavors, 10 fl.oz	200	0.5	39
Powder, 2 scoops, 32g (1.1 oz)	100	1	25
Synergy: Mystic Mango, 16 fl oz	100	0	24
Other flavors, 16 fl.oz	70	0	16
Tahitian Noni: Shake, 2 scoops	120	2.5	14
Protein Energy, 2 scoops	140	3	7
Thermo Force, 16 oz	260	0	65
The Juice, 11 fl.oz	260	0	65
Tiger's Milk (mix) Energy, 3 Tbsp	120	0	30
Total Balance, 9.5 oz can	230	7	25
Twin Lab: Ultra Fuel, 16 oz	400	0	100
RxFuel, 1 pkt	250	0	62
Ultima Replenisher, 12g pkt	40	0	10
Ultra Slim-Fast – see Slim-Fast			
Upper Deck, all flavors	80	0	19
Usana: Nutrimeal, 2 scoops, 43g	150	4	20
Fibergy, 2 scoops, 33g	90	1	23
SoyaMax, 2 scoops, 1 oz	105	1	1
Venom Energy (Elements), 8.2 fl.oz	130	0	29
Vitamin Water (Glaceau), 8 fl.oz	50	0	13
Vita-Trim Shake (Mkt America) 57g	210	2	26
Walgreens Nutritional Supplements:			
Advanced Formula, 8 oz can	250	6	40
Plus, 8 oz can	355	13	47
Light, 8 oz can	200	3	33
Weider (Powders):			
Creatine ATP, 1/2 cup, 1.7 oz	210	0	37
Complete Rx, 70g pkt, 2.5 oz	240	2.5	27
Lean Pro, 1/2 cup, 1.7 oz	160	0	20
Ultra Whey Pro, 1/2 cup, 1 oz	110	1	4
Women's Natural Replace., 33g	120	1	13
Dynamic: Body Shaper, 35g	140	0.5	22
Muscle Builder, 2 scoops, 45g	190	0	27
Weight Gainer, 4 scoops, 85g	330	0.5	62
Victory Pure Protein, 2 scoops	140	0	14
Victory Mass 1000, 7 oz	740	2.5	148
Mega Mass 4000, 3 scoops	1640	4	319
Worldwide: Carbo Rush, 20 fl.oz	280	0	60
Fat Shredder, 20 fl.oz bottle	0	0	0
Pure Protein, 22 fl.oz bottle	170	0	0
Thermo 525, 20 fl.oz bottle	5	0	1
XS Energy: Citrus/Energy, 8.4 fl.oz	8	0	0

Quick Guide

Cola Soda Drinks

Average All Brands
Coca-Cola and Pepsi

	C	F	Cb
8 fl.oz Cup	100	0	25
12 fl.oz Can	150	0	37
16 fl.oz Bottle	200	0	50
20 fl.oz Bottle	250	0	63
24 fl.oz *(Pepsi)*	300	0	75
1 Liter Bottle	400	0	100
2 Liter Bottle	800	0	200

Other Soda Drinks

	C	F	Cb
Club Soda, 12 fl.oz	0	0	0
Club Soda Cream, 12 fl.oz	170	0	42
Diet Soft Drinks, aver., 12 fl.oz	0	0	0
Ginger Ale, 12 fl.oz	120	0	30
Lemon Lime, 12 fl.oz	220	0	55
Orange, 12 fl.oz	180	0	45
Root Beer, 12 fl.oz	165	0	41
Tonic Water, 12 fl.oz	135	0	34
Mineral Water: Plain, 12 fl.oz	0	0	0
Sweetened/flavored, 12 fl.oz	150	0	37
w. Fruit Juice, 12 fl.oz	120	0	30
Seltzers: Plain/Diet, 12 fl.oz	0	0	0
Sweetened/flavored, 12 fl.oz	150	0	37
w. Fruit Juice, 12 fl.oz	120	0	30

Movie Theater & Take-Out

Average All Flavors (Figures allow for 25% Ice)

	C	F	Cb
Small, 12 fl.oz	110	0	27
Regular, 16 fl.oz	150	0	37
Medium, 22 fl.oz	210	0	5
Large, 32 fl.oz	300	0	75
Cinnabon: Icescapes, 16 fl.oz			
Orange Cream	360	16	50
Root Beer	470	22	63
Mochalatta	390	12	62

Soda Brands

Per 12 fl.oz Unless Indicated

	C	F	Cb
A&W: Cream Soda	165	0	41
Diet Cream Soda/Root Beer	1	0	0
Root Beer	180	0	45
Albertson's: Cola	160	0	43
Lemon Lime	140	0	38
Other flavors, average	170	0	47

Soda Brands (Cont)

Per 12 fl.oz Unless Indicated

	C	F	Cb
Arizona: Lemonade, 8 fl.oz	110	0	28
Arnold Palmer Lite, Half & Half:			
1 cup, 8 fl.oz	55	0	14
1 can, 23.5 fl.oz	170	0	52
Barq's: Root Beer	165	0	41
Barrelhead: Rootbeer	165	0	41
Big Red: 12 fl.oz	150	0	38
Bodyworks (Shasta), all flav.	90	0	23
Cactus Cooler	150	0	40
Canada Dry: Birch Beer; Cactus	165	0	41
Club Soda	0	0	0
Collins Mixer	120	0	30
Ginger Ale, all flavors	135	0	37
Diet, all flavors; Seltzer	0	0	0
Half & Half; Hi-Spot; Wild Cherry	165	0	41
Lemon Sour	150	0	37
Sour Mixer	135	0	34
Tahitian Treat	225	0	56
Tonic Water/Twist Lime	150	0	37
Diet	0	0	0
Clearly Canadian, 11 fl.oz, aver.	120	0	30
Coca-Cola: Classic	140	0	35
Coke II	160	0	40
Diet Coke/w. Lemon Twist	0	0	0
Cherry Coke/Vanilla Coke	150	0	40
Cragmont: Cola	165	0	41
Cherry	180	0	45
Diet, all flavors	0	0	0
Crush, all flavors	210	0	52
Crystal Light, all flavors	8	0	2
Diet Rite, all flavors	1	0	0
Doc Shasta	160	0	40
Dr Diablo, Cola	140	0	35
Dr Nehi	150	0	41
Dr Pepper: Regular	150	0	40
Diet (Reg.; Caffeine Free)	3	0	0.5
Fanta: Orange; Grape	180	0	45
Ginger Ale	130	0	33
Root Beer	165	0	41
Fresca	4	0	1
Frutopia: See Page 150			
Hansen's: Signature Soda			
Average all flavors, 8 fl.oz	110	0	30
1 bottle, 14 fl.oz	195	0	53
Natural Lemonade(s), 16 fl.oz	200	0	52

Soft Drinks • Soda (Cont)

Per 12 fl.oz Unless Indicated	C	F	Cb
Health Valley: Wild Berry	140	0	35
Ginger Ale; Sarsp. Root Beer	150	0	41
Rootbeer Old Fashioned	120	0	30
Hires: Cream; Root Beer	180	0	45
IBC: Root Beer	110	0	29
Diet	0	0	0
Jolt Cola	150	0	41
Kick (Royal Crown)	180	0	45
Knudsen: Spritzers, average	170	0	43
Lights, all flavors	110	0	28
Lucozade, 7 fl.oz	136	0	34
Mello Yello: Regular	180	0	45
Diet	5	0	0
Minute Maid: Diet Orange	3	0	0.5
Berry; Black Cherry; Orange	165	0	41
Fruit Punch; Grape; Strawberry	180	0	45
Lemonade	160	0	40
Peach; P'apple; R'berry; Grapefr.	165	0	42
Mountain Dew, 24 fl.oz bottle	170	0	46
Mr Pibb: Regular	150	0	37
Mug: Root Beer	160	0	43
Natural Brew: Apple, Cream	170	0	43
Cafe Mocha, Cherry Amaretto	160	0	40
Ginseng Cola, Ginger Ale	170	0	43
Nehi (Royal Crown): Cream	180	0	45
Ginger Ale, Quinine Water	135	0	45
Other flavors, average	195	0	45
Orangina, 10 fl.oz bottle	120	0	45
Orbitz, 300ml bottle, average	130	0	30
Pepsi: Regular/Blue/Caffeine Free	150	0	41
Diet Pepsi/Twist	0	0	0
One	1	0	0
Sierra Mist Lemon Lime	150	0	39
Twist w. Lemon	150	0	40
Wild Cherry	160	0	43
Perrier: Regular or flavors	0	0	0
Ramblin' Root Beer	180	0	45
RC Cola: Regular; Cherry	160	0	40
Diet Cola	1	0	0
Royal Mistic: Punch, 16 fl.oz	230	0	57
'N Juice, average	155	0	38
Sparkling, average, 11.1 fl.oz	115	0	28
Santa Cruz: Sparkling, all types	150	0	37
Orange	195	0	48
Schweppes: Bitter Lemon	165	0	41
Ginger Ale, regular; Raspberry	120	0	30
Ginger Beer; Lemon Lime	150	0	37
Grapefruit; Lemon Sour	165	0	41

Per 12 fl.oz Unless Indicated	C	F	Cb
Schweppes (Cont): Seltzer	0	0	0
Tonic: Regular	120	0	30
Sensa (Guarana flavored)	135	0	34
7UP: Regular	140	0	38
Cherry, Gold	155	0	38
Shasta: Black Cherry	170	0	46
Cherry Cola; Doc Shasta	160	0	40
Club Soda; Diet, all flavors	0	0	0
Cola, regular	170	0	46
Caffeine Free	160	0	40
Fruit Punch, Pineapple	200	0	50
Ginger Ale	130	0	33
Shasta Plus: all flavors	170	0	46
Slice: Lemon Lime	150	0	38
Diet Lemon Lime	0	0	0
Dr. Slice	140	0	40
Fruit; Grape; Pineapple; Red	190	0	51
CherryLime; Slice Cola	160	0	43
Snapple: Average all flavors	180	0	45
Spree (Shasta): all flavors	170	0	43
Sprite: Regular	150	0	37
Diet	4	0	1
Squirt: Regular Soda Citrus	150	0	40
Ruby Red Soda	170	0	46
Sunkist: Average all flavors	210	0	52
Diet Citrus	0	0	0
Diet Orange	7	0	1.5
Surge Citrus	170	0	46
TAB	0	0	0
Think!: Root Beer, 8.4 fl.oz	118	0	27
Sparkling Citrus, 8.4 fl.oz	130	0	31
Cola, 8.4 fl.oz	112	0	29
Upper 10 (RC): Regular	150	0	37
Diet	4	0	1
Vernor's: Ginger Ale	150	0	37
Diet, 10 fl.oz	0	0	0
Welch's: Sparkling, average	180	0	45
Wild Oats: Down to Earth	150	0	37
Wink	195	0	48

Kool-Aid, Tang

	C	F	Cb
Bright & Early, 6 fl.oz	90	0	23
Kool-Aid: Unsweetened, 6 fl.oz	2	0	0.5
Sugar, sweetened, 6 fl.oz	80	0	20
Sugar Free (NutraSweet), 6 fl.oz	5	0	1
Tang: All flavors, 6 fl.oz	90	0	23
Sugar-Free, 6 fl.oz	5	0	1

Instant Coffee

	C	F	Cb
Powder/Granules: Regular or Decaffeinated,			
1 level tsp	2	0	0.5
1 rounded tsp	4	0	1
Ground, 1 Tbsp	5	0	1
Brewed/Percolated, 1 cup, 8 fl.oz	5	0	1

Coffee With Milk/Cream/Creamers:

1 Cup Coffee (8 fl.oz):

	C	F	Cb
w. Whole Milk: Dash, 1 Tbsp	10	0.5	1
2 Tbsp, 1 fl.oz	20	1	1.5
w. 2% Milk, 2 Tbsp	15	0.5	1.5
w. 1% Milk, 2 Tbsp	12	0.3	1.5
w. Fat Free Milk, 2 Tbsp	10	0	1.5
w. Half & Half: 2 Tbsp	45	4	1
w. Cream (light coffee): 2 Tbsp	65	6	1
w. *Coffee Mate:* Liquid, reg., 1T.	40	2	5
Liquid Fat Free, 1 Tbsp	15	0	2
Powder, 1 heaping tsp	20	1	2
Sugar ~ Add Extra: 1 heaping tsp	25	0	6
Single portion, 1 pkt	25	0	6

Flavored Coffee Mixes

	C	F	Cb
Caffé D'Vita: 1 tsp	20	1	4
Coffee Essence, 1 tsp	16	0	4
General Foods, Cafe Intl: Regular	60	3	10
Sugar-free, average	30	2	3
Maxwell House: Mocha, 1 envelope	100	2.5	17
Mocha, sugar-free, 1 envelope	60	3	7
Van., Irish Cream, 1 envelope	90	1	20
Nescafé: Frothé, all flavors, average	90	1.5	19
Chicory: Instant Coffee, 1 tsp	6	0	1
Coffee Essence, 1 tsp	16	0	4

Coffee Substitute Mixes

Roasted Cereal Beverages: (No Caffeine)

	C	F	Cb
Cafix Instant Beverage, 1 tsp	6	0	1
Kaffree Roma (Natural Touch), 1 tsp	6	0	1
Postum, Instant Hot Beverage, 1 tsp	12	0	3
Revival Soy "Coffee", 1 Tbsp	5	0	1
Teeccino Caffe, 1 tsp	10	0	2

Vending Machine

	C	F	Cb
Cappuccino, 1 cup, 8 fl.oz	70	4	6

Coffee Shops/Restaurants

Per 8 fl.oz Cup (Unless Indicated)

	C	F	Cb
Coffee (Regular/Percolated/Filtered)	5	0	1
Americano Drip Coffee, 1 cup	5	0	1
Cafe Au Lait: 1 cup, 8 fl.oz	65	2.5	6
Nonfat Milk, 1 cup	45	0	7
Caffe Latté:			
8 fl.oz cup: w. Whole Milk	100	5	8
w. 2% Milk	80	2.5	8
w. Nonfat Milk	60	0	8
12 fl.oz: w. Whole Milk	180	10	14
w. Nonfat Milk	110	0.5	15
16 fl.oz: w. Whole Milk	200	10	16
w. Nonfat Milk	120	0	16
Cafe Mocha (Mochaccino): 1 c.	120	3	15
12 fl.oz	180	4.5	15
16 fl.oz	240	6	15
Cappuccino:			
8 fl.oz cup: w. Whole Milk	70	4	6
w. 2% Milk	60	2	6
w. Nonfat Milk	40	0	6
12 fl.oz: w. Whole Milk	110	6	9
w. 2% Milk	80	3	9
w. Nonfat Milk	60	0	9
16 fl.oz: w. Whole Milk	140	7	12
w. Nonfat Milk	80	0	12
Mocha, with Cream			
8 fl.oz: w. Whole Milk	180	12	16
w. Nonfat Milk	150	8	16
Tall, 12 fl.oz: Whole Milk	290	18	25
w. Nonfat Milk	230	11	26
Iced Mocha (no cream)			
Tall, 12 fl.oz: w. Whole Milk	190	9	24
w. Nonfat Milk	140	2	24
Espresso: Regular	4	0	1
Doppio (Double)	8	0	2
Espresso Con Panna			
(w. dollop whipped cream)	30	3	1
Espresso Macchiato	15	0.5	2
Frappuccino: Tall, 12 fl.oz	200	3	39
Grande, 16 fl.oz	270	4	52
Frappuccino Mocha:			
Large/Tall, 12 fl.oz	230	3	44
Grande, 16 fl.oz	310	4.5	59
Iced Latte: Similar to Caffe Latte			
Intellicino: 12 fl.oz	150	7	15
Lowfat (2% Milk)	120	3.5	5
Starbucks: *See Page 240*			

Hot Chocolate • Caffeine Counter

Irish & Liqueur Coffees

	C	F	Cb
Irish Coffee (no sugar)	175	10	0
Liqueur Coffee, aver. all types	200	10	16

Cocoa & Hot Chocolate

	C	F	Cb
Cocoa:			
8 fl.oz cup: w. Whole Milk	210	14	19
w. Nonfat Milk	80	8	21
Tall (12 fl.oz): w. Whole Milk	300	20	26
w. Nonfat Milk	120	11	5
Hot Chocolate:			
8 fl.oz cup: w. Whole Milk	200	10	25
w. Nonfat Milk	140	2	25
Tall (12 fl.oz): w. Whole Milk	300	15	38
w. Nonfat Milk	210	3	38
Cinnabon: Mocholatta Chill, 16 oz	410	18	54

Coffee Extras

	C	F	Cb
Chocolate (Cocoa) Topping, 1/2 tsp	10	0	2
Flavored Syrups, 2 Tbsp	80	0	20
Sugar-free, 2 Tbsp	0	0	0
Hershey's Chocolate Syrup, 2 Tbsp	100	0	24
Half & Half Cream, 2 Tbsp	40	3	3
Light Whipped Cream, 2 Tbsp	30	2	3
Marshmallows, miniature, 2	20	0	5

Bottled Coffee (Chilled)

Ready-To-Drink: Per Bottle

	C	F	Cb
Blue Luna: Cafe Latte 12 1/2 fl.oz	195	3	36
Lite Cafe Mocha, 12 1/2 fl.oz	114	3	15
Jakada (Folgers) Coffee Latte:			
French Roast, 10 1/2 fl.oz	170	3.5	31
Mocha, 10 1/2 fl.oz bottle	180	3.5	33
Vanilla, 10 1/2 fl.oz	180	3.5	32
Jaradelic (Planet Java), 9 1/2 fl.oz	180	3	34
Main St Cafe:			
French Van. Ice Latte, 12 fl.oz	190	33	31
Nescafe: Caffe Latte	140	3.5	23
Mocha	140	3	26
Starbucks: Per 9.5 fl.oz Bottle			
Frappuccino: Caramel	200	3	37
Coffee	190	3.5	35
Hazelnut	200	3.5	37
Mocha	200	3.5	37
DoubleShot, 6.5 fl.oz can	140	6	18

Caffeine Counter

Moderate caffeine intake is not harmful to healthy adults. However, regular large amounts (over 350mg/day) may cause dependency ('caffeinism') and adversely affect health. To be safe, limit caffeine to 200mg/day. Avoid if pregnant; breast feeding; a child under 8; or have heart arrhythmias.

	Caffeine (mg)
Coffee: Instant, Weak, 1 level teaspoon	45
Medium, 1 rounded teaspoon	70
Strong, 1 heaping teaspoon	100
Decaffeinated, 1 round teaspoon	2
Bags (Folgers), 1 bag (6-8 fl.oz)	115
Ground, 1 Tbsp, 6g	60
Bottled (Ready-To-Drink), 9.5 fl.oz	70
Coffee Shop: Brewed, 8 fl.oz	110-150
Cappuccino: 1 cup, 8 fl.oz	80
Tall, 12 fl.oz	120
Large, 16 fl.oz	160
Decappuccino (decaffeinated)	5
Espresso: Regular/Solo	80
Double (Doppio) Espresso	160
Iced Coffee, 12 fl.oz	80
Latte, 1 cup, 8 fl.oz	80
Mocha, 8 fl.oz	90
Hot Chocolate, 8 fl.oz	10
Tea (Black/Green): Weak, 1 cup	20
Medium Strength, 1 cup	40
Strong, 1 cup	70
Herbal Tea	0
Iced Tea, Tall Glass/Can, 12 fl.oz	25
Soda Drinks: Per 12 fl.oz Can	
Coca-Cola (Classic/Van./Cherry); Pepsi (Reg./Diet)	35
Diet Coke; TAB; RC Cola	45
Dr. Pepper; Sunkist Orange Soda; Mr PiBB	40
Jolt Cola; SunDrop; RC Edge	65-70
Pepsi One; Mtn Dew; Mellow Yellow; Surge	55
Chocolate Bars: Milk Chocolate, 2 oz	12
Dark Chocolate, 2 oz	30
Cocoa/Hot Choc. Mix, 1 oz pkt	5
Chocolate Milk, 1 cup, 8 fl.oz	3
Choc Chip Cookies, 1 medium, 1 oz	3
Chocolate Cake, 3 oz	5
Chocolate Icecream, 1/2 cup	2
Chocolate Syrup, 2 Tbsp, 1.4 oz	7

Extensive Caffeine Counter ~ www.CalorieKing.com

Tea & Iced Teas

Teas

	C	F	Cb
Regular: Bag, Loose or Instant			
Brewed, 1 cup, 8 fl.oz	1	0	0
(Add extra for sugar/milk)			
Herbal: Average all varieties, 1 cup	1	0	0
Bigelow: Apple Orchard, 1 cup	5	0	1
Other Varieties	2	0	0.5
Celestial Seasonings:			
Bengal Spice; Spearmint	5	0	0.5
Lemon Zinger	4	0	1
Roastaroma	10	0	2
Other varieties	2	0	0.5
Chai Tea Latté (Starbucks): See Page 240			

Quick Guide

Iced Tea

Average All Brands

	C	F	Cb
Pre-Sweetened: 8 fl.oz	100	0	25
12 fl.oz	150	0	38
16 fl.oz	200	0	50
Unsweetened: 8 fl.oz	2	0	0

Iced Tea Mixes

Per Serving (1 Cup, Made-Up)

	C	F	Cb
4C Instant	90	0	22
Bigelow, Nice Over Ice	1	0	0.5
Celestial Seasonings, Iced Delight	4	0	1
Crystal Light, Sugar Free	3	0	0
Kool-Aid Fruit T's	70	0	17
Lipton: Instant	0	0	0
Instant Lemon/Raspberry	3	0	1
Lemon	55	0	14
Peach/Raspb, Sugar Free	5	0	1
Nestea: 100% Instant	2	0	0
Decaffeinated	6	0	1
Ice Teasers, all flavors	6	0	1
Peach, Raspberry	90	0	22

"A woman is like a teabag. You never know her strength until she's in hot water."

~ Nancy Reagan

Bottled & Canned Teas

Per 8 fl.oz Unless Indicated

	C	F	Cb
Arizona:			
Original Iced Tea	100	0	25
Green Tea(s)/Asian Plum	70	0	18
Diet Green/Lemon	0	0	0
Iced Tea w. Ginseng Extract	60	0	15
Herb Tea w. Honey	70	0	17
Peach/Raspberry	90	0	22
Brisk: 1 liter Bottle, avg, 1 cup	90	0	24
12 fl.oz Can: Raspberry, 1 can	120	0	33
Raspberry, 1 can	130	0	35
24 fl.oz Bottle: Lemon, 1 cup	80	0	22
Hansen's: Natural Iced Tea, 8 fl.oz	70	0	21
Low Calorie Blueberry/Raspberry	10	0	3
Knudsen: Coolers, all flavors	90	0	23
Lipton (16 fl.oz Bottle): *Per 8 fl.oz*			
No Lemon	70	0	18
Lemon	90	0	21
Peach; Raspberry	110	0	26
Mistic: Tropical Cooler, 8 fl.oz	45	0	12
Nantucket: Blueberry Tea, 8 fl.oz	80	0	20
Original Lemon Tea; Half & Half	90	0	23
Diet Lemon Tea	10	0	2
Nestea Iced Tea: Diet Lemon	3	0	0.5
Cool from Nestea, 1 cup, 8 fl.oz	80	0	20
Diet Cool from Nestea	2	0	0.5
Lemon/Peach/Raspberry	90	0	22
Sweetened Ice Tea	65	0	17
Oregon Chai: Herbal Bliss, 1/2 cup	70	0	18
Nirvana/Kashmir Green, 1/2 cup	80	0	20
Royal Mistic: Regular, 12 fl.oz	145	0	36
Diet, 12 fl.oz	8	0	2
Schweppes, 8 fl.oz	90	0	22
Shasta, 8 fl.oz	80	0	20
Snapple: Regular, sweetened	70	0	17
Diet/Unsweetened	0	0	0
Lemon; Peach, Raspberry	100	0	25
SoBe: Green/Lemon Tea, 8 fl.oz	90	0	23
20 fl.oz bottle	225	0	57
Ssips (Johanna Farms), 8.45 fl.oz	100	0	25
Tropicana: Lemonfruit	100	0	25
Diet Lemon Fruit	15	0	4
Peach/Rasp./Tangerine, 8 fl.oz	120	0	28
11.5 fl.oz can	160	0	40
Twister: Apple Berry, 8 fl.oz	100	0	28
Turkey Hill: Regular	90	0	22
Raspberry Cooler	110	0	28

Alcohol Guide

▶ **Health Hazards: Excess alcohol** contributes to obesity, high blood pressure, stroke, heart and liver disease, some cancers, and even impotence.

Concentration and short-term memory are reduced as well as sporting performance.

Other alcohol hazards include stomach upsets, menstrual problems, anxiety, headaches, insomnia, work absenteeism, risky behaviors, and family arguments.

▶ **Alcohol contributes to obesity** through its high calories and by lessening the body's ability to burn fat. Fat storage is promoted, particularly in the belly - a health danger zone. Alcohol can also stimulate appetite.

▶ **Alcohol is potentially more harmful while dieting.** Blood sugar levels may drop with resultant tiredness and further impairment of concentration, reflexes and driving skills - and maybe even the dieter's resolve!

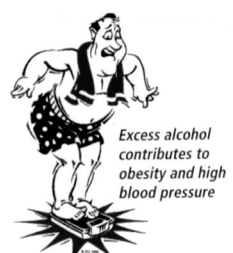

Excess alcohol contributes to obesity and high blood pressure

---

 SAFE ALCOHOL LIMITS

Women: No more than **1 drink** per day.
Men: No more than **2 drinks** per day.
(At least 2 days a week should be alcohol-free.)

1 Drink = 12 fl.oz regular beer, or 5 fl.oz wine, or 1½ fl.oz spirits (80 proof).
Each drink contains approximately 14g alcohol.

For some people, **safe drinking** will mean no alcohol drinks at all. (Even one drink may impair driving skills, particularly if tired; and 3-4 drinks daily has been linked to brain shrinkage in some social drinkers.)

▶ **It is advisable not to drink at all if you are:**
- pregnant or trying to conceive
- taking drug medication (unless approved by your doctor or pharmacist)
- have a condition such as liver or heart disease
- planning to drive, use machinery or play sport
- studying or needing to concentrate
- a child or adolescent

▶ **Women and adolescents are more prone** to alcohol's ill-effects due to their lower body weight, smaller livers and lesser capacity to metabolize alcohol.

Note: You cannot save daily drinks for one occasion.
    Binge drinking is particularly harmful ~
    4 drinks 'in a row' for males or 3 drinks for females.

Extra Information: www.CalorieKing.com

HOW TO CALCULATE ALCOHOL CONTENT

Percent alcohol on label refers to alcohol volume (ml alcohol/100ml).

100ml = 3½ fl. oz

To convert to grams (weight) of alcohol, multiply the percent volume by 0.8 - since 1 ml of alcohol weighs only 0.8 grams (actually 0.789g).

EXAMPLE
12 fl.oz Can Beer (5% alcohol)

5% alc.volume = 5% of 12 fl.oz
            = 0.6 fl.oz
            = 18ml alcohol
            (1 fl.oz = 30ml)

Weight (18ml x 0.8) = 14.4g alc.

GOVERNMENT WARNING

(1) According to the Surgeon General, women should not drink alcoholic beverages during pregnancy because of the risk of birth defects.

(2) Consumption of alcoholic beverages impairs your ability to drive a car or operate machinery, and may cause health problems.

Beers ◆ Ales ◆ Malt Liquors

Quick Guide

Beer (Alc) ~ Alcohol (Grams)

Beer Contains Zero Fat

	C	Alc	Cb
Malt Liquor/Ale (5.6% Alc. Vol.)			
12 fl.oz Can/Bottle/Glass	180	16	17
22 fl.oz Can/Bottle/Glass	330	29	32
Regular Beer (5% Alc. Vol.)			
7 fl.oz Glass	80	8.5	4
12 fl.oz Bottle/Can/Glass	140	14	10
16 oz. Bottle/Can	185	19	11
22 fl.oz Bottle	260	26	20
32 fl.oz Bottle	370	37	28
40 fl.oz Bottle	470	47	35
Light Beer (4.2% Alc. Vol.)			
7 fl.oz Glass	65	7	4
12 fl.oz Bottle/Can/Glass	110	12	6
16 fl.oz Bottle/Can	145	16	8
22 fl.oz Bottle	200	22	11
Low Alcohol Beer (2.3% Alc. Vol)			
(Example: Blatz LA),12 fl.oz	75	7	6
Non-Alcoholic/Near Beer			
(Less than 0.5% alcohol by volume)			
Average All Brands, 12 fl.oz	70	1	16

Beer Brands

Per 12 fl.oz Serving (Alc) ~ Alcohol (Grams)
*Percentage alcohol listed below
is by volume - not by weight.*

	C	Alc	Cb
Amber Ice (5.3% alcohol)	130	15	6
Amstel Light (3.5%)	100	10	5
Anchor Steam (4.6%)	155	13	16
Anheuser Light (3.2% alcohol)	75	9	7
Artic Ice (5.3%)	150	15	8
Artic Ice Light 3.2 (3.9%)	100	11	6
Augsburger Bock (4.9%)	170	14	17
Ballard Bitter (4.7%)	180	14	19
Beck's (5%)	150	14	12
Big Sky (4.8%)	150	14	12
Big Sky Light (4.5%)	105	13	5
Black Label (5.6%)	155	16	11
Blackhook Porter (4.9%)	160	14	14
Blatz (4.6%)	145	13	13
Blatz Light (3.9%), 12 fl.oz	110	11	8
Bud Dry (4.9%)	130	14	8
Bud Light (4.2%)	110	12	7
Bud Ice (5.5%)	150	16	9
Bud Ice Light (4.1%)	110	12	7

Brands (Cont)

Beer Contains Zero Fat

	C	Alc	Cb
Budweiser (4.9%)	145	14	11
Natural Light (4.2%)	110	12	7
Natural Ice (5.8%)	160	16	10
Busch (4.6%)	135	13	10
Busch Ice (5.9%)	175	17	13
Busch Light (4.2%)	110	12	7
Carling (4.4%)	140	13	10
Carlsberg (5%)	135	13	10
Castlemaine XXXX (4.7%)	140	13	9
Colt 45 Malt (5.6%)	160	16	11
Coors (4.9%)	150	14	12
Coors Dry (4.9%)	120	14	6
Coors Light 3.2 (4%)	100	11	4
Corona Extra (4.6%)	130	13	9
Dos Equis Lager (5%)	130	14	13
Elk Mountain Amber Ale (5.5%)	190	16	18
Elk Mountain Red (4.9%)	160	14	13
Extra Gold (4.9%)	150	14	12
Extra Gold 3.2 (4%)	120	11	10
Faust (5%)	170	14	17
First Reserve (4.9%)	170	14	16
Fosters Lager (4.9%)	135	14	9
George Killian's: Irish Brown (5.2%)	185	15	15
Irish Red (5%)	160	14	13
Wilde Honey Ale (5.3%)	170	15	14
Goebel (4.1%)	130	12	12
Goebel Light (3.9%)	110	11	8
Grolsch Premium (5%)	140	14	10
Hamm's (4.7%)	145	14	12
Light (4.2%)	110	12	7
Heileman's Classic Draft (4.7%)	145	13	12
Heineken (5%)	150	14	12
Heineken Special Dark (5.2%)	175	15	16
Herman Joseph's Sp. Prem. (4.9%)	150	14	12
Highland Ale: Black (5.6%)	180	16	16
Amber (5.2%)	160	15	14
Hurricane (5.8%)	160	16	10
Hurricane Ice (7.4%)	200	21	12
Icehouse (5.0%)	135	14	8
Icehouse (5.5%)	150	16	10
Jacob Best Ice (5.8%)	160	17	11
Jacob Best Light (3.9%)	110	11	7
Keystone Regular/Dry (4.9% alc.)	125	14	6
Ice (5.3%)	145	15	8
Light, 3.2 (4%)	100	14	4
Amber Light (3.8%)	110	11	8

Beers ✦ Ales ✦ Malt Liquors

Brands (Cont)

Beer Contains Zero Fat
Per 12 fl.oz Serving

	C	Alc	Cb
Killarney's (5%)	200	14	23
King Cobra (5.9%)	170	17	12
Kirin Lager (4.9%)	145	14	11
Kirin Light (3.2%)	95	9	7
Labatt's Blue (5%)	145	14	14
Leinenkugel's: Original (4.6%)	150	13	14
Light (4.1%)	105	12	6
Lone Star: Regular (4.7%)	140	14	12
Light (3.9%)	110	11	8
Lowenbrau Dark/Special (4.9%)	160	14	15
Magnum Malt Liquor (5.9%)	155	17	10
Meister Brau (4.5%)	130	13	12
Memphis Brown (4.6%)	120	13	6
Michelob: Regular (5%)	155	14	13
Light (4.3%)	135	12	12
Dry (4.9%)	130	14	8
AmberBock (5.2%)	165	15	15
Golden Draft (4.7%)	150	13	13
Golden Draft Light (4.2%)	110	12	7
Hefeweizen (5%)	155	14	12
Honeylarger (4.9%)	175	14	18
ULTRA (4.2%)	95	12	2.6
Miller Genuine Draft (5%)	145	14	13
Light (4.5%)	110	13	7
Miller High Life (5%)	145	14	13
Miller High Life Ice (5.5%)	160	16	11
Miller High Life Light (4.5%)	110	13	7
Miller Lite (4.5%)	100	13	4
Milwaukee's Best (4.5%)	130	13	12
Milwaukee's Best Ice (5.5%)	135	16	7
Milwaukee's Best Light (4.5%)	100	13	4
Minnesota's Best (4.9%)	140	14	10
Moosehead (5%)	125	14	14
Newcastle Brown Ale (4.5%)	140	12	13
Northstone Amber Ale (4.9%)	150	14	8
Old Milwaukee (4.6%)	145	13	3
Light (3.9%)	110	11	8
Ice (5.9%)	180	17	15
Old Style (4.7%)	140	13	12
Old Style Light (4.2%)	115	12	7
Old Style LA (2.2%)	75	6	6
Pabst Blue Ribbon (4.7%)	145	14	12
Pabst Light (3.9%)	110	11	8
Pabst Extra Light (2.2%)	70	6	6

Alc ~ Alcohol (Grams)	C	Alc	Cb
Pete's Wicked Ale (5%)	180	14	20
Piels (4.3%)	125	12	9
Ranier (4.7%)	135	13	12
Ranier Light (3.8%)	110	11	8
Red Bull Malt (5.9%)	160	17	11
Red Dog (5%)	150	14	14
Red Hook ESB (5.7%)	180	17	16
Red River Valley (4.9%)	165	14	15
Red Wolf (5.4%)	150	15	10
Sam Adams Light (4%)	130	11	10
Samuel Adams (4.6%)	170	13	17
Samuel Adams Lager (4.7%)	180	13	19
Sapporo Draft (Japan) (4.5%)	140	12	12
Schaefer (4.6%)	145	13	12
Schaefer Light (3.9%)	110	11	8
Schlitz (4.6%)	145	13	12
Schlitz Light (3.9%)	110	11	8
Schlitz Malt (5.9%)	180	17	15
Schmidt's (4.6%)	145	13	13
Schmidt's Light (3.9%)	110	11	8
Sheaf Stout, 5.7%	180	16	17
Sierra Nevada: Pale Ale (5.6%)	200	16	12
Big Foot (9.6%)	295	28	25
Porter (5.6%)	200	16	16
Wheat Beer (4.4%)	150	13	12
Silver Thunder (5.9%)	165	17	11
Stella Artois, 5%, 330ml	135	14	9
Southpaw Light (5%)	125	14	7
Stroh's (4.6%)	145	13	12
Stroh's Light (4.2%)	115	13	7
Wheat Hook (4.8%)	150	14	12
Winterfest (5.7%)	185	16	18
Zeigenbock Amber (4.4%)	145	12	13
Zima Clear Malt (4.6%)	150	14	13

Home-Brewed Beer: Similar to regular beers, according to alcohol content.

Non-Alcoholic Brews

Less Than 0.5% Alcohol

	C	Alc	Cb
Average All Brands (Busch NA, Kaliber, Kingsbury, O'Douls NA, Old Milwaukee NA, Pabst NA, Stroh's NA, Sharp's, Haakebeck, Texas Select)			
12 fl.oz Can/Bottle	65	1	14

Hard Lemonade

	C	Alc	Cb
Average All Brands (5%), 12 fl.oz	250	14	39
Doc Otis Lemon (4.8%), 12 fl.oz	250	14	39
Henry's Hard Lem'ade (5%), 12 fl.oz	285	14	46
Hooch Hard (5.2%), 330ml	215	14	32
Hooch Ice (5.7%), 330ml	230	15	32
Mike's (5.2%), 11.2 fl.oz	250	14	38

Cider Alc ~ Alcohol (Grams)

	C	Alc	Cb
Alcoholic Cider: Average, 6% alcohol,			
Dry, 12 fl.oz	130	17	12
Sweet, 12 fl.oz	170	17	15
Hardcore Crisp Hard Cider (6%)	190	17	19
Hornsby's: Draft Cider (6%)	170	17	16
Hard Apple Cider (5.5%)	200	16	27
Woodchuck (5%) Amber, 12 fl.oz	200	15	21
Dark & Dry, 12 fl.oz	180	15	17
Granny Smith, 12 fl.oz	165	15	11
Wyder's (4%) Raspb., 11.5 fl.oz	140	11	15

Quick Guide

Table Wine
Average All Varieties (11.5% Alcohol)

	C	Alc	Cb
4 fl.oz (¹/₂ large wine glass)	85	11	2
6 fl.oz (³/₄ large wine glass)	125	16	3
¹/₂ Carafe/Bottle, 375ml	265	34	6
1 Bottle, 750ml	530	68	13

Table Wines

	C	Alc	Cb
Red: Claret/Burgundy/Chianti, 4 fl.oz	80	11	2
Sparkling Reds, 4 fl.oz	90	11	3
Rose: Medium, 4 fl.oz	80	11	1.5
White: Dry (Chablis/Hock/Riesling) 4 fl.oz	75	11	1
Zinfandel Sweet			
(Moselle/Sauterne), 4 fl.oz	85	11	2
Sparkling, 4 fl.oz	95	11	4
Champagne: *Per 4 fl.oz Serving*			
Average 1 glass, 4 fl.oz	85	11	2
w. Orange Jce (3:1 orange)	75	8	4
w. Orange Jce (1:1 orange)	65	5	7
Cold Duck, 4 fl. oz	108	11	8
Sake: Rice Wine (16% alc.), 4 oz	125	15	5
Mulled Wine: (Gluhwein), 4 oz	180	14	20
Non-Alcoholic Wine, aver., 4 oz	50	0	5
Reduced Alcohol Wine (6%):			
Average all types, 4 fl.oz	50	0	12

Dessert Wines

	C	Alc	Cb
Madeira (18% alc), 2 oz	85	9	5
Marsala (18%), 2 oz	110	9	11
Port, Muscatel, (18%), 2 oz	85	9	5
Sherry (18%), 2 oz			
Dry, 1 Sherry glass	65	9	0.5
Sweet/Cream, average	85	9	5
Vermouth: Dry (18%), 2 oz	65	9	0.5
Sweet (15%), 2 oz	85	7	8

Cooking Wine

Average All Brands

	C	Alc	Cb
Red/White, 2 Tbsp, 1 oz	20	3	1
1 cup, 8fl. oz	160	22	12
Marsala, 2 Tbsp, 1 oz	35	4	2
Sherry, 2 Tbsp, 1 oz	40	4	2

Cooking with Wine:

For alcohol to evaporate, sufficient heat and cooking time (at least 30 minutes) is required.

Red and white table wines would then contain negligible residual calories.

Sweetened wines (marsala/sherry) would contain 10 calories per 1 fl.oz used.

Flambé Desserts: Only surface alcohol is burnt off, so negligible reduction in alcohol or calories.

Quick Guide Alc ~ Alcohol (Grams)

Spirits/Liquors
All Contain Zero Fat

Includes Bourbon, Brandy, Gin, Rum, Scotch, Tequila, Vodka, Whiskey.
Note: All spirits with same proof (alcohol) have similar calories and zero fat.

Average All Brands

	C	Alc	Cb
80 Proof (40% Alcohol by Volume):			
1 fl.oz (1 shot)	65	9.5	0
¹/₂ Bottle, 375 ml	810	120	0
1 Bottle, 750 ml	1620	240	0
86 Proof (43% Alcohol):			
1 fl.oz (1 shot)	70	10	0
¹/₂ Bottle, 375 ml	870	125	0
1 Bottle, 750 ml	1750	250	0
100 Proof (50% Alcohol):			
1 fl.oz (1 shot)	82	12	0
¹/₂ Bottle, 375 ml	1025	150	0
1 Bottle	2050	300	0

Coolers ◆ Cocktails

Coolers & Premix Cocktails

Zero Fat Unless Indicated **C** **Alc** **Cb**

	C	Alc	Cb
Bacardi Silver (4.9%), 12 fl.oz	**235**	14	35
Bacardi Fruit Mixers (Frozen Conc.)			
Made up (2 oz mix + 1 oz Rum + Ice)			
Margarita	**160**	10	22
Pina Colada	**230**	10	40
Other varieties, average	**200**	10	32
(If 2 oz Rum used, add extra 70 cals/10g alcohol)			
Bartles & Jaymes			
Malt Based Coolers (3.9% alc): *Per 12 fl.oz*			
Black Cherry; Classic Original	**200**	11	30
Exotic Berry, Juicy Peach	**210**	1	33
Fuzzy Navel; Hard Lemonade	**230**	11	38
Kiwi Strawberry	**215**	11	34
Margarita, Pina Colada	**270**	11	48
Raspberry Daiquiri	**220**	11	38
Strawb. Cosmopolitan/Daiquiri	**230**	11	35
Tropical Burst, Luscious Blackb.	**230**	11	38
Capt. Morgan Gold (5%), 12 oz	**240**	14	36
Cruzan Island Cocktails (5% alc): *Per 12 fl.oz*			
Jumbie Brew	**230**	14	32
Mojito	**300**	14	50
Wazi Koki	**285**	14	46
Heublein Premium Classics			
Long Is. Ice Tea (15% alc), 2 oz	**130**	7	20
Manhattan (22.5%), 2 oz + ice	**160**	11	20
Mai Tai (22%), 2 oz + ice	**160**	11	20
Pina Colada, 4 oz (10g fat) + ice	**280**	4	40
Jack Daniels Country Cocktails (5.9%)			
Average all flavors, 200ml	**170**	10	25
Jack Daniels Hard Cola (5%) 12oz	**234**	14	34
Jose Cuervo Cocktails (5.9% alc)			
Margarita/ Lime.Strawb. 200ml	**180**	10	27
Sauza Diablo (5%), 12 fl.oz	**260**	14	40
Seagram's Coolers (3.2% alc)			
Wild Berries/Blackberry, 12 fl.oz	**230**	12	36
Skyy Blue (5% alc), 12 fl.oz	**280**	14	45
Sparks (6% alc), 16 fl.oz	**350**	23	48
Stolichnayar Citr. (5%), 12 fl.oz	**240**	14	36
Smirnoff Ice (5% alc), 330ml	**225**	13	33
TGI Friday's Frozen Cocktails (12.5% alc):			
Per Serving (3 fl.oz Premix & Ice)			
Margarita; Strawberry Daiquiri	**145**	9	20
Other flavors, average	**240**	9	31

Premix Cocktails (Cont)

The Club **C** **Alc** **Cb**
(Premix Cocktails): *Per 4 oz*

	C	Alc	Cb
Long Island Ice Tea; Manhattan	**220**	16	30
Margar.; Scr'driver; Vod. Martini	**210**	7	40
Mudslide (9g fat)	**270**	12	41
P. Colada; Or. Craze; Whisk. Sour	**260**	10	40

Shooters

Alc ~ Alcohol (Grams)

		Alc	
Kamakazi	**150**	20	2
Mud Slide	**160**	13	11
Fuzzy Navel	**120**	13	7
Pineapple Bomber	**130**	11	13
Turbo	**110**	14	3
Shots: Average all types, 1½ fl. oz	**110**	14	3

Flavorings/Syrups

Non-Alcoholic, Fat Free

Angostura Bitters, ¼ tsp	**3**	0	0
Grenadine/Cassis, 2 Tbsp, 1 oz	**70**	0	17
Lime Juice, 2 Tbsp, 1 oz	**10**	0	2
Sugar Syrup, 2 Tbsp, 1 oz	**70**	0	17
Sour Mix, 2 Tbsp, 1 oz	**10**	0	2
Tonic Water, 8 fl.oz	**90**	0	22

Cocktail Mix 'N Drinks

No Alcohol Added

Bloody Mary Mix (Mr & Mrs T), 8 fl.oz	**40**	0	9
Pina Colada Mix: *Daily's*, 3 fl.oz	**160**	0	37
Mr & Mrs T, 4.5 fl.oz	**180**	0	43
Margarita Mix (J.Cuervo), 4 fl.oz	**100**	0	24

"The doctor told him to cut down to just one glass a day."

Cocktails • Liqueurs

Cocktails   **Alc** ~ Alcohol (Grams)

Zero Fat Unless Indicated
(Made to Standard Recipes)

	C	Alc	Cb
Bloody Mary	120	14	5
Blushin' Russian (9g fat)	365	14	47
Bourbon & Soda	110	15	1
Brandy Alexander (16g fat)	300	16	11
Cerebral Hemorrhage (5g fat)	290	17	32
Chupa Naranjas (w. 1½ oz Tequila)	150	16	8
Collins (w. 2 oz Gin)	180	20	11
Daiquiri	110	14	3
Gin & Tonic	170	16	14
Harvey Wallbanger (2 oz Vodka)	250	30	11
Highball (1½ oz Whiskey)	110	14	3
Irish Coffee (contains 9g fat)	210	14	8
L.A. Sunrise	280	26	21
Leprechaun's Libation	285	31	17
Long Island Iced Tea (w. 8 oz Cola)	230	19	25
w. Diet Cola	130	19	0
Mai Tai (w. 2 oz Rum)	260	27	17
Manhattan	130	17	3
Margarita	170	21	4
Martini	160	22	1
Mind Eraser	160	17	10
Mint Julep	165	20	8
Mosito (w. 2 oz Rum)	170	19	10
Pina Colada (contains 12g fat)	260	14	12
Screwdriver	180	14	20
Spritzer (3 oz Wine)	70	8	3
Tequila Sunrise	190	20	14
Tom Collins	120	16	2
Whiskey Sour	125	15	5

Liqueurs/Cordials   *Per 1 fl.oz*

	C	Alc	Cb
Baileys Irish Cream (34 Proof; 5g fat)	95	4	5
Lite (30 Proof; 2g fat)	75	4	7
Cherry Brandy (48 Proof)	80	6	9
Coffee Liqueur (53 Proof)	90	6.5	11
Amaretto (56 Proof)	110	6	17
Benedictine (80 Proof)	90	10	5
Cointreau (80 Proof)	100	10	7
Creme de Cacao (54 Proof)	100	6	15
Creme de Menthe (60 Proof)	120	7	14
Drambuie (80 Proof)	105	10	9
Grand Marnier (80 Proof)	100	10	7
Kahlua (53 Proof)	90	6.5	11
Kirsch (68 Proof)	80	8	6
Midori (42 Proof), average all types	80	5	14

Ten Hints to Avoid Harmful Drinking

1. **Add up the alcohol** you typically drink each day and on social occasions. How does this compare with 'low risk' amounts?

2. **Compare the alcohol content** of different drinks and select the lowest. Request half ounces of alcohol in cocktails and mixed drinks. Dilute them and keep topping off with non-alcoholic drinks.

3. **Try low alcohol** or non-alcohol alternatives such as fruit juices and mineral water. Take your own to parties.

4. **Before drinking alcohol,** quench your thirst with water and non-alcoholic drinks - particularly after vigorous exercise or sport.

5. **Slow the rate of drinking.** Chugging or drinking fast is the major cause of illness and death from alcohol poisoning.

6. **Avoid drinking in 'rounds'.**

7. **Have a non-alcoholic 'spacer'** between drinks (e.g. mineral water, orange juice).

8. **Don't drink on an empty stomach.** Food slows the rate of alcohol absorption.

9. **Keep track of the number of drinks** and know when to stop. Stick to a set limit.

10. **Do not drive, swim, or operate machinery** while under the influence.

Note: Alcohol can be very dangerous when taken with prescription or street drugs or when you are very tired.

Liqueurs/Cordials (Cont)

Per 1 fl.oz

	C	Alc	Cb
Ouzo (80 Proof)	90	10	5
Sambuca (84 Proof)	100	10	7
Schnapps (80 Proof)	100	10	7
Southern Comfort (78 Proof)	75	9	3
Tia Maria (64 Proof)	90	8	9
Triple Sec (60 Proof)	80	7	4

Coffee Liqueurs: *Average All Types*
(Includes Benedictine, Cointreau, Kahlua):

	C	Alc	Cb
1 serving	200	10	10

Deli, Sandwiches, Wraps

Cafeteria-Style Foods

	C	F	Cb
Beef Stroganoff, 5 oz	195	13	7
Beef Stroganoff w. 4 oz noodles	350	14	36
Chicken Lasagna, 1 piece	300	11	32
Chicken Chop Suey w. 4 oz rice	245	4	37
Deep Dish Burrito, 7 oz	265	13	20
Grnd Beef Casserole, 2 scoop, 6 oz	245	13	17
Italian Meat Sce for Spagh., 5 oz	150	9	9
w. 5 oz Spaghetti	350	10	49
Lasagna, 1 piece	275	11	25
Meatloaf, 3 oz	205	13	4
Ranch Beans, 2 scoops, 6 oz	350	11	45
Red Beans & Rice, 7 oz	280	9	37
Scalloped Potato/Ham, 2 scp, 6 oz	160	6	20
Stuffed Shells in Sauce (1)	105	3	17
Swedish Meatballs (3)	205	12	9
Sweet & Sour Pork/Rice, 9 oz	240	3	40
Swiss Steak w/Mushr. Gravy, 6 oz	280	11	4
Tator Tot Casserole, 2 scoops, 6 oz	260	15	20
Tenderloin Tips/Mushr. Gravy, 5 oz	210	13	3
w. 5 oz noodles	395	15	38
Tuna Noodle Casserole, 2 scp, 6 oz	180	6	17
Turkey Tetrazini, 2 scoops, 6 oz	195	7	17
Vegetable Lasagna, 1 piece	250	13	21

Croissants

		C	F	Cb
Unfilled: Medium 1½ oz		180	10	21
Filled: w. Ham (2 oz), Salad		280	14	24
w. Ham (2 oz), Cheese (2 oz)		470	30	20
w. Chick (2 oz) Cheese (2 oz)		470	30	20
w. Turkey/Ham/Chse (2 oz ea.)		580	36	20
Au Bon Pain: Ham & Cheese		290	9	39
Spinach & Cheese		220	9	29

7-Eleven: Page 231

Bagels

	C	F	Cb
Plain: Large, 3 oz (no filling)	240	2	45
w. 2 Tbsp Cream Cheese	340	12	46
w. 2 oz Lox (Smoked Salmon)	320	4	45

Also see Bagels Section: *Page 103*

Au Bon Pain: Page 179
Breugger's: Page 184
Einstein Bros Bagels: Page 199
Other Fast-Foods Restaurants: Page 175

Sandwiches   C F Cb

No Spreads Unless Indicated
(Includes 2 Slices Bread ~ 3 oz)

	C	F	Cb
BLT (5 strips Bacon, 2 Tbsp Mayo)	600	40	46
Breaded Chicken & Salad	540	28	46
Chicken (5 oz) Salad w. Mayo.	580	30	49
Chopped Liver, Egg, Mayo.	630	45	44
Corned Beef (5 oz) w. Mustard	560	28	44
Cream Cheese w. Olives (5 large)	340	14	46
Egg Salad w. Mayonnaise	570	29	49
Egg Salad Club w. Bacon, Mayo.	780	53	49
Grilled Cheese (3 oz)	540	30	44
Ham (4 oz); Cheese (4 oz), Mayo.	910	56	44
Lobster Salad (4 oz) w. Mayo.	530	25	45
Overstuffed Tuna Salad (7 oz)	870	39	75
Philadelphia Cheese Steak S'wich	550	23	42
Reuben (6 oz Beef/Pastrami, 2 oz Cheese,			
2 Tbsp Dressing)	920	60	28
Roast Beef (4 oz) w. Mustard	460	12	45
Roast Pork (4 oz) w. Apple Sauce	500	16	55
Shrimp Salad Club w. Bacon, Mayo.	800	57	48
Sloppy Joe w. Sauce (7 oz)	600	30	45
Steak Sandwich (5 oz cooked)	680	32	41
Triple Cheese (4 oz) Melt	720	45	46
Tuna (5 oz) Salad w. Mayo.	610	30	49
Turkey Breast (5 oz) w. Mayo.	460	18	44
Turkey Breast (5 oz) w. Mustard	360	7	44
Turkey Club w. Bacon, Mayo.	830	38	31
Vegetarian w. Avocado, Cheese	820	49	72

Subs: *See Subway Page 242*
7-Eleven: Page 231

Wraps & Roll-Ups

Average All Types
(Meat/Chicken/Fish/Veges)

	C	F	Cb
Small size, approx. 9 oz	500	25	48
Regular, approx. 15 oz	830	40	80
Large, approx. 22 oz	1400	70	134

Au Bon Pain: See Page 179
Other Fast-Foods Restaurants: Page 175

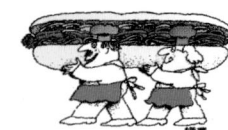

Restaurant & International Foods

Chinese & Asian Dishes

Appetizers	C	F	Cb
Curried Meat Triangles, 1 pce	150	5	12
Dumplings: Pork, steamed, 1	40	3	4
Pork, fried, 1 dumpling	75	7	4
Vegetable, steamed, 1	25	0.5	4
Egg Rolls, mini, 3 rolls	100	3	11
Spring Roll: Small, 1½ oz	100	7	10
Medium, 3 oz	200	12	20
Large, 5 oz	350	15	33
Wonton, 1 only	55	3	4
Soup: Clear, 1 bowl	30	1	4
with Noodles	100	3	12
Chicken & Corn	150	8	8
Rice: Plain, cooked, 1 cup, 6½ oz	245	0.5	53
Fried: 1 cup, 5 oz	320	13	42
Large dish, 16 oz	1010	40	134
Noodles: Chinese Egg, ckd, 1 cup	200	3	42
Entrees & Mains: Per Whole Dish			
Beef Satay, 17 oz	760	50	15
Beef in Black Bean Sce, 17 oz	530	33	17
Beef with Broccoli, 16 oz	650	30	31
Chicken & Almonds, 18 oz	685	50	18
Chicken (sliced) & Broccoli	280	12	13
Chop Suey: Chicken, 20 oz	560	37	12
Pork, 20 oz	680	50	12
Chow Mein: Beef/Chicken, 24 oz	940	60	50
Crab Rangoon, 1 dumpling	70	6	4
Crispy Fried Chicken, 8 oz	485	33	12
Egg Drop Soup, 1 cup, 8 fl oz	120	3	15
Lemon Chicken, 10 oz	580	32	25
Lo Mein (stir-fried)	620	29	61
Moo Shu Chicken, 2 wrapped crepes	430	16	43
Omelet, Chicken/Shrimp, 18 oz	990	82	10
Steamed Whole Fish, ½ Red Snapper	500	11	1
Sweet & Sour: Fish, 20 oz	1160	58	106
Pork, 18 oz	950	50	92
Vegetable Combination, w. oil, 6 oz	250	17	19
Vegetables, Steamed (no oil), 6 oz	120	1	25
Fortune Cookie: each	25	0.5	5
Extra Listings: See Frozen Meals			

Confucious say:

"Man who eat with one chopstick never have problem with obesity"

Cajun & Creole

	C	F	Cb
Alligator, 4 oz cooked	160	2	0
Baked Herb Chicken, 1 serving	850	53	2
Bouillabaisse	400	15	10
Cajun Fried Turkey, 1 serving	630	25	0
Cocktail Sauce, 1 Tbsp	15	0	3
Couche-couche, ½ cup	80	0	17
Crawfish Bisque, 1 serving	500	10	10
Crawfish, cooked, 2 oz	45	0.5	0
Creole Jambalaya, 1 serving	550	30	15
Dove, cooked, 1 oz	60	3.5	0
Frog's Legs, steamed (2)	45	0	0
Guinea Fowl, flesh, 1 oz, ckd	40	1	0
Hogshead Cheese, ¼ cup	80	5.5	0
Jambalaya, Shrimp & Crabmeat	520	14	12
Red Beans & Rice, 1 serving	400	17	52
Roasted Quail, w. Bacon on Toast	550	25	15
Remoulade Sauce, 1 Tbsp	55	5.5	1
Shrimp Creole, 1 serving	450	20	10
Stuffed Smothered Steak, w. 1 cup Rice	890	50	50
Squab, flesh, 1 oz cooked	60	3.5	0
Turtle, cooked, 1½ oz	60	1.5	0

French Foods

	C	F	Cb
Blanquette d'Agneau (Lamb Stew)	800	30	17
Brioche, 1 cake	280	14	34
Bouillabaisse (Fish Stew)	400	15	10
Coq au Vin (Chicken in Wine)	800	30	16
Coquilles St. Jacques, fried, 6 lge.	300	14	2
Crème Brulée, 1 serving	460	40	21
Creme Caramel (Caram. Custard)	260	10	38
Crepe Suzette, 1 x 6" crepe/sauce	220	10	13
Duck a l'Orange	780	35	47
Escargots (Snails), in garl. butter, (6)	200	10	4
French Stick Bread, 3 slices, 2.2 oz	150	1	35
Frogs Legs, fried, 4 med. pairs	400	20	10
Lamb Noisettes, fried, 2 chops	500	40	1
Mousse au Chocolat	380	15	33
Potage Creme Crecy (Carrot Soup)	360	18	14
Salade Nicoise (Tuna/Oliv./Veg.)	400	30	14
Veal Cordon Bleu (Veal/Ham/Ch)	650	25	18
Vichyssoise (Pot./Leek Soup), 1 c.	200	9	15
Baguette & French Stick: Page 102			
Croissants: Pages 112, 168			

Restaurant & International Foods

Cuban

	C	F	Cb
Bl. Beans w. Rice (Moros con Cristianos)	510	22	76
Blk.-eyed Pea Fritters (Bollitos de Carita)	80	5	6
Casserole Corn Tamale (Tammal en Cazuela)	445	20	55
Chkn w. Yellow Rice (Arroz con Pollo)	925	49	87
Cuban Bread (Pan Cubano)	80	1.5	15
Donuts in Syrup (Bunuelos)	170	5	10
with Melado	100	5	10
Grilled Plantains	145	0	40
Gypsy's Arm Cake (Brazo Gitano)	260	18	42
Roast Pork S'wich (Pan con Lechon)	640	30	62
Seasoned Beef w. Olives & Raisins (Picadillo)	435	36	10
Shredded Beef (Ropa Vieja)	550	35	10
Taro Root Mash (Pure de Malanga)	315	3	69
Yuca with Citrus Garlic Dressing (Yuca con Mojo)	190	9	25

German

	C	F	Cb
Bavarian Bread Dumpling, 3 small	330	10	28
Beef Goulash with Veges	520	20	46
Black Forest Cake, 1 slice	380	16	30
Bratwurst, grilled, 1 medium, 6 oz	450	37	2
Chicken: Fried, Viennese-style	530	20	28
Livers w. Apple/On., 6 oz	460	28	10
Herring, Pickled: Rollmops, 4 oz	260	16	3
with Sour Cream, 4 oz	310	20	3
Hot Sausage Curry	300	7	6
Kugelhupf Cake, 1 lge slice, 4 oz	400	23	40
Sauerbraten Pork (Pot Roast)	650	35	15
Torte: Linzer (Alm./Raspb. Jam)	430	18	58
Sacher (Choc./Apricot Jam)	260	12	23
Weiner Schnitzel, 1 medium	750	35	38

Greek

	C	F	Cb
Baklava Pastry, 1 only, 3 3/4 oz	400	21	45
Calamari, deep fried, 1 cup	300	13	17
Galactobureko, 1 serve (Filo, Custard, Pastry in Syrup)	360	15	48
Kataifi, (Filo, Nut, Pastry in Syrup)	350	11	56
Moussaka, 1 serve, 8 oz	350	22	22
Souvlakia (Lamb), each, 2 oz	120	6	1
Stuffed Tomatoes, 2 only	250	12	17
Taramosalata, 1 Tbsp, 1/2 oz	40	3	2
Tyropita (Filo/Egg/Cheese Pastry)	350	26	31
Tzatziki (Cucumber/Yog. Dip), 1 T.	20	1	1
Vine Leaves, stuffed, 3 rolls, 6 oz	200	5	13

Hawaiian

	C	F	Cb
Chicken Long Rice	250	15	12
Grilled Ahi Tuna (6 oz fillet)	450	28	2
Kalua: Chicken, 4 oz	280	16	0
Pork, 4 oz	350	24	0
Lau Lau: Chicken (1) 7 oz	260	21	3
Pork (1) 7 oz	320	26	5
Lomi Lomi Salmon, 1/2 cup, 4 oz	75	2	6
Poi (mashed ckd taro), 1 c., 8 1/2 oz	200	0.5	65
Mix, 1/3 cup, 3.2 oz (makes 2/3 c.)	70	0	18
Portugese Sausage, 2 oz	180	15	2
Spam Musubi: w. Regular Spam	265	11	34
(4 oz rice+1.3 oz Spam/7-Eleven Hawaii)			
Homemade: w. Lite Spam (50% less fat)	220	5	34
w. Turkey Spam (98% fat free)	200	3	34
Green Papaya Salad	160	0	40
Hawaiian Sweet Bread, 1/2 slice, 2 oz	180	4.5	29
Kal-bi (BBQ'd Short Ribs), 1 serving	1180	82	52
Kim Chee (pickled cabbage), 1/2 c, 4 oz	20	0	5
Loco Moco (rice/burger/egg/gravy)	650	27	63
Manapua (Char Siu Pork Bun), 2.3 oz	180	8	54
Potato Salad, 1/2 cup, 5 oz	170	10	17
Choc. Macadamia Nuts, 4 pces, 1 1/2 oz	270	20	20
Haupia (Coconut Pudd.), 1 pce (4"x 2 1/2")	120	6	17
Kulolo (Taro Pudding), 1 slice	125	5	19
Mochi (w. bean filling), 2.2 oz	195	5.5	32
Taro Pancake Mix, 1/3 cup (makes 2)	140	2	26
w. egg/oil, 2 pancakes	200	8	26
Plate Lunches:			
Chicken Katsu (9 oz): w. 2 scp Rice	1110	48	108
w. Macaroni Salad, 3/4 cup	1360	68	123
w. Tossed Salad + Fr. Dress. (2 T.)	1240	61	111
Hamburger (5 oz): w. 2 scoops Rice	710	24	81
w. Gravy + Macaroni Salad	1135	49	112
MahiMahi (7 oz): w. 2 scoops Rice	650	12	90
w. Macaroni Salad + Tartar Sce	1150	58	109
w. Macaroni Salad, no Tartar Sce	935	34	108
w. Tossed Salad + Fr. Dress. (3 T.)	815	27	96
w. Tossed Salad, no dressing	670	12	93
Teri Beef (5 oz): w. 2 scoops Rice	790	23	94
w. Macaroni Salad, 3/4 cup	1095	47	113
w. Tossed Salad, no dressing	800	23	95

Indian & Pakistani

(Meat dishes allow 4 oz meat/serving)

	C	F	Cb
Aloo Samosa, each	150	12	12
Alu Gosht Kari (Meat/Pot. Curry)	600	40	23
Bhona Gosht (Mint Broil Lamb)	560	28	5
Chicken Korma	500	35	6
Chicken Pilaf (Murgh Biriyani)	700	53	50

Restaurant & International Foods

Indian & Pakistani (Cont)

Per Serving	C	F	Cb
Chicken Tikka	260	16	2
Chicken Vindaloo	400	20	8
Chapati/Roti, 7" diam. piece	60	0.5	11
Dal (Lentil Puree): 1 cup, no oil	230	1	37
1 Tbsp Tadka (oil topping)	120	13	0
Dhakla (Lentil Dish), 1" sq., 1 oz	105	5	13
Dhansak, 1/2 cup	105	3.5	11
Gosht Kari (Meat Curry/Tom./Pot.)	460	25	17
Lamb Pilaf	520	35	40
Lassi (Sweet or Mango), 1 cup, 8 oz	160	4	24
Masala Gosht (Beef/Tom./Gravy)	400	25	18
Mulligatawney Soup, average	300	15	8
Murgh Tikka, 1 cup	300	4	7
Naan Bread, 1/4 (8" x 2"), 1 oz	75	2	11
Pappadum, 1 large/2 small	50	3	5
Pesrattu (Lentil Crepe), 9", 2.6 oz	130	5	15
Pork Vindaloo Curry	620	47	3
Rajmah (Kidney Bean Curry), 1 cup	225	5	35
Rogan Josh (Lamb/Yoghurt Sce)	500	30	3
Shahi Korma (Braised Lamb)	430	28	3
Tandoori Chicken: Breast	260	13	5
Leg/Thigh portion	300	17	6

Italian Dishes

	C	F	Cb
Bruschetta, 2 slices	380	17	53
Cannelloni, 1 tube, 6 oz	280	15	18
Chicken Cacciatore	370	22	4
Fettucine Alfredo w. Cream	910	63	60
Gnocchi, Spinach	300	18	17
Lasagne w. Meat, 10 oz	400	17	36
Linguini w. Red Clam Sauce	570	10	95
Manicotti, cheese/tomato	230	14	18
Minestrone Soup, 1 cup	260	6	28
Osso Buco (Veal/Tom./Mushr.)	550	28	5
Ravioli, 8 oz	300	12	30
Risotto (Chicken)	420	12	70
Spaghetti: Plain, 1 cup, 5 oz	185	1	44
Restaurant: 2 cups, plain	370	2	88
+ Bolognese (Meat Sce)	650	16	90
+ Marinara Sauce	540	13	105
Spaghetti & Meatballs	960	42	102
Saltimbocca (Veal/Ham/Cheese)	430	28	5
Shrimp Scampi (w. 8 large shrimp)	830	26	75
Tortellini, 20 pieces	530	20	74
Veal Marsala	400	20	11
Veal Parmigiana	350	20	5
Pizza: See Fast-Foods Section, Page 175			

Japanese

	C	F	Cb
Sushi Rice: cooked, 1 Tbsp	25	0	5
1 cup, 51/4 oz	380	3	82
Sushi (Maki) Rolls: Per Piece			
Average all types (California Rolls; Crm Cheese w. Crab; Eel; Salmon; Shrimp; Tuna; Yellowtail; Vegetable)			
Small (11/8" diam. x 11/8" high), 0.8 oz	22	0.5	0.5
Med. (13/4" diam. x 13/4" high), 1.6 oz	44	1	1
Large (21/4" diam. x 7/8" high), 2 oz	55	1.5	1.5
Sushi Packs: Per Pack			
Average all types: 6 large pces	335	7.5	7.5
9 medium pieces	405	9	9
12 small pieces	325	12	6
Futomaki (thick roll), 6 pieces	315	1.5	7
Hand Roll (Cone), 2, 6 oz	225	5	5
Inari (rice filled soybean pocket), 4 pce	260	5	46
Sushi-Nigiri (fish on rice):			
average all types, 1 piece	70	0.5	12
Sushi Plate: Assorted, 6 pieces	420	3	36
Combination (Sushi & Sushi Rolls)			
2 Sushi + 6 sm. & 3 med. rolls	400	7	72
Sashimi (Sliced Raw Seafood/Beef)			
Ika (Squid), 4 oz	105	2	0
Hamachi (Yellowtail), 4 oz	165	6	0
Naguro (Yellowfin Tuna), 4 oz	120	1	0
Niku (Beef), 5 oz	200	10	0
Saba (Mackerel), 4 oz	160	7	0
Suzuki (Sea Bass), 4 oz	110	0.5	0
Tako (Octopus), 4 oz	95	1	0
Dipping Sauces: Average, 2 Tbsp	30	0	7
Ginger Vinegar Dress., 2 Tbsp	20	0	5
Edamame (young green soybeans):			
Steamed/Salad (in pods), 4 oz	60	3	5
Boiled beans (no pods), 4 oz	160	7	12
Katsu-don Pork w. Rice	1100	39	141
Miso Soup w. Tofu pces, 1 cup	85	3	11
Seaweed Salad, 1.5 oz	20	2	0
Sukiyaki (Beef/Tofu/Veg.), 8 oz	400	24	32
Tempura (Batter-fried Shrimp & Veges.)			
3 large shrimp & veges	320	18	25
1 shrimp only	60	4	3
Teppan Yaki (Steak, Seafood & Veges.)			
10 oz serving	470	30	15
Teriyaki: Beef, 4 oz serving	350	25	4
Chicken, 4 oz serving	260	9	7
Salmon, medium, 6 oz serving	270	8	3
Sake Wine (16% alc.), 3 fl.oz	115	0	7
Yakatori, 1 skewer, 21/2 oz	140	5	1

Restaurant & International Foods

Kosher/Deli Foods

	C	F	Cb
Bagel/Bialy, 1 small, 2 oz	160	2	32
Beiglach (Cheese Knish)	350	17	35
Blintzes: Average, 1 only	120	1	25
w. Sour Crm. & Preserves	370	10	30
Borscht: (no cream), 1 cup	85	3	14
Diet/Reduced Cal., 1 cup	30	1	7
Cabbage Roll (meat/rice), 5 oz	170	6	21
Chicken Broth: 1 cup	80	8	0
with vegetables	100	8	5
with noodles	150	9	16
Lowfat, plain, 1 cup	25	1	0
Cholent, 1 med serve, 1 cup	350	16	48
Chopped Liver: 1 serve, 3 oz	110	6	5
with Egg Salad, 1/4 cup	100	7	3
Farfel, dry, 1/2 cup	90	0.5	21
Hallah (Bread), 1 sl., 1 oz	85	2	14
Gefilte Fish Balls:			
Regular, medium, 2 oz	55	2	4
with jelled broth	80	2	6
Cocktail size, 1 oz	30	1	2
Sweet, medium, 2 oz	65	2	4
with jelled broth	95	2	9
Herring: Smoked, 2 oz	120	8	0
in Sour Cream, 2 oz	150	10	0
Kasha, cooked, 1/2 cup	100	0.5	20
Kipfel (Vanilla/Almd. Cookie), 1 pce	60	2	7
Knaidlach, 1 ball	40	1	5
Knish: Kasha/Potato, 1 only	130	4	22
Cheese, 1 only	350	17	35
Knishette (Gabila's) Potato,			
4 piece, 4 oz	140	1	29
Spinach, 4 piece, 4 oz	110	1	20
Kreplach, beef, 1 piece	40	1	6
Kugel, potato/noodle, 1 serve	150	7	20
Latkes (Potato Pancake), 2 oz	200	11	22
3 Latkes w. Sour Cr./Apple Sce	750	25	95
Lochshen: Plain, 1 cup	130	2	26
Pudding, 1 cup	380	13	48
Lox (Smoked Salmon), 2 oz	65	2	0
Mandelbrot (Almond Bread),			
1 slice, 1/4" thick	45	2	5
Matzo (See Page 104): 1 oz board	110	0.5	21
Matzo Balls, 2 small, 1 large	90	3	12
Matzo Soup, with 1 large ball	180	7	24
New York Cheesecake, 4 oz	350	24	26
Pierogi, potato/cheese, 1 pce	90	4	11
Reuben Sandwich	920	60	28
Schmaltz (Rend'd chick. fat), 1 T.	90	10	0

Lebanese/Middle East

	C	F	Cb
Baba Ghannouj, 2 Tbsp, 1 oz	70	6	2
(Eggplant/Sesame Dip)			
Baklava, 1 pastry, 1 3/4 oz	245	18	18
(Pastry, Nuts, Syrup)			
Cabbage Rolls, 1 roll, 3 oz	100	3	12
(Cabbage Leaf, Meat, Rice)			
Cous Cous, 1 serve	400	21	43
(Semolina, Milk, Fruit, Nuts)			
Felafel (Chick Pea Fritter):			
Fried, 1 medium, 1 oz	60	4	4
Hummus, 1/4 cup, 2.2 oz	105	3	5
Fried Kibbi, 1 piece, 3 oz	180	8	15
(Wheat, Meat, Pinenuts)			
Kafta, 1 skewer, 1 1/2 oz	85	5	2
(Ground Lamb Saus. on Skewer)			
Kibbeh Naye, 1 cup, 9 oz	450	18	28
(Raw Lamb, Bulgur & Spices)			
Lebanese Omelet, 1 serving, 4 oz	200	12	13
(Egg, Spinach, Pinenuts, Onion)			
Pilaf, 1 cup	400	11	60
(Rice, Onion, Rais., Apr. Spice)			
Shawourma, 1 serve, 4 oz	280	15	2
(Spit Roast Beef)			
Shish Kabob, 1 stick, 2 1/2 oz	130	7	2
Spinach Pie, 1 piece, 3 1/2 oz	290	21	20
Sweet Almond Sanbusak, 1 pce	200	15	11
(Pastry, Almonds, Spices)			
Tabouli, 1 serve, 4 oz	170	14	7
Tahini Sauce, aver., 1 Tbsp	90	8	2

VISITING HOURS
6 A.M. TO 7 P.M.

Restaurant & International Foods

Mexican

	C	F	Cb
Black Bean Soup, 1 bowl	200	3	34
Bueso Fresco, 1/4 cup	80	4.5	8
Burritos *(Taco Bell):* Bean	370	12	54
Double Beef Supreme	510	23	52
Chili, plain, 1/4 cup	90	6	8
Chili con Carne: w. Beans, 1 cup	310	17	15
w/out Beans, 1 cup	370	28	10
Chimichangas, Beef, 5 oz	400	19	43
Chorizo Sausage, 2 oz	265	23	0
Churros, 1 1/2 oz	150	8	18
Corn Chips, 1/2 cup, 1 oz	160	10	17
Empanadas, average, 1 small	230	10	28
Enchilada, average	330	10	49
Fajitas, Chicken (Soft)	200	7	20
Guacamole, 2 Tbsp, 1 oz	120	12	2
Horchata: *Don Jose,* 1 cup, 8 fl. oz	140	4	25
Cacique, 1 pint bottle, 16 fl. oz	320	7	62
Margarita (w. 1 1/2 oz Tequila)	160	0	6
Menudo, 1/2 cup	55	1.5	10
Nachos: *Del Taco,* Regular	380	24	40
Macho Nachos	1100	63	113
Taco Bell: BellGrande	760	39	83
Supreme	440	24	44
Piloncillo (Brown Sugar): 1 Tbsp, 4g	15	0	4
Cone, small, 3", 3 oz	325	0	81
Quesadilla, Cheese *(Taco Bell)*	490	28	39
Refried Beans, 3/4 cup, 6 oz	160	3	26
Rice Pudding (Arroz Con Leche), 4 oz	140	3	24
Sopaipillas (flaky pastry puffs), 1 pce	100	7	10
w. Honey & Cream	200	14	18
Sopes (Gorditas), 2 oz	120	0	27
Taco *(Taco Bell):* Regular	210	12	18
Chicken	190	7	19
Taco Supreme	260	16	20
Double Decker Taco	380	17	43
Taco Salad w. Salsa	840	52	85
Taco Sauce, average, 1/4 cup	15	0	3
Taco Shell, regular	50	2	8
Tamales, Beef/Chicken, avg, 4.5 oz	250	11	27
Taquitos, Beef & Cheese, 4.5 oz	330	15	36
Tostada *(Taco Bell)*	250	12	27
Tortilla, Corn, 6" diam.	70	1	14
Tortilla Chips, 1 oz	150	8	18

Extra Listings of Mexican Dishes:
- Frozen Entrees/Meals: *See Page 58-69*
- Fast Foods Section *(Taco Bell, Del Taco)*
- Canned Bean/Chili Products: *See Page 72-78*

Polish

	C	F	Cb
Cabbage Rolls w. Sour Cr., 2 sm.	220	10	30
Chicken Casserole w. Mush., 1 c.	520	27	5
Kielbasa (Sausages, Onions, fried, 2 large.)	350	28	2
Meatballs in Sour Cream, 3 x 1 1/2" balls	300	16	11
Pierogi, Fruit/Veg, 3" ball	80	2	15
Pork Goulash (Pork/Veg. Stew)	550	21	38
Pot Roast with Vegetables	630	21	28

Soul Foods

	C	F	Cb
Breakfast Sausage, fried, 2 patties	250	17	0
Cornbread, homemade, 3 oz	200	7.5	28
Fatback, raw, 1/4 oz	60	6.5	0
Ham Hock, 1 oz	90	6.5	2
Hog Maw, 1 oz	45	2.5	0
Hominy, 3/4 cup	85	1	17
Hush Puppies, 5 pces, 3 oz	260	12	35
Neck Bones, Pork, 1 oz	65	4	0
Opossum, 1 oz	65	3	0
Oxtail, 1 oz	70	3.5	0
Pig Ear, 1/4 ear	50	3	0
Pig Foot, 1/2 foot	70	4.5	0
Pig Tail, 1/3 tail	115	10	0
Poke Salad, ckd, 1/2 cup	15	0.5	3
Pork Brains, 1 oz	40	2.5	0
Pork Cracklings, 1/2 oz	80	6	0
Pork Chitterlings, simmered, 3 oz	260	25	0
Pork Skin, 1 cup	70	4.5	0
Sousemeat, 1 oz	60	4.5	0
Succotash, 1/2 cup	80	1	17
Sweet Potato Pie, 1/8 of 9" pie	250	12	34
Tongue Pork, 1/3 tongue	75	5.5	0
Tripe, 2 oz	55	2	0
Vienna Sausage, 2 small, 1 oz	90	8	1

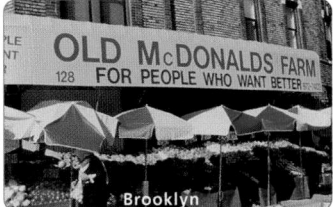

Brooklyn

Restaurant & Ethnic Foods

Thai Foods

	C	F	Cb
Appetizers: Satay Pork, 1 oz	100	4	2
Spring Roll, 1¼ oz	110	6	13
Soups: Tom Yam (Hot & Sour):			
Spicy Shrimp/Seafood, 1 cup	100	4	6
1 bowl	160	7	10
Vegetarian, 1 cup	50	0	11
Curries: Chicken w. Ginger, 1 cup	390	34	4
Thick Red Curry w. Beef, 1 cup	600	50	7
Thai Chicken Curry, 1 cup	340	23	4
Massaman Curry, 1 cup	680	57	8
Green Curry w. Pork, 1 cup	480	44	5
Pad Thai, Large serving, 18 oz	990	38	125
Fish: Steamed w. Spicy Thai Sce	450	8	46
Crispy Fried, 5 oz	290	15	9
Spicy Chicken (w. veges), stir-fry	450	22	14
Spicy Garlic Tofu w. veges, stir-fry	340	18	18
Sticky Thai Rice, plain 1 cup, 6oz	170	0.5	36
w. Coconut & Sesame Seeds, 1 cup	880	28	120
Stir-fried Rice Noodles, 1 c., 5½ oz	270	9	40
Stir-fried Vegetables, 1 cup	100	3	18
Salads: Green Papaya Salad	160	0	40
Spicy Prawn, 9 shrimp	170	3	15
Thai Chicken, 1 serving	330	9	17
Thai Beef Salad, 1 serving	260	9	15
Thai Noodle, 1 serving	410	13	45
Satay Chicken & Peanut Sauce:			
1 satay stick	390	24	20
Sauces: Peanut Satay, ½ cup, 4 oz	160	10	13

Spanish

	C	F	Cb
Arroz Abanda (Fish with Rice)	340	8	31
Arroz Con Pollo (Rice/Chick. Sal)	500	23	50
Clams Marinera, 8 clams	330	16	22
Cochifrito (Lamb w. Lemon/Garlic)	650	25	5
Cochinillo Asado, 2 sl. (Rst Suckling Pig)	300	15	3
Cocido Madrileno			
(Madrid-Style Boiled Dinner)	450	27	18
Flan de Leche (Caramel Custard)	325	9	52
Fritadera de Ternera (Sauteed Veal)	450	27	2
Gazpacho, 1 bowl	60	0	15
Paella a la Valenciana			
(Chicken & Shellfish Rice)	900	42	70
Pollo a la Espanola (Chicken)	475	30	4
Ternera al Jerez (Veal w. Sherry)	660	29	6
Zarzuela (Fish & Shellfish Medley)	530	27	40

Vietnamese

	C	F	Cb
Bo Xao Dau Phong	*Per Whole Dish*		
(Ginger Beef w.Onion, Fish Sce.)	750	30	10
Bo Nuong (Beef Satay), 2 sticks	265	9	4
Ca Chien Gung (Whole Snapper/Ging.)	600	16	6
Canh Chay (Veg./Tofu Soup)	80	3	13
Chicken & Rice Noodle Soup	400	3	55
Cuu Xao Lan (Curried Lamb,			
Veges in Coconut)	900	40	80
Ga Chien (Crisp Chick + Plum Sce)	900	40	105
Ga Nuong (Chicken Satay + Sce)	240	10	4
Ga Xao Rau(Marinated Chicken			
Braised w. Veg.)	800	26	100
Rau Cai Xao Chay			
(Stir Fried Vege., Soy Sauce)	400	15	65
Thit Heo Goi Baup Cai, each			
(Spicy Cabbage Rolls w. Pork)	200	7	11

Gourmet & Miscellaneous

	C	F	Cb
Ants Eggs/Larvae, 1 Tbsp	20	0	0
Ants, Choc. coated, 3 Tbsp	140	7	2
Bee Maggots, canned, 3 Tbsp	65	2	0
Caviar, black/red, 1 Tbsp	40	3	0
Caterpillars, canned, 2 oz	60	2	0
Frogs Legs, fried, 1 pair (large)	125	7	0
Haggis, boiled, 4 oz	350	24	22
Locusts, raw, 1 oz	35	1	0
Silkworms, raw, 1 oz	60	2	0
Snails in garlic butter, 6 large	200	10	4
Snake, roasted, 4 oz	160	6	0

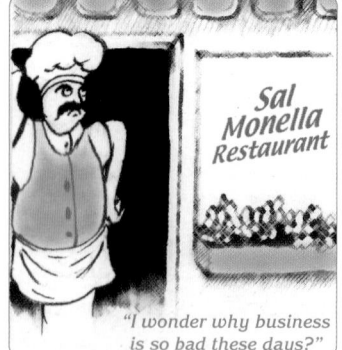

Sal Monella Restaurant

"I wonder why business is so bad these days?"

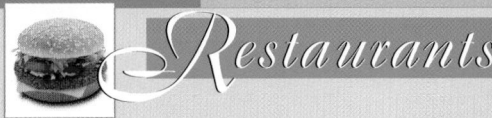

©2003
Allan Borushek

A & W®

Burgers

	C	F	Cb
Baby Burger	265	10	28
Mama Burger	480	28	36
Papa Burger	700	40	36
Grandpa Burger	910	55	36
Add Cheese to the above	55	4	0
Teen Burger Burger	565	33	36
Double Teen Burger	790	48	36
Mozza Burger	630	36	38
Double Mozza Burger	830	53	38

Chicken: Chicken Grill
	C	F	Cb
Chicken Grill	350	11	40
Chubby Chicken Burger	490	23	48

Chubby Chicken Pieces

	C	F	Cb
Thigh	410	31	9
Breast	330	19	10
Wing	205	14	6
Drumstick	140	8	5
Chubby Chicken Strips, 1	110	5	10

Chicken Strip Dipping Sauces

	C	F	Cb
Dijon Honey Mustard, 1 oz	105	6	11
Barbeque, 1 oz	35	0	7
Sweet and Sour, 1 oz	45	0	11

Hot Dogs: Hot Dog
	C	F	Cb
Hot Dog	375	22	31
Whistle Dog	490	30	39

Fries & Sides

	C	F	Cb
A&W Fries: Small, 2.9 oz	225	10	33
Regular, 4.75 oz	375	16	54
Large, 6 oz	470	20	68
Poutine: Small	420	24	38
Large	750	44	62
Fresh Onion Rings	380	25	37
Gravy, small	80	5	6

Salads

	C	F	Cb
Coleslaw, Individual	85	6	71
Potato Salad, Individual	160	8	22
Macaroni Salad, Individual	175	9	22

Breakfast

	C	F	Cb
Bacon 'n Egger	510	35	32
Sausages & Egger	600	42	34
Bacon & Eggs	515	40	28
Hash Brown	175	11	18
Toast, wholewheat, 2 pces, 3½ oz	365	15	52
French Toast, 2 pces, 10 oz	800	34	98
Cinnamon Bun	390	11	65
Apple Turnover	195	8	29

A & W® cont...

Desserts

	C	F	Cb
Cookies, average all types, 2	250	11	36
Soft Icecream Cone: Regular	220	11	30
Large	300	14	40

Fountain Beverages: Per Regular Size

	C	F	Cb
A&W Root Beer	215	0	36
Diet A&W Root Beer	3	0	0
Coco-Cola	190	0	53
Diet Coke	3	0	0
Sprite	195	0	50
Minute Orange Maid Soda	240	0	60
Hestea Iced Tea	195	0	50

Beverages

	C	F	Cb
Orange Juice, 10 fl.oz	135	0	33
Apple Juice, 10 fl.oz	140	0	35
2% Milk, 250 ml	125	5	12
Chocolate Milk, 250 ml	190	5	28
Hot Chocolate, 8 fl.oz	105	3	18
Coffee, 8 fl.oz	4	0	1

Milkshakes & Floats: Per Regular Size

	C	F	Cb
Chocolate Milkshake	460	13	75
Strawberry Milkshake	455	11	76
Vanilla Milkshake	450	13	74
A&W Root Beer Milkshake	455	11	78
A&W Root Beer Float	300	5	60

Applebee's®

Low Fat & Fabulous

	C	F	Cb
Asian Chicken Salad	645	9.5	108
Asian Chicken Salad, Half Portion	370	5.5	64
Blackened Chicken Salad	410	5	38
Blackened Chkn Salad, Half Portion	290	3	28
Chicken Fajita Quesadilla	520	11	63
Chicken Quesadilla	510	10	62
Chicken Rancho Rollup	590	12	80
Chicken Roma Rollup	550	10	75
Garlic Chicken Pasta	590	8	89
Lemon Chicken Pasta	530	11	78
Veggie Quesadilla	345	8	46
Whitefish w. Mango Salsa	435	10	53

Desserts, Sundaes

	C	F	Cb
Low Fat Brownie Sundae	415	2	82
Low Fat Marble Cheesecake	260	2	50
Low Fat Strawberry Shortcake	250	2	48

Arby's®

Breakfast Items	C	F	Cb
Biscuit: w. Butter	280	17	27
w. Bacon	360	24	27
w. Ham	330	20	28
w. Sausage	460	33	28
Croissant: Plain	220	12	25
w. Bacon	340	23	28
w. Ham	310	20	29
w. Sausage	440	32	29
Sourdough: w. Bacon	420	10	66
w. Ham	390	6	67
w. Sausage	520	19	67
French-Toastix, no syrup	370	17	48
French Toast Syrup	130	0	32
Swiss Cheese, 1 slice	45	3	0
Roast Beef Sandwich: Arby-Q®	360	14	40
Arby's Melt w. Cheddar	340	15	36
Beef 'N Cheddar	480	24	43
Big Montana®	630	32	42
Giant Roast Beef	480	23	42
Junior Roast Beef	310	13	34
Regular Roast Beef	350	16	34
Super Roast Beef	470	23	47
Sub Sandwiches: French Dip	440	16	45
Hot Ham 'N Cheese	530	27	45
Italian	780	53	49
Philly Beef 'N Swiss	700	42	46
Roast Beef	760	48	47
Turkey	630	37	51
Other Sandwiches			
Chicken Bacon 'N Swiss	610	33	49
Chicken Breast Fillet	540	30	47
Chicken Cordon Bleu	630	35	47
Grilled Chicken Deluxe	450	22	37
Hot Ham 'N Swiss	340	13	35
Roast Chicken Club	520	28	38
Market Fresh™ Sandwiches			
Roast Beef & Swiss	810	42	73
Roast Chicken Caesar	820	38	75
Roast Ham & Swiss	730	34	74
Roast Turkey & Swiss	760	33	75
Market Fresh™ Salads (no dressing)			
Caesar Salad	90	4	8
Caesar Side Salad	45	2	4
Chicken Finger Salad	570	34	39
Grilled Chicken Caesar Salad	230	8	8
Turkey Club Salad	350	21	9

Arby's® cont...

Light Menu	C	F	Cb
Garden Salad	70	1	14
Grilled Chicken	280	5	30
Grilled Chicken Salad	210	4.5	14
Roast Chicken Deluxe	260	5	33
Roast Chicken Salad	160	2.5	15
Roast Turkey Deluxe	260	5	33
Side Salad	25	0	5
Sides			
Cheddar Curly Fries w. Sce	460	24	54
Chicken Finger 4-Pack	640	38	42
Chicken Finger Snack	580	32	55
Curly Fries, small	310	15	39
Homestyle Fries, small	300	13	42
Jalapeno Bites™	330	21	30
Mozzarella Sticks	470	29	34
Onion Petals	410	23	43
Potato Cakes (2)	250	16	26
Baked Potato: Plain	355	0	82
w. Butter & Sour Cream	500	24	65
w. Broccoli 'N Cheddar	540	24	71
Deluxe Baked Potato	650	34	67
Desserts/Shakes			
Apple Turnover (Iced)	420	16	65
Cherry Turnover (Iced)	410	16	63
Chocolate Chip Cookie	125	6	16
Shakes: Chocolate, 14 oz	480	16	84
Jamocha/Vanilla, 14 oz	470	15	82
Strawberry, 14 oz	500	13	87
Condiments			
Arby's Sauce	15	0	4
Au Jus Sauce	5	0	1
BBQ Vinaigrette	140	11	9
Bronco Berry Sauce™	90	0	23
Buttermilk Ranch Dressing	360	39	2
Reduced Calorie	60	0	13
Caesar Dressing	310	34	1
Croutons: Cheese & Garlic	100	6	10
Seasoned	30	1	1
German Mustard	5	0	1
Honey French Dressing	290	24	18
Horsey Sauce®, packet	60	5	3
Italian Dressing, Reduced Calorie	25	1	3
Marinara Sauce	35	1	4
Mayonnaise	90	10	0
Light Cholesterol Free	20	1.5	1
Tangy Southwest Sauce™	250	26	3

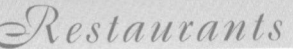

Atlanta Bread Company®

Bagel: Per Bagel	C	F	Cb
Asiago; Banana	350	3	67
Blueberry; Plain	340	1.5	68
Cherry	365	3.5	65
Chocolate Chip	330	3	62
Cinnamon Raisin	340	1.5	69
Everything	310	1.5	61
Honey Wheat; Jalapeno	330	1.5	66
Onion; Pumpernickel	300	1.5	60
Poppy Seed	310	2	60
Sesame Seed	310	2.5	60

Bread: Per Thick Slice (2 oz)	C	F	Cb
Asiago	150	2.5	26
Cinnamon Raisin	170	2.5	31
Cracked Wheat	160	2	30
French	140	0.5	29
Honey Wheat; Nine Grain; Rye	150	1.5	29
Pesto	150	0.5	29
Pumpernickel	150	1	28
Sourdough	140	0	29
Sundried Tomato	150	0	30

Muffins: Each	C	F	Cb
Apple Cinnamon	400	19	52
Banana Walnut	440	22	53
Blueberry	430	20	55
Chocolate Chip	460	21	60
Chocolate Mocha	470	23	61
Cranberry Apple	390	18	51
Cranberry Orange Walnut	440	23	51
Honey Raisin Bran	460	21	65
Lemon Poppy Seed	460	23	57
Low Fat Apple Cinnamon	310	5	60
Low Fat Banana/Low Fat Blueberry	310	5	60
Low Fat Chocolate	340	6	64
Low Fat Pumpkin	290	4.5	58
Peaches/Creme	530	25	68
Pumpkin	370	13	58
Zucchini	480	24	60

Muffin Tops: Blueberry	C	F	Cb
Blueberry	320	15	41
Banana Walnut	330	16	40
Chocolate Chip	340	16	45
Chocolate Mocha	350	17	45
Pumpkin	280	10	43

Rolls: French	C	F	Cb
French	180	0.5	37
Sourdough	190	0	38

Salads	C	F	Cb
Caesar, no dressing	35	0	8
Chicken	310	21	1
Chicken Caesar, no dressing	115	2.5	8
Chicken Curry	340	24	10
Chicken House, no dressing	115	2.5	8
Chopstix Chicken, no dressing	470	24	38
Fruit	140	1	32
Greek Chicken, no dressing	210	10	12
Greek, no dressing	120	8	12
House	35	0	8
Tuna	240	16	0

Sandwiches (sourdough)	C	F	Cb
ABC Special, no dressing	450	6	67
Avocado, no dressing	630	32	75
Chicken Curry, no dressing	630	25	70
Chicken Salad, no dressing	600	23	61
Honey Maple Ham, no dressing	310	4.5	66
Pastrami, no dressing	440	7	62
Roast Beef, no dressing	450	5	62
Tuna, no dressing	530	18	61
Turkey Breast, no dressing	420	4.5	60
Veggie, no dressing	290	1	60

Soup: Per Cup	C	F	Cb
Baked Potato	210	13	20
Black Bean & Rice; Chkn Gumbo	110	3	14
Black Bean w/Ham	200	7	32
Chicken 'n Dumpling	240	13	21
Chicken Chili	220	6	27
Chicken Noodle	110	4	12
Chicken Tortilla	140	7	15
Chili w. Beans	280	11	24
Clam Chowder	270	16	22
Country Bean	140	1.5	24
Cream of Broccoli	150	9	14
French Onion	60	2	9
Garden Veg.; Mushr., Barley & Sage	80	1	15
Italian Style Wedding	120	3	19
Lentil & Roasted Garlic	200	2.5	33
Pasta Fagioli	160	6	17
Seven Bean w. Ham	240	12	27
Southwest Chicken	180	9	20
Szechuan Hot & Sour	80	2	12
Tomato Florentine	120	3	17
Tomato, Fennel & Dill	100	7	8
Vegetable Chili	180	3.5	31
Wisconsin Cheese	210	11	20

Au Bon Pain®

Bagels: Per Bagel	C	F	Cb
Plain	300	1.5	72
Asiago Cheese	340	5	57
Cheddar & Scallion	310	4	51
Cinnamon Crisp	450	6	103
Cinnamon Raisin	300	1	65
Cranberrry Walnut	400	7	73
Dutch Apple Walnut	380	3	80
Everything	330	2	64
Foccacia Bagel	320	4	61
French Toast Bagel, 4.6 oz	360	7	64
Honey 9 Grain	310	1	66
Jalapeno Cheddar	320	6	50
Onion Bagel	320	1	67
Sesame Seed	340	4	64
Wild Blueberry	280	1	58

Spreads	C	F	Cb
Plain Cream Cheese, 2 oz	130	11	1
Honey Walnut, 2 oz	150	10	10
Sundried Tomato, 2 oz	140	12	3
Veggie, 2 oz	140	12	3

Breakfast Sandwiches: Per Sandwich	C	F	Cb
Bagel & Egg	500	5	83
Bagel & Egg w. Bacon or Cheese	580	12	83
Bagel & Egg w. Bacon & Cheese	660	19	83

Sandwiches: Per 1/2 Sandwich	C	F	Cb
Arizona Chicken	300	7	28
Chicken & Mozzarella Foccacia	400	7	36
Chicken Tarragon w. Field Onions	435	23	32
Croque Madame	285	11	26
Croque Monsieur	295	12	26
Fresh Mozzarella, Tomato & Pesto	395	21	30
Garden Vegetable Goat Cheese w. Artichoke	285	10	37
Hickory Smoked Ham & Brie	310	13	36
Honey Dijon Chicken	375	12	32
Smoked Turkey & Swiss	405	21	34
Smoked Turkey Club	315	14	26
Wraps: Chicken Caesar	320	13	30
Fields & Feta	310	9	50
Honey Smoked Turkey	260	3	42
Southwestern Tuna	355	15	34

Brownies: Blonde	C	F	Cb
	570	36	57
Cheesecake	470	26	55
Chocolate Chip	480	25	61
Peanut Butter	490	28	53
Pecan	510	31	55

Soups: Per 8 oz Serving	C	F	Cb
Black Bean	180	0	33
Broccoli Cheddar	250	18	14
Chicken Noodle	100	2	12
Clam Chowder	220	15	16
Corn Chowder	270	15	28
Curried Rice & Lentil	140	1	24
Garden Vegetable	50	1	8
Old Fashioned Tomato	140	6	19
Potato Leek	200	13	18
Split Pea	160	1	27
Tomato Florentine	120	3	17
Vegetarian Chili	170	1	31

Breads	C	F	Cb
Average, 1.75 oz slice	115	1.5	22
Bread Bowl, 1 bowl	600	2	118
Foccacia (1)	430	16	61
Four Grain Bread, 1 slice	400	4	74
French Sandwich Roll (1)	260	1	53
Rosemary Garlic Breadstick	200	2	37
Bread Rolls:			
Hearth (1)	210	2	38
Petit Pain (1)	180	0	37

Yogurt & Fruit Cups: Per Serving	C	F	Cb
Yogurt, average all types	220	3	43
Fruit Cup: Small, 1 cup	60	0	16
Large, 1 cup	130	1	32

Salads	C	F	Cb
Per Serving (Container)			
Caesar Salad	240	12	19
Charbroiled Salmon Filet, Yellow Peppers	220	11	9
Chef's Salad	290	15	11
Chicken	170	3	11
Chicken Caesar	380	18	19
Garden Salad, large	160	4	26
Garden Salad, small	90	2	14
Mediterranean Chicken	290	16	11
Pear, Field Greens, Gorgonzola	350	26	23
Tomato, Mozzarella w. Basil Pesto	280	19	11
Tuna Garden	440	24	28
Watercress, Chicken & Gorgonzola	250	15	3

Cookies: Per Cookie	C	F	Cb
Chocolate Chip; English Toffee	230	7	39
Choc Macadamia; Walnut Raisin	250	13	31
Oatmeal Raisin	210	6	38
Shortbread	240	7	44

Au Bon Pain® cont...

	C	F	Cb
Cakes & Bars			
Apple Strudel	400	23	46
Cinnamon Scone, 4.4 oz	440	17	82
Cherry Strudel	360	23	37
Orange Scone w. Icing	370	13	56
Pecan Roll	620	24	94
Croissants: Ham & Cheese	290	9	39
Spinach & Cheese	220	9	29
Filled: Plain	220	6	38
Almond	480	25	58
Apple	200	3	40
Chocolate	330	10	53
Cinnamon Raisin	300	4	60
Raspberry	290	9	47
Sweet Cheese	320	12	46
Muffins: Blueberry	470	15	79
Carrot Walnut Spice	520	25	67
Chocolate Chip; Double Choc	530	23	77
Old Fashioned Corn	390	16	56
Pumpkin	510	18	74
Raisin Bran	400	12	77
Lowfat: Chocolate Cake	280	2	64
Triple Berry	270	2	58
Drinks			
Mocha Blast, large, 24 oz	480	4	96
Iced Cappuccino, medium, 12 fl.oz	150	6	15
Iced Tea, medium, 12 fl.oz	130	0	33
Frozen Mocha Blast, 16 oz	320	3	64

"My new diet allows me a small saucer of anything I want for lunch."

Auntie Anne's®

	C	F	Cb
Pretzels: With Butter			
Almond	400	8	72
Cinnamon Sugar	450	9	83
Garlic	350	4.5	68
Glazin' Raisin®	510	4	107
Jalapeno	310	4.5	59
Kidstix, 4 sticks	250	3	48
Original	370	4	72
Parmesan Herb	440	13	72
Sesame	410	12	64
Sour Cream & Onion	340	5	66
Whole Wheat	370	4.5	72
Pretzels: Without Butter			
Almond Pretzel; Whole Wheat	350	1.5	72
Cinnamon Sugar	350	2	74
Garlic Pretzel; Sour Crm & Onion	320	1	66
Glazin' Raisin®	470	0.5	104
Jalapeno Pretzel	270	1	58
Kidstix, 4 sticks	230	7	48
Original Pretzel	340	1	72
Parmesan Herb	390	5	74
Sesame Pretzel	350	6	63
Dipping Sauces			
Caramel Dip	135	3	27
Cheese Sce; Hot Salsa Chse, aver.	100	8	4
Chocolate Flavored Dip	130	4	24
Light Cream Cheese	70	6	1
Marinara Sauce	10	0	4
Strawberry Cream Cheese	110	10	4
Sweet Mustard	60	1.5	8
Beverages: Per Serving			
Auntie Anne's Lemonade, 22 fl.oz	180	0	43
Dutch Ice (20 fl.oz): Kiwi-Banana	270	0	63
Blue Raspberry	230	0	55
Lemonade	450	0	110
Mocha	570	15	105
Orange Crème	400	0	92
Pina Colada	535	0	125
Strawberry	315	0	72
Wild Cherry	300	0	69
Dutch Ice (14 fl.oz): Kiwi-Banana	190	0	44
Blue Raspberry	165	0	38
Lemonade	315	0	77
Mocha	400	10	74
Orange Crème	280	0	64
Pina Colada; Strawberry	220	0	53
Wild Cherry	210	0	48

Back Yard Burgers® | Baja Fresh®

Burgers	C	F	Cb
Back Yard Burger 3/4 lb., 9 oz	560	31	30
Bacon Cheddar, 9 oz	660	39	35
Bar-B-Que, 8 oz	550	29	35
Blackened, 7 oz	580	33	35
Chilli, 8 oz	580	31	35
French Dip, 8 oz	570	45	35
Gardenburger®, 6 oz	330	5.5	45
Great Little Burger®, 6 oz	280	15	30
Hawaiian, 8 oz	570	31	35
Mexicali, 8 oz	550	30	40
Miz Grazi's, 9 oz	580	31	35
Mushroom, 8 oz	570	33	35
Worcestershire, 9 oz	570	35	40

Charbroiled 1/4 lb. Chicken Sandwiches	C	F	Cb
Bar-B-Que, 7 oz	290	7	30
Blackened, 7 oz	320	11	30
Hawaiian, 7 oz	310	11	30
Honey Mustard, 7 oz	380	8.5	40
Lemon Butter, 6 oz	300	11	30
Mexicali, 7 oz	350	9	35
Miz Grazi's, 7 oz	290	4	35
Savory, 7 oz	270	4	35

Specialities: BLT, 5 oz	261	12	30
Cup of Chilli, 8 oz	230	12	17

Baked Potatoes	C	F	Cb
Chilli & Cheddar, 14 oz	390	13	43
Ranch, 11 oz	470	29	43
Salsa, 11 oz	263	5	43
Traditional/Plain, 9 oz	196	0	42

Fries: Chilli Cheese Fries, 12 oz	400	21	70
Seasoned-Fries: Regular, 4 oz	310	16	38
Large, 7 oz	540	27	67
Waffle Fries: Regular, 3 oz	280	15	32
Large, 5 oz	420	22	53

Salads (No Dressing)	C	F	Cb
Charbroiled Chicken, 6 oz	175	2	15
Garden Fresh, 4.5 oz	65	0	15

Cobblers: Apple, 6 oz	340	13	52
Blackberry; Peach, 6 oz	320	12	48
Cherry, 6 oz	390	16	57

Shakes	C	F	Cb
Chocolate/Vanilla, 16 oz	540	25	68
Strawberry, 16 oz	520	25	64

Note: Carbohydrate figures are author estimates only

Burritos: Includes Cheese	C	F	Cb
Baja Burrito: Chicken	810	36	59
Steak	845	41	60
Burrito Mexicano: Chicken	895	20	120
Steak	935	25	120
Bean & Cheese	865	31	100
w. Chicken/Steak	1070	38	100
Burrito Ultimo w. Sour Crm: Steak	1110	50	90
Chicken	1070	45	90
Grilled Vegetarian w. Sour Crm	835	37	84
Burrito "Dos Manos": Chicken	1610	60	173
Steak	1645	65	173

Tacos: Includes Cheese & Sour Cream	C	F	Cb
Baja Style Tacos: Steak	105	3	20
Chicken or Shrimp	90	2	20
Tres Tacos Combos: 3 Steak	500	20	78
2 Steak, 1 Chicken	485	20	78
3 Chicken	455	18	78
2 Chicken, 1 Fish	505	25	80
3 Fish	615	39	82
Baja Mahi Mahi Taco	215	11	24
Baja Fish Taco	145	9	21
Baja Taco Combos: 2 Steak	345	6	50
1 Steak, 1 Chicken	340	5	50
1 Steak, 1 Fish	385	12	51
Taco Chilito: Chicken; Steak	370	14	35

Taquitos: Includes Sour Cream & Guacamole	C	F	Cb
Taquitos: Chicken	515	45	65
Steak	485	45	65

Baja Fajita Combo: Tortillas Not Included	C	F	Cb
Chicken	775	31	101
Steak	840	36	101

Quesadilla: Includes Sour Cream	C	F	Cb
Quesadilla	1010	62	59
Steak	1210	70	60
Chicken	1170	66	59
Mini-Quesadita	635	22	94
Steak or Chicken	690	25	94

Nachos: w. Sour Cream	C	F	Cb
w. Sour Cream	1735	98	154
Steak w. Sour Cream	1960	107	154
Chicken w. Sour Cream	1920	102	154

Torta: Steak/Chicken, average	890	46	72

Baja Ensalada:	C	F	Cb
Steak w. Dressing	905	63	37
Chicken w. Dressing	855	57	38

Tostada: Steak/Chicken	830	39	60
Mini Tostadita	785	29	91

Extras: Corn Chips (15), 1 oz	140	7	18
Baja Fresh Salads, no dress., 2 oz	15	0	2

Fast–Foods & *Restaurants*

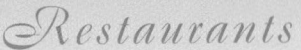

Banana's®

	C	F	Cb
Frosty: Per 8 oz Serving			
Banana Berry Cream	180	0.5	40
Citrus Blend	110	0	26
Mango Magic	150	0	38
Melon Banana	140	0.5	36
Orange Swirl Creamy	170	0.5	37
P-nut Butter Cup Creamy	380	20	35
Raspberry Creamy	170	2	31
Strawberry	50	0.5	12
Strawberry Creamy	150	0	32
Smoothie: Per 8 oz Serving			
Banana Berry	130	1	32
Chococino	350	19	39
Cookies N Cream	300	4	57
Mocha ala Orange	160	1	37
Pina Colada	170	0	44
Raspberry Flavored Lemony Batch	290	0	73
Strawberry Flavored Lemony Batch	250	0	66

Ben & Jerry's®

Icecream & Frozen Yogurt ~ See Page 30
Novelty Bars ~ See Page 34

Big Apple Bagels®

	C	F	Cb
Bagels			
All types, 5 oz	380	2	77
1/2 bagel, 2, 4 oz	190	1	38
My Favorite Muffin Bagels: Per Bagel (4 oz)			
Blueberry	320	1.5	66
Cinn. Raisin Sour Dough	310	1	66
Plain; Sour Dough	310	1	64
Honey Grain	310	3	61
Russian Black Bread	320	1	67
Whole Wheat	310	1.5	66
My Favorite Muffin Muffins: Each (6 oz)			
Plain; Blueberry	590	18	75
Plain, Fat Free	390	0	120
Chocolate	510	24	69
Chocolate, Fat Free	360	0	87
Cream Cheese: Per 2 Tbsp (1 oz)			
Plain; Garden Vegetable, average	100	10	1
Onion Chive	100	10	1
Honey Cinnamon; Very Berry, aver.	130	12	3
Lite varieties, average	70	5	2
Salsa Ole	90	8	1

Baskin Robbins®

	C	F	Cb
Hard Scooped Icecream			
Per Regular Scoop			
Cherries Jubilee	240	13	29
Chocolate: Regular Scoop	270	16	31
Small Scoop	180	10	20
Chocolate Chip	270	17	26
Chocolate Chip Cookie Dough	300	17	35
Chocolate Fudge	290	15	34
Cookies 'N Cream	300	19	29
French Vanilla	280	18	25
German Choc Cake	310	15	39
Gold Medal Ribbon	270	13	35
Jamoca	250	15	25
Jamoca Almond Fudge	280	16	30
Mint Choc Chip	270	18	26
Old Fashion Butter Pecan	290	20	23
Peanut Butter 'N Chocolate	330	22	29
Pink Bubblegum	270	14	34
Pistachio-Almond	300	21	23
Pralines 'N Cream	280	15	33
Quarterback Crunch	290	17	32
Reeses Peanut Butter	310	19	30
Rocky Road	300	17	34
Vanilla: Regular Scoop	250	16	24
Small Scoop	160	10	15
Very Berry Strawberry	220	10	30
World Class Chocolate	280	16	32
Lowfat Icecream: Espresso 'N Crm	180	2.5	31
No Sugar Added Icecrm, average	160	4	27
Ices, Sherbets, Sorbets: Regular Scoop			
Ices: Daiquiri	130	0	33
Sherbets: Rainbow	160	2	34
Sorbets: Average all flavors	115	0	29
Lowfat Yogurt (Hard): Regular Scoop			
Maui Brownie Madness	250	9	38
Nonfat Yogurt (Soft Serve): Small Scoop			
Nonfat Frozen Yogurt, 5 oz	190	0.5	39
Truly Free Yogurt, Cafe Mocha	140	0.5	27
Shakes, Smoothies, Blasts: Regular (16 fl.oz)			
Shakes: Chocolate Icecream	750	43	80
Vanilla Icecream	630	35	69
Smoothies: Average all flavors	320	1	70
Blasts: Cappuccino w/whipped crm	340	16	44
Cones: Sugar Cone	60	3	7
Cake Cone	25	0.5	4
Waffle Cone: Large	120	1.5	14
Fresh Baked	145	2	30

Restaurants & Fast-Foods

Big Boy®

Sandwiches	C	F	Cb
Big Boy	600	26	35
Brawny Lad™	420	21	30
Buddie Boy	760	34	80
Fish Sandwich	690	48	41
Small Hamburger	445	30	30
Super Big Boy™	830	66	34
Swiss Miss	635	44	28
Tuna Salad Sandwich	545	40	30
Sides & Salad			
French Fries	360	19	45
Chili	315	18	19
Onion Rings	580	41	45
Tartare Sauce, 2 oz	370	40	1
Trio Salad	620	46	18

Blimpie®

Cold Subs: Per 6" Sub on White	C	F	Cb
Blimpie Best	410	13	47
Cheese Trio	490	23	48
Club Sub	370	10	48
Ham & Swiss	410	14	46
Ham, Salami, Provolone	480	20	49
Roast Beef	390	7	47
Turkey Sub	330	6	48
Hot Subs: Per 6" Sub on White			
Grilled Chicken	400	9	52
Grille Max	415	6	72
Italian Meatball	500	22	52
Mexi Max	395	4.5	66
Roast Turkey Cordon Bleu	430	14	43
Steak & Cheese	550	26	51
Vegi Max	405	7	61
Salads: Chef	150	6	8
Coleslaw, 1/2 cup	180	13	13
Potato Salad, 2/3 cup	270	19	19
Turkey Salad	90	0.5	8
Dressings: Fat Free Italian, 1 fl.oz	20	0	5
Blimpie Dressing, 1 fl.oz	120	8	16
Blimpie Special Sub, 3/4 fl.oz	70	7	2
Wraps: Zesty Italian	530	22	59
Chicken Caesar	610	31	56
Soup: Chicken Noodle, 1 cup	140	3	20
Desserts: Oatmeal Raisin Cookie	190	8	27
Donuts, 2.6 oz each	340	22	28
Fudge Brownie, 1 brownie	245	11	34
Banana Nut Muffin	470	23	55

Bojangles®

Cajun Spiced Chicken	C	F	Cb
Breast	280	17	12
Leg	265	16	11
Thigh	310	23	11
Wing	355	25	11
Cajun Roast Chicken			
Breast, skin free	145	5	0
Leg, skin free	160	8	0
Thigh, skin free	215	15	0
Wing, skin free	230	15	3
Southern Style Chicken			
Breast	260	16	12
Leg	255	15	11
Thigh	310	21	14
Wing	335	21	19
Sandwiches/Snacks			
Buffalo Bites	180	3	5
Cajun Filet: w/out Mayo	335	11	41
w. Mayo	435	22	41
Cajun Steak Sandwich	435	26	39
Chicken Supremes	335	16	26
Grilled Filet, no mayo	235	5	25
w. Mayo	335	16	25
Biscuit Sandwiches			
Bacon	290	17	29
Bacon, Egg & Cheese	550	42	27
Biscuit (plain)	245	12	29
Cajun Filet	455	21	46
Country Ham	270	15	26
Egg	400	30	26
Sausage	350	23	26
Smoked Sausage	380	26	27
Steak	650	49	37
Fixins': Bo Rounds	235	11	31
Cajun Pintos	110	0	18
Corn on the Cob	140	2	34
Dirty Rice	165	6	24
Green Beans	25	0	5
Macaroni & Cheese	200	14	12
Marinated Cole Slaw	135	3	26
Multi-Grain Rolls	150	3	26
Potatoes, no Gravy	80	1	16
Seasoned Fries	345	19	39
Sweet Biscuits			
Apple Cinnamon	330	13	48
Bo Berry™	220	10	29
Cinnamon	320	18	37

Fast–Foods & *Restaurants*

Boston Market®

Entrees	C	F	Cb
1/4 Chicken:			
White meat w. skin, wing	280	12	2
No skin or wing	170	4	2
1/4 Chicken: Dark meat w. skin	320	21	2
No skin	190	10	1
1/2 Chicken w. skin	590	33	4
Chicken Pot Pie, 1 pie	750	46	57
Chunky Chicken Salad, 6.4 oz	480	39	4
Honey Glazed Ham (lean), 5 oz	210	8	10
Meatloaf, 5 oz	290	17	15
Meatloaf & Brown Gravy	340	21	18
Meatloaf & Chunky Tom Sauce	310	17	21
Rotisserie Turkey Breast: no skin	170	1	1
w. Stuffing & Gravy	600	18	67
Soup: Chicken Noodle, 6 oz	100	4.5	8
Chicken Tortilla, 6 oz	170	8	18
Turkey Tortilla, 6 oz	160	7	18
Salads: Caesar Side Salad, 4 oz	200	17	7
Caesar Salad Entree, 11 oz	670	57	24
no dressing, 8 oz	230	12	14
Chicken Caesar, 15 oz	810	60	25
Old Fashion Potato Salad, 3/4 cup	200	12	22
Sandwiches: BBQ Chicken	540	9	84
Chicken Salad	680	30	63
Chicken w. Cheese & Sauce	630	28	61
No Cheese or Sauce	390	5	60
Ham w. Cheese & Sauce	650	31	67
No Cheese or Sauce	410	8	65
Meatloaf w. Cheese	690	27	83
Open-Faced	730	36	74
Turkey: Bacon Club	780	38	64
Open-Faced	720	20	93
Turkey w. Cheese & Sauce	620	25	64
No Cheese or Sauce	390	3.5	61
Side Dishes: Rice Pilaf, 2/3 cup	180	5	32
Herb Buttered Corn, 3/4 cup	180	4	30
Hot Cinnamon Apples, 3/4 cup	250	4.5	56
Macaroni & Cheese, 3/4 cup	280	11	33
Mash Potatoes (3/4 c.) & Gravy	230	9	32
Savory Stuffing, 3/4 cup	310	12	44
Creamed Spinach, 3/4 cup	260	20	11
Baked Goods: Brownie	310	10	51
Corn Bread, 1 loaf	200	6	33
Nestle® Toll House Choc Cookie	390	19	51

Bob Evans®

Menu Items	C	F	Cb
Biscuits, plain	380	18	60
Chicken & Noodles Entree	335	20	18
Chicken Salad Platter w. fruit	600	39	43
Chicken Stir-Fry	790	6	142
Hamburger plus bun	565	34	23
Home Fries	225	11	30
Pot Roast Sandwich	1155	46	125
Sausage Gravy	445	33	26
Sausage Patty	170	15	0
Vegetable Stir-Fry	620	2.5	134
Wildfire Chicken Salad w. dressing	1660	98	125

Breugger's Bagels®

Bagels: Per Bagel	C	F	Cb
Classic Blueberry/Cranberry Orange	330	2	68
Classic Cinnamon Raisin	320	2	68
Classic Egg	320	2.5	64
Classic Everything	320	2	64
Cream Cheese: Per Serving (1 oz)			
Bacon Scallion	100	8	4
Chive; Cucumber Dill	100	9	2
Garden Veggie	90	8	3
Honey Walnut	110	8	5
Jalapeno; Pumpkin	100	9	3
Light Garden Veggie	60	4	2
Light Herb Garlic; Light Plain	70	4.5	3
Light Strawberry	70	4	4
Olive Pimento; Smoked Salmon	100	9	2
Plain	90	8	4
Sandwiches: Per Sandwich			
Deli-Style Ham w. Honey Mustard	440	4.5	77
Garden Veggie	390	6	70
Grilled Chicken Breast	590	11	74
Grilled Chicken Club w. Mayo	750	31	65
Herby Turkey	530	14	73
Hot Shot Turkey	430	6	70
Leonardo da Veggie	460	11	69
Mediterranean	540	19	74
Olivia De Hamiland	560	17	71
Roadhouse Chicken	710	20	77
Santa Fe Turkey	480	10	71
Turkey Club with Mayonnaise	590	23	65
Turkey with Mayonnaise	480	14	65

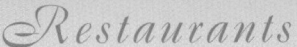

Burger King®

Burgers	C	F	Cb
Whopper® Sandwich	760	46	52
without Mayonnaise	600	28	52
Whopper® w. Cheese Sandwich	850	53	55
without Mayonnaise	690	36	53
Double Whopper® Sandwich	1060	69	52
without Mayonnaise	900	51	52
Double Whopper® w. Cheese	1150	76	53
without Mayonnaise	990	59	53
Whopper JR® Sandwich	390	22	32
without Mayonnaise	310	13	31
Whopper JR® w. Cheese	440	28	33
without Mayonnaise	360	19	32
Hamburger	310	16	30
Double Hamburger	450	24	30
Cheeseburger	360	19	31
Double Cheeseburger	540	31	32
Bacon Double Cheeseburger	580	34	32
BK Homestyle Griller™	480	27	35
BK Smokehouse Cheddar™ Griller	720	48	32
King Supreme™ Sandwich	550	34	32
BK ¼ lb Burger	490	21	50
BK Veggie™ Burger	330	10	45
w. Reduced Fat Mayo	290	7	44

Chicken & Fish Sandwiches	C	F	Cb
BK Big Fish® Sandwich	710	38	67
Chicken Sandwich	560	28	53
without Mayonnaise	460	17	52
Chicken Whopper	580	26	48
without Mayonnaise	420	9	47
Chicken Whopper Jr	350	14	30
without Mayonnaise	270	6	30
Chicken Tenders®: 4 pieces	170	9	10
5 pieces	220	12	13
6 pieces	250	14	15
8 pieces	340	19	20
Dipping Sauces (1 oz): Barbecue	35	0	9
Honey Flavored	90	0	23
Honey Mustard	90	6	9
Ranch	140	15	1
Sweet & Sour	40	0	10
Zesty Onion Ring	150	15	3

French Fries (Salted)	C	F	Cb
Small, 2.6 oz	230	11	31
Medium, 4 oz	370	17	49
Large, 5.6 oz	500	25	63
King Size, 6 oz	600	30	76

Salad Dressings: Per ½ oz	C	F	Cb
Kraft® Catalina	180	16	10
Kraft® Ranch	220	23	2
Kraft® Thousand Island	110	9	7
Light Done Right® Light Italian	50	4.5	4
Signature® Creamy Caesar	140	13	4
Salads: Chicken Caesar, no dress.	160	6	5
Garden Salad, no dressing	25	0	5
Onion Rings: Small, 1.8 oz	180	9	22
Medium, 3.2 oz	320	16	40
Large, 5 oz	480	23	60
King Size, 5.6 oz	550	27	70
Sides/Condiments: Croutons, ¾ oz	90	3	14
American Cheese, 2 slices, 25g	90	8	1
Bacon, 3 pieces, 8g	40	3	0
Ketchup, ½ oz	15	0	4
Parmesan Cheese, ½ oz	45	3.5	0
Breakfast: Biscuit, 3 oz	300	15	35
Egg'wich™: w. Bacon, Egg & Chse	420	23	36
w. Bacon & Egg	380	19	35
w. Egg & Cheese	410	23	36
Croissan'wich®:			
w. Egg & Cheese	320	19	24
w. Sausage & Cheese	420	31	23
w. Sausage, Egg & Cheese	520	39	24
French Toast Sticks (5), 4 oz	390	20	46
Hash Brown Rounds: Small, 2.6 oz	230	15	23
Large, 4.5 oz	390	25	38
Cini-Minis: 4 Rolls w/out Icing	440	23	51
Vanilla Icing only, 1 oz	110	3	20
Grape/Strawberry Jam	30	0	7
Desserts: Dutch Apple Pie, 4 oz	340	14	52
Hershey's® Sundae Pie, 2.6 oz	310	18	33
Hot Fudge Brownie Royale	440	19	62
Fresh Baked Cookies	440	21	57
Beverages: Sprite, med., 22 fl.oz	220	0	55
Coca-Cola®, medium, 22 fl.oz	230	0	56
Tropicana® Orange Juice, 10 fl.oz	140	0	33
Reduced Fat Milk, 1% Fat, 8 fl.oz	110	2.5	12
Chocolate Shake (syrup added),			
Small, 11 fl.oz	620	32	72
Medium, 14 fl.oz	790	42	89
Strawberry Shake (syrup added),			
Small, 11 fl.oz	620	32	71
Medium, 14 fl.oz	790	42	89
Vanilla Shake: Medium, 14 fl.oz	720	41	73
Small, 11 fl.oz	560	32	56

Fast–Foods & Restaurants

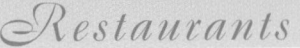

Captain D's Seafood® **C F Cb**

Platters: Per Platter

	C	F	Cb
Broiled Shrimp	720	8	131
Broiled Chicken	800	10	131
Broiled Fish	735	7	131
Broiled Fish & Chicken	775	10	131

Lunches Per Lunch

	C	F	Cb
Broiled Shrimp	420	7	64
Broiled Chicken	505	9	65
Broiled Fish	435	7	65
Broiled Fish & Chicken	480	8	68
Stuffed Crab	95	7	1

Sandwiches: Per Sandwich

	C	F	Cb
Broiled Chicken	450	19	29

Desserts: Per Slice

	C	F	Cb
Carrot Cake	435	23	49
Cheesecake	420	31	30
Chocolate Cake	305	10	49
Pecan Pie	460	20	64

Carvel Icecream®

Soft Serving Icecream

	C	F	Cb
Chocolate: Regular	420	22	48
Vanilla: Regular	440	22	46
No Sugar Added: Regular	285	6.5	13
Large	365	8.5	70
No Fat, Regular, aver. all flavors	265	0	58

Sherbet

	C	F	Cb
Sherbet, all flavors: Regular	310	2	68

Cakes & Novelties

	C	F	Cb
Blue Ribbon Cakes,			
Average all types, 4 oz	220	11	27
Flying Saucers,			
Chocolate; Vanilla	240	10	33
Lil' Love/Piece of Cake: 4 oz	260	13	31
Sheet Cake; Small Round: 4 oz	210	11	25

Carl's Jr.® **C F Cb**

Burgers/Sandwiches

	C	F	Cb
Bacon Swiss Crispy Chicken	760	38	72
Carl's Catch Fish Sandwich™	530	28	55
Charbroiled BBQ Chicken S'wich™	290	3.5	41
Charbroiled Chicken Club S'wich™	470	23	37
Charbroiled Santa Fe Chkn S'wich™	540	31	37
Charbroiled Sirloin Steak	550	24	52
Dble Sourdough Bacon Chseburger	880	59	37
Dble Western Bacon Chseburger®	920	55	65
Famous Bacon Cheeseburger™	700	41	51
Famous Star® Hamburger	590	32	50
Hamburger	280	9	36
Ranch Crispy Chicken Sandwich	660	31	71
Sourdough Bacon Cheeseburger	640	41	37
Sourdough Ranch Bacon Chseburger	720	46	43
Spicy Chicken Sandwich	480	26	47
Southwest Spicy Chicken S'wich	620	41	48
Super Star® Hamburger	790	47	51
Western Bacon Cheeseburger®	660	30	64
Western Bacon Crispy Chkn S'wich	750	28	91
Cheese: American Cheese, large	60	5	1
Swiss-style Cheese	50	4	0
Great Stuff Potatoes: Plain	290	0	68
Bacon & Cheese	640	29	75
Broccoli & Cheese	530	21	76
Sour Cream & Chives	430	14	70
Breakfast: Breakfast Burrito	550	32	36
Breakfast Quesadilla	370	17	38
English Muffin w. Margarine	210	9	28
French Toast Dips, no Syrup	370	20	42
Sourdough Breakfast	410	20	33
Scrambled Eggs	180	14	1
Sunrise Sandwich, no Bacon/Saus.	360	21	28
Bakery/Desserts			
Cheese Danish	400	23	49
Blueberry Muffin	340	14	49
Bran Raisin Muffin	370	14	61
Chocolate Chip Cookie	350	18	46
Strawberry Swirl Cheesecake	290	17	30
Side Orders: Chicken Stars, 6 pces	260	16	14
CrissCut Fries®, 5 oz	410	24	43
French Fries, small, 3 oz	290	14	37
Hash Brown Nuggets, 4 oz	330	21	32
Onion Rings, 4.5 oz	430	22	53
Salads: Per Serving (no dressing)			
Charbroiled Chicken Salad-to-Go™	200	7	12
Garden Salad-to-Go™	50	2.5	4

'...and could you please cut the pizza into only 6 pieces - I couldn't possibly eat 8!

Cheesecake Factory®

Per Slice	C	F	Cb
Adam's P. B. Cup Fudge Ripple	940	59	95
Banana Cream Cheesecake	860	61	70
Brownie Sundae Cheesecake	960	62	96
Choc Chip Cookie Dough	1080	71	100
Dulce de Leche Caramel Ch/cake	1000	70	83
Kahlua Cocoa Coffee	840	55	80
Keylime Cheesecake	700	48	63
Original Cheesecake	640	45	55
Vanilla Bean Cheesecake	870	62	69
White Choc. Raspberry Truffle	900	60	80

Chick-Fil-A®

Breakfast: Per Serving	C	F	Cb
Plain Biscuit	260	11	38
Hot Buttered Biscuit	270	12	38
Biscuit and Gravy	320	15	44
Biscuit: w. Bacon	300	14	38
w. Bacon & Egg	390	20	38
w. Bacon, Egg & Cheese	430	24	38
Biscuit: w. Egg	340	16	38
w. Egg & Cheese	390	21	38
Biscuit:			
w. Sausage	410	23	42
w. Sausage & Egg	500	29	43
w. Sausage, Egg & Cheese	540	33	43
Chicken Biscuit	400	18	43
w. Cheese	450	22	43
Danish	430	17	63
Hashbrowns	170	9	20

Chick-Fil-A Sandwiches: Per Sandwich			
Chicken Sandwich	410	16	38
no butter	380	13	37
Chicken Deluxe	420	16	39
Chicken, 1 fillet (no bun/pickles)	230	11	10
Chargrilled Chicken Sandwich	280	7	29
no butter	240	3.5	28
Deluxe	280	7	30
Chargrilled Chicken, 1 fillet			
(no bun/pickles)	100	1.5	1
Club Sandwich	360	13	31
Chicken Salad Sandwich	350	15	32

Cool Wraps®			
Spicy Chicken	390	7	51
Chargrilled Chicken	390	7	53
Chicken Caesar	460	11	51

Chick-Fil-A® cont...

Salads	C	F	Cb
Chick-n-Strips® Salad	340	16	19
Chargrilled Chicken Garden	180	6	8
Chicken Caesar Salad	240	10	6

Strips, Nuggets: Per Serving			
Chick-n-Strips® (4-count)	250	11	12
Nuggets (8-pack)	260	12	12

Salad Dressing: Per 1.25 oz			
Caesar	200	21	1
Basil Vinaigrette	210	21	4
Bleu Cheese; Buttermilk Ranch	190	20	2
Fat Free Dijon Honey Mustard	60	0	14
Light Italian	20	0.5	3
Spicy	210	22	2
Thousand Island	170	16	6

Sides: Per Serving			
Carrot & Raisin Salad, small	130	5	22
Coleslaw, small	210	17	14
Garlic and Butter Croutons, 1/2 oz	90	4	11
Roasted, Unsalted Sunflower Kernel,			
1/2 oz serving	80	7	3
Tossed Salad	80	5	6
Waffle Potato Fries™, small	280	14	37
Soup: Hearty Breast of Chicken	110	1.5	13

Sauces			
Polynesian, 1 oz	110	6	13
Dijon Honey Mustard, 1/2 oz	50	5	2
Barbecue, 1 oz	45	0	11
Honey Mustard, 1 oz	45	0	10

Desserts			
Cheesecake, 3.3 oz	340	21	30
Icedream® Cup, small	230	6	38
Icedream® Cone, small	160	4	24
Lemon Pie, 4 oz	320	10	51
Fudge Nut Brownie, 2.6 oz	330	15	45

Drinks			
Lemonade, 9 fl.oz	170	0.5	41
Diet Lemonade, 9 fl.oz	25	0	5
Iced Tea, sweetened, 9 fl.oz	80	0	19
Iced Tea, unsweetened, 9 fl.oz	0	0	0
Coca-Cola Classic®, 9 fl.oz	110	0	28
Diet Coke®, 9 fl.oz	0	0	0
Dr Pepper®, 9 fl.oz	110	0	30
Coffee, 10 fl.oz	10	0	2

Fast–Foods & *Restaurants*

Chili's®

Burgers (no Fries)	C	F	Cb
Old Timer Burger	790	45	52
Ranch Burger	1070	66	64
Chipotle Bleu Chse Bacon Burger	1120	75	54
Mushroom Swiss Burger	910	48	62
Ground Pepercorn Burger w. Strings & Dressing	1200	79	78
Lettuce Wraps w. Dipping Sauce	730	37	60
Awesome Blossom w. Sauce	2880	222	191
1/4 Whole w. Blossom Sauce	720	55	48
Chicken Crispers w. fries, corn, dressing	1630	95	105

Fajitas (includes 3 tortillas & garnishes)			
Mushroom Jack	1270	60	103
Chicken	1020	41	97
Steak	1070	51	93

Meals			
Grilled Margarita Chicken	725	25	72
Maragarita Grilled Tuna	880	25	97
Grilled Baby Back Ribs	1130	54	109
Citrus Fire Chicken & Shrimp	660	12	73
Sirloin Stack	1230	61	96
Flame Grilled Rib Eye	1080	66	70
Ranch Hand Filet	1190	81	62
South Western Egg Rolls	830	40	86
Wings over Buffalo w. Dressing	760	58	6
Boneless Buffalo Wings	1140	74	64
Bottomless Tostada Chips w. Salsa	910	46	109
Veggie & Smoked Chse Quesadilla	1160	67	95
Cajun Chicken Pasta	1190	56	103
Grilled Shrimp Alfredo	1290	53	142
Cheese Steak Sandwich (no Fries)	740	29	67
Chicken Caesar Pita (no Fries)	520	19	33

Fajita Nachos: Chicken	995	36	94
Beef	1130	50	100

Desserts: Molten Choc Cake	1505	67	207
Choc Chip Paradise Pie	1250	47	188

Chuck E. Cheese®

Appetizers	C	F	Cb
Blended Pizza Sauce, 1/4 cup	35	0	7
Buffalo Wings, 4 pieces	220	15	1
Lamb Wesson French Fries, ckd	285	10	43
Sargento Mozzarella Sticks, 2	380	24	26

Sandwiches: Fries Not Included			
Grilled Chicken Sub	740	39	57
Ham & Cheese	770	41	60
Hot Dog	430	29	27
Italian Sub	770	47	52

Pizza (Medium): Per 2 Slices			
BBQ Chicken	410	13	51
Beef	410	17	43
Cheese	330	10	43
Pepperoni	370	14	43
Sausage	385	15	44

Salad Dressings: Per 2 Tablespoons			
Kraft Catalina	35	0	8
NF Bleu Cheese	170	18	1
NF Lite Ranch	80	8	2
NF Olive Oil & Vinegar	90	9	2
NF Thousand Island	110	10	4

Birthday Items: Per Slice (1/12 Cake)			
8" Chocolate Cake w. Whip Cream	210	11	25
8" White Cake w. Whip Cream	210	11	26

Breakfast: Per Serving			
Kellogg's Snack Um's: Cinn. Blast	140	5	24
Froot Loops; Rice Krispy, aver.	125	1	26
PCB Banana Loaf Cake, 1	350	11	50
PCB Cinn. Crumb Pound Cake, 1	385	17	55

Desserts: Per Serving			
PCB Brownie	380	18	46
PCB Choc Chunk Cookie	410	19	56
PCB Original Krispy Treat	340	9	50

CinnaMonster®

Cinnamon Roll			
Caramel Pecan	210	8	30
Original	220	6	25

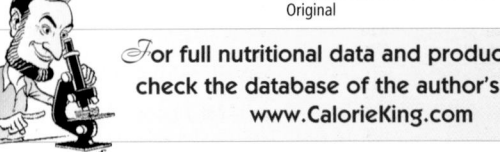

For full nutritional data and product updates check the database of the author's website www.CalorieKing.com

Church's Fried Chicken®

Fried Chicken

	C	F	Cb
Breast, 1 piece	200	12	4
Leg, 1 piece	140	9	2
Thigh, 1 piece	230	16	5
Wing, 1 piece	250	16	8
Krispy Tender Strips™, 1 piece	140	5	11
Tender Crunchers™, 6-8 pces	410	15	32
Chicken Fried Steak w. White Gravy	470	28	36

Side Items: Per Serving

	C	F	Cb
Apple Pie, 1 piece	280	12	41
Honey Butter Biscuits	250	16	26
Cajun Rice, regular	130	7	16
Cole Slaw, regular	90	6	8
Corn on the Cob, 1 ear	140	3	24
French Fries, regular	210	11	29
Okra, regular	210	16	19
Mashed Potatoes & Gravy, reg.	90	3	14

Coldstone Creamery®

Icecream & Sorbet

	C	F	Cb
Sweet Cream Icecream, 4 oz	260	16	24
Yogurt, 4 oz	140	0	24
Chocolate Icecream, 4 oz	240	16	20
Italian Sorbet, 4 oz	110	0	32
Waffle Cone	100	1	22

Cousin's Subs®

Italian 7 1/2" Subs: Per Sub

	C	F	Cb
Cappocolla & Cheese/Genoa	630	40	48
Special	800	53	48
Genoa & Cheese	730	49	48
Regular	685	44	48

Mini 4" Subs

	C	F	Cb
Chicken Salad	320	13	37
Italian Special	430	27	31
Provolone (Cheese)	420	27	30
Ham & Cheese	380	23	30
Meatball & Cheese	330	14	32
Seafood w. Crab	310	16	33
Tuna	475	33	30
Turkey Breast	350	19	31

Cousin's Subs® cont...

Cold 7 1/2" Subs

	C	F	Cb
BLT	615	42	45
Club Sub	745	43	48
Club Sub, no mayo/cheese	370	6	48
Cold Veggie	365	11	49
Cold Veggie, no mayo/cheese	245	2	49
Chicken Salad	570	26	61
Ham	310	5	47
Ham & Cheese	640	40	47
Provolone (Cheese) Sub	685	45	46
Roast Beef	620	34	46
Roast Beef, no mayo/cheese	365	6	46
Seafood with Crab	555	32	53
Tuna	830	60	46
Turkey Breast	560	32	48
Turkey Breast, no mayo/cheese	305	3	48

Hot 7 1/2" Subs

	C	F	Cb
Cheese Steak	540	24	46
Double Cheese Steak	850	46	46
Chicken Breast	620	34	46
Chicken Breast, no mayo/cheese	365	6	46
Gyro	680	40	55
Hot Veggie	490	23	49
Italian Sausage	480	22	50
Meatball & Cheese	585	27	50
Pepperoni Melt	785	52	47
Philly Cheese Steak	680	36	50
Steak	420	15	46
French Fries: Medium	400	19	55
Large	525	24	72
Extras: Hot Dog	300	16	29
Italian/Wheat Bread, half loaf	210	3	42

Soups: Per Regular Serving

	C	F	Cb
Cheese Broccoli	190	12	15
Cheese	240	16	18
Chicken w. Wild Rice	230	12	21
Chicken Dumpling	170	5	19
Chili	250	9	26
Clam Chowder	150	5	19
Cream of Potato	190	9	24
Salads: Chef Salad	190	10	7
Garden	135	8	7
Italian	295	20	7
Seafood	175	8	12
Side Salad	70	4	4
Tuna Salad	310	23	7
Cookies: Choc Chip	210	11	25

Culver's®

Butterburgers		C	F	Cb
Bacon Deluxe	710	45	30
Cheese, Single	385	19	32
Deluxe, Single	415	22	30
Double	460	21	32
Double Cheese	590	33	32
Mushroom & Swiss	570	33	25
Single	320	13	32
Sourdough Melt	655	32	44
Wisconsin Swiss Melt	635	31	40
Favorite Sandwiches: Chkn Filet	515	21	54
Chicken Tenders	465	25	28
Grilled Chicken Breast	310	9	35
Grilled Ham & Swiss	405	20	32
Norwegian Cod Filet	605	10	52
Philly Ribeye Steak	345	13	34
Pork Tenderloin	530	17	65
Roast Beef	405	15	27
Stacked Turkey	315	9	33
Turkey Sourdough BLT	525	20	44
Garden Fresh Salads: Chef	405	20	17
Grilled Chicken Caesar	410	20	21
Grilled Chicken Cashew	525	33	28
Taco: w. Shell	1130	89	59
w/out Shell	490	36	24
Tossed Salad, small	105	6	7
Seafood & Chicken: Shrimp Boat	520	27	50
CheckerBasket Chicken	1050	64	40
Norwegian Cod	510	27	37
Fries, Rings & Things: Dinner Roll	90	1	16
Cheese Curds	600	40	35
Chili Cheddar Fries	620	32	64
French Fries, regular	355	15	48
Mashed Potatoes & Gravy, small	100	2.5	17
Onion Rings	395	23	40
Frozen Custard: Cake Cone, Single	340	19	37
Dish, Single	310	18	31
Waffle Cone, Single	410	19	52
Desserts: Lemon Ice	210	0	52
Caramel Cashew, small	575	33	60
Hot Fudge Sundae, small	405	21	47
Old Fashioned Soda, Chocolate	445	19	64
Raspberry Cooler	480	0	116
Root Beer Float	465	16	77
Smoothie, Raspberry	615	17	107
Smoothie, Vanilla	555	17	92
Turtle, small	625	42	54

Dairy Queen®

Burgers/Sandwiches		C	F	Cb
Chicken Breast Fillet Sandwich	500	26	48
Chili 'n' Cheese Dog	330	21	22
DQ® Homestyle: Hamburger	290	12	29
Cheeseburger	340	17	29
Double Cheeseburger	540	31	30
Bacon Double Cheeseburger	610	36	31
Ultimate Burger	670	43	29
Grilled Chicken Sandwich	310	10	30
Hot Dog, regular	240	14	19
Super Dog™	580	37	39
Super Dog™, Chili 'n Cheese	710	47	42
BBQ Beef Sandwich	300	9	37
BBQ Pork Sandwich	280	8	36
Sides: Chkn Strip Basket w. Gravy	1000	50	102
Onion Rings	320	16	39
French Fries: Medium	440	23	53
Icecream Cones/Soft Serve				
DQ® Vanilla Soft Serve, 1/2 cup	140	4.5	22
DQ® Choc. Soft Serve, 1/2 cup	150	5	22
Vanilla Cone, medium	330	9	53
Chocolate Cone, medium	340	11	53
Dipped Cone, medium	490	24	59
Novelties: Buster Bar®	450	28	41
Chocolate Dilly® Bar	210	13	21
DQ® Fudge Bar, No Sugar Added	50	0	13
DQ® Sandwich	200	6	31
DQ® Vanilla Orange Bar, NAS	60	0	17
Lemon DQ Freez'r®, 1/2 cup	80	0	20
Starkiss®	80	0	21
Blizzards® & Sundaes				
Choc. Chip Cookie Dough, medium	950	36	143
Choc. Sandwich Cookie, medium	640	23	97
Chocolate Sundae, medium	400	10	71
*DQ® Treatzza Cake®*1/8 cake	370	13	56
*DQ® Treatzza Pizza™,*1/8 pizza	190	7	29
Royal Treats®: Banana Split	510	12	96
Peanut Buster® Parfait	730	31	99
Strawberry Shortcake	430	14	70
Frozen Yogurt				
Cup of Yogurt, medium	230	0.5	48
DQ® Nonfat Frozen Yogurt, 1/2 cup	100	0	21
Heath® Breeze®, medium	710	18	123
Strawberry Breeze®, medium	460	1	99
Yogurt Cone, medium	260	1	56
Yogurt Strawberry Sundae, medium	280	0.5	61
Misty® Slushes, medium	290	0	74

D'Angelo's®

	C	F	Cb
Sandwiches			
#9 Steak S/wich: Small	610	24	57
Large	1220	48	114
Chicken Stir Fry D'Lite: Pokket	360	4.5	45
Sub, Small	490	11	57
Sub, Large	940	22	114
Classic Vegetable D'Lite Pokket	340	9	52
Ginger Chkn Stir Fry D'Lite Pokket	400	5	49
Italian: Small	640	35	55
Large	1280	70	110
Roast Beef D'Lite: Pokket	290	3.5	39
Sub, Small	350	5	50
Sub, Large	700	10	100
Spicy Steak D'Lite Pokket	415	10	57
Steak D'Lite Pokket	380	10	48
Turkey D'Lite: Pokket	300	3	39
Sub, Small	360	4	50
Sub, Large	720	8	100
Salads			
Asian Chicken Salad	650	24	48
Caesar Salad	350	39	18
Chef Salad (no dressing)	210	12	17
Chicken Stir Fry (no dressing)	170	3.5	10
Roast Beef (no dressing)	150	3	9
Tuna (no dressing)	120	2.5	9
Turkey (no dressing)	160	2	9
Cookie: Choc Chunk, 3 oz	340	11	56

Davanni's

Hoagies: Per Half Hoagy (6")			
Chicken Breast	495	33	23
Without Mayonnaise	395	22	22
Chicken Parmigiana	385	19	23
Club: Regular	400	27	22
Without Mayonnaise	300	16	21
Italian Sausage	520	37	28
Meatball	465	31	31
Roast Beef: Regular	385	25	21
Without Mayonnaise	285	14	20
Pastrami: Regular	460	27	22
Without Mayonnaise	360	16	21
Turkey: Regular	370	24	22
Without Mayonnaise	270	13	21
Assorted: Regular	400	31	21
Without Mayonnaise	300	20	20

Davanni's® cont...

Hoagies (6") Cont.	C	F	Cb
Ham: Regular	380	25	22
Without Mayonnaise	280	14	21
Salami: Regular	485	38	21
Without Mayonnaise	385	27	20
Tuna: Regular	565	44	24
Without Mayonnaise	465	33	23
Vegie: Regular	445	29	28
Without Mayonnaise	345	18	28
Pizza	315	18	23
Cheese: Regular	400	29	21
Without Mayonnaise	300	18	20
Without Butter ~ Deduct	35	5	0
Without Cheese ~ Deduct	40	3	0

Grain Bun ~ Negligible difference except for extra fiber.

Pizzas			
Canadian Bacon & Vegetables:			
Thin, 1 slice	200	7	20
Traditional, 1 slice	250	7	30
Solo	630	18	75
Deep Dish, 1 slice	260	9	29
Pepperoni & Vegetables:			
Thin, 1 slice	210	10	19
Traditional, 1 slice	260	10	29
Solo	630	23	73
Deep Dish, 1 slice	270	12	28
Solo	790	33	99
The Works:			
Thin, 1 slice	250	14	18
Solo	600	32	43
Traditional, 1 slice	300	14	28
Solo	740	33	71
Deep Dish, 1 slice	310	16	27
Solo	900	43	85
Vegie Works:			
Thin, 1 slice	210	9	18
Solo	500	22	42
Traditional, 1 slice	260	9	28
Solo	630	22	70
Deep Dish, 1 slice	270	11	27
Solo	790	32	85

If no extra cheese ('light') deduct per slice on Vegie Works — 50 | 4 | 0

Sauce Type: Above figures are for red sauce

White Sauce (Olive Oil & Garlic) ~			
Add Per Slice	45	5	0

Davanni's® cont...

Extras	C	F	Cb
Garlic Cheese Bread:			
Half Order with Sauce	530	38	24
Lasagne: Garlic Toast	105	7	9
Half Lasagne with Toast	550	36	31
Whole Lasagne, with Toast	990	64	51
Potato Chips: Parmesan Garlic	230	36	31
Plain	230	14	25
Salad Dressings: Ranch, 1 oz	60	6	0
French, 1 oz	120	10	8
Italian, 1 oz	15	0	2
Bleu Cheese, 1 oz	180	6	0
Croutons, 1/4 oz	30	1	5

Drinks	C	F	Cb
Barq's Root Beer: 16 fl.oz	165	0	45
20 fl.oz	222	0	60
32 fl.oz	333	0	90
Milk, 10 fl.oz	120	3	14
Iced Tea, unsweetened	0	0	0

Daylight Donuts

Raised Donuts: Glazed, 1.35 oz	140	9	20
Chocolate Iced, 1.75 oz	190	9	23
Cholesterol Free: Glazed, 1.35 oz	140	6	20
Iced, 1.75 oz	190	6	23

Cake Donuts			
Plain, no topping, 2 oz	210	10	27
Chocolate Iced, 3 oz	340	15	48
Low Cholesterol, no topping, 2 oz	210	10	27

(The) Different Twist Pretzel Company®

Pretzels: Average All Types			
Regular: with Butter	325	8	56
without Butter	250	0	54
Pretzel Dip, 1 Tbsp	125	14	0

Dippin' Dots

Icecream: Average all types, 5 oz	190	9	22
Red. Fat/No Sugar Vanilla, 5 oz	120	6	17
Fat-Free/No Sugar Fudge, 5 oz	60	0	14
Nonfat Yogurt, 5 oz	110	0	23
Flavored Ice, 5 oz	50	0	13
Flavored Sherbet, 5 oz	100	1	21

Del Taco®

Breakfast	C	F	Cb
Breakfast Burrito	250	11	24
Bacon & Egg Quesadilla	450	23	40
Egg & Cheese Burrito	450	24	39
Macho Bacon & Egg Burrito™	1030	60	82
Steak & Egg Burrito	580	34	41
Tacos: Big Fat Chicken Taco™	340	13	38
Big Fat Crispy Chicken Taco™	620	38	52
Big Fat Steak Taco™	390	19	38
Big Fat Taco™	320	11	39
Chicken Soft Taco	210	12	16
Taco; Soft Taco, average	160	10	11
Ultimate Taco	260	17	13
Burritos: Combo Burrito™	530	22	61
Bean & Chse Red/Green Burrito	270	8	38
Chicken Works Burrito	520	23	57
Del Beef Burrito™	550	30	42
Del Classic Chicken Burrito™	560	36	41
Deluxe Combo Burrito™	570	25	64
Deluxe Del Beef Burrito™	590	33	45
Half Pound Red/Green Burrito	430	12	65
Macho Beef Burrito™	1170	62	89
Macho Combo Burrito™	1050	44	113
Spicy Chicken/Veggie Works, aver.	490	18	69
Steak Works Burrito	590	31	58
Quesadillas: Chicken	580	31	41
Regular	500	27	39
Spicy Jack Chicken	570	30	40
Spicy Jack Regular	490	26	38
Salads: Deluxe Chicken Salad™	740	34	77
Deluxe Taco Salad™	780	40	76
Taco Salad	350	30	10
Burgers: Cheeseburger	330	13	37
Double Del Cheeseburger™	560	35	35
Del Cheeseburger™	430	25	35
Nachos: Regular	380	24	40
Macho Nachos®	1100	63	113
Sides: Beans 'n Chse Cup, 7.7 oz	260	3	44
Rice Cup, 4 oz	140	2	27
Fries: Chili Cheese, 10.5 oz	670	46	50
Deluxe Chili Cheese™, 12 oz	710	49	53
Large, 7 oz	490	32	47
Regular, 5 oz	350	23	34
Shakes: Choc., small, 11.5 fl.oz	520	12	89
Vanilla; Strawb., sm., 11.5 fl.oz	420	7	77
Chocolate, large, 15 fl.oz	680	16	117
Vanilla; Strawb., large, 15 fl.oz	550	10	97

Denny's®

Breakfast	C	F	Cb
All American Slam®, no bread	710	62	9
Dagwood Breakfast, no bread	1250	90	35
Farmer's Slam, no syrup	1200	80	82
French Slam®, no syrup	1135	82	70
Grand Slam Slugger, no bread/pot.	790	46	58
Lumberjack Slam, no syrup	1130	68	79
Moons Over My Hammy	920	59	42
Original Grand Slam®	795	50	65
w. Syrup & Margarine	1030	60	101
Shamrock Slam, no bread	865	72	16
Slim Slam (no topping/sides)	440	6	56

Breakfast Skillets (no bread)	C	F	Cb
Big Texas Chicken Fajita	1220	70	25
Meat Lover's Skillet	1150	93	24

Breakfast Sides	C	F	Cb
Applesauce	60	0	15
Bacon, 4 strips	160	18	0
Bagel, 1 only	235	1	46
Biscuit: Buttered	270	11	40
w. Sausage Gravy	400	21	45
Country Fried Potatoes, 5 oz	395	20	23
Cream Cheese, 1 oz	100	10	1
Egg: 1 only	120	10	1
Two Egg Breakfast	825	67	24
Egg Beaters® (Egg Substitute)	70	5	1
English Muffins, each	125	1	24
Flour Tortillas and Salsa	290	8	50
Grits, 4 oz	80	0	18
Ham, grilled slice, 3 oz	95	3	2
Hashed Browns, 4 oz	220	14	22
Covered, 6 oz	320	23	21
Covered & Smothered, 8 oz	360	26	26
Dble Covered & Smother., 13 oz	460	26	48
Kellogg's® Dry Cereal, aver., 1 oz	100	0	23
Oatmeal N' Fixins, no bread	460	6	95
Quaker® Oatmeal, 4 oz	100	2	16
Sausage, 4 links	355	32	0
Sausage Gravy, 4 oz	125	10	6
Syrup: Blueberry/Strawberry, aver.	100	0	23
Maple-flavored, 3 Tbsp	145	0	36
Sugar-free, 3 Tbsp	25	0	9
Toast, 1 slice dry	90	1	17
Toppings, average, 3 oz	105	0	26
Whipped Cream, dollop, 2 oz	25	2	1
Whipped Margarine, 1/2 oz	90	10	0

French Toast	C	F	Cb
Plain	505	24	54
Cinnamon Swirl	1030	49	124

Omelette (no extras)	C	F	Cb
Ham'n Cheddar	580	45	4
Ultimate	565	47	9
Vegge-Cheese	480	39	9

Waffles (no extras)	C	F	Cb
Plain Belgian	305	21	23
w. Syrup & Butter	540	31	59

Buttermilk Hot Cakes: Plain (3)	490	7	95
w. Syrup & Butter	725	17	130

Steak & Eggs (no extras)	C	F	Cb
Country Fried Steak	430	36	10
Pork Chop	675	47	6
Sirloin Steak	620	49	1
T-Bone Steak	990	77	1

Soup: Per Cup (8 oz)	C	F	Cb
Chicken Noodle	60	2	8
Chili w. Cheese topping	400	19	21
Clam Chowder	215	11	22
Cream of Broccoli	195	12	15
Cream of Potato	220	12	23
Split Pea	145	5	18
Vegetable Beef	80	1	11

Sandwiches (no fries/sides)	C	F	Cb
Albacore Tuna Melt	640	39	42
BBQ Chicken	1070	46	124
BLT	610	38	50
Bacon Cheddar Burger	875	52	58
Big Texas BBQ Burger	930	58	53
Boca Burger®	615	28	66
Buffalo Chicken Sandwich	805	45	67
Chicken Burger	630	32	53
Classic Burger	675	40	42
w. Cheese	835	53	43
Club Sandwich	720	38	62
Double Decker Burger	1375	92	81
Garden Burger	665	33	75
Garlic Mushroom Swiss Burger	870	51	58
Grilled Chicken	520	14	64
Ham & Swiss on Rye	535	31	40
Patty Melt	790	50	37
Rueben	585	32	38
The Super Bird® Sandwich	620	32	48
Turkey Breast w. Multigrain	475	26	39

Denny's® cont...

Appetizers	C	F	Cb
Buffalo Chicken Strips (5)	735	42	43
Buffalo Wings (12)	855	54	1
Chicken Strips (5)	720	33	56
Mozzarella Sticks (8)	710	41	49
Onion Rings, 4 oz	380	23	38
Sampler, no condiments	1405	80	124

Entrees (no sides)	C	F	Cb
Chicken Strips, 10 oz	635	25	55
Fried Shrimp Dinner	220	10	18
Country Fried Steak	265	17	14
Fried Shrimp & Scampi	345	20	15
Shrimp Scampi Skillet Dinner	290	10	18
Grilled Chicken Breast Dinner	130	4	0
Pot Roast Dinner w. Gravy	290	11	5
Roast Turkey & Stuffing w. Gravy	390	3	38
Sirloin Steak Dinner	340	28	1
Steak & Shrimp Dinner	645	42	31
T-Bone Steak Dinner	860	65	0

Sides: Bread Stuffing, plain	C	F	Cb
Bread Stuffing, plain	100	1	19
Broccoli in Butter Sauce	50	2	7
Carrots in Honey Glaze	80	3	12
Corn in Butter Sauce	120	4	19
Fries: Unsalted, 6 oz	425	20	57
Seasoned, 6 oz	260	12	35
Smothered Cheese, 9 oz	765	48	69
Gravy, all types, average	15	0.5	2
Green Beans w. Bacon	60	4	6
Green Peas in Butter Sauce	100	2	14
Potato: Baked, plain w. skin	220	0	51
Mashed	105	1	21
Vegetable Rice Pilaf	85	1	16

Salads (no dressing/bread unless indicated)	C	F	Cb
Garden Deluxe Salad: w. Chkn Brst	265	11	10
w. Buffalo Chicken Strips	515	35	26
w. Fried Chicken Strips	440	26	26
w. Tuna	445	29	12
w. Turkey and Ham	320	11	12
Grilled Chkn Caesar w. Dressing	600	41	20
Side Caesar w. Dressing	360	26	20
Side Garden Salad, no Dressing	115	4	16

Dressings	C	F	Cb
BBQ Sauce, 1.5 oz	50	1	11
Blue Cheese, 1 oz	165	18	1
Caesar, 1 oz	135	14	1
French, regular, 1 oz	105	10	3
Honey Mustard, 1 oz	160	15	20
Italian Dressing, Low Calorie	15	0.5	3
Marinara Sauce, 1.5 oz	50	2	7
Ranch, 1 oz	130	14	1
Salsa, 2 oz	10	0	2
Sour Cream, 1.5 oz	90	9	2
Tartar Sauce, 1.5 oz	230	24	5
Thousand Island, 1 oz	120	11	5

Desserts: Per Serving	C	F	Cb
Banana Royale	550	25	80
Chocolate Layer Cake, 3 oz	275	12	42
Hot Fudge Cake Sundae, 7 oz	620	35	73
Pies: Per 1/6 Whole			
Apple, 7 oz	470	24	64
Cheesecake, no topping, 4 oz	470	27	48
Chocolate Peanut Butter	655	39	64
Hershey's Chococolate Chunks N' Chips	600	36	58
Oreo® Cookies & Creme, 6 oz	650	40	67

Sundaes	C	F	Cb
Single Scoop, no topping	190	14	14
Double Scoop, no topping	375	27	29
Banana Split	895	43	112
Grasshopper Sundae, 14 oz	730	34	97
Grasshopper Blender Blaster	735	37	92

Dessert Toppings: Per 2 oz	C	F	Cb
Blueberry, 2 oz	70	0	17
Chocolate, 2 oz	320	25	27
Fudge, 2 oz	200	10	30
Strawberry, 2 oz	80	1	17

Drinks	C	F	Cb
Cappuccino, 8 oz, average	100	2	38
Floats, Rootbeer/Cola	280	10	47
Malted Milkshake, van/choc.	585	26	82
Ruby Red Grapefruit Juice, 10 oz	160	0	41
Raspberry Iced Tea, 16 fl.oz	80	0	21

Feedback welcome

Please send comments to: Allan Borushek
POB 1616, Costa Mesa CA 92628
Email: allan@calorieking.com

Domino's® Pizza

	C	F	Cb
Buffalo Chicken Kickers™:			
1 average piece, 24g	47	2	3
1 order, 10 pieces, 240g	470	21	32
Hot Sauce, 1.5 oz Cup	15	0	4
Blue Cheese; Ranch, 1.5 oz	220	23	2

Classic Hand Tossed Pizza
Medium (12") Pizza: *Per 2 Slices (¹/₄ Pizza)*

	C	F	Cb
Cheese Pizza (base only)	375	11	55
America's Favorite Feast	510	22	57
Bacon Cheeseburger Feast	550	26	55
Barbeque Feast	505	20	62
Deluxe Feast	465	18	57
Hawaiian Feast	450	15	58
MeatZZa Feast	560	26	57
Pepperoni Feast	535	25	56
Vegi Feast	440	16	57

Large (14") Pizza: *Per 2 Slices (¹/₄ Pizza)*

	C	F	Cb
Cheese Pizza (base only)	515	15	75
America's Favorite Feast	700	30	78
Bacon Cheeseburger Feast	760	36	75
Barbeque Feast	690	27	85
Deluxe Feast	630	24	78
Hawaiian Feast	620	22	80
MeatZZa Feast	750	34	78
Pepperoni Feast	730	34	76
Vegi Feast	605	22	78

Crunchy Thin Crust Pizza
Medium (12") Pizza: *Per 2 Slices (¹/₄ Pizza)*

	C	F	Cb
Cheese Pizza (base only)	275	12	31
With Topping: Bacon	375	20	31
Beef	350	19	31
Cheddar Cheese	330	17	31
Pepperoni	350	19	31
X-tra Cheese & Pepperoni	400	23	32
Ham	300	13	31
Italian Sausage & Mushroom	360	18	34
Vegi (olive/mushr./onion/peppers)	340	17	34

Large (14") Pizza: *Per 2 Slices (¹/₄ Pizza)*

	C	F	Cb
Cheese Pizza (base only)	380	17	43
With Topping: Bacon	530	30	43
Beef	490	27	44
Cheddar Cheese	450	23	44
Pepperoni	480	25	44
X-tra Cheese & Pepperoni	550	30	45
Ham	415	18	44
Italian Sausage & Mushroom	500	25	48
Vegi (olive/mushr./onion/peppers)	470	23	47

Ultimate Deep Dish Pizza

	C	F	Cb
Medium (12') Pizza: *Per 2 Slices (¹/₄ Pizza)*			
Cheese Pizza (base only)	480	22	56
With Topping: Bacon	580	30	56
Beef	560	29	56
Cheddar Cheese	540	27	56
Pepperoni	555	29	56
Ham	505	23	56
Italian Sausage & Mushroom	565	28	59
Vegi	550	27	58

Large (14") Pizza: *Per 2 Slices (¹/₄ Pizza)*

	C	F	Cb
Cheese Pizza (base only)	675	30	80
With Topping: Bacon	830	43	80
Beef	785	40	80
Cheddar Cheese	745	36	80
Pepperoni	775	39	80
X-tra Cheese & Pepperoni	845	44	82
Ham	705	31	80
Italian Sausage & Mushroom	795	39	85
Vegi	765	36	83

Sides

	C	F	Cb
Breadstick, 1 stick, 37g	115	4	18
Cheesy Bread, 1 stick, 43g	140	6	18
Barbeque Wings, 1 piece	50	2.5	2
Hot Wings, 1 piece	45	2	0.5
CinnaStix®, 1 stick	120	6	15

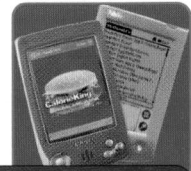

Don Pablos®

Appetizers: Per Serving	C	F	Cb
Acapulco Nachos	1460	104	63
Beef Fajita Nachos	1665	118	80
Chicken Fajita Nachos	1315	83	65
Chile Con Queso	155	11	5
Chips & Salsa	340	17	43
Cholula Buffalo Wings	1045	84	24
Don's Fiesta Sampler	1555	85	141
Prairie Fire Bean Dip	150	9	11
Queso Blanco	670	45	55
Spinach & Artichoke Jalapeno Dip	845	63	63
Burritos: Beef & Bean	1390	73	123
Chicken	1250	54	133
Chimichangas: Beef	1190	63	109
Chimi de Oro w. Queso	1400	78	116
Pollo (Chicken)	1090	49	117
Combinations: Conquistador	1975	87	179
El Matador	1405	76	110
El Presidente	940	46	77
Mexican Dinner	1045	57	75
Primo Combo	1184	62	90
Primo Combo All Chicked	1134	54	93
Dressings: Per 4 oz			
Blue Cheese	600	64	3
Chipolte Ranch	340	35	5
Creamy Cilantro	545	59	4
Don's House Vinaigrette	475	42	19
Honey Mustard	420	35	22
Italian	395	27	32
Low-Fat-French	200	5	40
Enchiladas: Mama's Skinny	580	15	57
Chicken Fajita Enchiladas	1350	81	77
Real Enchiladas Beef	1135	77	64
Real Enchiladas Chicken	855	49	52
Real Enchiladas Combo	995	63	58
Steak Fajita Enchiladas	1105	56	67
Three Amigos	990	53	63
Fajitas: BBQ Chicken Melt	1685	71	180
Classic Chicken	1350	61	139
Classic Steak	1770	104	157
Pepper Cheese Steak	1945	114	167
Peso Valley Vegetables	1355	70	155
Shrimp	1140	72	144
Shrimp & Chicken	1400	67	142
Shrimp & Steak	1610	88	151

Favorites	C	F	Cb
Chipolte BBQ Ribs	1890	122	103
Flautas Y Taquitos	1145	61	103
Parilla Chicken	530	6	63
Steak & Enchiladas	1375	81	68
Steak & Shrimp	1170	65	71
Lunch Specials: El Favorito	760	38	59
Cheese Quesadilla Salad	840	51	63
Dos Enchilladas	730	33	63
Vegetable Quesadilla Salad	855	49	76
Quesadillas: Beef Fajita	1700	103	128
Cheese	1460	87	110
Chicken Fajita	1420	75	116
Vegetable	1490	84	136
Salads: Grilled Chicken	470	22	26
Grilled Chicken Caesar	1455	106	95
Grilled Steak Caesar	1735	134	107
Soup & Salad Infinito	1420	83	136
Taco	1390	84	103
Tortilla Tossed	1050	63	101
Desserts: Chocolate Volcano	1380	77	161
Iron Skillet Pie	740	42	86
Sopapillas	525	29	6

Donato's® Pizza

Pizza: Per Slice (1/8 Large)	C	F	Cb
Chicken Vegy Medley	240	10	25
Classic Trio	360	22	26
Founders Favorite	380	27	27
Hawaiian	310	15	29
Mariachi Beef/Mariachi Chicken	305	16	26
Original Pepperoni	320	19	25
Serious Cheese	325	18	25
Serious Meat	420	25	26
The Works	370	22	27
Vegy	280	14	28
Vegy (without Cheese)	185	6	27
Salads: Garden w. Lite Italian Dr.	270	15	18
Side Salad w. Lite Italian Dressing	140	8	10
Subs: Big Don w. Italian Dressing	780	45	63
Big Don w. Lite Italian Dressing	645	30	63
Grilled Chicken Club	650	31	64
Ham & Cheese w. Italian Dressing	650	31	64
Ham & Cheese/Lite Italian	530	16	64
Vegy w. Lite Italian Dressing	445	12	59

Dunkin Donuts®

Donuts: Each	C	F	Cb
Apple/Blueberry Crumb Donut	230	10	34
Apple N' Spice Donut	200	8	29
Black Raspberry/Strawberry Donut	210	8	32
Blueberry Cake Donut	290	16	35
Boston Kreme Donut	240	9	36
Butternut Cake Donut	300	16	36
Chocolate Coconut Cake Donut	300	19	31
Chocolate Frosted Cake Donut	300	16	38
Chocolate Frosted Donut	200	9	29
Chocolate Glazed Cake Donut	290	16	33
Cinnamon Cake Donut	270	15	31
Coconut Cake Donut	290	17	33
Double Chocolate Cake Donut	310	17	37
Dunkin' Donut	240	15	25
Glazed/Powdered Cake Donut	270	15	33
Glazed Donut	180	8	25
Jelly Filled Donut	210	8	32
Jelly Stick Donut	290	12	44
Kreme Filled (Choc./Vanilla)Donut	270	13	35
Lemon Donut	200	9	8
Maple/Marble Frosted Donut	210	9	29
Old Fashioned Cake Donut	250	15	26
Strawb./Van. Frosted; Bavarian	210	9	30
Sugar Raised Donut	170	8	22
Toasted Coconut Cake Donut	300	17	35
Whole Wheat Glazed Cake Donut	310	19	32

Muffins			
Apple Danish, 3 oz	250	10	36
Banana Nut	530	23	72
Blueberry: Regular	490	17	76
Reduced Fat	450	13	74
Blueberry Scone, 4 oz	410	19	55
Cheese Danish, 3 oz	270	14	32
Chocolate Chip	605	24	88
Coffee Cake Muffin, 6.5 oz	710	29	102
Corn	500	16	78
Cranberry Orange	470	15	76
Honey Raisin Bran	480	14	79
Maple Walnut Scone, 4 oz	470	22	62
Raspberry White Chocolate, 4 oz	450	22	59
Strawberry Cheese Danish, 3 oz	250	12	33

Crullers: Glazed Cruller	C	F	Cb
Glazed Chocolate Cruller	280	15	35
Plain Cruller	240	15	25
Powdered Cruller	270	15	30
Sugar Cruller	250	15	30

Sandwiches: Per Sandwich	C	F	Cb
Biscuit Sandwiches:			
Egg/Cheese Sandwich	380	22	30
Sausage/Egg/Cheese Sandwich	590	42	31
Croissant: Plain, USA, each	290	18	26
Pizza; Spanish Cheese, average	520	35	33
Eng. Muffin S'wich:Ham/Egg/Chse	320	12	31

Bagels: Biscuit Bagel			
Garlic; Everything; Poppyseed	280	14	32
Onion	360	2.5	68
Sesame	350	4	66
Other types, average	380	4.5	74
Cream Cheese (Per Packet): Lite	340	3	69
	130	11	3
Average of other flavors	180	17	3

Cake Munchkins			
Plain (4)	220	14	22
Cinnamon; Powdered; Sugared (4)	250	14	29
Coconut; Coconut Toasted (3)	200	12	23
Sugar Raised (7)	220	12	26
Yeast Munchkin, Jelly Filled (5)	210	9	30
Yeast Lemon Filled (4)	170	8	23
Other types, average (3)	200	10	26

Fancies, Buns, Rolls, Fritters			
Apple Fritter	300	14	41
Bismark Chocolate Iced Donut	340	15	50
Bow Tie Donut	300	17	34
Cinnamon Bun	510	15	85
Coffee Roll: Regular	270	14	33
Frosted (Choc./Maple/Vanilla)	290	15	36
Eclair Donut	270	11	39
Glazed Fritter	260	14	31

Cookies			
Chocolate varieties, average (1)	220	11	26
Oatmeal Raisin Pecan	220	10	29

Drinks: Dunkacinno, 10 fl.oz	250	11	34
Hot Chocolate, 10 fl.oz	210	7	36
Iced Coffee, 16 fl.oz:	5	0	0
w. Cream, 16 fl.oz	60	6	2
w. Milk, 16 fl.oz	25	1	3
Vanilla Chai, 10 fl.oz	220	8	37

Coolatta®: Per 16 fl.oz			
Coffee Coolatta®: w. Cream	370	16	48
w. Milk	260	3	49
w. 2% Milk	240	1.5	49
Orange Mango Frt Coolatta®	280	0	69
Strawberry Fruit Coolatta®	270	0	68
Vanilla Bean Coolatta®	440	17	73

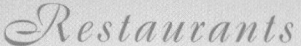

Breakfast	C	F	Cb
Cornbeef Hash, 7.5 oz	340	23	16
Egg Beaters® Breakfast	75	0	5
Eggs Benedict	600	31	35
Fruit Cup	60	0.5	15
Hash Browns, 6 oz	235	12	28
Homefries, 6 oz	210	12	24
Omelette: Bacon & Cheese	500	39	2
Cheese	390	30	2
Ham & Cheese	465	32	3
Supreme	420	30	8
Western	345	21	7
Pancake, Plain, 1	225	3	42
Waffle, Apple	960	45	125
Burgers: American Grill	785	50	36
Amer./Swiss/Provolone Gourmet	775	47	36
Bacon & Cheese	615	36	32
Cheeseburger	540	29	32
Garden	355	6.5	60
Hamburger	495	26	32
Southwest	680	36	56
Super	705	49	37
Swiss	580	32	34
Turkey	500	21	37
Sandwiches: BLT	290	14	27
Bacon Turkey Swiss	525	37	16
Chicken Bacon Deluxe	565	23	50
Chicken Breaded	515	19	50
Chicken Chargrill/Spicy	330	6	35
Chicken Fiesta	325	12	21
Cod	670	25	67
Croissant			
Grilled Cheese	505	36	26
Chicken Salad; Tuna	595	39	36
Turkey	390	18	31
Dutch Ham & Swiss	570	30	35
Hot Roast Beef	280	5.5	25
Pita: Chicken Fajita	620	18	68
Tuna	640	25	72
Turkey	445	5	67
Reuben	720	49	31
Shredded Pot Roast	530	30	27
Steak'n Cheese	765	50	42
Tuna Melt	610	41	35
Turkey Club	775	46	50
Turkey Pastrami	715	46	40
Whitefish (Breaded)	790	35	69

Appetizers	C	F	Cb
Cheese Fries	880	50	93
Cheese Sticks	410	24	17
Onion Rings	210	13	19
Wings	400	28	0.5
Dinners: Chicken Breast, stuffed	370	16	27
Chicken Fillets, 5	530	26	28
Chicken Milano	215	10	4
Chicken Naturelle	140	3.5	0
Chicken Parmigiana: Marinara	840	32	90
Meat	900	38	86
Chicken Stir-Fry	555	24	47
Chicken'n Biscuits	495	20	30
Chicken, 3 piece	1195	70	57
Cod, breaded	925	45	56
Floridian Scrod	120	1.5	4
Spaghetti Marinara	620	8	20
Veal Parmigiana w. Meat Sauce	820	26	105
Whitefish (Breaded)	790	35	69
Ziti w. Meat Balls & Meat Sauce	960	42	102
Salads & Dressings: Chef Salad	460	28	10
Chicken Salad	440	19	29
Chicken Caesar Salad	270	9	15
Chicken Portabella Salad	345	12	22
Fruit w. Sherbert	310	3	73
Garden Salad	100	3	16
Steak Salad	615	39	29
Taco Salad	385	19	36
Dressings: Bleu Cheese	90	7	7
French Fat Free	70	0	17
Fruit Salad	145	14	5
Italian Fat Free	10	0	3
Light Burgundy Vinaigrette	35	1.5	6
Thousand Island	95	9	3
Desserts: Cheesecake	505	36	40
Banana Fudge Sensation	975	44	47
Grilled Sticky Loaf	485	28	53
Icecream	285	15	33
Pies: Apple Reduced Fat	340	10	61
Peach Lite	300	10	50
Pudding (Sugar Free)	90	2.5	12
Strawberry Shortcake	685	26	14

**More extensive menu listings
in website database
www.calorieking.com**

Restaurants & **Fast-Foods**

Einstein Bros®

	C	F	Cb
Bagels: Average all types, 4 oz	330	1	70
Chocolate Chip Bagel, 4 oz	370	3	76
Egg Bagel, 3$\frac{1}{2}$ oz	340	3	69
Sesame Dip	380	5	75
Cream Cheese: Plain, 2 Tbsp	70	7	1
Plain Lite, 2 Tbsp	60	5	2
Smoked Salmon, 2 Tbsp	60	5	3
Flavors, average, 2 Tbsp	70	5	5
Spreads: Fruit, 2 Tbsp	75	0	19
Honey Butter, 1 Tbsp	90	8	4
Peanut Butter, 2 Tbsp	190	15	8
Sandwiches: BBQ Chicken	550	11	83
Baguette, Our Big Hero	920	39	98
Chicago Bagel Dog Asiago	740	34	78
Classic NY Lox & Bagel	660	27	79
Egg Santa Fe	650	24	78
Ham Deli	450	6	74
Holey Cow	900	50	77
Mediterranean Hummus	540	13	89
Roast Beef Deli	460	4	76
Roast Chicken & Smoked Gouda	520	11	68
Smoked Turkey Deli	420	1.5	75
The Veg-Out	490	13	77
Tuna Salad Deli	500	7	77
Turkey Pastrami Deli	440	2	76
Turkey Pastrami Reuben Deli	660	19	83
Bagel Shtick: Asiago	450	9	72
Cinnamon Sugar	570	24	79
Everything; Potato	380	4.5	73
Sesame Bagel Shtick	420	8	75
Bagel Chips: Plain, 1 oz serving	90	3	13
Flavors, average, 1 oz	90	3	13
Roll-Ups: Albuquerque Turkey	790	39	81
Baja Shaved Beef	720	36	67
Pacific Smoked Salmon	590	31	55
Cookies: Big Brownie	500	21	76
Chocolate Chunk, 4 oz	600	28	78
Oatmeal Raisin, 4 oz	550	21	82
Muffins: Banana Nut	520	29	59
Blueberry	460	24	57
Chocolate Chip	240	13	67
Lowfat Lemon Poppyseed	370	7	69
Mocha Chocolate Chip	550	29	66
97% Fat Free Apple Cinnamon	560	2	77
Scones: All types, 5 oz	490	17	75
Coffee: Cafe Latte, regular	140	5	13
Cappuccino	90	3.5	9

El Pollo Loco®

	C	F	Cb
Flame Broiled Chicken			
Breast	160	6	0
Leg	90	5	0
Thigh	180	12	0
Wing	110	6	0
Tortillas			
6" Corn	70	1	14
6.5" Flour	110	4	13
Burritos			
Bean, Rice & Cheese	505	16	73
Chicken Lover's	475	19	47
Classic	580	22	66
Mexican Chicken Caesar	735	35	65
Ranch	615	30	45
Spicy	635	21	80
Ultimate	635	23	66
Tacos: Chicken Soft Taco	235	12	15
Taco Al Carbon	180	8	20
Bowls			
Flame Broiled Chkn Salad	355	13	39
Mexican Chicken Caesar Salad	495	30	32
Nacho Pollo Bowl	765	33	64
Pollo Bowl	470	11	66
Smokey Black Bean Pollo Bowl	605	23	75
Specialties			
Chicken Nachos	1420	91	105
Chicken Quesadilla	595	29	48
Chicken Sticks (Kids), 4 oz	225	12	15
Chicken Tamale	180	8	21
Chicken Taquito	370	17	43
Chicken Tostada Salad	990	52	91
Tortilla Chips, unsalted	425	24	48
Tostada Salad, w/out shell & sour cr.	545	24	55
Tostada, shell only	440	27	42
Side Dishes			
Cole Slaw	205	16	12
Corn Cobbette (3")	80	1	18
French Fries	445	19	61
Garden Salad	105	7	7
Macaroni & Cheese	245	12	24
Pinto Beans	185	4	29
Potato Salad	255	14	30
Smokey Black Beans	305	16	35
Spanish Rice	130	3	24

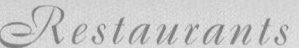

El Pollo Loco® cont...

	C	**F**	**Cb**
Dressings			
Bleu Cheese; Ranch	230	24	2
Creamy Cilantro	265	29	1
Hidden Valley Ranch	110	11	1
Light Italian	20	1	2
Thousand Island	220	21	7
Condiments: Guacamole	30	2	3
House/Spicy Chipotle Salsa	6	0	2
Jalapeno Hot Sauce, 1 pkt	5	0	1
Sour Cream	60	5	1
Pico de Gallo Salsa	11	0.5	1.5
Desserts			
Banana Split	715	28	107
Churros	180	11	18
Foster's Freeze without cone	180	5	30
Smoothies, all types	365	7	68

Fazoli's® Italian Food

	C	**F**	**Cb**
Soup; Bread			
Minestrone Soup	120	1	23
Breadstick, dry	90	1	17
Breadstick	140	6	18
Salads: No Dressing Unless Indicated			
Chicken & Pasta Caesar Salad	370	13	33
Chicken Finger Salad	190	9	8
w. Bacon Honey Mustard Dress.	400	28	17
Chicken Caesar Salad	420	29	17
Garden Salad	30	0	6
Italian Chef Salad	260	21	13
Pasta Salad	590	25	70
Side Pasta Salad	240	10	29
Dressings: Per 1 oz			
Honey French	150	12	9
House Italian	110	9	5
Reduced Calorie Italian	50	5	3
Ranch	150	17	1
Thousand Island	130	13	4
Submarinos: Per 1/2 Sandwich			
Original	1160	55	124
Meatball	1260	59	128
Turkey	990	34	121
Club	1100	44	121
Ham & Swiss	1000	37	120
Pepperoni Pizza	1060	40	133

Fazoli's® cont...

	C	**F**	**Cb**
Pizza: Per Double Slice			
Cheese	460	15	58
Combination	570	25	63
Pepperoni	530	22	61
Pasta: Per Serving			
Fettucine Alfredo: Small	530	15	80
Regular	800	22	119
Peppery Chicken Alfredo	610	16	80
Small Spaghetti: w. Marinara	420	6	74
w. Meat Sauce	450	8	74
w. Meatballs	720	31	80
Regular Spaghetti: w. Marinara	620	8	111
w. Meat Sauce	670	11	111
w. Meatballs	1020	42	119
Italian Specialties: Per Serving			
Baked Chicken Alfredo	790	29	82
Baked Chicken Parmesan	740	20	99
Baked Spaghetti Parmesan	700	25	76
Baked Ziti: Small	490	17	56
Regular	750	26	87
Cheese Ravioli: w. Marinara	480	15	65
w. Meat Sauce	510	17	65
Fettucine Broccoli	560	15	85
Lasagna: Regular	440	19	41
Broccoli	420	18	45
Pizza Baked Spaghetti	750	31	78
Sampler Platter	710	21	97
Shrimp & Scallop Fettucine	610	16	81
Paninis: Per Serving			
Chicken Caesar Club	660	35	51
Chicken Pesto	510	20	51
Four Cheese & Tomato	720	43	55
Ham & Swiss	600	30	53
Italian Deli	660	35	61
Italian Club	670	37	54
Smoked Turkey	710	38	57
Desserts: Per Serving			
Cheesecake: Plain	290	22	17
Turtle	420	34	24
Chocolate Chip	300	22	22
Lemon Ice	190	0	45
Milk Chocolate Chunk Cookie	360	15	54
Strawberry Topping, 1 oz	35	0	8

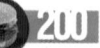

Restaurants & Fast–Foods

Freshens®

	C	F	Cb
Yogurt Smoothies: *Per 21 oz*			
Blueberry Sunset	385	0.5	84
Jamaican Jammer	475	1	110
Peachy Pineapple	405	1	91
Pina Collider	560	4	126
Raspberry Rapture	515	1	121
Raspberry Rocker	490	1	113
Strawberry Squeeze	390	0.5	88
Tropical Fruit Juice Smoothies: *Per 21 oz*			
Blueberry Wave	330	0.5	82
Caribbean Craze	330	0.5	84
Peach Sunset	365	0.5	93
Pineapple Passion	420	4	100
Raspberry Rhapsody	345	0.5	88
Raspberry Rumba	375	0.5	95
Strawberry Shooter	245	0	63
Orange Smoothies: *Per 21 oz*			
Aruba Orange	420	3.5	97
Orange Shooter	370	3	81
Orange Sunrise	415	3	90
Orange Wave	420	3	98
Coffee Smoothies: *Per 21 oz*			
Original Coffee	340	3.5	70
Caramel Coffee	425	4	89
Mocha Coffee	375	3.5	79
Oreo® Coffee	520	11	96
Decadent Smoothies: *Per 21 oz*			
Fudge Oreo® Supreme	640	11	126
Peanut Butter Cup	930	34	141
Pretzel Logic Pretzels, 1/2 Pretzel, 3 oz	255	3	49
Freshen® Farms Icecream, 1/2 Cup	150	6	21
MET-Rx® Performance Supplements			
Energy Booster, 1 sachet	3	0	1
Fat Burner, 1 sachet	5	0	1
Immune Booster, 1 sachet	4	0	1
Memory Booster, 1 sachet	6	0	1.5
Protein Booster, 1 scoop, 10g	35	0	0
Soy Booster, 1 scoop, 16g	60	0.5	5

Frisch's Big Boy®
~ Same Menu & Data as Big Boy ~

Godfather's™ Pizza

	C	F	Cb
Original Crust: *Per Slice*			
Cheese Pizza: Mini, 1/4 pizza	130	3	19
Medium, 1/8 pizza	230	5	34
Large, 1/10 pizza	260	6	36
Jumbo, 1/10 pizza	380	9	53
Combo Pizza: Mini, 1/4 pizza	175	7	21
Medium, 1/8 pizza	305	11	36
Large, 1/10 pizza	340	12	38
Jumbo, 1/10 pizza	505	18	56
Golden Crust: *Per Slice*			
Cheese Pizza: Medium, 1/8 pizza	210	10	26
Large, 1/10 pizza	240	9	28
Combo Pizza: Medium, 1/8 pizza	270	12	28
Large, 1/10 pizza	305	14	31

Golden Corral®

	C	F	Cb
Chicken			
Grilled	170	5	0
Fried	370	19	14
Shrimp, fried	250	12	24
Steak: *Per Serving*			
Ribeye, 6 oz	450	35	0
Sirloin, 5 oz	230	14	0
Chopped, 4 oz	320	23	0
Tips w. Onions	290	13	8
Sides: *Per Serving*			
Baked Potato	225	2	46
Texas Toast	170	6	26

Gretel's Pretzels®

	C	F	Cb
Pretzels			
Cinnamon/Sugar	195	3	38
Original	170	3	31
Poppy Seed	175	3.5	31
Raisin Danish/Icing	350	2	79
Sesame Seed	175	3.5	31
Sweet Dough	115	0.5	23

Fast-Foods & *Restaurants*

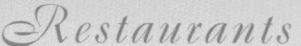

(The) Great American Bagel Co®   C F Cb

Bagels: Per Bagel

	C	F	Cb
4-Grain Honey; Cinn. Raisin	420	1.5	88
Apple/Blueberry Crumb, average	570	8	106
Banana Nut; Cheddar Herb, aver.	410	5	82
Blueberry; Onion; Strawberry	380	1	83
Cheddar Salsa	430	11	63
Cheese Twist	740	20	107
Chocolate Chip	390	4	75
Cinnamon Sugar; Egg	390	2	83
Cranb. Nut; P'nut Butter Choc Chip	400	6	72
Hot Tomazzo; Tomazzo	360	7	57
Jalapeno Cheddar	330	4.5	58
Plain	390	1.5	85
Pumpernickel; Pumpkin, average	330	1.5	72
Pumpkin Chocolate Chip	350	3.5	67
Spinach Herb	300	1	60
Stuffed Pepperoni	500	12	74
Stuffed Spinach	720	22	98
Sun-Dried Tomato Basil	390	1.5	77
Veggie; Whole Wheat; Salt	340	1	70
Other varieties, average	370	2	75

Hardees®

Breakfast Items

	C	F	Cb
Hash Rounds™, regular	230	14	24

Biscuits:

	C	F	Cb
Apple Cinnamon 'N' Raisin™	250	8	42
Bacon, Egg & Cheese	520	30	45
Biscuit 'N' Gravy™	530	30	56
Chicken Biscuit	590	27	62
Cinnamon 'N' Raisin™	370	18	48
Country Ham	440	22	44
Frisco™ Breakfast S'wich (Ham)	450	22	42
Ham	410	20	45
Jelly Biscuit	440	21	57
Made From Scratch® Biscuit	390	21	44
Omelet™	550	32	45
Pork Chop	530	22	56
Sausage	550	36	44
Sausage & Egg	620	40	45
Steak	580	32	56

Sunrise Croissant:

	C	F	Cb
Bacon	410	25	28
Ham	410	23	31
Sausage	560	40	28

Hardees® cont...   C F Cb

Hamburgers

	C	F	Cb
All Star	660	43	42
Bacon Swiss Crispy Chicken	670	44	45
Cheeseburger	320	15	30
Double Cheeseburger	480	28	31
Famous Star	570	35	42
Frisco™ Burger	740	51	38
Hamburger	270	10	29
Monster Burger®	990	72	37
Monster Roast Beef	610	39	26
Mushroom 'N' Swiss™	500	26	39
Six Dollar Burger	950	62	58
Super Star	790	53	42

Sandwiches

	C	F	Cb
Big Roast Beef™ Sandwich	410	24	26
Chicken Fillet Sandwich	430	18	42
Fisherman's Fillet™	520	28	47
Grilled Chicken Sandwich	350	16	28
Ham 'N' Cheese Supreme	490	27	45
Hot Dog w. Condiments	450	32	25
Hot Ham 'N' Cheese	300	12	34
Roast Beef Sandwich	310	16	26
Roast Beef Supreme	500	31	38
Turkey Supreme	480	25	40

Fried Chicken (edible portion)

	C	F	Cb
Breast, each	370	15	30
Wing, each	200	8	23
Thigh, each	330	15	30
Leg, each	170	7	15

French Fries: Regular

	C	F	Cb
Regular	340	16	45
Large	440	21	60
Monster	510	24	67

Sides: Coleslaw, small

	C	F	Cb
Coleslaw, small	240	20	13
Chicken Strips: 3 pieces	120	5	8
5 pieces	200	8	13
Crispy Curls: Regular	340	18	41
Large	520	28	62
Monster	590	31	70
Gravy, 1.5 oz	20	0.5	3
Honey Mustard, 1 oz	50	0	12
Mashed Potatoes & Gravy, small	90	0.5	17

Desserts & Drinks

	C	F	Cb
Apple Turnover	270	12	38
Chocolate Chip Cookie	370	19	61
Peach Cobbler, small	310	7	60
Orange Juice, 10 oz	140	0	34

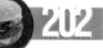

Restaurants & Fast−Foods

Haagen-Dazs®

Per 1/2 Cup	C	F	Cb
Baileys Irish Crm; Cookies & Crm	270	17	23
Bananas Foster	260	15	28
Belgian Chocolate; Pecan Pie	330	21	29
Butter Pecan	310	23	21
Cherry Vanilla; Strawberry	240	15	23
Chocolate	270	18	22
Chocolate Brownie w. Walnuts	290	19	25
Chocolate Cheesecake	300	18	29
Chocolate Chocolate Chip	300	20	26
Chocolate Cookies & Cream	270	17	24
Chocolate Peanut Butter	360	24	27
Chocolate Raspberry Gateau	270	15	29
Coffee	270	18	21
Coffee Almond Swirl	320	21	27
Coffee Mocha Chip; Vanilla Fudge	290	19	25
Cookie Dough Chip	310	19	29
Creme Caramel Pecan	320	20	29
Dulce De Leche	290	17	28
German Chocolate Cake	290	18	28
Macadamia Brittle; Mint Chip	300	20	25
Mango	250	14	28
Peanut Butter Fudge Chunk	340	23	25
Pineapple Coconut	230	13	25
Pistachio	290	20	22
Rocky Road	300	18	29
Rum Raisin; Vanilla	270	17	22
Strawberry Cheesecake	270	16	28
Vanilla Caramel Brownie	300	18	30
Vanilla Chocolate Chip	310	20	26
Vanilla Fudge Brownie	300	18	28
Vanilla Swiss Almond	300	20	24
Sorbet: Orchard Peach	130	0	33
Average other flavors	120	0	30
Gelato: Cappuccino; Raspberry	240	7	40
Chocolate; Coconut	240	8	37
Choc. Amaretto Almond Swirl	270	10	40
Hazelnut	260	12	33
Tiramisu	250	10	35
Frozen Yogurt: Choc. Choc. Chip	230	7	32
Apple Pie; Strawberry Chsecake	230	6	35
Coffee; Vanilla	200	4.5	31
Dulce De Leche	190	2.5	35
Lemon Pie	260	7	41
Peach Melba	210	3.5	37
Strawberry Non Fat	140	0	31
Vanilla Raspberry Swirl	170	2.5	31

Harvey's®

Main Menu	C	F	Cb
Original Hamburger	355	18	32
Original Cheeseburger	405	21	32
Original Patty by itself	190	16	2
Ultra Burger	410	19	33
w. Cheese	455	22	34
Ultra Patty by itself	240	7	0
Value Burger	300	13	30
w. Cheese	350	16	31
Value Patty by itself	135	11	0
Hot Dog	315	12	30
Fish Sandwich	350	10	49
Fish Patty by itself	185	8	16
Harvey's Grilled Chicken	300	5	35
Harvey's Crispy Chicken	380	10	48
Chicken Fajita	450	16	54
Chicken Nuggets	170	9	11
Veggie Burger, 3.2 oz	330	9	41
Crispy Fries: Junior, 3.2 oz	290	15	34
Regular, 4.2 oz	380	20	46
Large, 5.3 oz	475	25	57
Onion Rings: Regular, 2.8 oz	285	20	23
Large	430	30	34
Side Orders			
Poutine, 10 oz	700	40	67
Gravy, 3 oz	45	0.5	9
Garden Salad	120	6	11
Caesar Salad	55	1.5	5
Chicken Caesar Salad	145	4.5	6
Chicken Garden Salad	210	8	12
Soup: Harvest Vegetable, 1 cup	120	1.5	25
Beef Barley, 1 cup	105	1	20
Cream of Broccoli/Mushr., 1 cup	170	7	25
Chicken Noodle, 1 cup	100	1.5	17
Breakfast: Bagel	295	2	55
Breakfast Club Sandwich	310	15	26
Eggs (2): Fried	175	13	1
Scrambled Eggs	165	11	2
Hashbrowns	130	7	15
Home Fries	270	11	38
Orange Marmalade; Strawb. Jam	55	0	14
Muffins: Blueberry	375	19	62
Bran Muffin	435	17	57
Pancakes (2)	225	3	42
Pancake Syrup	165	0	42
Sausage	135	11	3
Toasted Western Sandwich	370	15	52

203

Fast-Foods & *Restaurants*

Harvey's® cont...

	C	**F**	**Cb**
Dressings & Sauces			
Sauces: Ketchup	10	0	2.5
Plum Sauce, 2 Tbsp	70	0	17
Honey Mustard, 2 Tbsp	80	0.5	19
B.B.Q/Sweet & Sour Sce, 2 Tbsp	55	0	14
Dressings: Balsamic Vinaigrette	65	7	1
Creamy Caesar/Ranch	70	7	1
Creamy Thousand Island; French	60	6	2
Light Caesar/Italian	35	2.5	3
Oriental Vinaigrette	60	6	1
Drinks			
Apple/Orange Juice	85	0	22
Coca-Cola Classic®, 12 fl.oz	150	0	39
Diet Coke, 12 fl.oz	1	0	0
Minute Maid Orange Soda, 12 fl.oz	170	0	44
Sprite, 12 fl.oz	135	0	35
Shakes: Choc.; Vanilla, 14.5 fl.oz	370	10	59
Strawberry, 14.5 fl.oz	355	9	56
Desserts: Apple Turnover, 3 oz	245	15	25

Hot Dog on a Stick®

Menu Items			
Fries, 1 order	400	24	41
American Cheese on a Stick	240	13	21
Hot Dog on a Stick	250	14	23
Lemonade, regular, 16 fl.oz	240	0	58
Pepper Jack on a Stick	260	14	23

I Can't Believe It's Yogurt®

Original Frozen Yogurt: Regular Serving (9 fl.oz)			
Awesome Amaretto	280	6	51
Cookies 'N Cream	260	3	54
French Vanilla	260	6	47
Peanut Butter Bliss	310	12	46
White Chocolate Mousse	280	7	49
Nonfat Frozen Yogurt			
Average all flavors: Regular	220	0.5	48
Small, 6.2 fl.oz	160	0	32
Nonfat (w. NutraSweet)			
Average all flavors: Regular	190	0.5	40
Small, 6.2 fl.oz	140	0.5	29

In-N-Out Burger®

	C	**F**	**Cb**
Burgers			
Hamburger	390	19	39
w. Mustard/Ketchup, no Spread	310	10	41
Protein Style, no Bun	240	17	10
Cheeseburger	480	27	39
w. Mustard/Ketchup, no Spread	400	18	41
Protein Style, no Bun	330	25	11
Double Double® (2 patty/2 sl. chse)	670	41	40
w. Mustard/Ketchup, no Spread	590	32	42
Protein Style, no Bun	520	39	11
French Fries, 125g	400	18	54
Drinks: Milk, 10 fl.oz	180	6	18
Coca-Cola®; Dr. Pepper, 16 fl.oz	200	0	54
Diet Coca-Cola®, 16 fl.oz	0	0	0
Lemonade, 16 fl.oz	180	0	40
Root Beer, 16 fl.oz	220	0	60
Seven-Up®, 16 fl.oz	220	0	52
Shakes: Chocolate, 15 fl.oz	690	36	83
Strawberry, 15 fl.oz	690	33	91
Vanilla, 15 fl.oz	680	37	78

International House of Pancakes®

Pancakes: (Syrup/Butter extra)			
Buttermilk, 1 (1.7 oz)	110	3	17
Short Stack, 3	330	9	51
Full Stack, 5	550	15	85
Buckwheat, 1 (1.7 oz)	110	4	15
Country Griddle, 1 (2 oz)	120	3.5	19
Harvest Grain 'N Nut, 1 (2¼ oz)	180	9	20
Crepes (Egg Pancakes), 1 (2 oz)	120	6	14
Syrup: 1 Tbsp	50	0	12
Whipped Butter, 1 Tbsp	80	9	0
Waffles (Plain)			
Regular, 1 (3 oz)	310	15	37
Belgian: Regular, 1 (4 oz)	390	19	48

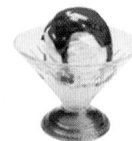

Restaurants & Fast–Foods

Jack in the Box®

Breakfast	C	F	Cb
Biscuit	190	9	24
Breakfast Jack®	310	14	34
Extreme Sausage Sandwich	720	53	35
French Toast Sticks, 4 pces	430	18	57
Hash Brown	150	10	13
Sausage Biscuit	380	27	25
Sausage Croissant	680	50	41
Sausage, Egg & Cheese Biscuit	760	60	33
Sourdough Breakfast Sandwich	450	26	36
Supreme Croissant	570	37	41
Ultimate Breakfast Sandwich	730	40	46
Country Crock Spread	25	3	0
Grape Jelly, 1 packet	35	0	10
Syrup	130	0	32

Burgers	C	F	Cb
Hamburger	250	9	30
Bacon Bacon Cheeseburger	910	58	58
Bacon Ultimate Cheeseburger	1120	75	59
Big Cheeseburger	700	40	59
Big Texas Cheeseburger	610	32	55
Ultimate Cheeseburger	990	66	59
Hamburger w. Cheese	300	13	31
Jack's Western Cheeseburger	660	37	59
Jumbo Jack®: Regular	600	31	58
w. Cheese	690	38	60
Sourdough Jack®	700	49	36

Teriyaki Bowls: Chicken	550	3	103
Soy Sauce	5	0	1

Mexican Food: Monster Taco	280	17	22
Salsa	10	0	2
Taco	180	10	16

Snacks: Onion Rings	500	30	51
Bacon/Cheddar Potato Wedges	750	50	55
Cheese Sticks: 3 piece	240	12	21
5 piece	400	21	35
Chicken Breast Pieces, 5 piece	360	17	24
Curly Fries: Chili Cheese, 8.3 oz	630	40	54
Seasoned, 4.4 oz	400	23	45
French Fries: Regular	330	16	44
Jumbo Fries	410	20	55
Super Scoop	580	28	77
Egg Rolls: 1 piece	130	6	15
3 piece	400	19	44
Fish & Chips	610	31	66
Stuffed Jalapenos: 3 piece	230	13	22
7 piece	530	30	51

Sandwiches	C	F	Cb
Chicken Fajita Pita	330	11	35
Chicken Sandwich	410	21	39
Chicken Supreme	710	39	62
Grilled Chicken Fillet	430	24	34
Jack's Spicy Chicken®	650	31	67
Sourdough Grilled Chicken Club	520	28	33

Salads: No Dressing	C	F	Cb
Garden Chicken	200	9	8
Side Salad	50	3	5

Salad Dressings	C	F	Cb
Blue Cheese, 2 oz	260	26	5
Buttermilk House, 2 oz	310	33	3
Low Calorie Italian, 2 oz	15	0	4
Thousand Island, 2 oz	160	12	12
Croutons, 1/2 oz	60	2	10

Condiments	C	F	Cb
Cheese: American, 1 slice	45	4	1
Swiss-style, 1 slice	40	3	1
Dipping Sauce: Barbeque, 1 oz	45	0	11
Buttermilk House, 1 oz	130	13	3
Frank's Red Hot Buffalo®, 1 oz	10	0	2
Marinara, 1 oz	15	0	3
Sweet & Sour, 1 oz	45	0	11
Tartar	210	22	2
Packet Sauce: Ketchup	10	0	2
Mayonnaise	150	17	0
Mustard	5	0	1
Sour Cream	60	6	1

Desserts	C	F	Cb
Apple Turnover	320	16	41
Cheesecake	310	16	34
Double Fudge Cake	310	11	49
Strawberry Banana Icecream	700	28	100

Icecream Shakes	C	F	Cb
Cappuccino, 16 fl.oz	640	28	85
Chocolate, 16 fl.oz	660	29	89
Oreo Cookie Classic, 16 fl.oz	670	33	81
Strawberry, 16 fl.oz	640	28	84
Vanilla, 16 fl.oz	570	29	65

Drinks	C	F	Cb
Barq's Root Beer®, 20 fl.oz	180	0	50
Coca-Cola Classic®, 20 fl.oz	170	0	46
Dr Pepper®; Minute Maid, 20 fl.oz	190	0	49
Lowfat Milk (2%) 8 fl.oz	140	5	14
Orange Juice, 10 fl.oz	140	0	32
Sprite®, 20 fl.oz	160	0	41

Jamba Juice®

Smoothies: Per 24 fl.oz

	C	F	Cb
Aloha Pineapple™	470	1.5	89
Banana Berry™	470	1.5	112
Berry Lime Sublime™	450	2	104
Caribbean Passion®, Orange-A-Peel	440	2	102
Chocolate Moo'd™	690	8	141
Citrus Squeeze®	450	2	93
Coldbuster™	430	2.5	100
Cranberry Craze®	420	2	97
Grapeberry Crush	390	1.5	91
Jamba Powerboost™	440	1.5	103
Kiwi-Berry® Burner	470	0	104
Mango-A-Go-Go™	500	2	117
Orange Berry Blitz™	410	2.5	94
Orange Dream Machine	540	2.5	112
Peach Pleasure®	460	2	108
Peanut Butter Moo'd™	840	22	139
Peenya Kowlada®	650	5	118
Protein Berry Pizazz™	440	1.5	102
Razzmatazz™	480	2	112
Strawberries Wild™	450	0	105

Jimmy John's®

French Bread Sandwiches: No Mayonnaise.

Big John	330	3	na
Bootlegger Club	435	3.5	na
Bootlegger Club w. Cheese	485	8	na
Ham & Cheese	200	12	na
Roast Beef	365	3	na
The Pepe w. Cheese	370	10	na
Turkey	355	0.5	na
Turkey Tom	320	1	na
Turkey w. Cheese	465	8	na
Turkey Tom w. Cheese	425	8	na

Slim Jims: Figures based on 8" French Bread;
without Mayonnaise or Sauce.

Baked Turkey Breast	355	0.5	60
Double Provolone	515	15	62
Ham & Cheese	405	10	61
Rare Roast Beef	365	3	60
Salami & Capicola	550	18	61
Tuna Salad w. Mayonnaise/Sauce	615	25	67

Gargantuan™ Sandwich
Made on 8" French Bread

w. Cheese, Mayonnaise, Sauce.	890	46	65

Jimmy John's®cont...

Gourmet Subs
Made on 8" French Bread.

	C	F	Cb
Big John w. Mayonnaise	485	20	52
Sorry Charlie w. Mayo/Sauce	575	25	60
The Pepe w. Mayo/Cheese	525	27	53
Turkey Tom w. Mayo	475	18	52
Vegetarian w. Mayo/Cheese	670	36	56
Vito w. Italian Dressing/Cheese	560	23	55

Gourmet Club Sandwiches
Made on 8" French Bread w. Cheese.

Beach Club w. Mayo	775	36	66
Billy Club w. Mayo	650	30	64
Bootlegger's w. Mayo, no Cheese	700	28	63
Country Club w. Mayo	630	27	63
Hunter's Club w. Mayo	710	30	63
Italian Night w. Dressing/Mayo	770	43	65
Smoked Ham Club w. Mayo	575	29	63
Tuna Club w. Mayo/Sauce	845	40	72
Veggie Club w. Mayo	935	51	68

Gourmet Club Sandwiches
Made on 7-Grain Wheat Bread w. Cheese.

Beach Club w. Mayo	825	41	67
Billy Club w. Mayo	695	34	65
Bootlegger's w. Mayo, no Cheese	640	25	63
Country Club w. Mayo	680	32	64
Hunter's Club w. Mayo	760	35	64
Italian Night w. Dressing/Mayo	820	47	66
Smoked Ham Club w. Mayo	625	33	64
Tuna Club w. Mayo/Sauce	895	45	73
Veggie Club w. Mayo	985	55	69

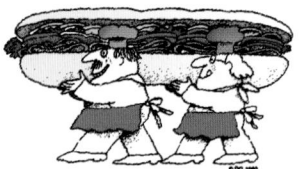

© DG 1992

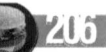

KFC ®

Original Recipe®	C	F	Cb
Breast	340	19	11
Drumstick	140	8	4
Thigh	250	18	6
Whole Wing	145	9	5
Extra Crispy™ : Breast	470	28	19
Drumstick	160	10	5
Thigh	370	26	12
Whole Wing	190	12	10
Hot & Spicy Chicken			
Breast	450	27	20
Drumstick	140	9	4
Thigh	390	28	14
Whole Wing	180	11	9
Other Entrees			
Chunky Pot Pie	770	42	69
Colonels Crispy Strips:			
3 pieces	340	16	20
Blazin, 3 pieces	315	15	21
Honey BBQ, 3 pieces	375	15	33
Spicy, 3 pieces	335	15	23
Popcorn Chicken: Small, 3.5 oz	360	23	21
Large, 6 oz	620	40	36
Wings: Hot Wings™, 6 pieces	470	33	18
Honey BBQ Wings, 6 pces	605	38	33
Sandwiches			
Original Recipe®: w. Sauce	450	22	33
without Sauce	360	13	21
Honey BBQ Crunch Melt	555	26	48
Honey BBQ Flavored Chicken	310	6	37

Sandwiches	C	F	Cb
Triple Crunch®: w. Sauce	490	29	39
without Sauce	390	15	29
Triple Crunch® Zinger: w. Sauce	550	32	39
without Sauce	390	15	36
Tender Roast®: w. Sauce	350	15	26
without Sauce	270	5	23
Twister®	600	34	52
Blazin Twister®	720	43	56
Crispy Caesar Twister®	745	41	66
Side Dishes: Biscuit, 2 oz	180	10	20
BBQ Baked Beans, 5.5 oz	190	3	33
Coleslaw, 5 oz	230	14	26
Corn on the Cob, 5.7 oz	150	1.5	35
Green Beans, 4.7 oz	45	1.5	7
Macaroni & Cheese, 5.4 oz	180	8	21
Mashed Potatoes w. Gravy, 4.8 oz	120	6	17
Mean Greens, 5.4 oz	70	3	11
Potato Salad, 5.6 oz	230	14	23
Potato Wedges, 5.5 oz	375	15	53
Desserts			
Double Choc Chip Cake, 2.7 oz	320	16	41
Little Bucket Parfaits:			
Choc Cream	290	15	37
Fudge Brownie	280	10	44
Lemon Creme	410	14	62
Strawberry Shortcake	200	7	33
Colonels Pies: Apple Pie Slice, 4 oz	310	14	44
Pecan Pie Slice, 4 oz	490	23	66
Strawb. Creme Pie Slice, 2.7 oz	280	15	32

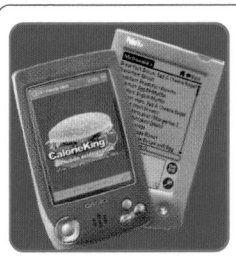

Kenny Rogers Roasters®

	C	F	Cb
Chicken			
1/2 Chicken: No Skin or Wing	315	10	1
w. Skin	515	28	2
1/4 Dark Meat: No Skin	170	7	1
w. Skin	270	17	1
1/4 White Meat: No Skin or Wing	145	2	1
w. Skin	245	11	1
Pies: Chicken Pot Pie	710	33	78
Pitas: BBQ Chicken	400	7	51
Chicken Caesar	605	35	34
Roasted Chicken	685	35	42
Turkey: Sliced Breast	160	2	0
Salads (No Dressing): Per Serving			
Chicken Caesar	285	9	18
Pasta	230	12	28
Roasted Chicken	290	10	19
Side	25	0	5
Sour Cream & Dill Pasta	230	16	20
Tomato Cucumber	125	2	10
Sandwiches: Turkey	385	12	30
Side Dishes: Per Serving			
Cinnamon Apples	200	5	41
Cole Slaw	225	16	18
Corn: on the Cob	70	0.5	14
Cornbread Stuffing	325	19	34
Muffin	175	8	24
Sweet Corn Niblets	115	0.5	28
Creamy Parmesan Spinach	120	6	10
Honey Baked Beans	150	1	32
Italian Green Beans	115	8	10
Macaroni & Cheese	200	6	24
Potatoes: Baked Sweet	265	0	62
Garlic Parsley	260	12	37
Potato Salad	390	27	34
Real Mashed	295	14	39
Rice Pilaf	175	5	43
Steamed Vegetables	50	0	8
Zucchini & Squash Santa Fe	70	5	8
Soup: Chicken Noodle, 1 bowl	90	2	12
Chicken Noodle, 1 cup	55	1	7

Kilwin's®

	C	F	Cb
Icecream: Per 1/2 Cup			
Black Cherry; Caramel Revel	90	0	23
Butter Pecan	190	13	16
Butter Pecan Yogurt	130	6	17
Chocolate	170	10	17
Chocolate Chip Cookie Dough	190	10	22
Chocolate Ripple	100	0	23
French Silk; Mud	190	11	20
Lemon/Raspberry Sorbetto	100	0	25
Old Fashioned Vanilla	180	9	20
Toppings: Caramel, 40g	160	4.5	31
Fudge, 40g	110	6	28
Fudge: Per Piece (40g)			
Butter/Vanilla Pecan	160	5	29
Chocolate	150	4.5	30
Chocolate Peanut Butter	160	5	29
Chocolate Pecan/Walnut; P. Butter	160	6	28
German Chocolate	160	7	27
Heavenly Hash	200	11	24
Walnut Maple	160	5	29
Chocolate Bars: Per 1 oz Bar			
Chocolate Sea Foam, Dark/Milk	190	9	28
Happy Birthday; Teacher; Thank You	160	9	17
Kilwin's Molded	270	13	24
Clusters: Per Serving			
Almond Cluster: Dark (4)	250	19	20
Milk (4)	210	19	17
Cashew Cluster: Dark (4)	190	13	16
Milk (3)	250	16	20
Coconut Cluster: Dark (4)	230	15	24
Milk (4)	210	13	21
Peanut Cluster (3)	220	16	16
Dark/Milk (4)	230	16	19
Pecan Cluster: Dark (4)	240	11	20
Milk (4)	250	18	21
Raisin Cluster: Dark (3)	190	9	28
Milk (4)	170	1	25
Chocolate-Coated Candy: Per Serving			
Coated Almonds: Dark (5); Milk (6)	220	15	20
Coated Brazils: Dark (6)	230	19	14
Milk (7)	250	20	15
Coated Cashews: Dark (6)	220	16	16
Milk (7)	240	17	17
Coated Pecans: Dark (7)	230	20	14
Milk (8)	270	23	17

Koo•Koo•Roo®

Rotisserie Chicken	C	F	Cb
Leg & Thigh, 4.8 oz	300	18	1
Breast & Wing, 6.5 oz	355	16	1
Half Rotisserie Chicken, 11.3 oz	655	34	2

Original Skinless Flame Broiled Chicken™

	C	F	Cb
3 Piece Original Dark	260	15	0
Breast & Wing (skin on wing)	210	8	0
Original Breast, 3.4 oz	155	4	0
Half Original Chkn (skin on wing)	390	16	6

Fresh Roasted Carved Turkey

	C	F	Cb
Turkey Breast S'wich w. Lite Mayo	540	24	31
$^1/_2$ Turkey Brst S'wich w. Lite Mayo	270	12	16
$^1/_4$ lb Sliced White Meat	155	1	0
$^1/_4$ lb Sliced Dark Meat	210	8	0
Open-Faced Turkey Sandwich w. potato, stuffing, gravy, sce	760	35	60
Hand-Carved Turkey Dinner w. pot., veges, stuffing, gravy, sce	880	36	83
Turkey Pot Pie, 5.5 oz	905	45	83

Salads: Per Regular (no dressing)

	C	F	Cb
BBQ Chicken Salad, 15$^1/_2$ oz	370	16	23
Caesar Salad, 9$^1/_3$ oz	105	4	13
Chicken Caesar Salad, 12 oz	180	7	15
Chinese Chicken Salad, 17 oz	420	13	56
Koo Koo Roo House Salad, 16 oz	165	6	21
Chicken Chop Salads:			
Chargrilled: w. Curry Sauce	865	39	65
w/out Sauce	580	11	66
Southwestern, w/out Sauce	635	11	79

Pasta Salads: Pesto Pasta, 4 oz

	C	F	Cb
Pesto Pasta, 4 oz	190	5	24
Tomato Basil Pasta, 4 oz	110	2	19

Soup: Chili Chicken, 4 oz

	C	F	Cb
Chili Chicken, 4 oz	100	2	13
Ten Vegetable, 8 oz	120	3	21
Turkey Dumpling, 8 oz	165	4	14

Sandwiches: Per Sandwich

	C	F	Cb
BBQ Chicken w. Sce	500	16	46
Original Chkn Breast w. Dressing	655	27	64
Chicken Caesar w. Dressing	790	36	65
Turkey Breast w. Lite Mayo	540	24	31
Wraps: Caesar Chicken	840	47	60
Greek Chicken	720	30	66
Firecracker	860	38	87

Cold Sides

	C	F	Cb
Cucumber Salad, 4.5 oz	30	0	7
Creamy Cole Slaw, 5 oz	235	20	14
Lentil Salad, 4.5 oz	175	5	24
Tangy Tomato Salad, 4.5 oz	45	3	6

Hot Sides

	C	F	Cb
Baked Yams, 6 oz	200	0	47
Black Beans, 6 oz	210	3	34
Creamed Spinach, 5 oz	100	7	10
Hand-Mashed Potatoes, 6.5 oz	185	5	32
Macaroni & Cheese, 6 oz	310	11	35
Roasted Garlic Potatoes, 5 oz	145	3	28

Dressings: Per Serving

	C	F	Cb
BBQ, 2 Tbsp	45	2	7
Balsamic Vinaigrette, 2 Tbsp	60	4	4
Caesar, 2 Tbsp	170	19	1
Chinese Chicken Salad, 2 Tbsp	100	8	8
Cranberry Sauce, 1 oz	45	0	11
Gravy, 2 oz	95	10	3
Lahvash (flatbread), each	60	0	12

Kohr Bros®

Frozen Custard: Per $^1/_2$ Cup

	C	F	Cb
Chocolate	140	6	18
Orange Sherbet	105	2	21
Vanilla	130	6	16

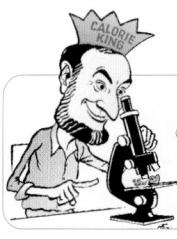

For full nutritional data and product updates check the database of the author's website www.CalorieKing.com

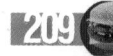

Krispy Kreme®

	C	F	Cb
Yeast Doughnuts			
Per Donut Unless Indicated			
Glazed Rings: Doughnut	200	11	23
Chocolate Iced w. Sprinkles	260	12	36
Chocolate Iced	280	14	6
Maple Iced	250	12	34
Cinnamon Bun	260	16	28
Sugar Doughnut (3)	200	12	1
Cinnamon Twist	230	9	3
Glazed Twist	210	9	8
Cake Doughnuts: Per Donut Unless Indicated			
Traditional Cake Doughnut	220	13	25
Chocolate Iced	270	13	36
Powdered Sugar	260	13	33
Glazed Cruller	240	14	26
Chocolate Iced	280	15	35
Old Fashioned: Sour Cream	280	11	41
Glazed Blueberry	300	15	37
Glazed Devil's Food	390	24	41
Honey & Oat	270	13	36
Vanilla Iced Cake w. Sprinkles	280	13	39
Mini Cake: Plain (4)	250	14	27
Powdered Sugar (3)	210	10	26
Chocolate Enrobed (3)	270	17	26
Filled Doughnuts: Per Donut			
Apple-Filled Cinn. Sugar Coated	280	13	35
Blueberry-Filled Sugar Coated Yeast	270	13	33
Chocolate Iced: Crème-Filled	340	18	39
Custard-Filled	310	16	39
Glazed: Cherry-Filled Yeast	290	14	36
Crème-Filled	350	20	39
Raspberry-Filled	350	21	36
Yeast: Powdered Raspberry-Filled	300	16	36
Vanilla Iced Crème-Filled	360	19	41
Vanilla Iced Custard-Filled	290	16	33
Glazed Lemon-Filled	290	16	34
Glazed Custard-Filled	290	16	34
Powdered Strawberry-Filled	260	16	9
Other Doughnuts/Pies: Honey Bun	410	24	44
Doughnut Holes: Powder Sugar (3)	220	13	23
Glazed (3)	220	13	25
Chocolate Enrobed (3)	270	17	27
Glazed Mini Cruller (1)	230	10	32
Pies: Coconut Crème (1)	450	21	61
Peach (1)	370	17	51
Cherry (1)	410	19	56
Apple (1)	400	19	54

Krystal®

	C	F	Cb
Breakfast			
Biscuit: Plain	260	15	27
Bacon, Egg & Cheese	390	25	28
Chik	340	17	34
Sausage	440	32	27
Country Breakfast	660	42	46
Hash Browns	190	13	17
Sunriser	240	14	14
Sandwiches			
Krystal: Regular	160	7	17
Double	260	13	24
Bacon Cheese	190	10	16
Cheese	180	9	16
Double Cheese	310	16	26
Chik	240	11	24
Chili	200	7	22
Chili Cheese Pup	210	12	17
Corn Pup	260	19	19
Plain Pup	170	9	15
Fries			
Regular	370	18	49
Chili Cheese	540	28	59
Desserts/Drinks			
Chocolate Shake	380	11	58
Krystal Chill	200	7	22
Apple Turnover	220	10	31
Lemon Meringue Pie	360	10	60

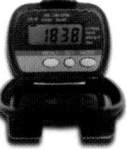

La Rosa's®

Pan Crust Small Pizza: Per Slice	C	F	Cb
Blanca, small	250	16	18
Cheese	220	13	19
Deluxe/Pepperoni Topper	260	17	19
Meat Topper	280	18	19
Veggie Topper	250	15	21

Pan Crust Medium Pizza: Per Slice	C	F	Cb
Blanca, medium	350	22	28
Cheese	300	16	30
Deluxe/Pepperoni Topper	370	21	31
Meat Topper	400	23	30
Veggie Topper	320	16	32

Pan Crust Large Pizza: Per Slice	C	F	Cb
Blanca, large	570	34	45
Cheese	480	24	49
Deluxe Topper	590	23	50
Meat Topper	630	37	49
Pepperoni Topper	590	34	49
Veggie Topper	510	25	52

Traditional Crust Small Pizza: Per Slice	C	F	Cb
Blanca, small	220	13	15
Cheese	180	9	17
Deluxe/Pepperoni Topper	230	14	17
Meat Topper	250	15	17
Veggie Topper	190	9	19

Traditional Crust Medium Pizza: Per Slice	C	F	Cb
Blanca, medium	260	16	17
Cheese	200	10	19
Deluxe/Pepperoni Topper	280	16	20
Meat Topper	300	18	20
Veggie Topper	220	11	21

Traditional Crust Large Pizza: Per Slice	C	F	Cb
Blanca, large	280	17	18
Cheese	210	10	20
Deluxe/Pepperoni Topper	290	17	21
Meat Topper	310	19	21
Veggie Topper	230	11	22

Focaccia Style Small Pizza: Per Slice (1/6 Pizza)	C	F	Cb
Cheese/Florentine, small	150	9	13
Roma	180	12	13

Focaccia Style Med. Pizza: Per Slice (1/10 Pizza)	C	F	Cb
Cheese, medium	230	12	23
Florentine	240	13	24
Roma	300	18	23

Calzones: Per Slice (1/3 Whole)	C	F	Cb
3 Meat & 3 Cheese	1080	55	102
3 Veggie & 3 Cheese	438	34	105
Cheese	840	34	101
Cheese & Pepperoni	960	45	101
Cheese Steak	1020	54	93

Focaccia Style Large Pizza: Per Slice (1/12 Pizza)	C	F	Cb
Cheese, large	310	17	31
Florentine	330	17	33
Roma	400	24	21

Super Crust Small Pizza: Per Slice	C	F	Cb
Blanca, small	230	11	22
Cheese	200	7	24
Deluxe/Pepperoni Topper	250	12	25
Meat Topper	270	14	24
Veggie Topper	210	8	26

Super Crust Medium Pizza: Per Slice	C	F	Cb
Blanca, medium	270	15	23
Cheese	220	8	25
Deluxe/Pepperoni Topper	290	15	26
Meat Topper	310	16	25
Veggie Topper	230	9	27

Super Crust Large Pizza: Per Slice	C	F	Cb
Blanca, large	430	23	36
Cheese	340	13	40
Deluxe/Pepperoni Topper	450	23	41
Meat Topper	490	26	40
Veggie Topper	370	14	43

Hoagy (no cheese/dressing)	C	F	Cb
Baked Buddy	710	40	53
Chargrilled Chicken Hoagy	540	10	62
Double Royal Hoagy	920	55	55
Double Steak Hoagy	440	49	54
Filet of Haddock	630	25	62
Meatball Hoagy	590	28	57
Royal Hoagy	610	30	55
Steak Hoagy	560	27	52
Tuna Fish Hoagy	630	32	61
Hoagy Dressing: Chse on Hoagy	230	18	0
Italian Dressing	320	34	3
Mayonnaise	100	11	0
Mushroom Sauce	20	0.5	3
Pizza Sauce	50	2	7
Tartar Sauce	260	24	11

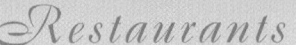

La Rosa's® cont...

C **F** **Cb**

Lite & Low Fat Menu

	C	F	Cb
Grilled Chicken Hoagy, low fat	540	10	62
Grilled Chicken Salad, low fat	380	10	40
Lite Deluxe Pizza: Small, 1 slice	170	5	25
Medium, 1 slice	190	6	27
Large, 1 slice	300	13	26
Minestrone Soup, 1 bowl	80	1	15

Pasta Dinner (Entree): Per Serving

Cheese Ravioli	460	19	53
Lasagna	610	33	48
Meat Ravioli	440	16	54
Spaghetti: w. Meat Sauce	680	18	104
w. Meatballs	890	33	113
w. Sauce	580	10	106

Chicken Wings: Per Serving

Special Recipe Wings (12)	1160	94	16
Spicy Hot Wings (12)	1180	94	22
Dressing: Blue/Ranch, 1.5 oz	230	24	2

Fresh Baked Bread: Per Serving

Garlic Bread, 2 slices	240	9	35
w. Cheese (2)	390	21	35
Garlic Bread Sticks (5)	740	26	109
w. Cheese (5)	1030	49	109
Sauces: Garlic Dipping Sauce	360	40	0
Pizza Sauce	50	2	7
Rolls: Plain Dinner Roll	150	0.5	31
Seasoned Garlic Roll	230	8	32

Salad (No Dressing)

Antipasto Meal	260	19	8
Chargrilled Chicken Salad Meal	380	10	40
Tossed Garden Salad	210	13	14
Tuna Salad Meal	760	48	50

Salad Dressing: Per Packet

La Rosa's Italian	230	26	2
Marzetti Blue Cheese	220	24	2
Marzetti Buttermilk Ranch	260	29	1
Marzetti Creamy Caesar	200	22	2
Marzetti Fat Free Honey Dijon	70	0	16
Marzetti Fat Free Italian	20	0	5
Marzetti Fat Free Ranch	40	0	10
Marzetti Honey French	210	18	14
Marzetti Thousand Island	220	21	7

Soup

Minestrone, 12 oz	130	2	22

La Salsa Fresh Mexican Grill®

C **F** **Cb**

Burritos: Includes Cheese, Sauce, Salad

	C	F	Cb
Baja Fish Burrito	490	12	6
Bean & Cheese	630	19	87
California Burrito	780	30	100
El Champion	460	19	20
Fajita Burrito Chicken	760	29	81
Grande Chicken	870	32	102
Los Cabos Shrimp Burrito	790	36	86
Original Gourmet: Chicken	600	25	61
Steak	600	27	60
Sonoran Fish Burrito	190	8	3

Taco Baskets: Includes Cheese, Sauce, 2 Tacos

Baja Style: Fish	790	48	59
Shrimp	490	10	9
Chicken Taquitos, 1 plate	780	41	57
La Salsa: Chicken	500	15	55
Beef	500	19	54
Mexico City: Chicken	380	6	53
Beef	380	10	52
Sonoran Style Fish	430	17	34

Favorites: Includes Cheese & Sauce

Caesar Salad	780	30	100
Chile-Lime Salad	630	19	87
Classic Quesadilla	600	25	61
Nachos, 1 order	760	29	81
Taco Salad	870	32	102

Platters: Burrito Ranchero

Burrito Ranchero	950	33	120
Carne Asado Platter	720	20	96
Enchilada Platter: Cheese	990	51	91
Chicken	810	28	92
Pollo Asado Platter	720	15	97
Taquitos & Quesadilla	1700	89	147
Two Soft Tacos Platter:			
Mexico City Beef	690	16	107
Mexico City Chicken	690	13	108

By Themselves

Baja Style Fish Taco w. Cheese	400	24	29
Baja Style Shrimp Taco w. Cheese	400	27	30
Black Beans, 1 cup	310	3	54
Chicken Taco La Salsa w. Cheese	250	8	28
Mexico City Chicken Taco w. Chse	190	3	27
Rice, Seasoned, 1 cup	220	3	43
Rice & Black Beans, 1 portion	320	2.5	60
Sonoran Style Fish Taco w. Cheese	210	9	17

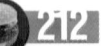

Lamar's®

	C	F	Cb
Bars			
Caramel Iced, Unfilled	430	18	59
Chocolate Iced: Unfilled	540	22	81
Bavarian Cream Filled	600	22	96
Chocolate Fluff Filled	800	35	118
White Fluff Filled	810	35	120
Bizmarks			
Bavarian Cream	620	22	101
Blueberry/Lemon Filled	530	21	80
Cherry Filled	550	19	88
Donuts			
Apple Spice Cake	340	17	44
Bluberry Cake	350	17	47
Chocolate Iced Cake	330	18	37
Old Fashioned Sour Cream	420	18	60
Ray's Chocolate Glazed	290	11	44
Ray's Original Glazed	220	10	31
Other Menu Items			
Apple Fritter	650	26	91
White Iced Cake	320	17	38
German Chocolate Knot	480	27	54
Cinnamon Roll	690	25	106
Cinnamon Roll Raisin Nut	850	27	137
Cinnamon Twist	770	26	120

Little Caesar's®

	C	F	Cb
Pizza: Per Slice			
12" Round: Cheese	160	6	22
Pepperoni	180	8	21
12" Square: Cheese	140	5	19
Pepperoni	160	6	19
12" Thin: Cheese	120	6	12
Pepperoni	150	8	12
14" Round: Cheese	170	6	23
Meatsa	220	10	24
Pepperoni	200	8	23
Supreme	230	10	25
Veggie	190	7	25
14" Square: Cheese	140	5	19
Pepperoni	160	7	19
14" Thin: Cheese	130	6	13
Pepperoni	160	9	13
16" Round: Cheese	230	8	30
Pepperoni	260	11	31
18" Round: Cheese	240	8	30
Pepperoni	270	11	32
Baby Pan! Pan!	310	15	32
Pizza By The Slice: Cheese	290	10	39
Pepperoni	340	14	39
Sandwiches (Cold): Italia	690	32	68
Ham & Chse; Turkey	600	22	68
Tuna	820	39	71
Veggie	720	38	71
Sandwiches (Hot): Meatsa	960	53	72
Pepperoni	980	56	71
Supreme; Cheeser	900	49	74
Vegetarian	760	36	74
Salads: Antipasto	130	7	10
Caesar; Greek	80	3	7
Tossed Salad	50	0.5	9
Dresssings: Caesar, 1 oz	230	25	1
Buttermilk Ranch, 1 oz	270	29	1
Crmy Caesar; Golden Ital.; Blue Chse	220	23	2
Fat Free Italian, 1 oz	25	0	5
Honey French, 1 oz	220	18	14
Thousand Island, 1 oz	220	21	7
Sides: Chicken Wings, 1 piece	50	4	0
Crazy Bread, 1 stick, 1.2 oz	90	2.5	14
Crazy Sauce, 4 oz	45	0	9
Italian Cheese Bread, 1 piece	120	6	12
Cinnamon Stick	340	9	57

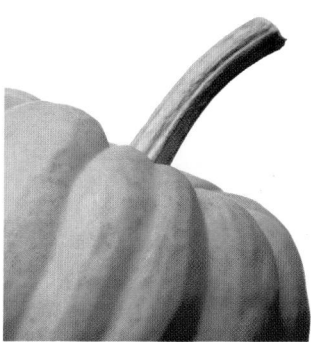

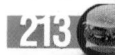

Fast-Foods & *Restaurants*

Long John Silver's®

Sandwiches	C	F	Cb
Ultimate Fish	480	25	46
Fish Sandwich	430	20	46
w. Cheese	480	25	46
Chicken Sandwich	340	14	40
w. Cheese	390	19	40

Side Items	C	F	Cb
Fries: Regular	250	15	28
Large, 5 oz	420	24	46
Cheese Sticks (3)	160	9	12
Coleslaw, 4 oz	170	7	23
Corn Cobbette: no butter	80	0.5	19
w. butter	140	8	19
Hushpuppy, 1 piece	60	2.5	9
Rice, 4 oz	180	4	34

Soup: Broccoli Cheese, 8 oz bowl	180	12	13
Clam Chowder: 1 cup	260	12	26
1 bowl	520	24	52

Salads: Garden Salad	45	0	9
Grilled Chicken Salad	140	2.5	11
Ocean Chef Salad	130	2	15
Side Salad, no dressing	20	0	3
Dressing: Italian, 1 pkt	90	9	2
Ranch, 1 pkt	170	18	1
Ranch, Fat Free, 1 pkt	40	0	9
Thousand Island, 1 pkt	120	10	5
French, Fat Free, 1 pkt	40	0	10

Chicken: Battered Plank, 1 piece	140	8	9

Fish	C	F	Cb
Breaded Clams, 1 order	250	14	26
Battered Shrimp, 1 piece	45	2.5	3
Country Style Breaded Fish, 1 pce	200	10	17
Crabcake, 1 cake	150	9	12
Lemon Crumbed: Regular, 2 pces	240	12	10
A-la-carte, 2 pces w. rice	480	17	52
Add-A-Piece (1) w.rice	150	7	9
Fish Meal, 1 meal	730	29	89
Popcorn Shrimp, 1 serving	320	15	33

Condiments	C	F	Cb
Honey Mustard Sauce, 1 pkt	20	0	5
Ketchup, 1 pkt	10	0	2
Malt Vinegar, 1 pkt	0	0	0
Shrimp Sauce, 1 pkt	15	0	3
Sweet & Sour Sauce, 1 pkt	20	0	5
Tartar Sauce, 1 pkt	40	3.5	2

Desserts: Per Piece	C	F	Cb
Banana Split Sundae Pie	300	17	34
Chocolate Créme Pie	280	17	29
Double Lemon Pie	350	18	41
Dutch Apple Pie	290	13	44
Pecan Pie	390	19	53
Pineapple Créme Cheesecake	310	17	36
Strawberries N' Créme Pie	280	15	32

Beverages: Per Medium	C	F	Cb
Coca-Cola	270	0	62
Diet Coke	0	0	0
Dr Pepper	250	0	69
Hi-C Pink Lemonade	260	0	62
Minute Maid Lemonade	260	0	69
Sprite	260	0	62

Maggie Moo's Icecream & Treatery®

Icecream: Per 1/2 Cup	C	F	Cb
No Sugar Added 10%	140	8	18
Non Fat	100	0	21

Sorbet: Per 1/2 Cup	C	F	Cb
Non Fat Non Dairy	90	0	22

Yogurt: Per 1/2 Cup	C	F	Cb
Non Fat	100	0	20
Non Fat No Sugar Added	60	0	11

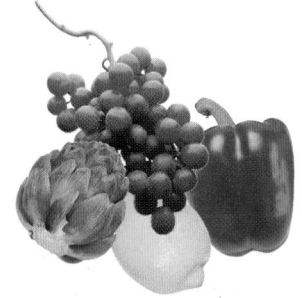

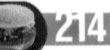

Restaurants & Fast-Foods

McDonald's®

Burgers/Sandwiches	C	F	Cb
Big Mac®	590	34	47
Big N' Tasty®	540	32	39
with Cheese	590	37	40
BBQ Chicken Sandwich	340	8	48
Cheeseburger	330	14	36
Chicken Fajita: w. Cheese	190	7	21
w/out Cheese	170	6	19
Chicken McGrill®	400	17	37
Plain (no mayo)	300	6	37
Crispy Chicken	500	26	46
Double Cheeseburger	480	27	37
Filet-O-Fish®	470	26	45
Hamburger	280	10	35
Homestyle Burger	450	20	44
McChicken Sandwich	520	23	54
w/out Cheese	390	12	52
w/out Cheese or Sauce	330	6	51
w/out Sauce	460	16	53
Quarter Pounder®	430	21	37
with Cheese	530	30	38
Sourdough Crispy Chicken	580	29	54
Sourdough Supreme Burger	660	40	44

French Fries	C	F	Cb
Small, 2.4 oz	210	10	26
Medium, 5 oz	450	22	57
Large, 6 oz	540	26	68
Super Size, 7 oz	610	29	77

Chicken McNuggets®/Sauces	C	F	Cb
Chicken McNuggets®: 4 pieces	210	13	12
6 pieces	310	20	18
9 pieces	460	29	27
Chicken Select Strips: 4 pieces	310	16	19
6 pieces	470	23	29
Sauce: BBQ, 1 oz pkg	50	0	11
Honey (1 pkg), $^{1}/_2$ oz	45	0	12
Honey Mustard (1 pkg), $^{1}/_2$ oz	50	4.5	3
Hot Mustard (1 pkg), 1 oz	60	3.5	7
Light Mayonnaise (1 pkg)	45	4.5	1
Sweet 'N' Sour	50	0	11

Muffins/Danishes: Per Serving	C	F	Cb
Apple Danish	340	15	47
Cheese Danish, 3.7 oz	400	21	45
Cinnamon Roll, 3.4 oz	390	18	50
Lowfat Apple Bran Muffin, 4 oz	300	3	61

Breakfast Menu: Per Serving	C	F	Cb
Bacon, Egg & Cheese Biscuit	480	31	31
Biscuit, 2.7 oz	240	11	30
Breakfast Sourdough	560	33	41
Chorizo & Egg Breakfast Burrito	290	16	24
Egg McMuffin®	300	12	29
English Muffin, 2 oz	150	2	27
Ham, Egg & Cheese Bagel	550	23	58
Hash Browns, 2 oz	130	8	14
Hotcakes: Plain, (3)	340	8	58
w. Margarine, 2 pats	420	17	56
w. Margarine, 2 pats & Syrup (1)	600	17	104
Sausage Biscuit	410	28	30
with Egg	490	33	31
Sausage Breakfast Burrito, 4 oz	290	16	24
Sausage McMuffin®	370	23	28
with Egg	450	28	29
Sausage Patty, 1.5 oz	170	16	0
Scrambled Eggs (2), $3^{1}/_2$ oz	160	11	1
Spanish Omelete Bagel	690	38	60
Steak, Egg & Cheese Bagel	700	35	57

McSalad Shaker™ Salads/Dressings	C	F	Cb
Chef Salad	150	8	5
Garden Salad	100	6	4
Grilled Chicken Caesar Salad	100	2.5	3
Croutons (1 pkg)	50	1	9
Dressings: Caesar (1 pkg), $1^{1}/_2$ oz	150	13	5
Fat-Free Herb Vinaigrette (1 pkg)	35	0	8
Honey Mustard (1 pkg)	160	11	13
Ranch Dressing (1 pkg)	170	18	3
Red French Red. Calorie (1 pkg)	130	6	18
Thousand Island (1 pkg)	130	9	11

Desserts/Cookies	C	F	Cb
Baked Apple Pie, $2^{3}/_4$ oz	260	13	34
Chocolate Chip Cookies, 1 bag	280	14	37
Fruit 'n Yogurt Parfait:			
w. Granola	380	5	76
w/out Granola	280	4	53
McDonaldland® Cookies, 2 oz bag	230	8	38
McFlurry™: Butterfinger®	620	22	90
M&M®	630	23	90
Nestlé Crunch®	630	24	89
Oreo®	570	20	82

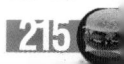

Fast-Foods & *Restaurants*

McDonald's® cont...

	C	**F**	**Cb**
Sundaes/Cone			
Sundae: Hot Caramel Sundae	360	10	61
Hot Fudge Sundae, 6.3 oz	340	12	52
Strawberry Sundae	290	7	50
Nuts (Sundae/Topping), 1/4 oz	40	3.5	2
Cone: Vanilla Reduced Fat	150	4.5	23
Drinks			
1% Lowfat Milk, 8 fl.oz ctn	100	2.5	13
Orange Juice, 16 fl.oz	180	0	42
Root Beer Float, 16 fl.oz	310	7	57
Thick Creamy Shakes:			
Chocolate, 16 fl.oz cup	580	17	94
Strawberry, 16 fl.oz cup	560	16	89
Vanilla, 16 fl.oz cup	570	16	89
Coca-Cola Classic® (25% Ice):			
Childs, 12 fl.oz	110	0	29
Small, 16 fl.oz	150	0	40
Medium, 21 fl.oz	210	0	58
Large, 32 fl.oz	310	0	86
Super Size, 42 fl.oz	410	0	113
Diet Coke (25% Ice):			
Childs, 12 fl.oz	1	0	0
Small, 16 fl.oz	2	0	0
Medium, 21 fl.oz	3	0	0
Large, 32 fl.oz	4	0	29
Sprite(25% Ice): Small, 16 fl.oz	150	0	39
Childs, 12 fl.oz	110	0	28
Medium, 21 fl.oz	210	0	56
Large, 32 fl. oz	310	0	83
Super Size, 42 fl.oz	410	0	109
Hi-C Orange Drink:			
Small, 16 fl.oz	160	0	44
Childs, 12 fl.oz	120	0	32
Medium, 21 fl.oz	240	0	64
Large, 32 fl.oz	350	0	94
Super Size, 42 fl.oz	460	0	124

Mazzio's® Pizza

	C	**F**	**Cb**
Pizza: Per Slice (1/8 Medium Pizza)			
Cheese: Thin Crust	160	9	18
Original Crust	180	6	29
Deep Pan Crust	310	16	37
Large Pizzeria Crust	320	15	42
Pepperoni: Thin Crust	160	10	18
Original Crust	230	11	29
Deep Pan Crust	320	16	37
Large Pizzeria Crust	330	15	42
Sausage: Thin Crust	190	12	19
Original Crust	250	12	30
Deep Pan Crust	350	19	38
Large Pizzeria Crust	380	20	43
Combo: Thin Crust	200	13	20
Original Crust	250	12	31
Deep Pan Crust	350	19	39
Large Pizzeria Crust	370	19	44
Supremebuster: Thin Crust	190	11	19
Original Crust	240	11	30
Deep Pan Crust	340	18	38
Large Pizzeria Crust	360	18	43
Meatbuster: Thin Crust	220	14	19
Original Crust	270	14	30
Deep Pan	370	21	38
Large, Pizzeria Crust	410	22	43
Chicken Club: Thin Crust	180	8	19
Original Crust	250	10	30
Deep Pan Crust	350	17	38
Large Pizzeria Crust	360	15	40
California Alfredo: Thin Crust	210	14	17
Original Crust	260	13	28
Deep Pan Crust	370	20	36
Large Pizzeria Crust	390	20	41
Mexican: Thin Crust	280	14	25
Original Crust	330	13	36
Deep Pan Crust	440	22	44
Large Pizzeria Crust	490	21	52
"Mazzio's Works": Thin Crust	220	14	20
Original Crust	270	14	31
Deep Pan Crust	380	21	39
Large Pizzeria Crust	410	22	44
Appetizers: Per Serving			
Cheese Nachos, 1/2 container	440	10	19
Cheese Dippers, 1/4 container	330	16	38
Wings of Fire: Large	370	28	2
Small	360	26	3

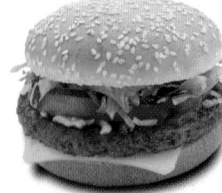

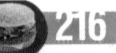

Mazzio's® cont...

C F Cb

Appetizers (Cont): Per Serving

	C	F	Cb
Cinnamon Sticks, 3.2 oz	350	16	45
Breadsticks, 2.8 oz	120	2.5	25
Meat Nachos, 5 oz	520	18	20

Pasta: Per Serving

	C	F	Cb
Calzone: Pepperoni, 1/10 whole	240	8	33
Ham-Bacon-Cheddar, 1/10 whole	280	8	32
Fettuccine Alfredo, 14.7 oz	1320	42	195
Italian Sampler, 24 oz	1640	57	218
Lasagne w. Meat Sauce, 16 oz	700	36	60
Spaghetti: w. Meatballs, 21 oz	1560	53	206
w. Meat Sauce, 17 oz	1210	26	200
w. Marinara, 16 oz	940	10	208

Mimi's Cafe®

Menu Items: Per Serving

Broiled 10 oz Halibut Steak	625	16	51
Capellini w. Tomatoes & Basil	680	8	130
EggBeater Fitness Omelette	655	8	110
Half-A-Turkey Sandwich	410	6	55
Maggie's Chicken and Fruit	545	9	59
Roasted Turkey Breast	540	8	52
Two "AA" Large Eggs	395	8	62

Mrs Winners Chicken®

Menu Items

Biscuit	245	5	45
Chicken: Baked Chicken Fillet	120	2	0.5
Breaded Chicken Sandwich	205	10	12
Chicken Fillet Sandwich	380	7	45
Chicken Salad	585	8	39
Chicken Salad Sandwich	315	6	33
Coleslaw	190	16	9
Potato Fries	225	9	27
Seafood Salad	555	9	41
Steak Sandwich	540	11	43

Mrs Fields Cookies®

C F Cb

Per 1 Cookie, 1.7 oz

	C	F	Cb
Butter; Butter Toffee	220	10	30
Chewy Fudge	220	11	30
Cinnamon Sugar	300	12	41
Coconut Macadamia	280	13	39
Debra's Special	280	12	39
Milk Choc	230	11	29
Milk Choc w. Walnuts/Macadamia	320	18	36
Milk Chocolate Chip	280	13	38
Oatmeal Chocolate Chip	280	13	40
Oatmeal Raisin	180	7	29
Peanut Butter	310	16	36
Peanut Butter Milk Chocolate	300	17	35
Pumpkin Harvest	200	10	24
Semi-Sweet Chocolate	280	14	32
w. Pecans/Walnuts	310	16	38
Triple Chocolate	220	10	31
White Chunk Macadamia	310	17	37

Bite Size Nibbler™: Per 2 Cookies, 1 oz

Butter	110	4.5	15
Chewy Chocolate Fudge	110	5	15
Cinnamon Sugar	120	4.5	17
Debra's Special	100	4.5	13
Milk Choc w. Walnuts	120	6	14
Peanut Butter; Triple Choc	110	6	13
Milk/Semi-Sweet Chocolate	110	5	15
White Chunk Macadamia	120	7	13

Brownies: Each (76g)

Double Fudge	360	19	49
Frosted Fudge	440	21	62
Pecan/Walnut Fudge	380	23	45
Pecan Pie Brownie	390	24	40

Bundt Cakes: Per Piece (83g)

Banana Walnut	350	21	35
Banana Walnut w. Choc Chip	370	22	39
Blueberry	270	12	36
Raspberry	270	12	36

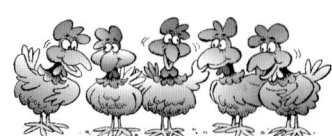

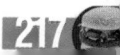

Mr Sub®

Breads and Wraps	C	F	Cb
Cheese Tortilla, 2.6 oz	235	8	34
Harvest Wheat, reg., 4.9 oz	380	4.5	70
Hearty Multi-Grain, reg., 5 oz	370	5	69
Mozza Cheddar, reg., 5.6 oz	435	8	70
Spinach Tortilla, 2.6 oz	225	5.5	37
Sundried Tomato Tortilla, 2.6 oz	220	5	37
Traditional, regular, 4.9 oz	370	3	70
Whole Wheat Tortilla, 2.6 oz	215	5.5	37
Cheese (Processed), 1 slice	85	6	3

Classic Subs: Per Regular Sub	C	F	Cb
Assorted	665	20	82
Ham	500	6	87
Meatball	735	26	78
Pizza	590	21	72
Salami	570	18	74
Vegetarian	395	3	73

Premium Subs: Per Regular Sub	C	F	Cb
Breaded Chicken	755	20	100
Canadian Club	555	11	78
Grilled Chicken	570	7	80
Louisiana Chicken	585	14	71
Seafood with Crab	515	5	89
Steak & Cheese	615	16	70

Specialty Subs: Per Regular Sub	C	F	Cb
BBQ Rib	695	26	73
BLT	540	14	75
Corned Beef	230	3.5	35
Roast Beef	500	9	70
Tuna	565	9	81
Turkey	235	2.5	37

Wraps: Louisiana Chicken	C	F	Cb
Louisiana Chicken	360	12	39
Roast Beef	300	8	38
Seafood with Crab	325	5.5	52
Steak & Cheese	370	12	38
Tuna	365	9	46
Turkey	285	5.5	41

Sauces: Per 1/2 oz	C	F	Cb
BBQ Sauce	17	0	44
Louisiana	9	0	2
MR SUB Secret Sauce	80	9	0
Mayo Lite	60	5	2
Meatball	13	0	3
Pizza	12	0.5	2
Steak	18	0	5

Soups and Chili	C	F	Cb
Bean and Spring Vegetable	124	1	23
Caribbean and Black Bean	111	0.5	22
Chicken Noodle	95	2	14
Chili with Beef	185	1	31
Clam Chowder	175	8	21
Cream of Mushroom	65	1	10
Cream of Potato and Leek	170	8	20
French Canadian Pea	145	2.5	23
Garden Vegetable	50	0.5	11
Italian Wedding Style	125	3	21
Minestrone	80	0.5	15
Pasta Fagioli	140	1	25
Vegetable Beef and Barley	85	1	16

Salads	C	F	Cb
Garden, 5.6 oz	30	0	2
Julienne, 7.2 oz	95	3	8
Louisiana Chicken, 7.5 oz	160	8	1
Seafood with Crab, 8.6 oz	130	1.5	16
Tuna Salad, 8.6 oz	160	4.5	8

Cookies	C	F	Cb
Gourmet Choc. Chunk	180	10	21
Gourmet Double Chocolate Chip	180	10	21
Gourmet Oatmeal Raisin	160	6	24

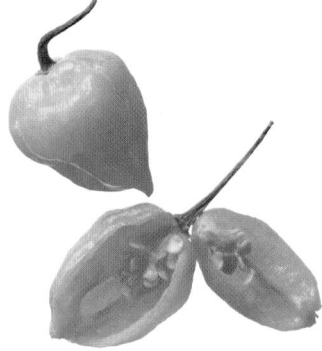

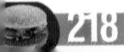

Restaurants & Fast-Foods

Nathan's Famous®

Hamburgers	C	F	Cb
Regular	435	23	32
Double Burger	670	41	32
Super Burger	535	32	34

Sandwiches			
Chicken Salad	155	4	9
Breaded Chicken Sandwich	510	25	48
Charbroiled Chicken S'wich	290	6	35
Cheese Steak Sandwich	485	26	37
Fillet of Fish S'wich	405	15	46
Pastrami Sandwich	325	12	34
Turkey Sandwich	270	2	34

Platters			
Fried Clam	1025	51	119
Chicken: 2 pieces	1095	66	72
4 pieces	1790	109	99
Fillet of Fish	1455	74	137
Fried Shrimp	795	34	100

Sides			
French Fries	515	26	62
Frank Nuggets (7)	360	24	25
Frankfurter	310	19	22

Olive Garden®

Lunch			
Capellini Pomodora, 13 oz	350	11	52
Chicken Giardino, 15.5 oz	350	7	40
Linguine alla Marinara, 10.6 oz	280	6	48
Shrimp Primavera, 19 oz	490	15	65

Dinner			
Chicken Giardino, 21.5 oz	460	8	59
Capellini Pomodora, 21 oz	560	18	84
Linguine alla Marinara, 17 oz	450	9	79
Shrimp Primavera, 26 oz	730	25	84

Extras			
Minestrone Soup, 6 fl.oz	100	1	18
Breadstick, plain, 1 stick	140	1.5	26

(The) Old Spaghetti Factory®

Entrees	C	F	Cb
Fettuccine Alfredo	1140	87	61
Spaghetti Pot Pourri	990	40	110
Spaghetti: w. Clam Sauce	720	33	82
w. Clam/Meat Sauce	620	22	84
w. Clam/Mushroom Sauce	580	20	83
w. Meat Sauce	520	11	85
w. Meatballs/Tomato Sauce	720	18	95
w. Mizithra Cheese	910	57	76
w. Mizithra/Clam Sauce	810	45	79
w. Mizithra/Meat Sauce	720	34	80
w. Mizithra/Mushr./Tomato Sce	680	32	79
w. Mushroom/Meat Sauce	490	9	84
w. Mushroom/Tomato Sauce	450	6	83
w. Sausage/Meat Sauce	730	25	86
w. Tomato Sauce	440	5	84
w. Tomato/Clam Sauce	570	19	83
w. Tomato/Meat Sauce	480	8	84

Salad Dressing: Per 1 1/2 oz			
1000 Island Dressing	180	17	5
Balsamic Vinaigrette	160	17	5
Blue Cheese; Crmy Pesto Dressing	205	21	2
Caesar Dressing	270	29	1
Honey Mustard	40	0	9

Panda Express®

Chicken: Black Pepper, 5 oz	210	10	11
Orange Chicken, 5 oz	310	13	31
Chicken w. Mushrooms, 5 oz	170	9	9
Chicken w. String Beans, 5 oz	180	9	12
Spicy Chicken w. Peanuts, 5 oz	510	29	28
Beef: Beef & Broccoli, 5 oz	180	11	13
Pork: Sweet & Sour Pork, 4 oz	310	20	8
Sweet & Sour Sauce, 2 oz	60	0	16
Vegetables: Mixed Veges, 5 oz	80	3	11
Soups: Hot & Sour Soup, 12 oz	110	4	13
Egg Flower Soup, 12 oz	80	0	18

Chow Mein & Rice: Per 8 oz Serve			
Vegetable Fried Rice	410	19	47
Steamed Rice	220	0	48
Lo Mein	270	10	37
Vegetable Chow Mein	300	10	43
Egg Rolls: 2 pieces, 3 oz	190	6	30

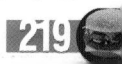

Fast-Foods & *Restaurants*

1-Potato-2®

Per Baked Potato (No Skin)

	C	F	Cb
Ultra-Lites			
Chicken Stir-Fry	330	3	62
Chicken Fajita; Carribean Chicken	270	1.5	49
Chick, Mushroom, Rst Red Pepper	245	2	45
Crab & Broccoli DeLite	335	2.5	57
Vegie & Herb Cheese	240	1.5	44
Lite Potatoes			
Chicken Caesar & Broccoli	375	12	50
Herb Roasted Vegetable	260	6	48
Fresh Mex Chckn; Spinach Souffle	320	9	45
Gourmet Potatoes			
BBQ Chick, Cheddar, Bacon	685	43	44
Bacon & Cheese	660	47	39
Bacon Double Cheeseburger	765	54	40
Broccoli & Cheese	545	36	45
Chicken Broccoli & Chedd.; 3 Chse	590	37	45
Chicken Caesar & Broccoli	710	51	53
Crab, Broccoli & Cheese	595	35	45
Mexican	670	46	50
Philly Steak & Cheese	675	40	45
Potato Skins (with Sour Cream)			
Bacon 'n Cheddar, 9 oz	975	53	100
Southwestern, 11 oz	910	46	105
Fries: Fresh Cut Fries, Small, 13 oz	615	39	60
Fresh Fries 'n Chicken Tenders	920	50	92
Topped Fries, Nacho Cheese	840	54	80
Soups: Baked Potato Soup, 13 oz	640	26	81
Broccoli & Chse Potato Soup, 13 oz	665	29	80
Country Skillets			
Idaho "Nachos"	1010	60	88
BBQ Chick, Cheddar & Bacon	890	57	70
Bacon, Ranch & Cheddar	1090	74	87

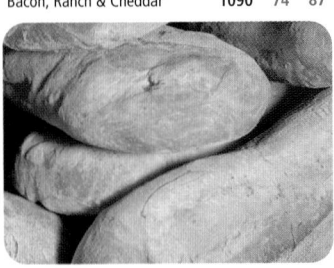

Panera Bread®

	C	F	Cb
Bagels			
Asiago	330	5	57
Blueberry; Cinnamon Raisin	330	1	70
Chocolate Chip	360	6	67
Cinnamon Crunch	510	9	95
Dutch Apple & Raisin	350	2.5	73
Everything	300	1.5	60
Morning Glory	380	7	71
Plain; Multigrain; Sesame	300	1.5	61
Salad: Per Container			
Caesar Salad	380	25	22
Caesar w. Chicken	480	27	24
Chicken Oriental	550	33	39
Classic Cafe	400	36	12
Fandango	400	28	23
Greek	480	45	15
Sandwiches: Cheese	730	44	48
Asiago Roast Beef	730	35	54
Bacon Turkey Bravo	860	34	84
Chicken Salad	480	24	37
Grilled Chicken	590	16	47
Italian Combo	1040	39	110
Peanut Butter & Jelly	440	16	64
Sierra Turkey	760	44	68
Smoked Ham & Cheese	640	33	47
Smoked Turkey	460	15	46
Tuna Salad	760	44	63
Tuscan Chicken	950	57	82
Veggie	440	16	56
Soup: Per Container			
Baked Potato	240	15	20
Beef & Three Bean Chili	250	9	27
Broccoli Cheddar	220	17	13
Chkn Noodle; Sirloin Steak & Veg	110	2.5	15
Cream of Chicken w. Wild Rice	210	13	18
Fire Roasted Vegetable Bisque	180	11	16
Forest Mushroom	140	8	14
French Onion	80	3	11
Mesa Vegetable & Bean	100	0.5	18
Potato Cream Cheese	190	10	21
Potato Leek	220	14	21
Savory Vegetable Bean; Vege Lentil	120	2	21
Sirloin Beef	210	10	20
Vegetarian Black Bean	180	0.5	32
Vegetarian Vegetable Gumbo	110	3	18
White Chicken Chili	180	6	24

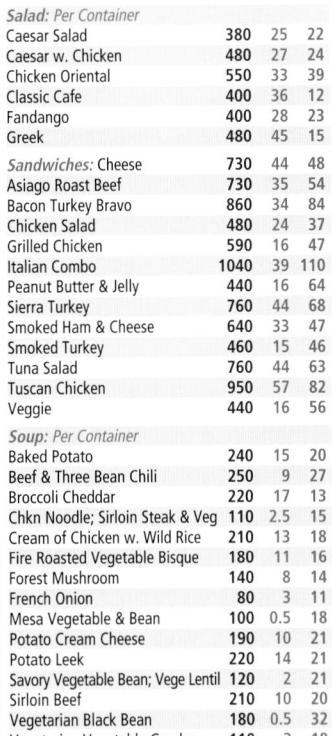

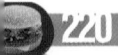

Papa John's®

	C	**F**	**Cb**
Original Large Pizza (14")			
Per Slice (¹/8 Whole)			
All the Meats	390	19	37
Cheese; Garden	280	10	38
Pepperoni	305	12	37
Sausage	325	14	37
Six Cheese	425	21	38
Spinach Alfredo	335	14	35
The Works	345	15	38
Thin Large Pizza (14"): Per Slice (¹/8 Whole)			
All the Meats	395	26	22
Cheese	235	13	22
Garden Special	225	12	24
Pepperoni	265	16	22
Sausage	285	17	22
Six Cheese	375	24	23
Spinach Alfredo	295	17	20
The Works	320	20	24
Extras: Bread Stick (1)	140	2	26
Cheese Sticks (2)	180	8	20
Cheese Sauce, 1 Tbsp, ¹/2 oz	30	2	0
Garlic Sauce, 1 Tbsp, ¹/2 oz	75	8.5	0
Pizza Sauce, 1 Tbsp, ¹/2 oz	10	0.5	1

Peter Piper® Pizza

	C	**F**	**Cb**
Cheese Pizza			
Small Pizza (10"), 1 Slice	160	5	19
Personal Pizza (7"), 1Slice	105	3.5	12
Medium Pizza (12"), 1 Slice	175	5.5	20
Large Pizza (14"), 1 Slice	235	8	28
Extra Large Pizza (16"), 1 Slice	205	6.5	24
Pepperoni Pizza			
Small Pizza (10"), Small Slice	185	8	18
Personal Pizza (7"), 1 Slice	150	6.5	15
Medium Pizza (12"), 1 Slice	200	8.5	20
Large Pizza (14"), 1 Slice	270	12	27
Extra Large Pizza (16"), 1 Slice	235	10	24
Sides			
Chicken Wings, 4 wings	210	16	1
Breadsticks (1)	120	4.5	17

Perkin's® Family Restaurant

	C	**F**	**Cb**
Entrees			
Chicken Dinner	620	13	60
Fish Dinner	470	7	60
Fruit Cup	50	0.5	12
'Lite & Healthy'	105	2	15
Omelettes			
Country Club	930	79	6
Deli Ham & Cheese	960	79	8
'Everything' Omelette	695	54	9
Granny's Country Omelette	940	82	7
w. 9 oz Hash Browns	1245	90	57
Salads: Chef's, Mini	215	11	7
Muffins			
Banana Nut	585	29	75
Blueberry	505	23	71
Carrot	560	23	88
Choc Choc Chip	545	26	73
Cranberry Nut	560	28	71
Oat Bran: Regular	515	16	87
98% fat-free	495	1	111
Pancakes: Buttermilk, (3)	440	12	70
Harvest Grain:			
w. Low-Cal Syrup (5)	475	3.5	93
Short Stack (3)	270	2	56
Pies: Per Slice			
Apple Pie	520	26	72
Cherry Pie	570	24	84
Coconut Cream Pie	440	21	56
French Silk Pie	550	34	59
Lemon Meringue Pie	395	15	63
Peanut Butter Brownie	455	27	4

Feedback welcome

Please send comments to:
Allan Borushek
POB 1616,
Costa Mesa CA 92628
Email: allan@calorieking.com

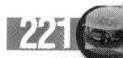

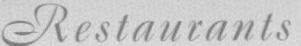

Petro's®

	C	F	Cb
Baked Potatoes			
#1 Lite	365	0.5	74
#2 Butter Sour Cream	480	18	74
#3 Loaded	680	33	78
#4 Loaded w. Chili	780	37	90
#5 Broccoli 3 Cheese	655	30	77
Chili			
Chicken: Small	175	3	27
Medium	275	4	43
Large	375	6	58
Original: Small	235	9	26
Medium	370	14	42
Large	505	19	57
Veggie: Small	245	7	37
Medium	385	11	58
Large	525	15	79
Garden Salads: Small	45	0.5	8
Large	85	1	16
Hot Dogs: Chili	315	17	28
Chili/Cheese; Loaded	350	19	30
Plain	265	14	22
Slaw	350	16	23
Loaded Tostitos™			
Ultimate Nachos	880	51	79
Lite Pasta Petro®: Small	335	2.5	52
Medium	495	3.5	80
Large	680	4.5	108
Lite Petro®: Small	380	12	48
Medium	530	16	66
Large	785	24	99
Pasta Petro®: Small	405	16	45
Medium	625	26	67
Large	850	36	91
Petro Salads: Grilled Chicken	740	41	42
Original	570	36	42
Petro®: Chicken, Small	465	24	43
Medium	665	36	59
Large	970	52	88
Original: Small	515	30	43
Medium	735	43	58
Large	1075	63	87
Veggie: Small	525	28	52
Medium	745	41	70
Large	1090	60	105
Tostitos™ Chips: Queso	500	27	60
Ransalsa	560	35	61
Salsa	415	18	62

Pick-Up-Stix®

	C	F	Cb
California Rolls	200	8	27
Beef Dishes: Beef and Broccoli	510	27	37
House Special	875	27	48
Mongolian	350	20	20
Szechwan	340	20	20
Bowls			
Teriyaki Chicken	1155	22	148
Teriyaki Vegetable	450	1.5	96
Buddah's Feast: Dark	105	0.5	16
Light	80	0.5	16
Chicken Dishes (Per Cup): Cashew	360	16	33
Garlic	285	12	24
House	755	34	58
Kung Pao	440	22	33
Lemon Twisted	260	3	37
Orange Peel	535	15	76
Sweet n Sour	475	22	60
w. Vegetables	195	3	20
Chow Mein: Per Cup			
Beef	350	10	50
Chicken	355	9	52
House Special	360	9	52
Shrimp	310	5	51
Vegetable	270	3.5	49
Fried Rice (Per Cup): Beef	505	16	68
Chicken	475	13	70
Egg	420	8	74
House	480	14	69
Shrimp	430	10	68
Vegetable	390	8	67
Rice: White, 1 cup	205	0.5	45
Salad: Per Serving			
Chicken Salad w/out Dressing	470	20	35
Chinese Chicken Salad w. Lime Dressing	675	20	35
Chinese Chicken Salad w. Original Dressing	650	22	75
Shrimp: Per Cup			
Black Bean	190	5	23
Garlic	185	5	23
Orange Peel	310	5	54
Szechwan	180	5	21
w/Vegetables	170	5	19
Soup: Per 2 Cup Bowl			
Hot & Sour	290	5	38
Wonton	290	13	27
Vegetables: Szechwan, 1 cup	105	1	21

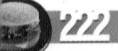

Pizza Hut®

Pan Pizza: *Per Slice, Med Pizza*	C	F	Cb
Beef Topping	330	18	29
Cheese	290	14	28
Chicken Supreme	270	12	29
Ham	260	12	28
Italian Sausage	340	20	29
Meat Lover's®	360	21	29
Pepperoni	280	14	28
Pepperoni Lover's®	330	18	29
Pork Topping	320	17	29
Super Supreme	340	18	30
Supreme	320	17	29
Veggie Lover's®	270	12	30

Personal Pan Pizza: *Per Pizza*	C	F	Cb
Beef Topping	710	35	71
Cheese	630	28	71
Ham	580	23	70
Italian Sausage	740	39	71
Pepperoni	620	28	70
Pork Topping	700	34	71

Stuffed Crust *Per Slice, Large Pizza*	C	F	Cb
Beef Topping	390	18	40
Cheese	360	16	40
Chicken Supreme	350	13	41
Ham	330	13	39
Italian Sausage	400	20	40
Meat Lover's®	470	25	40
Pepperoni	360	16	39
Pepperoni Lover's	420	21	40
Pork Topping	380	18	40
Super Supreme	430	22	41
Supreme	410	20	41
Veggie Lover's®	340	14	42

Thin 'n Crispy®: *Per Medium Slice*	C	F	Cb
Beef Topping	270	15	22
Cheese	200	9	22
Chicken Supreme	200	7	23
Ham	170	7	21
Italian Sausage	290	17	22
Meat Lover's®	310	19	22
Pepperoni	190	9	21
Pepperoni Lover's®	250	13	22
Pork Topping	270	14	22
Super Supreme	280	15	23
Supreme	250	13	23
Veggie Lover's®	190	7	24

Hand Tossed: *Per Medium Slice*	C	F	Cb
Beef Topping	330	17	29
Cheese	240	10	28
Chicken Supreme	230	7	29
Ham	260	10	28
Italian Sausage	340	18	28
Meat Lover's®	320	17	28
Pepperoni	280	13	28
Pepperoni Lover's®	250	11	27
Pork Topping	320	16	29
Super Supreme	290	14	29
Supreme	270	12	29
Veggie Lover's®	220	8	29

The Big New Yorker™: *Per Slice*	C	F	Cb
Beef/Pork Topping	480	26	42
Cheese	380	17	41
Ham	340	13	41
Pepperoni	370	16	41
Italian Sausage	570	33	42
Supreme	450	23	43
Veggie Lover's®	450	22	52

The Edge: *Per Square*	C	F	Cb
Chicken Supreme	90	3.5	9
Meat Lover's®	160	11	8
The Works	110	6	9
Veggie Lover's®	70	3	9

The Insider: *Per Slice, Medium Pizza*	C	F	Cb
Cheese	370	17	35
Pepperoni	360	17	35
Supreme	420	21	36

The Sicilian: *Per Slice*	C	F	Cb
Beef Topping	260	11	31
Cheese	290	13	31
Chicken Supreme	270	11	32
Ham	255	10	30
Italian Sausage	335	18	31
Meat Lovers	350	19	31
Pepperoni	280	13	31
Pepperoni Lovers	320	16	31
Pork Topping	320	16	31
Super Supreme	340	18	32
Supreme	310	15	32
Veggie Lovers	270	11	32

Twisted Crust: *Per Slice, Large Pizza*	C	F	Cb
Cheese	450	16	58
Pepperoni	440	15	58
Supreme	470	18	59

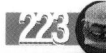

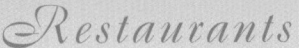

Pizza Hut® cont...

	C	F	Cb
Ultimate Lovers Pan: Per Slice			
Cheese, 1 slice	330	17	29
Meat	370	22	29
Pepproni	300	16	29
Veggie	270	12	30
Ultimate Lovers Personal Pan: Per Pan			
Cheese, 1 slice	740	35	72
Meat	840	45	72
Pepperoni	780	39	72
Veggie	610	24	75
Ultimate Lovers Stuffed Crust: Per Slice			
Cheese, 1 slice	400	19	41
Meat	470	26	41
Pepporoni	430	22	40
Veggie	350	15	42
Ultimate Lovers Thin n' Crispy: Per Slice			
Cheese, 1 slice	250	12	22
Meat	320	19	22
Pepperoni	250	13	22
Veggie	200	8	24
Ultimate Lovers Hand Tossed: Per Slice			
Cheese, 1 slice	280	13	28
Meat	330	17	28
Pepperoni	290	14	28
Veggie	230	8	30
Ultimate Big NewYorker: Per Slice			
Cheese, 1 slice	470	22	47
Meat	580	33	47
Pepperoni	480	23	47
Veggie	400	16	50
Sandwiches: Ham & Cheese	550	21	57
Supreme Sandwich	640	28	62
Dessert Pizza: Apple, 1 slice	250	4.5	48
Cherry, 1 slice	250	4.5	47
Pasta: Cavatini Pasta	480	14	66
Cavatini Supreme Pasta	560	19	73
Spaghetti: w. Marinara Sauce	490	6	91
w. Meatballs	850	24	120
w. Meat Sauce	600	13	98
Sides: Breadsticks, 1 serving	130	4	20
Breadstick Dipping Sce, 1 oz	30	0.5	5
Garlic Bread, 1 slice	150	8	16
Hot Buffalo Wings (4)	210	12	4
Mild Wings (5)	200	12	0
Sauce: Marinara (container)	60	1	12
Ranch (container)	440	48	4

Pizzeria Uno®

	C	F	Cb
Entrees			
Veggie Burger Meal	610	15	104
Tomato Basil Chicken	570	8	83
Zesty Pasta Marinara	380	3.5	75
Thin Crust Pizza: 9" Individual			
Vegetarian: w. Cheese	850	22	127
No Cheese	620	5	124
Soup			
Tomato Garden Vegetable	125	1	25
Light Lunch w. Soup	745	6	150
Salads			
Special House	90	1	17
Light Lunch w. Salad	710	6	141
Pasta Green Salad	410	9	69
Veggie Dip Platter	460	11	77

Pollo Tropical®

(na) ~ not available

Grilled Chicken:

	C	F	Cb
1/4 Chicken White, 5 oz	295	14	1
1/4 White no Skin, 4 oz	170	3	0
1/4 Chicken Dark, 4.5 oz	300	18	0.5
1/4 Dark no Skin, 3.5 oz	170	7	1
Bananas Tropical, 7 oz	500	13	90
Black Beans (combo portion), 5 oz	150	2	24
Black Beans, side, 8.5 oz	270	4	43
Boiled Yucs, 12 oz	330	0	81
Boneless Breast, 5 oz	140	1	1
Chicken Caesar S'wich, 6.5 oz	460	10	36
Chicken Sandwich, 8 oz	440	19	35
Chicken TropiChop	560	10	na
Congri, 7 oz	440	13	69
Corn, 3 oz	140	1.5	34
Grilled Chicken Salad (No Dressing)	210	4	na
Grilled Tropical Shrimp, 1 Skewer	90	1	0
Island Park, 5 oz	210	10	1
White Rice, 7 oz	340	6	65
Yucatan Fries, 5.3 oz	440	24	54

Restaurants & Fast–Foods

Popeye's®

Chicken	C	F	Cb
Chicken Breast: Mild/Spicy	530	31	18
Chicken Leg: Mild/Spicy	200	12	7
Chicken Thigh: Mild/Spicy	390	29	12
Chicken Wing: Mild/Spicy	220	15	10
Sides			
Biscuit, 2 oz	225	12	25
Cajun Rice	180	7	23
Cinnamon Apple Pie, 3 oz	250	10	37
Coleslaw	235	17	20
Corn on the Cob	255	4	48
French Fries, 4.5 oz	380	18	50
Mashed Potatoes: no Gravy	95	2	17
w. Gravy	120	4	18
Onion Rings, 4 oz	380	20	43
Red Beans & Rice	340	19	33

Quizno's Subs®

Subs with less than 7 grams Fat			
Honey Bourbon Chicken, small	330	6	45
Turkey Lite, small	335	6	52
Tuscan Chicken Salad, small	325	6.5	45
Veggie Lite, small	300	6	40

Quincy's®

Steak	C	F	Cb
Chopped, 8 oz	500	42	0
Country Style Steak w. Gravy	530	25	44
Cowboy Steak, 14 oz	580	33	9
Filet w. Bacon	340	17	2
N.Y. Strip Steak, 10 oz	450	26	1
Porterhouse Steak	680	46	0
Ribeye, 10 oz	450	29	0
Sirloin: Large	370	20	2
Regular	285	16	0
Sirloin Junior	195	10	0
Sirloin Tips	205	8	4
Smothered Strip Steak	620	41	12
T-Bone, 13 oz	520	35	0
Soups: Chili with Beans	235	11	21
Clam Chowder	180	9	21
Cream of Broccoli	170	10	18
Vegetable Beef	90	2	14
Entrees: Grilled Chicken	125	2	1
Homestyle Chicken Filet	220	9	21
Grilled Salmon	230	4	1
Sth Breaded Shrimp	545	31	47
Steak & Shrimp	680	39	33
Roasted Herb Chicken	875	65	4
Roasted BBQ Chicken	940	65	21
Grilled Trout	300	12	2
Sandwiches: No Mayo/Extras			
Bacon Cheeseburger	665	41	33
Grilled Chicken Sandwich	325	4	39
Philly Cheese Steak	590	30	38
Smothered Steak	430	15	36
Spicy BBQ Chicken	370	5	45
Breads: Banana Nut	165	7	22
Biscuit	270	15	29
Cornbread	140	5	17
Yeast Roll	160	4	29
Sides: Baked Potatoes	300	0	86
Corn on the Cob	140	1	33
Rice Pilaf	105	2	20
Desserts: Banana Pudding	240	12	30
Brownie Pudding Cake	310	5	66
Chocolate Chip Cookie	60	3	8
Apple Cobbler	255	8	49
Cherry Cobbler; Peach Cobbler	310	8	55
Frozen Yogurt	135	2	25
Sugar Cookie	60	3	8
Fudge Topping; Caramel	105	4	15

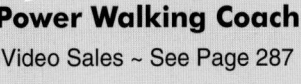

Rally's Hamburgers®

Burgers/Sandwiches	C	F	Cb
Rallyburger	435	22	35
with Cheese	490	27	35
Big Buford	745	48	35
Chicken Fillet Sandwich	400	15	43
Chili w. Cheese & Onion: 7 oz	360	22	20
13 oz size	670	41	37
Super Barbecue Bacon	595	31	49
Super Double Cheeseburger	760	48	37
French Fries			
Regular	210	11	26
Large	320	16	39
X-Large	425	21	52
Shakes			
Vanilla, small	320	11	49
Other flavors, small	410	12	73

Ranch 1®

Salads	C	F	Cb
Chicken on Gourmet Greens	350	11	31
Gourmet Greens	220	7	31
Zesty Caesar Salad	180	3	31
Zesty Chicken Caesar Salad	290	6	31
Sandwiches			
American Ranche	390	10	51
Club Sandwich	470	16	53
Grilled Chicken Philly	450	14	53
Ranch Classic	370	5	53
Spicy Grilled Chicken	420	11	58
Side Kicks			
Fruit Cup	90	0.5	18
Ranch Fries	350	14	51
Specialties			
Baked Potato: w. Broccoli	510	0.5	117
w. Cheese	790	25	118
w. Chicken	610	4	114
Chicken Tenders (all white meat)	370	15	7
Grilled Chkn & Vegetable Platter	790	7	129
Grilled Chicken Fajita	330	16	25
Grilled Chicken Hot Pasta	590	10	86

Rax®

Sandwiches	C	F	Cb
Regular Rax	390	22	31
Deluxe	520	35	34
BBC	715	51	36
Grilled Chicken	525	33	32
Jr. Deluxe	365	25	25
BBQ Beef	400	20	43
Mushroom Melt	600	37	35
Turk/Bacon Club	680	46	37
Turkey	485	32	32
Cheddar Melt	345	23	26
Philly Melt	535	32	35
Potatoes: Plain	205	0	60
Cheese/Broccoli	280	0	71
Cheese	270	0	70
Cheese/Bacon	335	18	70
w. Butter	305	11	60
w. Sour Topping	255	4	62
Soups: Cream of Broccoli	95	4	14
Chicken Noodle	115	1	20
Chili	160	9	11
Salads: Grilled Chicken	160	5	6
Side Salad	40	4	2
Garden	220	9	12
Salad Dressings: Fat Free: Ranch	30	0	6
Italian	12	0	2
Catalina	32	0	6
1000 Island	130	13	5
Buttermilk Ranch	175	20	1
Blue Cheese	145	16	1
Creamy Caesar	140	15	1
Honey French	140	5	9
Vinaigrette	30	2	4

Rocky Mountain Chocolate Factory®

Box: Per Piece			
English Toffee, 66g piece	350	24	34
Lucy Assorted, 16g piece)	220	12	29
Square, Happy Birthday, 22g pce	210	12	27
Truffle, regular, 36g pce	170	11	19
Tin: Per Piece			
Burgundy English Toffee, 17g pce	270	19	26

Restaurants & Fast–Foods

Red Lobster®

Fish
Per Lunch Portion (5 oz raw wt.)
(For **Dinner Portion** of 10 oz, double the figures.)
Prepared with No Added Fat
Add extra for butter sauce. [1 tsp = 30 cals; 3g fat (90%); 30mg sodium]

	C	F	Cb
Catfish	170	10	0
Cod (Atlantic)	100	1	0
Flounder	100	1	1
Grouper	110	1	0
Haddock	110	1	2
Halibut	110	1	1
Lemon Sole	120	1	1
Mackerel	190	12	1
Monkfish	110	1	0
Norwegian Salmon	230	12	2
Ocean Perch (Atlantic)	130	4	1
Pollock	120	1	1
Rainbow Trout	170	9	0
Red Rockfish	90	1	0
Red Snapper	110	1	0
Sockeye Salmon	160	4	2
Swordfish	100	4	0
Tilefish	100	2	0
Yellowfin Tuna	180	6	0

Shellfish

	C	F	Cb
King Crab Legs 16 oz	170	2	6
Snow Crab Legs, 16 oz	150	2	1
Calamari, breaded, fried, 5 oz	360	21	30
Langostino, 5 oz	120	1	2
Maine Lobster, 18 oz	240	8	5
Rock Lobster, 1 tail, 13 oz	230	3	2
Calico Scallops, 5 oz	180	2	8
Deep Sea Scallops, 5 oz	130	2	2
Shrimp, 8-12 pces., 7 oz	120	2	0

Steaks/Chicken

	C	F	Cb
Sirloin, 8 oz	350	15	0
Strip Steak, 7 oz	690	64	0
Hamburger, 1/3 lb	320	23	0
Filet Mignon, 8 oz	350	16	0
Rib Eye Steak, 12 oz	980	82	0
Skinless Chicken Breast, 4 oz	140	3	0

Rita's®

	C	F	Cb
Cream Ice:			
Small	205	3	45
Medium	325	4.5	72
Large	490	7	107
Quart	880	12	194
Gelati: Medium	380	12	66
Medium w. Cream Ice	410	14	70
Large	570	18	100
Large w. Cream Ice	615	22	105
Italian Ice: Small	170	0	45
Medium	270	0	70
Large	410	0	108
Quart	735	0	195
Misto: Large	415	7	90
Large w. Cream Ice	465	11	88
Super	620	10	135
Super w. Cream Ice	695	17	132
Frozen Custard: Small	275	14	31
Medium	370	20	42
Large	535	28	60

Rocky Rococco®

	C	F	Cb
Pizza: Per Regular Slice			
Cheese Pizza, 5.75 oz	380	9	54
Sausage Pizza, 7 oz	495	19	54
Pepperoni Pizza, 6.1 oz	430	13	54
Sausage & Mushroom, 7.6 oz	500	19	55
'Garden of Earth', 7.6 oz	390	10	56
Pizza: Per Super Slice			
Average all types	700	27	82

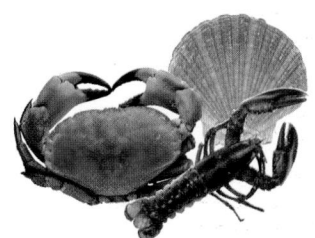

Round Table® Pizza

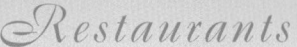

Large Pizza: Per Slice (1/12 Whole)	C	F	Cb
Cheese: Thin	210	8	23
Pan	290	10	37
Chicken & Garlic Gourmet™:			
Thin	230	9	24
Pan	320	11	38
Chicken Rostadoro™: Thin	250	10	25
Pan	330	12	39
Gourmet Veggie™: Thin	220	9	25
Pan	310	11	39
Guinevere's Garden Delight®:			
Thin	210	7	25
Pan	290	9	38
Hawaiian: Thin	210	7	25
Pan	290	9	38
Hearty Bacon Supreme™: Thin	270	14	22
Pan	360	16	36
Italian Garlic Supreme™: Thin	270	14	23
Pan	360	16	37
King Arthur's Supreme®: Thin	270	14	24
Pan	340	14	38
Maui Zaui™ (Polynesian Sce):			
Thin	240	9	27
Pan	330	11	41
Maui Zaui™ (Red Sce): Thin	240	9	25
Pan	320	11	39
Montague's All Meat Marvel®:			
Thin	290	17	24
Pan	350	16	37
Pepperoni: Thin	240	11	23
Pan	310	12	37
Pepperoni Rostadoro™: Thin	270	12	26
Pan	350	14	40
Roastin Toastin™ Chicken Club:			
Thin	260	12	25
Pan	350	14	39
Western BBQ Chicken™: Thin	240	9	23
Pan	320	11	37
16" Pizzas: Per Slice (1/8 WWhole)			
Aloha Vinnie Pepperoni™	430	14	55
Big Vinnie Pepperoni™	460	19	49
Maui Mama (Polynesian Sce)	570	22	63
Maui Mama (Red Sce)	560	22	61
Mama Zella Pizza	550	23	59

Personal Pizzas: Per Pizza	C	F	Cb
Cheese: Thin	580	24	60
Pan	810	36	106
Chicken Rostadoro™: Thin	680	29	66
Pan	910	31	112
Hawaiian: Thin	560	19	66
Pan	780	21	109
Gourmet Veggie™: Thin	590	23	67
Pan	820	25	114
Guinevere's Garden Delight®:			
Thin	550	20	66
Pan	760	21	110
Hearty Bacon Supreme™: Thin	700	35	59
Pan	940	37	105
Italian Garlic Supreme™: Thin	760	41	63
Pan	990	43	109
King Arthur's Supreme®: Thin	750	39	64
Pan	900	34	109
Maui Zaui™ (Polynesian Sce): Thin	620	23	71
Pan	850	25	117
Maui Zaui™ (Red Sce): Thin	590	22	66
Pan	820	24	111
Montague's All Meat Marvel®:			
Thin	780	44	61
Pan	1010	46	107
Pepperoni: Thin	640	31	60
Pan	840	29	106
Pepperoni Rostadoro™: Thin	740	35	70
Pan	970	37	116
Roastin Toastin™ Chicken Club:			
Thin	710	33	66
Pan	940	35	112
Western BBQ Chicken™: Thin	610	23	61
Pan	840	25	107
Sides/Sandwiches			
Garlic Bread	470	21	59
w. Cheese	630	33	59
Garlic Parmesan Twists, 3 pce	510	14	76
Buffalo Wings, 3 pce	210	14	1
6 pce	420	28	2
Honey BBQ Wings, 3 pce	190	13	4
6 pce	390	25	8
Sandwiches: Chicken Club	820	39	75
Ham Club	810	37	76
RT Pizza	690	34	65
RT Veggie	680	29	79
Turkey Club	800	37	75

Restaurants & Fast-Foods

Roy Rogers®

Breakfast Items	C	F	Cb
Biscuit	390	21	44
Cinnamon 'N' Raisin Biscuit	370	18	48
Sausage Biscuit	510	31	44
Sausage & Egg Biscuit	560	35	44
Bacon Biscuit	420	23	44
Bacon/Ham & Egg Biscuit	470	26	44
Ham & Cheese Biscuit	450	24	48
Ham, Egg & Cheese Biscuit	500	27	48
Sourdough Ham, Egg & Cheese	480	24	45
Big Country Breakfast: with Bacon	740	43	61
with Sausage	920	60	61
with Ham	710	39	67
3 Pancakes	280	2	56
with 1 Sausage	430	16	56
with 2 Bacon	350	9	56
Bagel, all types, average	300	2	60
Hashrounds	230	14	24
Burgers: Hamburger	260	9	33
Cheeseburger	300	13	34
1/4 lb Hamburger	430	18	41
1/4 lb Cheeseburger	470	22	42
Sourdough Bacon Cheeseburger	730	46	43
Sourdough Grilled Chicken	500	21	46
Bacon Cheeseburger	490	28	29
Sandwiches: Roast Beef	260	4	30
Chicken Fillet	500	24	49
Grilled Chicken	340	11	32
Fisherman's Fillet (seasonal)	490	21	56
Chicken: Fried: Breast	370	15	29
Wing	200	8	23
Thigh	330	15	30
Leg	170	7	15
1/4 Roy's Roaster: White Meat	500	29	3
No Skin	190	6	2
Dark Meat	490	34	2
No Skin	190	10	1
Nuggets: 6 piece	290	18	20
Salads: Grilled Chicken	120	4	2
Garden	190	14	3
Fries: Regular	350	15	49
Large	430	18	59
Baked Potato: w. Margarine	240	13	27
Cornbread	310	17	35
Coleslaw, 5 oz	295	25	16
Desserts: Hot Fudge Sundae	320	10	50
Strawberry Sundae	260	6	44

Rubio's Baja Grill®

HealthMex®
All HealthMex® items have less than 20% of calories from fat.

	C	F	Cb
Burrito w. Chicken	510	11	74
Burrito w. Grilled Fish	540	10	74
Combo	690	13	93
Taco Chicken	170	3	23
Taco w. Grilled Fish	180	3	24
Taco Combo: w. Chicken	480	8	68
w. Chicken & Mahi Mahi	490	7	69
w. Mahi Mahi	500	7	70
Tacos			
Carne Asada	250	11	24
Lobster	240	10	25
Fish Taco	300	16	30
Fish Taco Especial	370	21	29
Grilled Chicken	290	15	24
Grilled Fish	310	15	24
Shrimp	260	13	24
Quesadillas: Cheese	700	41	53
Grilled Chicken	810	44	54
Carne Asada	860	50	55
Shrimp; Lobster	770	42	55
Burritos			
Baja Carne Asada	700	36	58
Baja Chicken	650	30	56
Bean & Cheese	580	22	74
Bean & Rice	600	10	111
Carnitas	640	36	47
Especial: Carne Asada	830	40	81
Chicken	780	35	80
Carnitas	820	51	55
Fish	690	36	70
Lobster	770	39	89
Mahi Mahi	640	31	52
Shrimp	660	27	77
Los Otros: Chips	520	27	68
Nachos Grande	1270	77	117
w. Carne Asada	1430	86	119
w. Chicken	1380	80	118
In-Combo Chips & Beans	480	21	68
Chips	520	27	68
Beans	220	3	44
Rice	260	3.5	48
Chicken Taquitos (3)	410	20	38
Guacamole: Small	190	17	8
Large	370	34	16

Rubio's® cont...

Combos	C	F	Cb
Baja Grill Combo	1100	45	129
Cabo Combo	1190	55	137
Pesky's Combo	1170	61	115
Baja Bowls: Grilled Chicken	460	6	82
Carne Asada	490	8	83
Salsa: Regular	10	0	2
Verde	5	0	1
Picante	20	1	2
Kid Pesky® Meals: Taquitos	320	17	22
Bean & Cheese Burrito	570	21	72
Cheese Quesadilla	560	29	48
Fish Taco	300	16	27
Add Beans	130	3	22
Add Chips	210	11	28
Add Rice	110	1.5	21
Churro, mini	85	4	12
Desserts: Choco Taco	300	15	38
Churro	170	8	23

Note: Rubio's uses only skinless chicken breast & lean trimmed steak.

Canola oil is used – no lard or MSG.

Runza®

Sandwiches	C	F	Cb
Runza® Original Sandwich	545	20	66
Runza® Cheese Sandwich	605	25	68
BBQ Chicken Sandwich	370	11	36
Fish Sandwich	475	23	46
Polish Dog	405	25	25
Smothered Chicken Sandwich	280	9	25
Special Deluxe Chicken Sandwich	295	8.5	29
Kids-Size: Mini Corn Dogs	320	21	25
Chicken Nuggets	310	20	15
Runza® Sandwich	275	10	33
Hamburger	200	10	15
Hamburgers: Deluxe Hamburger	455	19	50
1/4 lb Hamburger	345	14	28
1/4 lb Cheeseburger	405	18	29
1/2 lb Double Hamburger	510	23	30
1/2 lb Double Cheeseburger	625	23	30
Bacon Cheeseburger Deluxe	515	28	30
Swiss Cheese Mushroom Burger	415	20	30

Runza® cont...

Onion Rings & Fries	C	F	Cb
Fries: Regular, 3.3 oz	315	17	35
Large, 3.6 oz	345	19	39
Jumbo, 6.8 oz	640	35	72
Onion Rings: Regular, 4.3 oz	465	29	45
Large, 6.7 oz	715	44	69
Onion Ring Dip, 2 oz	90	6.5	4

Salads & Dressings	C	F	Cb
Tossed Salad	90	4	4
Tossed Salad w. Chicken	210	8.5	5
Dressing: Ranch, 2.6 oz	290	30	4
Reduced Calorie Ranch, 2.6 oz	175	15	5
French, 2.6 oz	150	0	35
Lite Italian, 2.6 oz	40	1	5
Thousand Island, 2.6 oz	325	30	15

Soups	C	F	Cb
Boston Clam Chowder	305	17	30
Broccoli Cheese	280	16	27
Wisconsin Cheese	365	25	27
Cauliflower Cheese	315	19	30
Potato w. Bacon	205	9	27
Chicken Noodle	110	1	16
Vegetable Cheese Medley	250	16	19
Homemade chili	250	8	21

Desserts & Drinks	C	F	Cb
Brownie w. Nuts	465	16	74
Vanilla Shake, regular	520	15	84
Oreo® Shake, regular	655	24	97
Pepsi®, medium, 12 fl.oz	160	0	40

Ryan's® Family Steakhouse

Butter Pecan Frozen Yogurt	C	F	Cb
Sugar Free/Non-Fat	90	0	21
Menu Items: Per Serving			
Chicken Pot Pie	150	14	21
Clam Chowder, 1 cup	160	6	18
Macaroni & Cheese	340	14	38
Mashed Potatoes	100	4.5	14
Yeast Roll	340	6	68

7-Eleven®

	C	F	Cb
Hot Dogs			
1/4 Pound Big Bite Hot Dog	550	34	24
Hot Dog Bun only	120	1.5	22
1/3 Pound Biggest Big Bite	600	47	25
Cheeseburger Big Bite	530	35	25
Burritos			
The Bomb (14 oz)	940	42	116
w. Green Chilies	910	42	114
Reynoldos Jumbo Burritos (10 oz):			
Beef & Bean	680	22	93
Beef & Potato	590	20	82
Red Hot Burrito	640	20	88
Green Burrito	710	26	93
Sandwiches (7-Eleven)			
Big Eats Deli Sandwiches:			
Chicken Salad, 7.3 oz	630	35	47
Classic Chicken Caesar, 8.3 oz	540	24	47
Hearty Ham, 8.3 oz	570	30	48
Roast Beef & Bacon, 8.5 oz	650	33	47
Smoked Turkey w. Chse/Mayo	560	27	45
Stacked Turkey & Ham, 7.8 oz	630	34	46
Tuna Salad, 7.5 oz	550	22	56
Stuffed Baguettes:			
Philly Steak, 8 oz	540	24	56
w. Ham & Cheese, 8 oz	500	18	58
Hot Pockets: Ham 'n' Cheese, 7 oz	480	19	55
Meatballs w. Mozzarella	490	18	59
Giggles To Go			
Grilled Cheese Sandwich, 2.8 oz	270	15	27
The Deli Market (7-Eleven)			
Breakfast Sandwiches:			
Beef, Chse & Bacon Bite w. Bun	390	23	23
Croissant w. Bacon, Egg & Chse	420	26	34
Croissant w. Ham, Egg & Chse	390	22	34
Engl. Muffin w. Saus., Egg, Chse	450	24	37
Sausage, Egg & Chse Biscuit	500	31	34
Snack Stix™ Treats: Per Stick (3.5 oz)			
BBQ Chicken	230	6	34
Cheese & Steak	290	12	31
Egg, Ham & Cheddar	280	11	35
Egg, Sausage & Cheese	290	12	35
Grilled Chicken & Cheese	270	11	30
Ham & Cheese; Supreme	280	12	32
Pepperoni & Cheese	340	18	30
Sausage & Cheese	300	13	32
Sushi			
California Rolls, 8-Pack	560	8	80

	C	F	Cb
Taquitos (Battered Tortilla)			
Beef Taco & Cheese, 3 oz	250	11	30
Chicken & Monterey Jack Cheese	280	14	30
Fiesta Chicken	220	12	22
Go-Go Taquitos:			
Beef Taco & Cheese, 3 oz (1)	250	11	30
Fiesta Chicken, 3 oz (1)	220	12	22
Monterey Jack Chkn, 3 oz (1)	280	14	30
Fountain Drinks (Figures Assume 1/4 Ice)			
Coca-Cola/Pepsi/Dr.Pepper/7Up:			
Gulp, 16 oz	150	0	38
Big Gulp, 32 oz	300	0	75
Super Gulp, 44 oz	410	0	102
Double Gulp, 64 oz	600	0	150
Diet Coke/Diet Pepsi, 16 oz	1	0	0
Slurpees: Average All Flavors,			
16 oz size	220	0	55
22 oz size	300	0	75
32 oz size	440	0	110
44 oz size	600	0	150
StrataCups: 28 oz size	390	0	95
40 oz size	550	0	137
Slurp & Gulp Combo,			
32 oz Big Gulp & 22 oz Slurpee	600	0	150
Café Coolers: Mocha, 12 oz	350	12	63
French Vanilla, 12 oz	380	16	58
Fruit Coolers			
Orange/Strawb. Creme, 12 fl.oz	280	1	68
16 fl.oz size	370	1	90
20 fl.oz size	470	2	113
Arizona Rasp. Green Tea, 12 fl.oz	230	0	56
Cafe Select: 12 fl.oz	7	0	2
16 fl.oz size	10	0	2
20 fl.oz size	12	0	3
24 fl.oz size	15	0	4
Fresh Fruit Salad, 1 bowl, 10 oz	140	0	32

Sammy's® Woodfired Pizza

	C	F	Cb
Healthy Dining Meals			
Chinese Chicken Salad	480	13	49
Chopped Chicken Salad	395	11	20
Grilled Shrimp Wrap	560	19	57
Grilled Vegetable Penne	610	20	84
Tomato Angel Hair Pasta	650	18	105
Vegetarian Pizza, 1/2 Pizza	885	21	130

231

Sbarro's®

Meals: Per Serving

	C	F	Cb
Baked Ziti, 1 serving	930	42	90
Chicken Parmigiana, 2 pces, 7 oz	365	20	13
Meat Lasagne, 1 serving	825	41	68
Spaghetti w. Sauce, 1 serving	910	23	144

Pizza: Per Slice

	C	F	Cb
Cheeze	485	18	55
Pepperoni	590	27	55
Sausage	640	29	56
Supreme	600	25	59

Stuffed Pizza: Per Slice

	C	F	Cb
Spinach/Broccoli	825	40	85
Sausage Pepperoni	965	47	83

Schlotzsky's®

Bread/Buns

	C	F	Cb
Dark Rye, regular	325	2	68
Sourdough, regular	335	2	68
Wheat, regular	335	3	66
Jalapeno Cheese, regular	355	4	66
Pizza Crust	330	2	68

Original Sandwiches: Per Sandwich

	C	F	Cb
The Original, regular	740	31	79
Large Original, family size	1390	58	152
Deluxe Original, regular	930	42	84
Ham & Cheese Original, regular	750	27	82
Turkey Original, regular	820	32	81

Sandwiches: Per Regular Sandwich

	C	F	Cb
Albacore Tuna	495	10	77
Albacore Tuna Melt	740	29	83
Albuquerque Turkey	920	41	85
All American Angus	900	39	82
BLT	580	24	70
Chicken Breast	500	4	80
Chicken Club	685	23	75
Corned Beef	595	12	78
Corned Beef Reuben	840	33	82
Dijon Chicken	495	6	74
Fiesta Chicken	840	36	79
Pastrami & Swiss	880	36	81
Pastrami Reuben	945	41	83
Pesto Chicken	510	9	73
Roast Beef	625	15	78
Roast Beef & Cheese	855	32	83
Santa Fe Chicken	605	14	81

Sandwiches (Cont): Per Regular Sandwich

	C	F	Cb
Smoked Turkey Breast	500	7	75
Texas Schlotzsky's	775	32	76
The Philly	840	29	86
The Vegetarian	480	11	79
Turkey & Bacon Club	835	35	79
Turkey Guacamole	645	19	84
Turkey Reuben	825	34	80
Vegetable Club	540	18	76
Western Vegetarian	610	28	76

Soups: Per Cup (8 oz)

	C	F	Cb
Boston Clam Chowder	235	15	24
Broccoli Cheese w. Florets	250	17	23
Chicken Gumbo	110	5	13
Chicken Tortilla	165	3	24
Chicken w. Wild Rice	380	28	24
Minestrone	90	1	17
Old-Fashioned Chicken Noodle	120	2	18
Pilgrim Corn Chowder	285	17	38
Potato w. Bacon	225	13	31
Ravioli; Santa Fe Vegetable	120	2	20
Red Beans & Rice	165	1	32
Schlotzsky's Vegetable	220	2	44
Steak & Black Bean	150	1	25
Seven Bean Medley	145	2	24
Timberline Chili	210	7	24
Vegetable Beef & Barley	100	3	12
Vegetarian Vegetable	140	6	20
Wisconsin Cheese	320	25	26

Deli Salads: Per 5 oz Container

	C	F	Cb
Potato	290	15	35
Mustard Potato	250	13	31
Homestyle Cole Slaw	190	10	24
Elbow Macaroni	275	19	23
California Pasta	60	3	10
Albacore Tuna, 4.4 oz	135	8	2

Leaf Salads
w/out Dressing/Croutons/Noodles

	C	F	Cb
Caesar	150	8	11
Chicken Caesar	255	10	13
Chinese Chicken	150	3	11
Garden Salad	60	1	8
Small	25	1	3
Greek	180	10	13
Ham & Turkey/Smkd Turkey Chef's	250	11	15

Schlotszky's® cont...

	C	F	Cb
8" Sourdough Crust Pizzas			
Bacon, Tomato & Mushroom	610	22	78
Barbeque Chicken	685	15	93
Chicken & Pesto; New Orleans	650	19	78
Double Cheese	580	19	76
Double Cheese & Pepperoni	720	32	77
Fresh Tomato & Pesto	540	16	76
Mediterranean	525	18	72
Smoked Turkey & Jalapeno	625	17	80
Southwestern	610	17	76
Thai Chicken	665	17	89
The Original Combination	625	23	79
Vegetarian Special	550	17	76
Salad Extras: Chow Mein Noodles	75	4	9
Garlic Chinese Croutons	45	2	5
Greek Balsamic Vinaigrette	170	17	2
Light Italian Dressing	90	8	3
Olde World Caesar Dressing	260	27	1
Ranch Dressing: Traditional	270	29	1
Spicy	230	25	2
Light	140	11	9
Schlotzsky's Deli Chips, 1.5 oz bag	210	11	26
Sesame Ginger Vinaigrette	170	15	8
Thousand Island Dressing	220	21	6
Kid's Deals: Cheese Pizza	460	11	72
Cheese Sandwich	400	15	49
Ham & Cheese Sandwich	430	16	50
PBJ Sandwich	470	16	71
Pepperoni Pizza	505	16	72
Desserts/Cookies			
Cookies: Oatmeal	150	5	24
Cookies w. Real M&M's	140	5	20
Other varieties, average	165	7	23
Cheesecake: Cookies & Crème	330	18	36
Fudge Brownie Cake	410	25	46
New York; Strawberry Swirl	310	18	31

Shakey's®

	C	F	Cb
Pizzas (12")			
Per Slice (1/10 Pizza)			
Cheese only:			
Thin Crust	135	5	13
Thick Crust	170	5	22
Homestyle Pan	305	14	31
Onion/Olives/Mushrooms:			
Thin Crust	125	5	14
Thick Crust	160	4	22
Homestyle Pan	320	15	32
Sausage Pepperoni:			
Thin Crust	165	8	13
Thick Crust	205	8	22
Homestyle Pan	375	20	31
Sausage Mushroom			
Thin Crust	140	6	13
Thick Crust	180	6	22
Homestyle Pan	340	17	31
Pepperoni:			
Thin Crust	150	7	13
Thick Crust	185	6	22
Homestyle Pan	345	15	31
Shakey's Special:			
Thin Crust	170	9	13
Thick Crust	210	8	22
Homestyle Pan	385	21	32
Other Items			
3-Piece Chicken & Potato	945	56	51
5-Piece Fried Chicken & Potato	1700	90	130
Hot Ham & Cheese Sandwich	550	21	56
Potato Wedges, 15 pieces	950	36	120
Shakey's Super Hot Hero	810	44	67
Spagh. w. Meat Sce/Garlic Bread	940	33	134

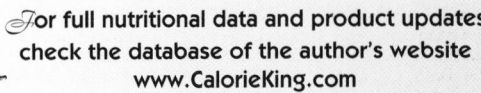

For full nutritional data and product updates
check the database of the author's website
www.CalorieKing.com

Fast – Foods & *Restaurants*

Shoney's®

Breakfast	C	F	Cb
All Star Breakfast, no extras	190	14	1
Deluxe Pancake Platter	1610	32	300
Half Stack Pancake Platter	930	14	187
Big Eater Steak Brkfast, no extras	630	41	1
Steak Breakfast	995	66	49
Sunrise Breakfast	970	60	88
Sausage Biscuit (1)	540	34	42
Sausage Biscuits (2)	1055	65	83

Burgers			
All-American: Burger	690	32	44
Bacon Cheeseburger	890	49	44
Mushroom Swiss Burger	970	58	49
Famous Patty Melt	945	60	40
Half Pound Burger	1350	53	130

Sandwiches			
Blackened Chicken	885	21	122
Charbroiled Chicken Sandwich	895	22	122
Chicken Parmesan Sandwich	750	30	80
Corned Beef Reuben	790	53	37
Fish Sandwich	830	17	126
Fried Chicken Sandwich	560	15	77
Original Slim Jim Sandwich	1005	34	123
Potatoes & Gravy Sandwich	770	24	95
Raymond's French Dip	500	14	53
Turkey Club/Whole Wheat	950	53	47
Ultimate Grilled Cheese S'wich	895	46	77

Steaks			
BBQ Ribs	1520	78	124
Choice Sirloin, 6 oz	1225	51	127
Half-O-Pound w. Grilled Onions	1335	52	133
Half-O-Pound w. Grilled Mushr.	1315	52	127
Ribeye, 8 oz	1480	75	127
Southwest Half-O-Pound	1305	69	83
T-Bone, 12 oz	1810	100	127
Surf & Turf:			
Ribeye & 5 Fried Shrimp	1640	82	138
Ribeye & 6 Grilled Shrimp	1590	81	128
Sirloin & 5 Fried Shrimp	1380	58	138
Sirloin & 6 Grilled Shrimp	1330	57	128
T-Bone & 5 Fried Shrimp	1965	107	138
T-Bone & 6 Grilled Shrimp	1920	105	128
Rib Combos, w. Fries:			
1/4 Rack & BBQ Chicken	1230	54	103
1/4 Rack & Tenderloins	1370	70	120
1/4 Rack & Fried Shrimp	1145	50	113
1/4 Rack & Grilled Shrimp	1125	52	103

Blue Plate Specials	C	F	Cb
Cajun Whitefish	480	11	56
Baked Whitefish	510	8.5	58
Grandma's Meatloaf w. Glaze	1090	47	93
Grandma's Meatloaf w. Gravy	1090	49	88
Original Country Fried Steak	1150	62	103
Grilled Liver 'n' Onions	710	22	79
Ham Steak Dinner (no veges)	670	26	60
Roast Beef Platter (no veges)	880	30	96
Pasta: Chicken Alfredo	1705	78	170
Italian Feast	1435	45	204
Pasta Ya-Ya	1850	81	176
Shrimp Alfredo	1780	85	171
Spaghetti	495	16	63
Seafood: Fish 'n' Shrimp	1100	39	129
Fried Fish Platter	1050	39	123
Grilled Cod/Salmon Lite	200	4	0
Grilled Salmon	750	19	95
Grilled Shrimp	720	20	96
Grilled Shrimp Lite	315	8	30
Shrimper's Feast	1035	39	128
Shrimp Stir Fry	875	19	131
Sides: Baked Potato, Plain	345	6.5	67
French Fries, 4 oz	210	11	25
Onion Rings, 1 order (7 rings)	500	14	83
Chicken: Chicken Stir Fry	1200	35	172
Charbroiled Blackened Chicken	830	26	100
Charbroiled Chicken Breast	795	23	99
Fried Chicken Tenderloins	1160	61	121
Monterey Chicken	910	40	84
Smothered Chicken	1035	39	128
Junior Meals: Fish 'N Chips	310	11	29
All-American Jnr Burger	235	11	20
Junior Chicken	190	10	12
Spaghetti	250	8	32
Desserts, Icecream, Sundaes			
Apple Pie: a la Mode	1205	53	174
w. NutraSweet	455	18	64
Cheesecake, 1 slice, 4 oz	365	26	23
Hot Fudge Sundae	600	30	75
Original Strawberry Pie, 1 slice	330	17	45
Ultimate Hot Fudge Cake	875	37	126
Cherry/Peach Pie w. Nutrasweet	450	21	68
Caramel Sundae	620	27	141
Chocolate/Vanilla Milk Shake	1085	51	141
Strawberry Sundae	610	27	85
Walnut Brownie a la Mode	575	34	61

Sizzler®

Hot Entrees	C	F	Cb
Hamburger	625	33	36
Dakota Ranch Steak: 6 oz	315	20	0
8 oz	420	27	0
9 1/2 oz	500	32	0
Hibachi Chicken Breast			
w. Pineapple	195	3	13
Lemon-Herb Chicken Breast	140	3	0
Malibu Chicken Patty, each	310	19	11
Salmon	250	12	0
Santa Fe Chicken Breast	150	3	0
Shrimp: Broiled	150	6	0
Fried, 4 only	225	2	35
Mini	150	1	24
Shrimp Scampi	145	3	0
Swordfish	315	14	0

Hot Bar	C	F	Cb
Broccoli Chse Soup, 4 oz	140	9	10
Chicken Noodle Soup, 4 oz	30	1	4
Chicken Wings, 1 oz	75	4	4
Clam Chowder, 4 oz	120	6	11
Focaccia Bread, 2 pces	110	7	9
Meatballs, 4 balls	155	11	5
Minestrone Soup, 4 oz	35	0	7
Pasta: Fettucine, 2 oz	80	1	15
Spaghetti, 2 oz	80	0	16
Potato Skins, 2 oz	160	8	22
Refried Beans, 1/4 cup	60	1	11
Saltine Crackers, 2 crackers	25	1	4
Taco Filling, 2 oz	105	9	3
Taco Shells, each	50	2	7

Dessert Bar: Chocolate Syrup, 1 oz	90	0	21
Choc/Vanilla Soft Serve, 4 oz	135	4	24
Strawberry Topping, 1 oz	70	0	18
Whipped Topping, 1 Tbsp	10	1	1

Salads & Toppings	C	F	Cb
Prepared Salads: Per 2 oz			
Carrot & Raisin	130	10	10
Chinese Chicken; Teriyaki Beef	55	2	6
Mediterranean Minted Fruit	30	0	7
Mexican Fiesta	55	1	10
Old Fashioned Potato	85	5	10
Red Herb Potato	120	9	9
Seafood	55	3	4
Seafood Louis Pasta	65	2	9
Spicy Jicama	15	0	4
Tuna Pasta	135	10	6

Sides	C	F	Cb
Cottage Cheese, 2 oz	50	1	2
Eggs, 1 oz	45	3	0
Garbanzo Beans, 1/4 cup	65	1	11
Kidney Beans, 1/4 cup	50	0	10
Olives, 1 oz	60	6	1
Peaches, 1/4 cup	35	0	9
Peas, 1/4 cup	30	0	6
Real Bacon Bits, 1 Tbsp	30	2	2
Turkey Ham, 1 oz	60	5	0

Dressings: Per 1 oz	C	F	Cb
Blue Cheese	110	12	1
Honey Mustard	160	16	4
Italian, Lite	15	0	2
Japanese Rice Vinegar, Fat Free	10	0	2
Parmesan Italian	100	10	2
Ranch	120	12	2
Ranch, Reduced-Calorie	90	8	4
Thousand Island	145	15	3

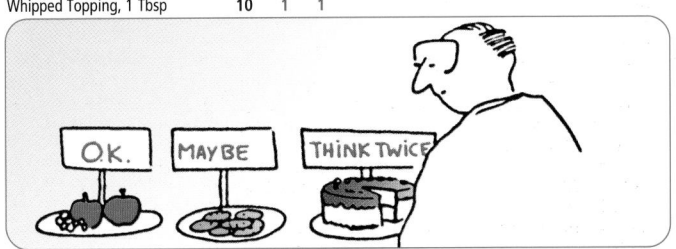

Fast–Foods & 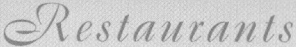 Restaurants

Skyline Chili®

Menu Items: Per Serving

	C	F	Cb
Chili (Regular): Plain, 1/2 pint	250	15	4
w. Beans, 1/2 pint	260	12	17
Chili Spaghetti: Regular	400	14	44
Jumbo	540	19	59
Chili Spaghetti w. Onions: Reg.	410	14	47
Jumbo	550	19	63
Chili Spaghetti w. Beans: Reg.	480	14	57
Jumbo	650	19	79
Chili Spaghetti w. Beans/Onions:			
Regular	490	14	60
Jumbo	660	19	82
Burritos: Regular	570	30	42
Deluxe Burrito	640	34	47
Skyliner Cheese Coneys: Regular	240	14	23
Cheese Coney	350	24	23
Chili Sandwich	190	9	25
w. Cheese	300	18	24
Black Beans and Rice	330	12	44
3-Way (Spagh., Chili, Chse): Reg.	710	42	39
Jumbo	1050	61	61
4-Way (3-Way + Onions): Reg.	720	42	41
Jumbo	1070	61	65
4-Way (3-Way + Beans): Reg.	780	42	52
Jumbo	1160	61	80
5-Way (3-Way + Onions + Beans):			
Regular	790	42	54
Jumbo	1180	61	84

Salads

	C	F	Cb
Garden Salads: Regular	80	5	4
Large	150	10	7
Greek Salads: Regular	370	36	9
Large	690	68	13
Nacho Salads: Regular	450	25	40
Large	750	42	66

Smoothie King®

Weight Gain Smoothies: Per 20 oz

	C	F	Cb
Hulk™: Chocolate/Vanilla	845	29	128
Strawberry	955	29	156
Malts	885	41	118
Peanut Power®	500	21	71
Peanut Power Plus™: Grape	705	21	119
Strawberry	630	21	105
Shakes	875	41	117

Smoothie King®

Lowfat Smoothies: Per 20 oz

	C	F	Cb
Angel Food™; Mangofest™	330	0.5	79
Blackberry Dream™	345	0.5	86
Blueberry Heaven™	260	1	59
Celestial Cherry High™	285	0.5	69
Cherry Picker™	360	0.5	98
Cranberry Cooler	540	0	132
Cranberry Supreme™	575	0.5	141
Grape Expectations™; Caribbean®	400	0.5	96
Grape Expectations II™	530	0.5	129
Hearty Apple™	380	2	91
Immune Builder™; Island Treat®	335	1	80
Instant Vigor™	360	1	87
Lemon Twist® Banana	340	0.5	82
Lemon Twist® Strawberry	400	0.5	97
Light & Fluffy®	390	0.5	98
Muscle Punch®/Plus™	340	1.5	80
Orange Ka-Bam™	320	0	104
Peach Slice™	340	0	80
Peach Slice Plus®	470	0	113
Pep Upper®	335	1	80
Pineapple Pleasure®	315	0.5	76
Pineapple Surf™	440	1	104
Raspberry Sunrise™	335	0.5	84
Slim & Trim™: Chocolate	270	1.5	50
Strawberry	355	1	78
Orange-Vanilla	200	0.5	43
Vanilla	225	1	51
Strawberry Kiwi Breeze™	300	0	70
Strawberry X-Treme™	370	0	91
Youth Fountain™	265	0.5	65

Specialty Smoothies: Per 20 oz

	C	F	Cb
Banana Boat™	520	14	93
Coconut Surprise™	455	6	99
Mo'cuccino™	420	12	71
Pina Colada Island™	550	11	102

Workout Smoothies: Per 20 oz

	C	F	Cb
Activator®: Banana/Choc./Vanilla	430	1	90
Strawberry	530	1	123
Power Punch™	430	1.5	102
Power Punch Plus®	500	2	113
Super Punch™	425	0.5	95
Super Punch Plus®	515	0.5	118

High Protein Smoothies: Per 20 oz

	C	F	Cb
Almond Mocha/Chocolate	400	13	45
Banana	410	14	44
Lemon/Pineapple	390	13	41

Snappy Tomato®

Large Pizza: Per 2 Slices	C	F	Cb
Cheese Pizza	320	10	42
Sausage	380	16	44
Pepperoni	400	18	42
Snappy Tomato Supreme	420	28	na

Sonic Drive-In®

Burgers: #1. Burger	C	F	Cb
#2. Burger	480	25	43
#1. Cheeseburger	645	42	44
#2. Cheeseburger	550	31	44
Bacon Cheeseburger	725	49	44
Super Sonic #1	930	66	45
Super Sonic #2	840	55	46
Jr. Burger	355	21	27

#1. Burger values: 575 | 36 | 43

Toaster Sandwiches: BLT	580	41	42
Bacon Cheddar Burger	675	38	60
Chicken Club	675	29	75
Country Fried Steak	710	45	55
Grilled Cheese	280	12	39

Sandwiches: Country Fried Steak	750	47	56
Breaded Chicken	580	23	66
Grilled Chicken	345	13	31

Wraps: Chicken Strip w. Dressing	575	29	55
w/out Ranch Dressing	430	13	53
Grilled Chicken: w. Ranch Dressing	540	27	40
w/out Ranch Dressing	395	12	38

Chicken: Chicken Strip Dinner	750	32	86
Chicken Strip Snack	270	13	22

Coneys: Plain: Regular	260	16	22
Extra Long	485	27	44
Cheese: Regular	365	24	24
Extra-Long	665	42	47
Corn Dog	260	17	23

Breakfast: Breakfast Burrito	730	47	47
Bacon Egg & Cheese Toaster®	500	29	40
Sausage Egg & Cheese Toaster®	570	36	44
Ham Egg & Cheese Toaster®	435	19	41
Fruit Taquitos	300	7	51
Sunrise Breakfast: Regular	225	0	60
Large	370	0	100

Drinks: Barq's® Root Beer, large	335	0	84
Coca-Cola®, large	290	0	72
Coca-Cola® Float, large	545	17	59

Faves & Craves

	C	F	Cb
French Fries: Regular	195	11	22
Large	250	13	30
Super Sonic	360	18	44
Ched 'R' Peppers®	255	12	29
Cheese Fries: Regular	265	17	23
Large	320	19	31
Chili Cheese Fries: Regular	300	19	24
Large	360	22	32
Fritos® Chili Pie	610	44	36
Mozzarella Sticks	380	19	35
Onion Rings: Regular	330	5	66
Large	505	7	102
Supersonic	705	10	144
Tater Tots: Regular	260	16	27
Large	365	21	40
Supersonic	485	28	53
Cheese Tater Tots: Regular	330	22	28
Large	435	27	41
Chili Cheese Tater Tots: Regular	365	25	28
Large	550	36	42
Blasts: Regular, all types	640	27	56
Large, all types, average	935	40	85
Slushes: Small, average	220	0	58
Regular, averge all flavors	330	0	85
Large, average all flavors	515	0	132
Wacky Pack®, average	195	0	50
Route 44®, average	700	0	180
Slush Floats/Flurry®: Reg., aver.	410	12	48
Large	600	17	70
Desserts: Banana Split	465	11	75
Chocolate Sundae	360	11	41
Dish of Vanilla	265	11	19
Hot Fudge Sundae	390	15	40
Icecream Cone	285	11	23
Pineapple Sundae	400	11	53
Strawberry Sundae	320	11	32

Souper Salad®

Menu Items: Cornbread, 1 portion	C	F	Cb
Blueberry Bread, 1 portion	255	5	49
Focaccia Bread, 1 portion	385	7	69
Gingerbread, 1 portion	295	11	46
Salad Dressings: Fat Free Ranch	30	0	9
Fat Free Cranberry Vinaigrette	50	0	12
Soft Serve Frozen Dessert	105	3	19

Cornbread, 1 portion values: 265 | 6 | 49

Souplantation®

Soups: Per 1 Cup	C	F	Cb
Low Fat: Chicken Tortilla	100	3	5
Chicken/Turkey Noodle	160	3	17
Vegetable Medley	90	1	14
Regular Soup:			
Chesapeake Corn Chowder	310	13	43
Cream of Mushroom	290	21	15
Irish Potato Leek	260	16	23
Minestrone w. Italian Sausage	210	11	14
Navy Bean w. Ham	340	10	30
New England Clam Chowder	330	20	21
Vegetarian Harvest	190	8	23
Chili: House Chili	230	3	26
Breads			
Buttermilk Corn	140	2	27
Sourdough	150	0.5	27
Focaccia: Garlic Parmesan	100	3	15
Pizza /Tomarillo	140	6	16
Fresh Tossed Salads: Per 1 Cup			
Antipasto Salad; BBQ, average	140	10	6
Classic Caesar Salad	190	14	10
Won Ton Chicken Salad	150	8	12
Prepared Salads: Per 1/2 Cup			
Artichoke Rice	160	8	21
Aunt Doris' Red Pepper Slaw	70	0	18
Baja Bean & Cilantro	180	3	29
BBQ Potato	160	8	20
Carrot Raisin	90	3	17
Chinese Krab	160	8	19
Confetti Pasta w. Cheddar & Dill	160	9	16
Dijon Potato w. Garlic Dill Vinegar	140	7	16
Greek Couscous w. Feta Cheese	170	9	19
Oriental Ginger Slaw w. Krab	70	3	8
Southern Dill Potato	120	3	20
Thai Noodle w. Peanut Sce	170	8	17
Dressing & Croutons: Per 2 Tbsp			
Blue Cheese Dressing	140	14	3
Blush Vinaigrette	120	12	3
Creamy Cucumber Dressing	80	7	4
Garden French Tomato	40	1.5	7
Honey Mustard Dressing	150	13	8
Fat Free	45	0	10
Ranch House Dressing	130	13	1
Fat Free	50	0	2
Thousand Island Dressing	110	11	3
Zesty Italian Dressing	160	18	1
Fat Free	20	0	5

Hot Tossed Pastas: Per Cup	C	F	Cb
Bruschetta	260	4	41
Creamy	360	16	43
Garden Vegetable: w. Meatballs	270	7	42
w. Italian Sausage	300	10	42
Italian Vegetable Beef	270	6	43
Vegetarian Marinara w. Basil	260	4	44
Muffins: Per Muffin			
Regular: Apple Raisin	150	7	22
Apricot/Banana/Cherry Nut	150	7	22
Carrot Pineapple w. Oat Bran	150	6	23
Chocolate Varieties	170	8	22
Georgia Peach Poppyseed	150	6	20
Lemon	140	4	19
Wild Maine Blueberry	140	5	22
Zucchini Nut	150	7	22
Desserts: Per 1/2 Cup			
Apple Medley	70	0	18
Banana Royale	80	0	20
Chocolate Chip Cookie, small	70	3	10
Jello, flavored	80	0	20
Rice Pudding	110	2	20
Tropical Fruit Salad	75	0	19
Vanilla Pudding	140	3	24
Vanilla Soft Serving	140	4	22
Chocolate Syrup, 2 Tbsp	70	0	18
Granola Topping, 2 Tbsp	110	4	16

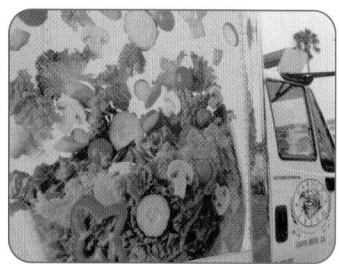

Southern Tsunami®

Sushi: *Per Serving*	C	F	Cb
California Roll, 9 pieces	290	5	54
California Roll & Inari, 7 pieces	325	6	58
California Salad Roll, 6 pieces	570	20	83
Combos: Seaside, 12 pieces	300	3.5	48
Shoreline, 10 pieces	475	5.5	84
Stardust, 11 pieces	305	3	58
Vegetable, 9 pieces	240	4	45
Cream Cheese Roll:			
w. Imitation Crab, 9 pces	530	25	60
w. Salmon, 9 pces	570	29	53
w. Tuna, 9 pces	550	26	53
Crunchy Shrimp Roll, 9 pieces	650	19	83
Dragon Roll, 9 pieces	645	34	63
Eel Roll, 9 pieces	465	18	55
Full Moon Combo, 6 pieces	305	7	50
Futomaki, 9 pieces	310	1.5	68
Futomaki & Inari, 6 pieces	355	4.5	68
Green River Roll, 9 pieces	490	20	55
Grilled Salmon Roll, 9 pieces	350	6.5	54
Inari, 4 pieces	260	5	46
Mix & Match (M & M) Roll:			
Eel & Carrot, 12 pieces	315	7	51
Imitation Crab & Carrot, 12 pces	245	0.5	53
Tuna & Cucumber, 12 pces	245	1	49
Shrimp & Avocado, 12 pces	280	4	50
Marina Plate, 6 pieces	280	4	48
Meteor Special, 11 pieces	370	3	67
Nigiri: *Per Piece*			
Eel	85	2	13
Octopus; Salmon; Yellowtail	65	0.5	12
Shrimp	90	1	12
Snapper; Squid; Tuna	60	0	12
Ocean Crab Roll, 9 pieces	370	3	67
Orange Roll, 9 pieces	395	8	65
Small Roll: *Per 12 Pieces*			
Avocado	295	7	52
Carrot	240	0.5	53
Cucumber	225	0.5	50
Eel	390	13	50
Imitation Crab	250	0.5	53
Salmon	330	6	47
Shrimp	265	1	49
Tuna	260	1.5	49
Yellowtail	290	3	49

Sushi (Cont): *Per Serving*	C	F	Cb
Snack Pack: *Per 12 Pieces*			
Avocado	295	7	52
Carrot-Cucumber	230	0.5	51
Carrot	240	0.5	53
Cucumber	225	0.5	50
Imitation Crab & Cucumber	240	0.5	51
Spicy Roll: *Per 9 Pieces*			
Shrimp	335	5.5	52
Yellowtail	365	8	52
Salmon	360	9	52
Tuna	290	6	45
Sunshine Platter, 15 pieces	815	13	154
Tofu Roll, 9 pieces	250	3	48
Tsunami Roll, 9 pieces	480	15	63
Salads			
Calamari Salad, 4 oz	180	2.5	20
Edamame (soybeans), 4 oz	170	7.5	12
Edamame Salad, 4 oz	60	3	4
Harusame Salad, 2 oz	60	0.5	13
Seabreeze Salad, 2 oz	55	1.5	11
Sauce			
AFC Spicy Sauce, 2 oz	50	4.5	2

Spaghetti Warehouse®

Lunch	C	F	Cb
Minestrone Soup	80	1.5	12
Grilled Chicken Marinara	530	8	65
Seafood Marinara	385	5	65
Spaghetti: w. Tomato Sauce	425	5	82
w. Marinara Sauce #12	440	5	84
Spicy Marinara Sce Spaghetti	280	4	52
Vegetable Primavera	340	4	65

Dinner			
Minestrone, 1 bowl	110	2	18
Grilled Chicken Marinara	640	10	85
Grilled Halibut	880	14	106
Grilled Marinated Chicken Breast	910	17	116
Marinara Sauce #12	520	6	99
Seafood Marinara	520	8	86
Spaghetti w. Tomato Sauce	525	6	101
Spicy Marinara Sce Spaghetti	330	6	60
Vegetable Primavera	610	8	116

Starbuck's®

Hot Beverages: *Grande (16 fl.oz)*	C	F	Cb
Caffe Americano	15	0	3
Caffe Latte: w. Whole Milk	270	14	22
w. Lowfat Milk (2%)	220	7	22
w. Nonfat Milk	160	1	23
w. Soy Milk	150	8	10
Breve	570	42	16
Caffe Misto/Au Lait: Whole Milk	150	8	12
Caffe Mocha: w. Whole Milk	370	21	40
w. Lowfat Milk (2%)	340	16	40
w. Nonfat Milk	290	11	40
w. Soy Milk	320	14	44
Breve	580	40	36
Cappuccino: w. Whole Milk	180	9	15
w. Lowfat Milk (2%)	140	5	15
w. Nonfat Milk	110	0	15
w. Soy Milk	100	5	7
Caramel Apple Cider	370	8	74
Caramel Macchiato: Whole Milk	250	9	36
w. Lowfat Milk (2%)	225	5	36
w. Nonfat Milk	190	1	36
w. Soy Milk	210	3	44
Breve	420	21	37
Chai Tea Latte: 16 fl.oz	320	13	36
w. Nonfat Milk	210	0.5	37
Egg Nog Latte: w. Whole Milk	500	27	49
w. Nonfat Milk	460	22	49
Drip Coffee	10	0	2
Espresso: Solo	5	0	1
Doppio	10	0	2
Espresso Con Panna: Solo	110	9	3
Doppio	115	9	4
Espresso Macchiato: Solo	15	0.5	2
Doppio	20	0.5	3
Hot Chocolate w. Whole Milk	450	24	49
Mocha Valencia w. Whole Milk	480	25	60
Steamed: w. Whole Milk, 16 fl.oz	300	16	23
w. Lowfat Milk (2%)	240	9	23
w. Nonfat Milk	170	1	24
w. Soy Milk	160	9	9
w. Breve	560	48	16
Steamed Cider	230	0	57
Tazo Chai	320	9	52
White Chocolate: w. Whole Milk	480	20	60
w. Lowfat Milk (2%)	450	18	61
w. Nonfat Milk	400	11	61
w. Soy Milk	430	13	65
Breve	690	40	56

Cold Beverages: *Grande (16 fl.oz)*	C	F	Cb
Iced Caffe Americano	15	0	3
Iced Caffee Latte: w. Whole Milk	160	8	13
w. Lowfat Milk (2%)	130	4.5	14
w. Nonfat Milk	100	0	14
w.Soy Milk	90	4.5	88
Iced Mocha: w. Whole Milk	310	16	35
White Choc. Mocha, Whole Milk	320	8	52
Iced Tazo Chai w. Whole Milk	320	5	66

Blended Drinks: *Grande (16 fl.oz)*	C	F	Cb
Frappuccino®: Caramel	350	9	61
Chocolate Brownie	490	14	88
Coffee	270	3.5	55
Eggnog	330	9	57
Expresso	230	3	46
Mocha	290	4	61
Tazo Berry®, Grande (16 fl.oz)	210	0	53
Tazo Berry® & Cream	600	23	63

Beverage Additions: *Per Serving*	C	F	Cb
Caramel Sauce	10	0	2
Fontana® Syrup, all flav., 4 pumps	80	0	21
Mocha Syrup	100	2	24
Power Packet	110	0	23
Sweetened Whipped Crm Topping	100	10	2

Bottled Frappuccino: *Per 9.5 fl.oz Bottle*	C	F	Cb
Caramel	200	3	37
Coffee	190	3.5	35
Hazelnut	200	3.5	37
Mocha	200	3.5	37

Starbucks Icecream (Grocery) ~
See Icecream Section

Icecream Bars	C	F	Cb
Coffee & Almond Bar	280	18	26
Coffee Frappuccino Bar	110	2	20
Mocha Frappuccino Bar	120	2	21
Java Icecream Bar	270	16	29

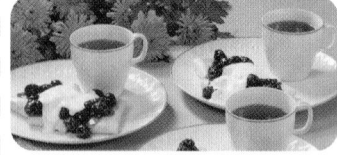

Steak Escape®

Small Sandwiches (7")	C	F	Cb
Grand Cobbler	220	9	22
Grand Escape	300	14	14
Grandest Chicken	250	9	14
Great Escape	300	14	15
Hambrosia	215	9	16
Ragin Cajun	235	7	18
Turkey Club	240	10	13
Vegetarian	220	12	12
Wild West BBQ	310	12	17

Large Sandwiches (12")	C	F	Cb
Grand Cobbler	465	14	32
Grand Escape	550	24	31
Grandest Chicken	450	14	31
Great Escape	545	24	30
Hambrosia	450	18	32
Ragin Cajun	455	14	35
Turkey Club	595	21	28
Vegetarian	410	20	33
Wild West BBQ	615	24	6

Fresh Salads & Potatoes	C	F	Cb
Side Salad	25	0	4
Grilled Salad: w. Chicken	215	7	6
w. Ham	285	14	5
w. Steak	265	12	6
w. Turkey	185	6.5	6
Smashed Potato: Plain	225	0	77
w. Chicken	420	7	79
w. Ham	490	14	78
w. Steak	465	12	79
w. Turkey	390	3.5	79

Fresh Cut Fries	C	F	Cb
Small	500	26	66
Medium	650	34	87
Large	920	48	123

Condiments	C	F	Cb
Mayonnaise, 1 oz	105	12	0
Bull's Eye BBQ Sauce, 1 oz	44	0	10

Steak 'N Shake®

Steakburgers & Sandwiches	C	F	Cb
Steakburger	275	7	33
with Cheese	355	13	33
Super	375	12	33
Super with Cheese	450	18	33
Triple	475	17	33
Triple with Cheese	625	30	34
Ham Sandwich	450	22	37
Grilled Cheese Sandwich	250	13	24
Grilled Chicken Sandwich	510	22	53

Other Items	C	F	Cb
Baked Beans	175	4	27
Chef Salad	315	18	6
Chili & Oyster Crackers	335	14	37
Chili Mac & 4 Saltines	310	12	34
Chili 3 Ways & 4 Saltines	410	16	45
Cottage Cheese, 1/2 cup	95	4	3
French Fries	210	10	28
Lettuce/Tom/ Salad/1oz 1000 Isl.	170	15	7

Desserts	C	F	Cb
Apple Danish	390	24	35
Brownie	260	12	39
Cheesecake	370	11	61
with Strawberries	385	11	65
Pies: Apple	405	18	61
Cherry	335	14	48
Apple, A La Mode	550	25	76
Cherry, A La Mode	475	22	63
Sundaes: Brownie Fudge	645	35	81
Hot Fudge Nut	530	34	51
Strawberry	330	22	29
Vanilla Ice Cream	250	12	23

Shakes & Drinks: Hot Chocolate	685	19	129
Floats: Coca-Cola	515	17	76
Orange	500	17	74
Lemon	555	19	82
Root Beer	530	17	78
Freezes: Lemon	550	25	69
Orange	515	24	63
Shakes: Chocolate/Vanilla	610	38	57
Strawberry	650	40	62

Feedback welcome

Please send comments to: Allan Borushek
POB 1616, Costa Mesa CA 92628
Email: allan@calorieking.com

Subway®

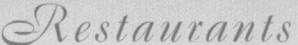

C F Cb

7 Under 6™ Sandwiches (6″)
Figures based on Italian bread and following toppings: Lettuce, tomato, onion, green peppers, olives and pickles.

	C	F	Cb
Ham	288	5	46
Roast Beef	293	5	45
Roasted Chicken Breast	318	5	47
SUBWAY Club®	323	6	46
Turkey Breast	280	4.5	46
Turkey Breast & Ham	293	5	46
Veggie Delite®	226	3	44

Breakfast Sandwiches (6″)
Figures based on Italian bread.

Bacon & Egg	320	16	34
Cheese & Egg	317	15	34
Ham & Egg	338	14	35
Western Egg	300	12	36

Classic Sandwiches (6″)
Figures based on Italian bread and following toppings: Lettuce, tomato, onion, green peppers, olives, pickles, cheese, oil, vinegar, salt and pepper.

BMT®	482	24	46
Cold Cut Trio™	440	21	47
Meatball	527	26	53
Seafood & Crab	405	16	52
Steak & Cheese	390	14	48
SUBWAY Melt®	410	16	47
Tuna	445	22	46

Deli Sandwiches (6″): Ham

Ham	210	4	35
Roast Beef	223	4.5	35
Tuna	325	16	36
Turkey Breast	215	3.5	36

Select Sandwiches (6″)
Figures based on Italian bread and following toppings: Lettuce, tomato, onion, green peppers and select sauce.

Dijon Horseradish Melt	465	22	47
Honey Mustard Ham	310	5	52
Red Wine Vinaigrette Club	350	6	53
Southwest Turkey Bacon	407	17	48
Sweet Onion Chicken Teriyaki	374	5	59
VegiMax w. Gardenburger	390	8	56

Select Sauces: Per Tablespoon

Asiago Caesar	77	8	1
Honey Mustard	20	0	5
Horseradish	100	9	2
Southwest	60	6	1

C F Cb

7 Under 6™ Salads:
Figures include lettuce, tomato, onion, green peppers, olives and pickles.

	C	F	Cb
Ham	112	3	11
Roast Beef	117	3	10
Roasted Chicken Breast	140	3	12
SUBWAY Club®	146	3.5	12
Turkey Breast	105	2	11
Turkey Breast & Ham	117	3	11
Veggie Delite®	50	1	9

Classic Salads:
Figures include lettuce, tomato, onion, green peppers, olives, pickles and cheese.

BMT®	275	19	11
Cold Cut Trio	234	15	11
Meatball	320	20	17
Seafood & Crab®	197	11	17
Steak & Cheese	182	8	12
SUBWAY Melt®	203	10	11
Tuna	238	16	10

Salad Dressings: Per 2 oz

Fat-Free French	70	0	17
Fat-Free Italian	20	0	4
Fat-Free Ranch	60	0	14

Soup: Per 1 Cup

Black Bean	180	4.5	27
Brown & Wild Rice w. Chicken	190	11	17
Cheese w. Ham & Bacon	230	16	13
Chicken & Dumpling	130	4.5	16
Cream of Broccoli	130	7	12
Cream of Potato w. Bacon	210	12	20
Golden Broccoli Cheese	180	12	12
Hearty Chili Beef	250	7	31
Minestrone	70	1	11
Potato Cheese Chowder	210	10	22
Roasted Chicken Noodle	90	4	7
Tomato Bisque	90	2.5	15
Vegetable Beef	90	1.5	14

Breads: 6″ Hearty Italian

6″ Hearty Italian	207	2.5	41
6″ Honey Oat	250	3.5	48
6″ Italian (White) Bread	195	2.5	38
6″ Monterey Cheddar	235	6	39
6″ Parmesan Oregano	210	3.5	40
6″ Roasted Garlic	225	3	45
6″ Sourdough	208	3	41
6″ Wheat Bread	205	2.5	40
Deli Style Roll	165	2.5	32

Subway® cont...

Condiments & Extras

	C	F	Cb
Bacon, 2 strips	45	4	0
Cheese: American; Pepperjack,			
2 triangles	40	3.5	0
Cheddar , 2 triangles	60	5	0
Provolone, 2 half circles	50	4	0
Swiss, 2 triangles	53	4	0
Mayonnaise: 1 Tbsp	110	12	0
Light Mayonnaise, 1 Tbsp	46	5	1
Mustard, all types, 2 tsp	7	0	1
Olive Oil Blend, 1 tsp	45	5	0
Vinegar, 1 tsp	1	0	0

Cookies: Per Cookie

	C	F	Cb
Choc. Chip; M&M	215	10	30
Chocolate Chunk	217	10	30
Double Chocolate	210	10	30
Peanut Butter	220	12	26
Oatmeal Raisin	200	8	30
Sugar	227	12	28
White Macadamia Nut	220	11	28

Fruizle Express (small)

	C	F	Cb
Berry Lishus	113	0	28
Berry Lishus w. Banana	140	3	35
Peach Pizazz	103	0	26
Pineapple Delight	133	0	33
Pineapple Delight w. Banana	160	0	40
Sunrise Refresher	120	0	29

Sub Station®

Sandwiches
Per 1/2 Sub (Incl. Oil, Vinegar, Salad)

	C	F	Cb
Ham & Cheese	505	30	40
Ham, Turkey & Cheese	510	30	40
Turkey & Cheese	525	31	40
Roast Beef & Cheese	525	31	39
Ham, Salami, Pepperoni, Cappicola,			
Bologna, Turkey & Cheese	635	42	40

Sweet Tomatoes®

~ Same Menu & Data as
Souplantation (See Page 238) ~

Taco Cabana®

Grilled Chicken

	C	F	Cb
1/4 Chicken White, 5 oz	295	14	1
No Skin, 4 oz	170	3	0
1/4 Chicken Dark, 4.5 oz	300	18	0.5
No Skin, 3.5 oz	170	7	1
Fajitas: Beef, 4 oz	245	12	4
Chicken White, 4 oz	190	6	4
Chicken Dark, 4 oz	240	11	2
Sides: Black Beans, 4 oz	110	0.5	21
Borracho Beans, 4 oz	110	2.5	17
Calabacita, 4 oz	80	5	7
Chips, 2 oz	290	14	36
Elotes, 1 ea	220	11	27
Guacamole, 1 oz	50	2	4
Queso, 3 oz	190	12	7
Refried Beans, 4 oz	170	6	21
Salsas, all types, 1 oz	10	0	2
Sour Cream, 1 oz	60	6	1
Spanish Rice, 4 oz	180	5	30
Tortillas: 6" Flour	130	3.5	22
6" Table Corn	70	1	11
Tortilla Soup: Small, 8.5 oz	250	8.5	26
Large, 19 oz	370	13	32

Tacos

	C	F	Cb
Bean & Cheese	290	12	35
Black Bean	220	5	37
Carne Guisada	200	8	20
Crispy Beef	150	7	13
Soft Chicken	220	9	21

Burritos

	C	F	Cb
Bean & Cheese	710	27	85
Beef	650	24	76
Black Bean	560	11	95
Chicken	670	26	74

Breakfast Tacos

	C	F	Cb
Bacon & Egg	250	12	22
Barbacoa	310	15	2
Chorizo & Egg	250	12	22
Potato & Egg	240	10	27

TCBY®
~ See Page 31 - Icecream Section ~

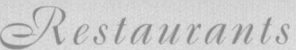

Taco Bell®

Tacos	C	F	Cb
Taco, regular	210	12	18
Taco Supreme®	260	16	20
Soft Taco Beef	210	10	20
Soft Taco Chicken	190	7	19
Soft Taco Steak	280	17	20
Double Decker® Taco	380	17	43
Double Decker® Taco Supreme	420	21	45

Gorditas			
Cheesy Gordita Crunch	560	33	44
Cheesy Gordita Crunch Supreme	610	37	47
Gordita Baja™ Beef	360	21	29
Gordita Baja™ Chicken; Steak	340	18	28
Gordita Supreme® Beef; Steak	300	14	27
Gordita Supreme® Chicken	300	13	28
Gordita Nacho Cheese Beef	310	15	30
Gordita Nacho Cheese Chkn; Steak	290	13	28

Chalupas			
Chalupa Baja® Beef	420	27	30
Chalupa Baja® Chicken; Steak	400	24	27
Chalupa Supreme® Beef	380	23	29
Chalupa Supreme® Chicken	360	20	28
Chalupa Supreme® Steak	360	20	27
Chalupa Nacho Cheese Beef	370	22	30
Chalupa Nacho Cheese Chkn; Steak	350	19	29

Specialities			
Tostada	250	12	27
Cheese Quesadilla	490	28	39
Chicken Quesadilla	540	30	40
Enchirito® Beef	370	19	33
Enchirito® Chicken; Steak	350	16	31
Meximelt®	290	15	22
Mexican Pizza, 7$^1/_2$ oz	540	35	42
Taco Salad w. Salsa & Shell	850	52	69
Taco Salad w. Salsa, w/out Shell	400	22	31
Southwest Steak Bowl	660	33	66
Taco Salad w. Salsa, w/out Shell	400	22	31
Zesty Chicken Border Bowl	720	45	58
w/out Dressing	460	19	55

Nachos and Sides: Nachos, 3.5 oz	320	18	34
Nachos Supreme®	440	24	44
Nachos BellGrande®	760	39	83
Mucho Grande Nachos	1320	82	116
Pintos 'n Cheese, 4.5 oz	180	8	18
Mexican Rice, 4.75 oz	190	9	23
Cinnamon Twists, 1.25 oz	150	4.5	27

Taco Bell® cont...

Burritos	C	F	Cb
7-Layer Burrito	520	22	65
Bean Burrito	370	12	54
Burrito Supreme® Beef	430	18	50
Burrito Supreme® Chicken/Steak	420	16	49
Chili Cheese Burrito	330	13	40
Double Burrito Supreme® Beef	510	23	52
Double Burrito Supreme® Chicken	460	17	50
Double Burrito Supreme® Steak	470	18	48
Fiesta Burrito Beef	380	15	49
Fiesta Burrito Chicken; Steak	370	12	48
Grilled Stuft Beef	730	35	75
Grilled Stuft Chicken; Steak	690	29	73

Taco John's®

Tacos			
Bravo	360	15	40
Burger	280	11	29
Crispy	190	12	13
El Grande	480	29	30
El Grande Chicken	330	18	24
Sierra Taco™ Beef	500	30	39
Sierra Taco™ Chicken	430	24	37
Softshell	230	10	23
Softshell Chicken	170	5	21

Burritos: Bean Burrito	380	11	53
Beefy Burrito	440	20	44
Chicken and Potato Burrito	450	18	56
Chicken Fajita Burrito	320	10	41
Combination Burrito	410	15	49
El Grande Burrito	450	19	51
El Grande Chicken	630	26	66
Meat and Potato Burrito	500	23	58
Ranch Burrito Beef	440	22	43
Ranch Burrito Chicken	380	17	41
Smothered Burrito	540	24	57
Super Burrito	450	19	51

Favorites: Bean Tostada	160	7	17
Cheese Crisp	220	16	9
Chilito	440	22	41
Double Enchilada	780	43	58
Mexi Rolls	670	40	53
Mexican Pizza	560	31	47
Quesadilla: Regular	460	24	41
Chicken	430	20	42
Tostada	200	12	13

Restaurants & Fast—Foods

Taco John's®

Specialities

	C	F	Cb
Chicken Festiva Salad (w. dressing)	690	50	39
Chicken Festiva Salad (no dressing)	370	20	27
Chicken Nachos	810	54	57
Potato Olés Bravo	570	35	55
Potato Olés w. Nacho Cheese	530	34	50
Sierra Chicken Sandwich	480	27	37
Super Nachos	925	62	70
Super Potato Olés	970	61	82
Taco Salad (with dressing)	770	50	55
Taco Salad (no dressing)	600	33	50

Platters

	C	F	Cb
Beef and Bean Chimi	740	33	82
Beef Enchilada	830	41	79
Chicken Enchilada	690	32	71
Smothered Burrito	880	36	101

Sides

	C	F	Cb
Green Chili	225	12	20
Mexican Rice	250	5	44
Nachos	440	30	35
Potato Olés: Small (Kid's Meal)	310	18	33
Regular	410	24	45
Large	540	32	59
Refried Beans	360	11	45
Side Salad	290	25	15
Texas Style Chili	380	22	23

Desserts

	C	F	Cb
Apple Grande	260	9	40
Choco Taco	310	17	37
Churros	160	11	13
Cookies (Kid's Meal), 1 bag	130	5	20
Taco John's Cinnamon Mint Swirl	60	0	14

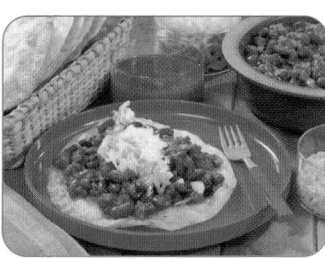

Taco Time®

Burritos

	C	F	Cb
Casita Burrito®, Beef	650	31	54
Crisp Burrito: Bean	425	18	53
Beef	550	30	39
Chicken	420	25	32
Veggie	490	16	70
Double Soft Bean Burrito	510	12	77
Double Soft Combination Burrito	615	23	66
Double Soft Beef Burrito	725	33	55
Value Soft Bean Burrito, Single	380	10	58
Value Soft Meat Burrito, Single	490	21	48
Veggie Burrito	490	16	70

Tacos: Crisp Taco

	C	F	Cb
Crisp Taco	295	17	16
Natural Super Taco, Meat	625	27	60
Rolled Soft Flour Taco	510	23	46
Soft Taco Chicken	390	16	41
Soft Taco Super Shredded Beef	370	11	38
Taco Cheeseburger, Meat	635	36	48
Value Soft Taco	315	15	23

Specialties: Crustos®, 3.5 oz

	C	F	Cb
Crustos®, 3.5 oz	375	15	47
Empanada, Cherry	250	9	37
Mexi Fries®: Regular, 4 oz	265	17	27
Large, 8 oz	530	34	54
Mexican Rice, 4 oz	160	2	30
Nachos: Regular, 10.5 oz	680	38	61
Deluxe, 15.25 oz	1050	57	91
Quesadilla, Cheese (Kid's Meal)	205	11	17
Refritos, 7 oz	325	10	44

Salads: Per Serving

	C	F	Cb
Chicken Taco (no dressing), reg.	370	21	27
Taco Salad (no dressing), regular	480	28	30
Tostada Delight® Salad, Meat	630	33	48

Fillings & Extras: Chips, 2 oz

	C	F	Cb
Chips, 2 oz	265	12	35
6" Taco Shell	110	6	14
7" Flour Tortilla	90	1	16
8" Fried Flour Tortilla	205	11	24
Cheddar Cheese, 3/4 oz	85	7	0
Chicken, 2.5 oz	110	6	2
Enchilada/Hot Sauce, 1 oz	12	0	3
Lettuce, 1/2 oz	2	0	0
Shredded Beef, 2.5 oz	70	0	1
Taco Meat, 2.5 oz	210	11	7

Tim Horton's®

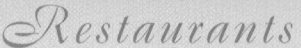

Bagels	C	F	Cb
Average all types	300	3	59

Cream Cheese: Per 1 1/2 oz	C	F	Cb
Plain	140	14	1
Plain Light	90	7	3
Garden Vegetable	150	13	3
Strawberry	150	12	7

Baked Goods	C	F	Cb
Butter Croissant	210	11	25
Cheese Croissant	240	12	27
Cherry Cheese Danish	380	23	33
Plain Tea Biscuit, 3 oz	220	6	36
Raisin Tea Biscuit, 3 oz	250	6	47
Southern Country Cran./Rasp., 6 oz	470	19	68

Cakes: Per 1/8 Whole	C	F	Cb
Black Forest	500	21	75
Celebration (white)	500	16	85
Chocolot Fantasy	420	15	72
Shadow, white & chocolate	430	19	63

Cookies: Per Cookie	C	F	Cb
Chocolate Chip	150	7	21
Oatcakes	190	10	22
Oatmeal Raisin	150	6	22
Peanut Butter, all types	170	10	18
Plain Macaroon	140	8	14

Donuts: Per Donut	C	F	Cb
Honey Stick	280	15	34
Sugar Twist	230	10	32
Walnut Crunch	320	18	36
Cake Donut: Chocolate Glazed	350	22	35
Old Fashion Glazed	270	12	39
Old Fashion Plain	220	12	24
Sour Cream Plain	280	18	25
Filled Donut: Angel Cream	280	13	36
Blueberry	220	8	33
Boston Cream	230	8	36
Canadian Maple	230	8	36
Strawberry	220	8	33
Yeast: Apple Fritter	300	14	40
Chocolate Dip	230	10	33
Dutchie	280	13	39
Honey Dip	230	10	32
Maple Dip	250	10	36

Timbits: Each	C	F	Cb
Yeast: Honey Dip	50	1	10
Dutchie	60	2	10
Filled: Banana Cream	45	1	8
Lemon	50	2	9
Spiced Apple; Strawberry	50	2	9
Cake: Old Fashion Plain	45	2	7
Chocolate Glazed	70	3	9

Muffins: Blueberry Bran	C	F	Cb
	300	9	51
Carrot Whole Wheat	410	22	52
Low Fat Carrot/Cranberry	260	2	60
Wild Blueberry	330	11	54
Chocolate Chip Plain	390	15	62
Raisin Bran	360	10	66
Oatbran 'n Apple	350	12	58
Oatbran Carrot 'n Raisin	340	11	57
Oatmeal Raisin	430	11	80
Lowfat Honey	290	2	66

Pies: Per 1/4 Whole	C	F	Cb
Apple	540	31	62
Banana Cream	440	26	57
Cherry	570	31	70
Chocolate Cream	490	31	52

Tarts: Fresh Strawberry (1)	C	F	Cb
	220	9	36
Raisin Butter Tart (1)	330	11	54

Sandwiches	C	F	Cb
Albacore Tuna Salad, no dressing	350	8	49
Black Forest Ham & Swiss w. Dress.	640	27	53
Chunky Chicken Salad, no dressing	380	10	50
Fireside Roast Beef w. Dressing	470	19	48
Garden Vegetable w. Dressing	460	24	50
Harvest Turkey Breast w. Dressing	470	18	53

Soup: Chili	C	F	Cb
	320	9	32
Cream of Mushroom	195	10	21
Hearty Vegetable; Minestrone	130	2	14
Potato Bacon	195	7	29
'Tim's Own' Chicken Noodle	100	3	15
Vegetable Beef Barley	110	2	18

Beverages	C	F	Cb
Cafe Mocha, 10 fl.oz	250	10	34
Cappuccino Ice, 16 fl.oz	430	23	54
Coffee, 10 fl.oz	80	4	10
French Vanilla Cappuccino, 10 fl.oz	130	5	20
Fruit Punch, 300ml	150	0	38
Hot Chocolate, 10 fl.oz	200	6	44

Togo's Eatery®

	C	F	Cb
Salads: Per Serving			
Caesar Salad, 11 oz	470	30	23
Garden Salad, 16.5 oz	255	10	32
Oriental, 11 oz	500	21	49
Potato Side Salad, 4 oz	215	13	25
Taco Salad, 17.8 oz	945	59	76
Dressings: Per 2.3 oz Packet			
Ranch	320	33	5
RC Italian	60	5	4
Oriental	220	14	24
Caesar; Thousand Island	240	23	8
RC Ranch	190	16	10
Sandwiches: Per 6" Sandwich on White Roll			
Albacore Tuna	700	30	79
Avocado & Turkey	675	28	80
Avocado, Cucumber & Alfalfa	635	28	85
BBQ Beef	725	22	95
California Roasted Chicken	510	15	73
Chunky Chicken Salad	635	26	72
Egg Salad w. Cheese	730	35	76
Ham & Cheese	660	26	76
Hot Pastrami	705	26	86
Hummus	670	21	102
Italian Dry: Salami & Cheese	770	33	78
Capicolla, Mort., Cotto; Provol.	735	32	74
Meatballs w. Pizza Sauce	710	28	78
Pastrami Reuben	875	45	85
Roast Beef (Hot or Cold)	550	11	73
Turkey & Bacon Club	665	26	73
Turkey & Cranberry	625	13	96
Turkey & Cheese	740	23	75
Turkey, Ham & Cheese	670	25	76

Treat Street®

	C	F	Cb
Yogurt			
Everything: Butter Pecan	90	0	19
Chocolate; Strawb./Vanilla	100	0	24
Everything Non Fat No Sugar Added:			
Chocolate	70	0	18
Other flavors	80	0	19
Everything Non Fat, all flavors	90	0	19
Plain Non Fat Pistachio Mix	90	0	20
Plain Non Fat No Sugar Added:			
Butter Pecan	80	0	18
White Chocolate	80	0	19

Una Mas®

	C	F	Cb
Burritos			
Bean & Cheese Burrito	650	25	80
El Cheapo	555	9	98
Fajita Burrito: Chicken	715	21	89
Steak	735	26	89
Fish Burrito Cabo Style	490	14	53
Gallito	590	30	62
Thai Chicken Burrito	500	16	62
Vegetariano Burrito	540	20	69
Una Mas Burrito: Chicken	585	15	76
Steak	605	20	76
Tacos: Crispy Chicken Taco	240	17	12
Fish Taco Cabo Style	265	6	36
Una Mas Taco: Chicken	340	9	48
Steak	345	11	48
Veggie	275	7	45
Favoritos: 5-Layer Dip	345	22	25
Chicken Enchiladas (2)	480	20	37
Nachos	1220	81	91
Quesadilla Grande	635	46	49
Quesadilla Chica	355	18	28
TJ Caesar Salad	355	18	29
w. Chicken	520	26	30
Tortilla Soup: Cup	200	13	4
Bowl	330	20	6
Tostada Salad	475	20	50
w. Chicken	640	29	53
Verde Salad	210	5	19
Side Orders: Beef, 3 oz	190	13	1
Black Beans, 5 oz	150	3	23
Chicken, 3 oz	165	8	1
Corn Tortilla	80	1	17
Fish, 4 oz	195	8	0
Flour Tortilla (12")	150	4	25
Fresh Guacamole, 2 oz	80	7	4
Monterey Jack Cheese, 1 oz	100	7	1
Pinto Beans, 5 oz	170	2	29
Refried Beans, 1/2 Cup	100	2	18
Rice, 5 oz	160	2	31
Sour Cream, 1 oz	60	6	1
The Works	160	14	5
Tortilla Chips, 1 oz	140	7	18
Salsa & Dressing: Chipotle Sce	5	0	1
Salsa Fresca/Ranchero, 1 oz	5	0	1
Mild Sauce; Salsa Verde, 1 oz	10	0	2
Caesar Dressing, 2 oz	140	12	2
Jalapeno Vinaigrette, 2 oz	140	1	16

247

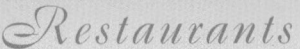
Weinerschnitzel®

(Carbohydrate figures - author estimates only)

Hamburgers	C	F	Cb
Deluxe: Hamburger	575	37	30
Cheeseburger	635	42	32
Bacon Cheeseburger	685	46	32
Breakfast: Breakfast Burrito	570	37	50
Breakfast Sandwich	540	32	38

Original or All Beef Hot Dogs	C	F	Cb
BBQ Bacon Dog	380	23	37
Chili Dog	295	16	38
Chili Cheese Dog	350	21	40
Corn Dog	290	23	25
Deluxe Dog	275	14	38
Kraut Dog	265	14	37
Mustard Dog	260	14	37
Relish Dog	280	14	37

Specialties	C	F	Cb
Italian Sausage	195	15	na
Chicken Deluxe	535	32	na
Apple Pie	240	12	32
Fries: Regular	270	10	36
Large	380	14	50
Chili Cheese Fries	465	36	na

Wendy's®

Sandwiches	C	F	Cb
Big Bacon Classic®	570	30	46
Chicken Breast Fillet	430	16	46
Chicken Club	470	20	47
Classic Single with Everything	410	19	37
Grilled Chicken Sandwich	300	7	36
Kids' Meal: Jr. Hamburger	270	9	34
Jr. Cheeseburger	310	12	34
Jr. Cheeseburger Deluxe	350	16	37
Jr. Bacon Cheeseburger	380	19	34
Spicy Chicken Sandwich	430	14	47

French Fries: Medium	C	F	Cb
	390	17	56
Biggie	440	19	63
Great Biggie	530	23	75
Kid's Meal	250	11	36

Chicken Nuggets: 5 Piece	C	F	Cb
	220	14	13
4 Piece Kid's Meal	180	11	10

Salads	C	F	Cb
Caesar Side Salad	70	3	9
w. Croutons/Dressing	290	23	12
Side Salad, no Dressing	35	0	7

Garden Sensations Salads	C	F	Cb
Chicken BLT Salad: no Dressing	310	16	10
w. Croutons/Dressing	690	47	31
Mandarin Chicken™: no Dressing	150	1.5	17
w. Dressing/Nuts/Noodles	620	36	52
Spring Mix Salad, no Dressing	180	11	12
w. Dressing/Pecans	530	44	26
Taco Supremo: no Dressing	360	17	29
w. Chips/Sour Cream/Salsa	670	34	61

Dressings & Sauce: Per Packet	C	F	Cb
Barbecue Sauce	40	0	10
Blue Cheese	290	30	3
Caesar	150	16	1
Creamy Ranch	250	25	5
Reduced Fat	110	9	7
French Fat Free	90	0	21
Honey Mustard Dressing	310	16	10
Lowfat	120	4	23
Honey Mustard Sauce	130	12	6
House Vinaigrette	220	20	9
Oriental Sesame Sauce	280	21	21
Sweet & Sour Sauce	50	0	12
Thousand Island	260	25	7

Hot Stuff Baked Potato™	C	F	Cb
Plain	310	0	72
Bacon & Cheese	580	22	79
Broccoli & Cheese	480	14	81
Sour Cream & Chives	370	5	72
Country Crock Spread	60	7	0
Chili: Per Serving			
Small	200	6	21
Large	300	9	31
Hot Chili Seasoning	5	0	2
Cheddar Cheese, shredded, 2 Tbsp	70	6	1
Saltine Crackers, 2	25	0.5	4

Frosty™ Dairy Dessert: Per Cup	C	F	Cb
Junior, 6 oz	170	4	28
Small, 12 oz	330	8	56
Medium, 16 oz	440	11	73

Whataburger®

Burgers/Sandwiches	C	F	Cb
Whataburger®	595	29	53
Small bun no oil	425	21	31
Double Meat Whataburger®	835	46	53
Justaburger®	295	12	27
WhataChick'N®	580	30	56
Whataburger Jr.®	305	15	29
Grilled Chicken S'wich: w. Dressing	455	18	49
No dressing	395	12	47
No bun oil or dressing	370	9	47
Small bun, mustard (no dressing)	335	8	30

Whatameals® Includes Drink & Fries	C	F	Cb
Whataburger® Meal	1255	50	169
Whataburger® w. Bacon & Chse	1420	62	170
Chicken Strips w. Toast & Gravy	970	48	132
Chicken Strips Kids Meal	740	38	92
Double Meat Whataburger®	1495	67	169
Grilled Chicken S'wich Meal	1115	39	165
Justaburger® Kids Meal	655	26	97
WhataChick'N® S'wich Meal	1240	51	172
Whataburger Jr.® Meal	705	29	110

Sides	C	F	Cb
French Fries: Small	240	14	37
Medium	420	21	51
Large	560	29	69
Onion Rings: Medium	305	17	36
Large	465	25	54

Chicken & Salads	C	F	Cb
Chicken Strips (2)	380	24	22
Garden Salad	55	0	11
w. Cheddar Cheese	225	15	11
Grilled Chicken Salad	215	5	19
w. Cheddar Cheese	385	19	19
Dressings: Ranch, 2 oz	310	33	3
Low Fat Ranch. 2 oz	70	4	10
Low Fat Viniagrette, 2 oz	35	2	6
Thousand Island, 2 oz	160	12	12

Shakes	C	F	Cb
Chocolate; Strawberry:			
Small, 20 fl oz	615	16	100
Medium, 32 fl oz	905	25	146
Vanilla: Small, 21 fl oz	560	17	82
Medium, 32 fl oz	835	26	122

Desserts: Hot Apple Pie	C	F	Cb
Desserts: Hot Apple Pie	250	12	34
Chocolate Chunk Cookie, 2 oz	140	8	35
White Choc Macadamia Cookie, 2 oz	240	12	31

Breakfast	C	F	Cb
Bacon, 2 slices	75	5	1
Biscuit: Plain	290	15	33
w. Bacon	365	20	34
w. Bacon, Egg, Cheese	490	29	35
w. Egg & Cheese	415	24	34
w. Sausage	505	34	34
w. Sausage Gravy	480	32	48
w. Sausage, Egg, Cheese	630	43	34
Breakfast-On-A-Bun®: w. Bacon	320	16	29
w. Sausage	460	30	29
Breakfast Platters (Biscuit/Eggs/Hash Brown):			
w. Bacon, 2 slices	665	39	52
w. Sausage, 1 patty	805	52	51
Cinnamon Roll, 4.6 oz	430	17	63
Egg Omelet Sandwich	290	15	28
Hash Brown Sticks (4)	140	8	16
Pancakes: Plain (3)	300	3	57
w. Bacon, 2 slices	375	8	58
w. Sausage, 1 patty	515	22	57
Scrambled Eggs (2)	160	11	2
Taquitos: Bacon & Egg	375	20	28
Potato & Egg	370	19	35
Sausage & Egg	380	22	28

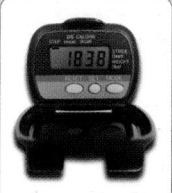

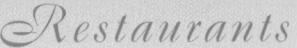

Fast–Foods & *Restaurants*

Winchell's®

Baked Products	C	F	Cb
Bagel	310	1	22
Banana Nut Muffin	535	28	63
Blueberry Muffin	440	25	54
Blueberry Muffin, Low Fat	410	3	42
Bran Muffin	425	20	48
Bran Muffin, Low Fat	405	3	44
Cheese Muffin	520	25	51
Chocolate Chip Muffin	480	22	54
Croissant	260	17	28

Cake Donuts: Per Donut Unless Indicated

	C	F	Cb
Buttermilk Bar Glazed	260	16	29
Cinnamon Crumb Cake	245	18	30
Glazed Old Fashion	250	18	28
Iced Cake	230	15	28
Iced French	220	13	24
Iced Old Fashion	260	19	28
Iced Donut Holes (4)	230	15	28
Plain Donut Holes (4)	215	14	26

Raised Donuts: | | | |

	C	F	Cb
Apple Fritter	670	41	55
Bear Claw	560	30	47
Chocolate Bavarian	325	18	36
Chocolate Rounds	240	16	29
Chocolate Twist	240	16	29
Glazed Cinnamon Roll	430	24	12
Glazed Jelly	320	17	36
Glazed Rounds	230	15	27
Glazed Twist	230	15	27
Glazed Rounds	230	15	27
Iced Bar	240	16	29
Sugar Rounds	225	15	27
Sugar Twist	225	15	27

Drinks: | | | |

	C	F	Cb
Frozen Orange Chilla	340	8	66
Frozen Mocha Cappuccino	490	19	74

Zantiago®

Burrito	C	F	Cb
Hot Cheese, Chilito	330	15	35
Mild Cheese, Chilito	335	15	36

Enchilada	C	F	Cb
Beef	315	15	26
Cheese	390	23	26

Taco	C	F	Cb
Burrito	415	19	41
Regular	200	12	13

White Castle®

Hamburgers	C	F	Cb
Hamburger	135	7	11
Cheeseburger	160	9	11
Bacon Cheeseburger	200	13	12
Double Hamburger	235	14	16
Double Cheeseburger	285	18	16

Sandwiches: Chicken	190	8	21
Fish Sandwich	160	6	18
Breakfast Sandwich	340	25	17

Sides: Cheese Sticks, 3 piece	290	17	19
Chicken Rings, 6 piece	310	21	14
French Fries, small	115	6	15
Onion Chips, small	180	9	25
Onion Rings, 8 piece	540	26	69

Drinks: Coca-Cola, 14 fl.oz	120	0	32
Chocolate/Vanilla Shake, 14 fl.oz	230	7	35
Iced Tea, 14 fl.oz	45	0	12

Yoshinoya®

Bowls	C	F	Cb
Beef Bowl: Regular, 15 oz	840	30	109
Large, 21 oz	1160	41	153
Kids, 9 oz	340	11	48
Chicken Bowl: Regular, 19 oz	760	15	125
Large, 30 oz	1110	22	180
Kids, 10 oz	370	9	53
Combo Bowl: Regular, 17 oz	750	19	117
Large, 27 oz	1220	36	171
Vegetable Beef Bowl: Reg.,18 oz	770	23	114
Large, 28 oz	1090	32	163
Vegetable Bowl: Regular 19 oz	530	3.5	116
Large, 32 oz	780	5	169

Tempura: Fish Tempura, 22 oz	990	24	168
Fish & Beef Tempura, 30 oz	1450	45	214
Fish & Chicken Tempura, 31 oz	1450	37	225
Shrimp Tempura, 20 oz	890	19	160
Shrimp & Beef Tempura, 28 oz	1350	40	206
Shrimp & Chicken Tempura, 29 oz	1340	32	217

Extras	C	F	Cb
Beef, 5^1/2 oz	370	28	6
Chicken & Vegetables, 9^1/2 oz	300	12	21
Rice, 10 oz	460	2.5	104
Vegetable, 9 oz	60	0.5	12

Note: Yoshinoya Beef Bowl Restaurants are based in California.

Notes on Cholesterol

- **Cholesterol** is a white waxy substance produced mainly by our liver. It is also found in animal food products. Plant foods have no cholesterol.

- **Cholesterol is essential to life.** It is a structural part of every body cell wall and is the building block for vitamin D, sex hormones, and bile acids which help in the digestion of dietary fats.

- **The body makes sufficient cholesterol** for its needs and does not rely on cholesterol in the diet. Dietary fats have a major influence on blood cholesterol levels - more so than dietary cholesterol.

- **A high blood cholesterol increases** the risk of atherosclerosis - the thickening of arteries that can reduce or block blood flow to the heart muscle, brain, eyes, kidneys, sex organs and other body parts.

  This in turn increases the risk of heart attack, stroke, blindness, kidney failure, impotence and other blood circulatory problems.

  Other risk factors which increase the risk of atherosclerosis include high blood pressure, tobacco smoking, obesity and diabetes (uncontrolled).

HEART ATTACK WARNING SIGNALS

Many victims die before reaching hospital by ignoring warning signals and delaying medical help.

Symptoms vary and commonly include:

- **Chest pain**, vice-like squeezing or burning sensation in centre of chest or between shoulder blades, or feeling of severe indigestion.

- **Pain** may spread to shoulders, neck, jaw or arms.

- **Sweating**, nausea, dizziness, shortness of breath, irregular pulse.

If you experience any of the above symptoms seek IMMEDIATE medical attention!

Every minute counts.

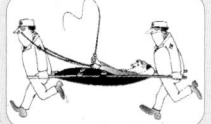

BLOOD CHOLESTEROL

Check Your Risk!

Cholesterol Level (mg/dL)	Risk of Heart Attack
240 and above	~ High Risk
200 - 239	~ Borderline/High
Below 200	~ Desirable

♥ Know your cholesterol level, particularly if there is a family history of heart disease or stroke. If high, see your doctor.

♥ All adults should have their cholesterol, HDL and triglycerides tested at least every 5 years.

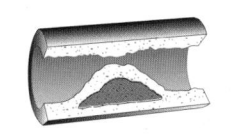

▲ Atherosclerosis can clog arteries and impede blood flow to the heart muscle or other body organs.

▼ A thrombus (blood clot) can form on unstable, festering atherosclerotic plaque and rapidly block blood flow.
A heart attack or stroke can result.

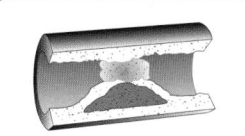

Fats & Cholesterol Guide

The amount and type of dietary fat has the greatest influence on blood cholesterol levels.

Fats in food are a mixture of 3 basic types: saturated, monounsaturated, and polyunsaturated. Animal fats are mainly saturated while plant oils and fish oils are mainly mono- and polyunsaturated.

Saturated fats have subgroups known as long chain, medium chain, and short chain fats. Most of the long chain fats raise blood cholesterol; and increase the risk of blood clots and thrombosis leading to artery blockage.

Long chain saturated fats are found mainly in full cream milk, cheese, butter, cream, fatty meats and sausages, and processed foods.

Monounsaturated fats tend to more selectively lower 'bad' LDL-cholesterol and maintain the protective 'good' HDL-cholesterol in the bloodstream - but only if they replace saturated fats in the diet.

Foods rich in monounsaturates include canola and olive oils, canola margarine, peanuts, and avocados.

Polyunsaturated fats consist of two main classes. **Omega-6** polyunsaturates tend to lower blood cholesterol. Rich sources include safflower, sunflower and corn oils.

Omega-3 polyunsaturated fats can lower blood cholesterol, and also confer extra benefits by lowering blood triglycerides, and reducing the risk of thrombosis, heart arrhythmias, and artery spasm.

Best practical omega-3 sources include canola oil and margarine, soybean oil and fish. (See adjoining chart)

A balanced intake of the two omega classes is important for optimal health. Increasing slightly omega-3 intake by Americans would help to attain a more ideal balance. Adequate vitamin E intake is also important.

> All fats are high in calories and need to be limited for weight control.

DIETARY FATS COMPARISON

■ Saturated Fat ■ Monounsaturated Fat
■ Linoleic (Omega-6) ■ Alpha-Linolenic (Omega-3)

OILS — PERCENTAGE CONTENT

Oil	Saturated Fat	Monounsaturated Fat	Linoleic (Omega-6)	Alpha-Linolenic (Omega-3)
CANOLA OIL	7	63	20	10
LINSEED/FLAX OIL	9	19	17	55
SAFFLOWER OIL	9	14	77	
GRAPESEED OIL	10	22	68	
SUNFLOWER OIL	11	23	66	
CORN OIL	14	32	52	2
OLIVE OIL	14	76	10	
SOYBEAN OIL	15	23	54	8
PEANUT OIL	19	45	34	2
COTTONSEED OIL	26	16	58	
PALM OIL	51	39	10	

SPREADS & FATS

Saturated Fat includes 'Trans Fats' ☐ WATER CONTENT

Spread	Saturated Fat	Monounsaturated Fat	Linoleic (Omega-6)	Alpha-Linolenic (Omega-3)	Water Content
LIGHT MARGARINE	14	14	21		51
CANOLA MARGARINE	18	45	12	6	19
POLYUNSATURATED MARG.	24	20	36		20
BUTTER	57	18	2		24
LARD	41	47			12
BEEF FAT	44	37	4		15

GOOD SOURCES OF OMEGA-3 FATS

Plant Sources	Omega-3 Fats (Grams)
Canola Oil, 1 Tbsp, 1/2 fl.oz	1.5g
Flaxseed Oil, 1 Tbsp	8g
Soybean Oil, 1 Tbsp	1.2g
Canola Margarine, 1 Tbsp, 1/2 oz	1g
Soybeans, cooked, 1/2 cup, 4 oz	0.5g
Walnuts, 1/2 oz	0.5g

FISH - Per 4 oz Serving
High Content: Salmon (Chinook), Tuna, Trout (Lake), Sardines, Herring, Mackerel — 3g
Medium Content:
Salmon (Pink/Red/Coho), 4 oz — 2g
Fair Content: Per 4 oz Serving
Bass, Catfish, Cod, Grouper, Hake, Halibut, Kingfish, Perch, Pollock, Shark, Trout (Rainbow), Tuna (Skipjack), Crab, Oysters, Blue Mussel, Shrimp, Squid } 0.5-1g

How Much is Needed?
As little as 1-2 grams daily of omega-3 fats may benefit general health. High doses of fish oil supplements should only be taken as directed by your doctor.

Dietary Cholesterol

Cholesterol in food varies in its effect on blood cholesterol level (BCL) from person to person. Much depends on the amount and type of fat, and fiber eaten at the same meal.

Any elevating effect of dietary cholesterol on BCL is more likely to occur when the diet is high in saturated fat. Little elevation, if any, generally occurs when dietary fats are balanced in favour of mono- and polyunsaturated fats (including omega-3 fats). For example, while fish does contain cholesterol, the omega-3 fats can prevent any increase in BCL. Conversely, a meal containing no cholesterol but rich in saturated fat, may see a significant increase in BCL.

Consequently, the need to be overly concerned about dietary cholesterol is being de-emphasised in favour of a stricter approach to limiting total fats, and saturated fat in particular.

The liver usually cuts back its own cholesterol production in response to cholesterol in the diet. Many people can consume normal amounts of high cholesterol foods without concern.

However, it is difficult to identify just who is at risk - the so-called 'hyper-responders' - and because over 50% of Americans have a BCL above ideal levels, the **American Heart Association** advises all Americans to be prudent and limit their cholesterol intake to less than 300mg daily.

This limitation still allows the inclusion of most foods regularly eaten - even the overly maligned egg.

Note: Eggs contain a modest 5 grams of fat per large egg of which barely 2 grams are saturated, the rest being mono- and polyunsaturated.

By comparison, a cup of whole milk has almost 10g fat of which 6g are saturated.

CHOLESTEROL COUNTER

Cholesterol is found only in foods of animal origin. Plant foods contain no cholesterol. AHA recommends limiting dietary cholesterol to less than 300mg/day.

	Chol
Meat - Average all types:	mg
Lean Meat, cooked, 4 oz	70
Fatty Meat, cooked, 4 oz	105
Fat, thick strip, 2 oz	35

(Note: While lean meat and fat have similar amounts of cholesterol, choose lean meat to limit fat intake.)

	Chol
Chicken/Turkey, average, 4 oz	90
Organ Meats: Liver, fried, 4 oz	500
Brains, beef, pan fried, 3 oz	1700
Sausages: Frankfurter, 1.5 oz	25
Salami, 2 slices, 2 oz	40
Bacon: 3 slices, cooked, 1 oz	20
Fish: Fish fillets, average, ckd, 4 oz	70
Tuna/Salmon, canned, 3 oz	30
Scallops, 9 medium, 3 oz	30
Shrimp, 12 large, raw, 3 oz	130
Oysters, raw, 6 medium, 3 oz	45
Lobster, Crab, raw, 3 oz	80
Eggs (Chicken), 1 large	210
1 medium	180
Egg White, *Egg Beaters*	0
Milk/Yogurt: Whole, 1 cup, 8 fl.oz	35
1% Milk, 1 cup	10
Skim/Non-fat, 1 cup	5
Soy Milk	0
Cheese: Natural/Hard/Cream 1 oz	30
Cottage, lowfat, 4 oz	5
Ricotta, part skim, 4 oz	25
Fats: Butter, 2 Tbsp, 1 oz	60
Margarine, Oils (vegetable)	0
Mayonnaise, 1 Tbsp	10
Cream: Heavy, whipping, 2 T, 1 oz	40
Half & Half/Sour, 2 Tbsp, 1 oz	10
Icecream: Regular, $1/3$ cup, 4 fl.oz	30
Fruit, Vegetables, Avocados	0
Nuts, Seeds, Grains	0
Coffee, Tea, Soda, Beer, Wine	0

Blood Cholestrol ~ Diet Hints

DIETARY HINTS TO LOWER BLOOD CHOLESTEROL

1. **Maintain a healthy weight.**
   If overweight, lose weight with lowfat eating and daily exercise.

2. **Reduce saturated fat intake by:**
   (a) eating less dairy fat. Choose lowfat or fat-reduced varieties of milk, yogurt, cheese, and icecream. Enjoy soy drinks.
   (b) replacing saturated fats with fats and oils rich in mono- and polyunsaturated fats; and carbohydrate-rich foods. Choose vegetable oils such as canola, olive, sunflower and soybean. Avoid solid frying fats. *Take Control* and *Benecol* (spreads) contain plant stanol esters which can lower total and LDL cholesterol.
   (c) eating less fat from meat and poultry. Choose lean cuts of meat and skinless chicken. Go easy on luncheon meats, salamis and fatty sausages. Enjoy fish.
   (d) eating less saturated fats from baked and fried fast-foods. Avoid deep-fried foods. Avoid donuts, cakes, pastries and cookies unless made with healthier fats and oils.

3. **Increase your 'soluble' fiber intake.**
   Foods rich in 'soluble' fiber include dried beans, baked beans, lentils, chick peas, hummus, nuts, seeds, psyllium seed husks and psyllium fiber supplements.
   Oat bran, rice bran and barley are also useful, as are fruit, veges and avocados.

4. **Eat more soya bean products** such as: soy drinks, tofu, tempeh (cultured soya beans), soy flour and soy vegetarian foods.
   Soy protein in place of animal protein can significantly decrease high blood cholesterol levels - as well as 'bad' LDL-cholesterol and blood triglycerides. Good' HDL-cholesterol is maintained. For best results, eat at least 25g of soy protein per day (from 3-4 servings)

5. **Eat more fruit and vegetables in place of high-fat foods.**
   Aim for 2 fruits and 5 servings of vegetables per day. They also contain valuable antioxidants.
   The fat of avocados (and most nuts and seeds) is mainly unsaturated and lowers blood cholesterol levels.

6. **Limit cholesterol to 300mg per day.**
   (Extra Notes ~ See Previous Page)

7. **Avoid brewed unfiltered coffee** (espresso; plunger-style). It contains oil compounds (diterpenes) which can raise blood cholesterol. American style filtered coffee is fine.

8. **Spread your food intake over the day.**
   Have 5-6 small meals per day rather than just 2-3 large meals. Nibbling, versus gorging, favors lower blood cholesterol.

ALCOHOL - WINE

Alcohol is a mixed bag. Moderate amounts of 1-2 drinks daily appear to reduce the risk of heart attack and ischaemic stroke in older persons.

However, larger amounts increase the risk of high blood pressure, obesity, heart failure and hemorrhagic stroke; and can aggravate hypertriglyceridemia - in addition to many other health hazards.
(See Alcohol Guide - p.163)

The over-riding harmful effects of excess alcohol do not allow its recommendation for any aspects of health promotion.

Notes On Wine:
Red wine (more so than white) contains antioxidants which may help protect cholesterol in the blood from becoming oxidized.

Most fruits, vegetables and tea also contain protective antioxidants.

Fats in the diet not only affect blood cholesterol levels. They can also strongly influence blood clot formation and thrombosis, as well as blood flow and ultimate oxygen delivery to body parts and organs.

While advanced atherosclerosis can impede blood flow to the heart and other organs, it is thrombosis (complete blockage by blood clots) or arterial spasm which commonly result in a heart attack or stroke.

Plant and fish oils rich in omega-3 fats lessen the risk of blood clots, thrombus formation and artery spasm by reducing platelet stickiness and adhesion to artery walls. This reduces the risk of atherosclerotic plaque becoming unstable and reactive.

Omega-3 fats also improve blood flow by reducing blood viscosity; and increasing the flexibility of red blood cells (**RBC**) that need to flex and twist on themselves in order to squeeze through tiny narrow capillaries often half their diameter.

A diet high in saturated fats has the opposite effect by stiffening RBC membranes and increasing blood viscosity thereby hindering blood flow. The stiffening of the RBC membrane also reduces its ability to release vital oxygen to body cells and take up carbon dioxide.

Stiff red blood cells may also form aggregates like coin stacks. In narrow blood vessels, this further impedes blood flow and impairs oxygen release through the much lessened surface area of red blood cell membranes exposed to blood. (Smoking, lack of exercise, and stress can have similar adverse effects on thrombosis, red blood cell flexibility and blood flow.)

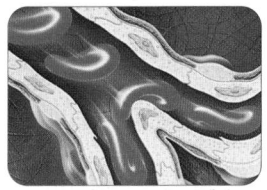

▲ Picture of Healthy Blood Flow

Flexible red blood cells twist and slide through tiny capillaries - often half the diameter of red blood cells.

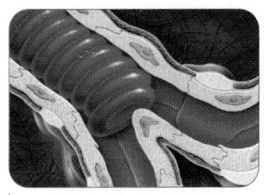

▲ A Not-So-Healthy Picture!

Red blood cells have lost their flexibility and ability to twist and slip through capillaries. They are stacked up thereby impeding blood flow.

A diet high in saturated fats can contribute to this picture - as can smoking, lack of exercise and stress.

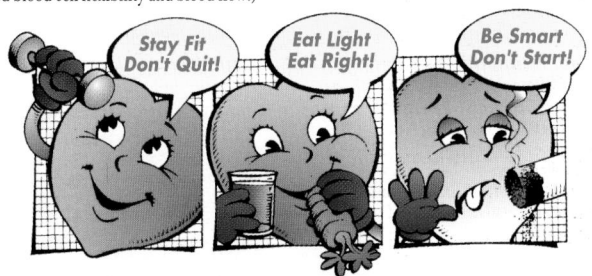

Osteoporosis Guide

Calcium's Role in the Body

Calcium plays a vital role in nerve and muscle function, clotting of blood, enzyme regulation, insulin secretion and overall bone strength. Bones and teeth store 99% of the body's calcium.

The calcium level in blood is kept at a steady level by the continual exchange of calcium between blood and bone. When insufficient calcium is obtained from food the body draws calcium out of the bones.

This bone loss over a period of years may lead to **osteoporosis** - thinning of the bones (*porous bones*).

The bones become weak, brittle and easy to fracture, particularly the bones of the wrist, hips and spine. Loss of height and curvature of the spine may also result, as may periodontal disease - the deterioration of the jaw bones that support the teeth.

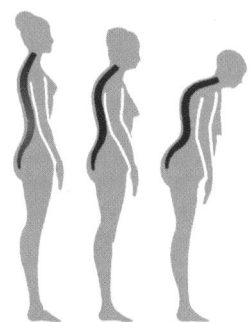

As osteoporosis progresses after menopause, vertebrae may collapse causing the spine to curve and shoulders to hunch.

Osteoporosis - Common in Women

While osteoporosis also occurs in men, women are particularly vulnerable (1 in 4 by age 60). They have about 30% less bone than men, and a greater bone loss at menopause when estrogen levels drop. Slender framed women are at greater risk. (A woman in her eighties can have lost up to two thirds of her skeleton.)

Insufficient dietary calcium during pregnancy and breastfeeding will see bone reserves drawn upon, increasing the risk of osteoporosis.

Causes of Osteoporosis

The major factors associated with the bone loss of osteoporosis appear to be:

- **Hormone changes of menopause.**

- **Insufficient calcium in the diet.**
  (Absorption decreases with age.)

- **Insufficient exercise (weight bearing -**
  such as walking, cycling.)

- **Family history of osteoporosis.**

- **Other contributing factors may include:** excess amounts of alcohol, protein and phosphorus (from meats and soft drinks); insufficient vitamin D and magnesium; and cigarette smoking.

RECOMMENDED DAILY INTAKE OF CALCIUM

	Calcium
Infants:	
0-6 mths ~	360mg
6-12 mths ~	540mg
Children:	
1-10 yrs ~	800mg
10-12 yrs ~	1200mg
Teenagers:	
13-18 yrs ~	1200mg
16-18 yrs ~	800mg
Adults: 19+ yrs ~	800mg
Women:	
Pre-menopausal ~	1000mg
Menopausal(beginning)~	1200mg
Post-menopausal ~	1500mg
Pregnancy/breastfeeding:	
10-18 yrs ~	1600mg
19+ yrs ~	1200mg

Early Prevention Important

Gradual loss of bone begins in the thirties after maximum bone mass is reached. The stronger the bones at that time, the less trouble is likely to occur later. The earlier that prevention or treatment begins the greater the benefit. **The key to prevention** is to build strong, dense bones early in life. **By age 16,** some 80% of peak bone mass is reached.

Young women may lessen the risk by eating high-calcium foods, not engaging in excessive dieting that results in menstrual period cessation (less estrogen), taking regular exercise and not smoking.

In menopausal women, hormone therapy as well as calcium supplements and exercise, can help retard osteoporosis. Your doctor can advise you.

Dietary Sources of Calcium

Milk, yogurt, calcium-enriched soy drinks and cheese are the richest sources of calcium. (Lowfat and nonfat varieties contain similar amounts of calcium.)

Canned fish with edible bones (salmon/sardines) are high in calcium. Tofu (calcium coagulant), tempeh, broccoli and dried beans are also good sources.

> ### Calculating Calcium ~ Food Labels
> The calcium content of packaged foods and drinks is shown in the Nutrition Facts label as a percentage of the DRI (dietary reference intake) of 1000 mg calcium. To convert this percentage into milligrams of calcium, simply mutiply the percent figure by 10 (or add a zero). Examples: 5% = 50 mg calcium; 35% = 350 mg calcium.

Extra Notes on Calcium

Soy drinks (calcium-enriched) may be preferable to cow's milk. Body calcium losses are much greater with animal protein. Soy protein is relatively 'bone-sparing'.

Persons who have difficulty eating sufficient calcium-rich foods should consider a **calcium supplement.** Prescribed high doses of calcium (1500-2000mg/day) may benefit persons with osteoporosis - as well as vitamins D and K, and magnesium.

Calcium in food reduces iron absorption by up to 60% when eaten with iron-containing foods. Ideally, consume calcium-rich foods/supplements at smaller meals and mid-meal snacks. Daily calcium above 2000mg is unlikely to provide any additional benefit.

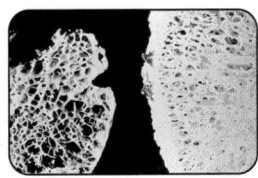

▲ Osteoporotic Fragile Bone   ▲ Healthy Dense Bone

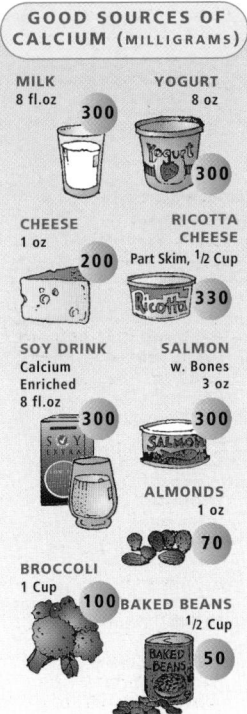

GOOD SOURCES OF CALCIUM (MILLIGRAMS)

MILK 8 fl.oz — 300	**YOGURT** 8 oz — 300
CHEESE 1 oz — 200	**RICOTTA CHEESE** Part Skim, 1/2 Cup — 330
SOY DRINK Calcium Enriched 8 fl.oz — 300	**SALMON** w. Bones 3 oz — 300
	ALMONDS 1 oz — 70
BROCCOLI 1 Cup — 100	**BAKED BEANS** 1/2 Cup — 50

Calcium Counter

Milk & Milk Drinks	Calcium (mg)
Milk Fluid:	
Whole: 1 cup, 8 fl.oz	300
1 small glass, 6 fl.oz	220
1% or 2%: 1 cup, 8 fl.oz	300
Lowfat/Skim: 1 cup, 8 fl.oz	300
Hi-Calcium (Borden), 1 cup	1000
Viva w. extra Calcium, 1 cup	500
Condensed Milk, sweet, 1 fl.oz	110
Evaporated Milk: Skim, 1 fl.oz	90
Whole/Lowfat	80
Dry/Powder: Whole, 1/4 cup	290
Skim/Nonfat, 1/4 cup	380
Other Milks & Milk Drinks	
Buttermilk, average, 1 cup	300
Chocolate Milk, average, 1 cup	300
Nesquik Double Chocolate, 1 cup	400
Goats Milk, 1 cup	320
Malted Milk, 1 cup	350
Milkshakes: Medium, 15 fl.oz	450
Café Latte, 1 cup, 8 fl.oz	220
Cappuccino, 1 cup, 8 fl.oz	150
Milk Drink Powders:	
Malted Milk, dry powder, 1 oz	80
Chocolate, Instant, 3 Tbsp	10
Cocoa Powder: Regular, 1 Tbsp	10
Cocoa Mix: Hershey, 1/3 cup	40
Alba High Calcium, 1 envelope	320
Soy & Grain Drinks	
Soy: Regular, non-fortified, 1 cup	60
Enriched/Calcium-fortified, 1 cup	300
Dry Powder, 1 oz	80
Rice/Oat Drinks: Average, 1 cup	10
Yogurt	
Average All Brands, 1 cup, 8 oz	350
Fruit-flavored: 1 cup, 8 oz	250
Small cup, 6 oz	200
4 oz cup	150
Plain: Average, 1 cup, 8 oz	300
Fat Free/Lowfat, 8 oz	350
Custard-style: 6 oz	100
Drinkery (Nouiche)	300
Frozen Yogurt, average, 1/2 cup	150
Fats/Oils	
Butter, Margarine, Spreads, Oils	0
I Can't Believe It's Not Butter	0
w. Sweet Cream and Calcium, 1 Tbsp	100
Country Crock with Calcium, 1 Tbsp	100

Cream	Calcium (mg)
Average: Unwhipped, 1 Tbsp	15
Whipped, 1 heaping Tbsp	15
Half & Half, 1 Tbsp	15
Non-dairy Creamers, 1 tsp	0
Ice Cream & Ices	
Ice Cream: Regular, 1 scoop	65
1/2 cup	90
Premium (Ben & Jerry's), 1/2 cup, 4 oz	150
Soft Serve, 1/2 cup	120
Lowfat, 1/2 cup, 4 oz	150
Ice Milk, average, 1/2 cup	100
Sherbet, average, 1/2 cup	50
Fruit Sorbet	0
Sundae, regular, 6 fl.oz	200
Soy/Tofu Ices, average, 1/2 cup	10
Cheese: Per 1 oz (1 1/2" Cube)	
Natural, Hard: Average, 1 oz	200
Processed Cheese: Average, 1 oz	150
Single-wrapped, 3/4 oz	120
Cheese Substitutes: Average, 1 oz	200
Specific Cheeses:	
Blue, 1 oz	150
Brie	50
Camembert	110
Cheddar	200
Cottage Cheese: 1 round Tbsp, 1 oz	20
1/2 cup, 4 oz	80
Cream Cheese	20
Dorman's Light, average 1 oz	200
Edam, Gouda	200
Feta	140
Goat, semi-soft	85
Gruyere	290
Kraft Light Naturals, average	250
Light-Line (Borden), singles	200
Monterey Jack	210
Mozzarella, average	170
Parmesan, grated, 1 Tbsp	70
Processed, average	160
Provolone	210
Ricotta, part skim, 1/2 cup, 4 1/2 oz	330
Swiss	270
Cheese Dishes: Souffle, 4 oz	240
Macaroni & Cheese, 1 cup, 8 oz	150
Ham & Cheese Crepes, 8 oz	350
Quiche, 1 serve, 6 oz	200

Eggs

	Calcium (mg)
1 large Egg	30
Scrambled, with Milk	50
Omelet w. Cheese ($1/2$ oz)	260

Fish & Seafood

Canned Fish: Tuna, canned, 3 oz	10
Salmon: with bones, 3 oz	190
without bones, 3 oz	10
Sardines, with bones, 3 oz	90
Fresh Fish: cooked, average, 4 oz	35
Seafood: Lobster, cooked, 4 oz	60
Mussels/Oysters (10), 4 oz	95
Crabmeat, cooked, 4 oz	50

Meats & Poultry

Average all types, cooked, 4 oz	20
Vegetarian Soy Burgers:	
Example: *BocaBurger*, 1 pattie, $2^1/2$ oz	100

Soups: *Average all types*

No Milk or Cheese added, 1 serve	30
with Milk, $1/2$ cup, 1 serve	180

Sauces: Non-Dairy, average, 2 Tbsp

	10
Cheese/White Sauce, 2 Tbsp	40

Spices: Average all types, 1 tsp

	5

Bread, Bagels

Bread: White, 1 slice, 1 oz	30
Wholewheat, Rye, 1 slice, 1 oz	30
Bagels, average	30
Buns/Rolls: Small	40
Large	90
English Muffins, 2 oz	90
Pita, $6^1/2$ " diameter, 2 oz	50
Tortillas, Corn, 1 oz	40

Breakfast Cereals

Ready To Eat: Average all types, 1 oz	20
with $3/4$ cup Milk/Soy (enriched)	250
All-Bran, $1/2$ cup, 1 oz	150
Kashi Heart to Heart, $3/4$ cup, 1.2 oz	500
Life (Quaker), 1 cup, 1 oz	100
Special K Red Berries, 1 cup	150
Total (General Mills), all types, 1 oz	1000
Wheaties (General Mills), 1 cup, 2 oz	350
Hot Type, cooked: Corn Grits, 1 cup	5
Cream of Wheat, 1 cup	50
Oatmeal/Rolled Oats: Regular, ckd, 1 cup	20
Instant, fortified, 1 pkt	100

Note: Breakfast cereals are a good medium for calcium-rich milk or soy drinks (150mg per $1/2$ cup).

Flours, Grains

	Calcium (mg)
Wheat Flour: All-purpose, 1 cup	20
Self-rising, 1 cup	330
Whole-wheat, 1 cup	50
Carob Flour, 1 cup, $3^1/2$ oz	360
Corn meal, 1 cup, 4 oz	20
Soybean Flour, 1 cup, 3 oz	170
Grains, Barley, Rice: Cooked, 1 cup	15

Pasta, Spaghetti

Average all types, cooked, 1 cup	15
Lasagne, average, 1 serve	300
Macaroni & Cheese, aver., 1 cup	150
Spaghetti w. Meat Sce, 1 serve	20
with 1 Tbsp Parmesan	90

Sugar & Syrups, Honey

Sugar: White	0
Brown, 1 Tbsp	10
Syrups: Table Syrup, 2 Tbsp	0
Choc., Thin type, 2 Tbsp	5
Fudge type, 2 Tbsp	40
Molasses: Light, 2 Tbsp	70
Blackstrap, average, 1 Tbsp, $3/4$ oz	270
Honey, Jam, Jelly	0

Cookies & Cakes, Desserts

Cookies: Average all types, 1 cookie	5
Crackers, average, 1 only	5
Cake: Plain, average, 2 oz	40
Carrot Cake with Icing	45
Cheesecake, 1 piece	80
Fruitcake, 1 piece	40
Croissants, average, 2 oz	20
Custard, average, $1/2$ cup	150
Danish pastry, average, 2 oz	60
Donuts, average, 2 oz	20
Gelatin, plain w. water, $1/2$ cup	2
Muffins: Regular, average, $1^1/2$ oz	40
English Muffins, 2 oz	90
Pancakes, 4" diameter, average, 1 oz	40
Pies: Apple/Fruit, average, 5 oz	20
Custard Pie, average, 5 oz	140
Pecan Pie, 1 piece, 5 oz	70
Pumpkin Pie, 1 piece, 5 oz	80
w. Icecream, 1 scoop: Add	70
Puddings: Canned, aver., 5 oz	80
Dry Mix, made w. milk, $1/2$ cup	150
Rice Pudding, $1/2$ cup	120
Waffles, 7" diameter average	160

Calcium Counter

Candy, Chocolate

	Calcium (mg)
Chocolate: Milk Chocolate, 1 oz	50
Plain/Fruit, 1 oz	65
with Almonds, 1 oz	80
Kit Kat Wafer (1 1/2 oz); Mars Bar (1.8 oz)	80
Milky Way Bar, 2 oz	60
Carob Bar, average, 2 oz	220
Sugar Candy, Jelly Beans, M'mallow, 1 oz	0

Snacks & Nutrition Bars

Breakfast Bars *(Carnation)*	20
Corn Chips; Tortilla Chips, 1 oz	40
Granola Bars, average	30
Popcorn, 1 cup	5
Potato Chips, 1 oz	10
Nutrition Bars: *Balance Oasis* Bars	350
Dr Soy Bars	350
GeniSoy 'Soy Nutty' Bar	250
Jenny Craig; Power Bars	300
MetRx, After Fx, Pure Protein Bars	500
Nature's Plus Calcium Almond Blitz	1200
Slim-Fast 'Meal On The Go'	300
TwinLab Protein Fuel Bars	350
Viactiv Bar	300
Wholefoods Everyday Bars	300

Nuts & Seeds (Shelled)

Almonds, 12-15 nuts, 1/2 oz	40
Brazil Nuts, 4 medium, 1/2 oz	30
Cashews, 6-8 nuts, 1/2 oz	5
Coconut, fresh, 1/2 oz	5
Filberts (Hazelnuts), 1/2 oz	40
Macadamias, 6 medium, 1/2 oz	10
Peanuts, raw, 1 oz	25
Walnuts, 1 oz	20
Seeds: Pumpkin, 1 oz	15
Sesame, 1 Tbsp	10
Sunflower, 1 oz	30
Tahini, 1 Tbsp, 1/2 oz	20

Drinks – Alcohol, Soda, Water

Beer, Cider, Wine, 1 glass	5
Spirits, Liqueurs	0
Coffee, Tea, Soda, Fruit Drinks	5
Water: Tap, average, 1 cup	5
Mineral Water *(Perrier)*, 1 glass, 6 oz	20

Fruit & Fruit Juice

	Calcium (mg)
Fresh Fruit: Average all types, 1 serve	20
Apple, 1 medium	10
Avocado, 1 medium	20
Banana, 1 medium	10
Orange, 1 medium	50
Pear, 1 medium	20
Rhubarb, cooked, 1/2 cup	170
(calcium largely not available to body)	
Dried Fruit: Average, 1 oz	20
Figs, 3 medium, 1 1/2 oz	55
Fruit Juice: Average, 1 cup, 8 fl.oz	25
Orange Juice, calcium fortified (8 fl.oz):	
Citrus Hill Plus Calcium, Hi-C	300
Donald Duck	350
Minute Maid (Premium Calcium)	300
Jui2ce, 8 fl.oz	200
Tropicana (Calcium)	350
Welch's Healthy Sensation, 1 cup	350

Vegetables

Average all types, 1 cup	40
Higher Calcium Content:	
Beans, dried: cooked, 1/2 cup	50
Baked/Refried Beans, 1/2 cup	60
Broccoli, chopped, 1 cup	100
Chickpeas, boiled, 1/2 cup	40
Collards, cooked, 1 cup	150
Dandelion Greens, cooked, 1 cup	150
Kale, 1 cup	130
Mustard Greens, 1 cup	100
Soybeans, cooked, 1/2 cup, 3 oz	60
Spinach, cooked, 1/2 cup	120
Potato: Plain, 1 large	20
Au Gratin, 1 cup	200
Mashed w. Milk, 1 cup	60
Tofu: *Mori Nu:* Silken, 4 oz	90
Azumaya: Silken, 3 oz	120
Firm/Extra Firm, 3 oz	150
Hinoichi: Regular, 1" slice, 3 oz	100
Firm/Extra Firm, 3 oz	150
Soft, 1" slice, 3 oz	60
Nasoya: Firm, Soft, 3 oz	120
Extra Firm, 3 oz	150
Silken, 3 oz	60
Tree of Life: Firm, 3 oz	150
Miso: 1/2 cup, 5 oz	100
Tempeh: 4 oz serving	100

Frozen Entrees/Meals	Calcium (mg)
Budget Gourmet: Ziti Parmesano	160
Three Cheese Lasagne	360
Healthy Choice:	
Cheddar Broccoli Potatoes (Solos)	200
Chicken Broccoli Alfredo (Bowl)	150
Meat Lasagna (Medley)	200
Lean Cuisine:	
Chicken Carbonara (Café Classics)	150
Chicken Fettucine (Dinnertime)	250
Creamy Chicken/Veges Bowl	250
French Bread Pizza, Cheese, 6 oz	300

Frozen Pizzas ~ Regular Large	
Average All Brands: Cheese, 1/4 pizza	350
Meats (Sausage/Pepperoni), 1/4 pizza	250

Nutritional Shakes/Drinks	
Atkins Shake, 11 fl.oz can	300
Balanced: Diet, 11 fl.oz can	500
High Protein, 11 fl.oz can	250
Boost, regular, 8 fl.oz can	300
Choice dm (Mead Johnson) 8 fl.oz	330
Ensure High Calcium, 8 fl.oz can	400
Genisoy Shake, 1 scoop, 35g	250
Jevity (w. Fiber) 8 fl.oz	215
Kashi GoLean Shake, 11 oz can	400
Kindercal	240
Met-Rx Protein Shake, 11 fl.oz	950
Myoplex (EAS) Nutrition Shake, 11 oz	400
Optifast 800, Powder or Can (RTD)	200
Slim-Fast Shakes, 325ml can	400
Spiru-Tein, Vanilla, 8 fl.oz can	600
Ultra Slim-Fast: Soy Protein Drink, 11.5 oz	350
Shake, 11 oz can	400
Mix, Meal, 1 scoop, 33g	150
Usana Nutrimeal, 2 scoops, 43g	400
Walgreens, Slim For Less, 11 oz can	400

Calcium Supplements	
Caltrate 600, 1 tablet	600
Citracal, 1 tablet	200
Maalox Soft Chews, 1	400
Nature's Life 'Super Cal-Mag', 1	500
Os-cal; 1 tablet	500
Posture Calcium, 1 tablet	600
Tums: Regular, 1 tablet	200
Extra Strength, 1 tablet	300
Viativ Soft Calcium Chews, 1 chew	500

Fast-Foods, Restaurants	Calcium (mg)
Chicken: Grilled/BBQ, 1/4 chicken	20
Battered & Fried, 2 pieces	80
Nuggets, 6 pack	20
Crispy Chicken Deluxe Sandwich	50
Croissant Sandwich: Plain	40
with Cheese, 1 oz	240
Fish Sandwich: no Cheese	60
with Cheese	140
Fish Filet Deluxe	70
Fish, fried, 2 pieces	20
French Fries: Small Serving	10
Hamburgers: Average all outlets,	
Regular, no Cheese	120
Cheeseburger, regular	120
McDonald's: Big Mac	160
Quarter Pounder w. Cheese	120
Egg McMuffin	120
Hot Dog: Plain	60
with Cheese	150
Mexican: Burrito	120
Enchilada	300
Nachos, regular	200
Taco, regular	140
Taco Bell Salad	400
Pizza: Average all types,	
Medium (12"), 2 slices	250
Double Cheese, 2 slices	350
Large (16"), 2 slices	350
Double Cheese, 2 slices	500
Pizza Hut:	
Cheese, medium, 2 slices	290
Pepperoni, medium, 2 slices	300
Potato: Plain, baked, 8 oz	20
Stuffed w. Cheese Topping	100
with Cheese Filling	300
Sandwiches: no Cheese	60
with 1 oz Cheese (regular)	260
with Cream Cheese	80
Subway: 6" Sandwich, average	100
Cheese & Egg Bkfst Sandwich	150
Steak & Cheese Wrap	150
Cheese (extra fixin'), 3 triangles	150
Pocket Sandwich, no Cheese	150
Salads (Classic), average	100
Salads: Chef, regular	300
Coleslaw, small	20
Shakes, average	330

Fiber Guide

Introduction

Fiber is the general term for those parts of **plant** food that we cannot digest (although bacteria in the large bowel partly digests fiber through fermentation). It is not found in foods of animal origin (meats, dairy products).

Fiber promotes intestinal health, bowel regularity, can benefit diabetes and blood cholesterol levels, and may help prevent colon cancer. High fiber foods also assist weight control.

Most Americans don't eat enough fiber - less than 20 grams/day - instead of a **healthier 25 to 35 grams/day.**

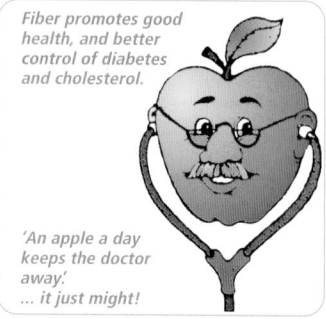

Fiber promotes good health, and better control of diabetes and cholesterol.

'An apple a day keeps the doctor away.'
... it just might!

Types of Fiber

Plant foods contain a mixture of different fibers in varying proportions. Insoluble and soluble fiber categories are based on their solubility in water. All types of fiber are beneficial to the body.

◆ **Insoluble fibers** (cellulose, hemi-celluloses, lignin) make up the structural parts of plant cell walls. The **best sources** are wheat bran, corn bran, rice bran, wholegrain cereals and breads, dried beans and peas, nuts, seeds and the skins of fruits and vegetables.

These fibers absorb many times their own weight in water. They create a soft bulk and hasten the passage of waste products through the intestines.

They promote bowel regularity, and aid in the prevention and treatment of uncomplicated forms of **constipation**, **diverticulosis and haemorrhoids.**

The risk of colon cancer may also be reduced by fiber's diluting effect of potentially harmful substances.

◆ **Soluble fibers** (pectin, gums, mucilages) are found mainly within plant cells, soy milk (whole bean) and products.

Types of Fiber (Cont)

Best Sources of Soluble Fiber:
Fruits and vegetables, oat bran, barley, dried beans and peas, psyllium and flax seed.

These fibers form a gel which slows both stomach emptying and the absorption of sugars from the intestines. This helps to control **blood sugar** levels.

Weight control is also aided by the slower emptying of the stomach and the feeling of **fullness provided by soluble fiber.**

Some soluble fibers can lower **blood cholesterol** by binding bile acids and excreting them. More body cholesterol must then be broken down to supply bile acids for emulsification of dietary fats. **Rice bran, while not high in soluble fiber can also lower blood cholesterol.**

◆ **Resistant starch** is that part of starchy foods (approx. 10%) which is tightly bound by fiber and resists normal digestion. Friendly bacteria in the large bowel ferment and change the resistant starch into short-chain fatty acids which are important to bowel health and may protect against colon cancer.

Starchy foods include bread, cereals, rice, pasta, potatoes and legumes.

Fiber & Weight Control

Fiber can assist weight control in several ways. Fiber-rich foods such as fresh fruit and vegetables, potatoes and whole-grain bread contain few calories for their large volume (due to their lowfat, high water content).

Their bulk fills the stomach and satisfies appetite much earlier than fiber-depleted foods. The extra chewing time also contributes to satiety, and gives the stomach time to register a feeling of fullness. Excessive calories are less likely to be consumed.

Fiber-depleted foods and drinks are more concentrated in calories; e.g. fats, sugar, candy, soft drinks, fruit juices, alcohol. They require little or no chewing. Large amounts with excessive calories can be consumed before appetite is satisfied.

Example: Whereas one fresh apple might satisfy our appetite, an apple juice drink with the equivalent sugars and calories of 2-3 apples does little to satisfy appetite. (See illustration below.)

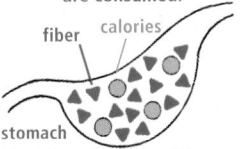

High Fiber Foods fill the stomach. Fewer calories are consumed.

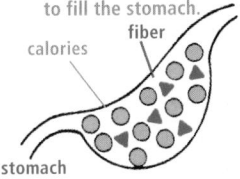

Low Fiber Foods are more concentrated in calories. More food must be eaten to fill the stomach.

EFFECTS OF REMOVING FIBER FROM FOOD

2-3 pieces of fresh fruit produces 1 glass of fruit juice. The removal of fiber concentrates the sugar and calories.

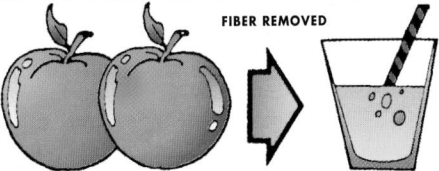

FIBER REMOVED

Fresh Fruit		Fruit Juice
High Fiber	←	Negligible Fiber
Low Calorie Density	←	High Calorie Density
Long Eating Time	←	No Eating Time (Drink)
Satisfies Hunger	←	Does Not Satisfy Hunger
Sugar Slowly Absorbed	←	Sugar More Quickly Absorbed
Less Insulin Required	←	More Insulin Required

Fiber Guide - Constipation

Constipation

Constipation can reasonably be defined as a failure to have a bowel movement at least every second day - and just as importantly, without straining or pain.

Typically, stools are too hard, too narrow, and too small . . . *sinkers* rather than *floaters*.

The **main cause** is simply a lack of dietary fiber. Other contributing factors include insufficient fluids, too little exercise, emotional stress, gastro-intestinal disease, lack of proper dentition to chew high-fiber foods, and some medications (e.g. some antacids, antidepressants, tranquilizers).

Note: Check with your doctor to rule out any underlying medical problem – especially if you have a change in bowel habits in middle-age or later years.

DESIRABLE FIBER INTAKE

Adults: 25-35gm per day
Children (under 18): Age + 5gm
Example: 6-year old (6 + 5)= 11gm

SAMPLE FOOD QUANTITIES
For 35 Grams of Fiber/Day `Fiber`

Breakfast Cereal (higher-fiber)	5g
plus 4 slices whole wheat Bread	6g
plus 3 servings fresh Fruit	9g
plus 1 medium Potato (w. skin) **or** 1 cup Brown Rice **or** 1/2 cup whole-wheat Pasta	4g
plus 3-4 servings Veges/Salad	6g
plus 1 cup Bean Soup **or** 1/4 cup Baked/Soy Beans **or** 1/2 cup Corn/Peas/Lentils **or** 1 1/4 oz Almonds (natural) **or** 3 medium Figs	5g

---

HINTS TO INCREASE FIBER AND AVOID CONSTIPATION

1. Breakfast is an important contributor to daily fiber intake. Eat high-fiber breakfast cereals (bran-based cereals, oatmeal etc.). Add 1-2 tablespoons of unprocessed bran (wheat/ barley/ rice) and wheat germ if required.

Dried fruits, chopped nuts, soy grits, and seeds are also excellent additions to cereals.

Note: A gradual increase in fiber will prevent bloating, gas or pain. Persons intolerant to bran may benefit from psyllium-based fiber supplements and cereals.

2. Drink 6-8 glasses of water daily. Fiber works by absorbing many times its own weight of water.

3. Eat wholegrain breads, or fiber-enriched breads. One slice of whole-wheat bread has over double the fiber of regular white bread.

4. Enjoy fruit as fresh fruit with skins rather than as fruit juice. Enjoy whole-wheat pasta, barley, brown rice, nuts and seeds.

5. Eat more vegetables, salads and legumes - especially dried beans, baked beans, lentils, potatoes with skins, avocado, broccoli, brussel sprouts, cabbage, carrots, celery, and peas.

6. Add bran (barley/rice/wheat) or soy grits to soups, casseroles, yogurt, desserts, biscuits, cakes. Also use wholemeal flour or soy flour in place of white flour. Use nuts and seeds.

7. Snack on fresh or dried fruits, carrot or celery sticks, popcorn, nuts or seeds, wholegrain crackers, high-fiber bars (low-fat). Limit amounts if overweight.

8. Exercise regularly to strengthen abdominal muscles and stimulate the gut. Keep up fluids, especially in warm weather.

9. Avoid indiscriminate and regular use of harsh laxatives. They can overstimulate the intestinal muscles and may make normal bowel activity impossible. It may take several weeks to restore normal bowel function.

Fiber Guide

FOODS WITH ZERO FIBER

- Dairy Products (Milk, Cheese, etc)
- Meats, Poultry, Fish, Eggs
- Fats/Oils, Sugar/Syrups

(Only foods of plant origin contain fiber.)

Breakfast Cereals **Fiber**

General Mills: Basic 4, 1 cup, 2 oz	3
Cheerios (Honey Nut; Multigrain), 1 c., 1 oz	3
Team Cheerios, ³/4 cup, 1 oz	1
Energy Crunch Wheaties, 1 cup, 1.95 oz	3
Fiber One, ¹/2 cup, 1 oz	13
Multi-Bran Chex, 1 cup, 2 oz	8
Oatmeal Crisp Almond, 1 cup, 2 oz	4
Raisin Nut Bran, ³/4 cup, 2 oz	5
Total, average all types, 1 oz	3
Wheat Chex; Wheaties, 1 cup	5
Wheaties Energy Crunch, 1 cup	4
Health Valley: 10 Bran O's, ³/4 cup, 1.95 oz	4
Amaranth Flakes, ³/4 cup	4
Corn Bran Flakes, ³/4 cup	4
Fiber 7 Flakes, ³/4 cup	4
Golden Flax, ¹/4 cup	6
Granola (Fat Free), ²/3 cup	6
Healthy Crunches & Flakes, ³/4 cup	4
Healthy Fiber Flakes, ³/4 cup	4
Oat Bran Flakes, all types, ³/4 cup	4
Real Oat Bran, ¹/2 cup	5
Kellogg's: All-Bran, ¹/2 cup, 1 oz	10
All-Bran w. Extra Fiber, ¹/2 cup, 1 oz	13
Bran Buds, ³/4 cup, 2 oz	12
Corn Flakes, Fruit Loops, Smacks, ³/4 cup	1
Cracklin' Oat Bran, ³/4 cup, 2 oz	6
Cocoa/Rice Krispies Treats, ³/4 cup, 1 oz	0
Complete: Wheatbran Flakes, ³/4 c., 1 oz	5
Oatbran Flakes, ³/4 cup	
Corn Pops, 1 cup, 1 oz	0
Frosted Mini Wheats, 1 cup, 2 oz	6
Healthy Choice, all types, 1 cup	5
Nutri-Grain Almond, 1¹/4 cup, 2 oz	4
Cereal Bars, 1 bar, 1.3 oz	4
Mueslix (Almond. Raisin Date), ²/3 cup	4
Raisin Bran, 1 cup, 2 oz	8
Smart Start Original, 1 cup	2
Soy Protein, 1 oz	2
Special K; Product 19, 1 cup	1
Special K Red Berries, 1 cup	4
Wheat Chex, 1 cup	5

Fiber ~ Fiber (grams)
Breakfast Cereals (Cont) **Fiber**

Kashi: GoLEAN Cereal, ³/4 cup, 1.4 oz	10
GoLEAN Crunch!, 1 cup, 1.8 oz	8
GoLEAN Bars, each	6
Breakfast Pilaf, ¹/2 cup, cooked, 5 oz	6
Good Friends, ³/4 cup, 1 oz	8
Cinna-raisin Crunch, 1 cup, 1³/4 oz	10
Heart to Heart, ³/4 cup, 1.2 oz	5
Puffed Kashi, 1 cup, 0.9 oz	1
Quaker: Cap'n Crunch, ³/4 cup	1
100% Natural Granola, average,¹/2 cup	3
Crunchy Corn Bran, 1 cup, 1 oz	5
Fruity Oh's, 1 cup	2
Honey Nut, 1 cup	3
Life Cereal (³/4 cup), Oat Squares (¹/2 c.)	2
Oat Bran, ¹/3 cup	6
Oatmeal, average, 1 packet	3
Puffed Rice, 1 cup	1
Puffed Wheat, 1 cup	2
Shredded Wheat, 3 biscuits	3
Post: 100% Bran, ¹/2 cup	8
Blueberry Morning, 1 cup, 2 oz	2
Cocoa/Fruity Pebbles, 1 cup	0
Cranberry Almond Crunch, 1 cup, 2 oz	3
Frosted Alpha Bits, 1 cup	1
Fruit & Fibre, 1 cup, 2 oz	5
Grape-Nuts, ¹/2 cup, 2 oz	5
Great Grains, ²/3 cup, 1.8 oz	4
Honey Bunches of Oats, ³/4 cup, 1 oz	1
Shredded Wheat 'n Bran, ¹/2 cup	3

Brans & Supplements

Oat Bran: 1 Tbsp (level)	0.8
¹/3 cup, (5¹/3 Tbsp), 1 oz	4.2
Rice Bran: ¹/3 cup, 1 oz	6
Wheat Bran: unprocessed: 1 Tbsp	1.6
2 Tbsp (level), ¹/4 cup	3.2
¹/4 cup, (4 Tbsp), ¹/2 cup	6.4
¹/2 cup, 1 oz	13
Corn Germ: ¹/4 cup, 1 oz	5
Wheat Germ: ¹/4 cup, 1 oz	3
Psyllium Seed Husks, 2 Tbsp	8
Metamucil, 1 dose	3.4

Hot Cereals, Oatmeal

Bulgur (cracked Wheat), ckd, 1 cup	8
Cream of Wheat, ckd, ²/3 cup	1
Hominy Grits, dry, 3 Tbsp, 1 oz	1.2
Oatmeal (uncooked ¹/3 cup), ckd, ²/3 cup	2.7

Fiber Guide

Breads & Crackers | **Fiber**

Bread: White, 1 slice, 1 oz	0.7
Whole-wheat, 1 slice, 1 oz	1.5
Whole-grain, 1 slice, 1 oz	2
Rye, Pumpernickel, 1 oz	1.5
Bagel/Roll/Bun, 1 medium, 2 oz	1.5
Pita, whole wheat, 5" pocket	4.5
Crackers: Graham, average, 2	1.4
Saltine, 4 crackers	0.3
Crispbreads (Rye), average, 2	4
Matzo 1 board, 1 oz	1
Rice Cakes: Average, 1 cake	0.3
Tortilla: Regular, 6"	0.5
Whole-wheat, 6"	1.3

Barley, Pasta, Rice & Flours

Barley, pearled, raw, $^{1}/_{4}$ cup, 1.7 oz	5
Rice: White, cooked, 1 cup, 7 oz	1.6
Brown, cooked, 1 cup	3.2
Rice-A-Roni, average, 1 cup	1.5
Spaghetti/Noodles: cooked, 1 cup	2
Whole-wheat, cooked, 1 cup	7
Amaranth *(Health Valley)*, 1 cup	9
Flour: Wheat, All-purpose, 1 cup, $4^{1}/_{2}$ oz	3.5
Whole-wheat, 1 cup, $4^{1}/_{2}$ oz	15
Cornmeal, stone ground, 1 cup, $4^{1}/_{2}$ oz	13
Carob Flour, 1 cup, $3^{1}/_{2}$ oz	13
Rye Flour, 1 cup, $3^{1}/_{2}$ oz	15
Soy Flour: Defatted, 1 cup, $3^{1}/_{2}$ oz	17
Full-fat, raw, 1 cup, 3 oz	8
Soy Meal, defatted, 1 cup, $4^{1}/_{2}$ oz	14

Frozen Entrees & Dinners

***Average All Brands:** Per Serving*	
Beans/Chili base, average	6-10
Potato/Pasta base, average	4-6
Vegetable base, average	3
Meat/Chicken base, average	2-3
Pizzas, $^{1}/_{4}$ large, average	3
Vegetarian Soy Burgers, 1 pattie	5

Soups

Chicken Noodle, 1 cup	0
Tomato Soup, average, 1 cup	0.5
Vegetable Soup, average, 1 cup	3
Health Valley: Per 1 Cup Serving	
Black Bean; Minestrone	10
Tomato	4
5-Bean Vegetable; Lentil & Carrots	13
Mushroom & Barley; Split Pea; Vegetable	7
Rotini & Vegetables	4

Fast Foods & Restaurants | **Fiber**

Hamburgers: Small, average	1.5
Large/Whopper, average	2.5
Hot Dog, Regular	1.5
French Fries: Small serving, $2^{1}/_{2}$ oz	2.5
Regular/Medium, $3^{1}/_{2}$ oz	3.5
Chicken Nuggets, 6 pack	0.5
Chicken Sandwich, average	2
Taco, average	4
Sundaes, Shakes, Soft Drinks	0
Arby's: Baked Potato w. Broccoli	9
Roast Beef Sandwich, regular	3
Denny's: Grilled Chicken Caesar Salad	3
Classic Burger w. fries	3
Club Sandwich	3
Grilled Chicken Sandwich	1
Domino's (Pizza): Veggie, 2 sl. (12")	4
Pepperoni, 2 slices (12")	2.5
Cheese., Saus/Mushr., 2 slices, (12")	3
McDonald's: Arch Deluxe; Crispy Chicken	4
Big Mac	3
Egg McMuffin	1
Salads: Garden; Grilled Chicken Caesar	2
Pizza Hut: Per 2 slices, Medium	
Pan Pizza: Cheese, Pepperoni	2
Supreme	4
Thin 'n Crispy: Supreme	4
Hand-Tossed, average	3
Personal Pizza, 1 whole	5
Subway: Sandwich, white roll	2.5
w. Honey Wheat Roll	3.2
Footlong, w. Wheat Roll	6.4
Salads, average	2

Cakes, Cookies, Snack Bars

Apple/Fruit Pie, 1 serving	2
Cake: w. plain flour, 1 serving	1
w. whole-wheat flour, 1 serving	3
Carrot Cake, 1 serving	2
Cookies, oatmeal, (3 small/1 large)	3
Donuts	0
Fruit Cake, 1 serving	3
Fig Bars, 2	1.3
Muffins, Oat Bran (2 small, 1 large), 4 oz	5
Granola Bars, average, 1 bar	1
Fi-Bar Nectar, 1 bar	4
Health Valley: Fruit/Granola Bars	4
Cereal Bars	7
IDN Snack Bar	3
SoBeBars (Mkt America), Peanut	3
Vita-Trim Bars (Mkt America)	5

Chocolate, Chips, Popcorn — Fiber

	Fiber
Cheese Balls/Curls/Twists	0
Chocolate, Hard Candy, Cheese Balls	0
Chocolate with nuts/fruit, 2 oz bar	1
Mars Bar	1
Potato Chips, corn chips, 1 oz	1
Popcorn, 3 cups	2
Pretzels, Twists, 6	1

Nuts, Seeds

Almonds: Natural, 25 kernels, 1 oz	4
Blanched (skins removed), 1 oz	3
Cashews, Filberts, Pecans, 1 oz	1.7
Peanuts, Mixed Nuts, Coconut, 1 oz	2.5
Peanut Butter, 2 Tbsp, 1 oz	1.8
Pistachio Nuts, dried, shelled, 1 oz	3
Walnuts, Black/English, dried, 1 oz	1.5
Seeds: Amaranth, $2^1/2$ Tbsp, 1 oz	3.5
Flax Seeds, 3 Tbsp, 1 oz	7
Psyllium Seed Husks, 5 Tbsp, 1 oz	20
Quinoa Seeds, 3 Tbsp, 1 oz	2.7
Sesame Seeds, whole, 1 oz	3
Sesame Butter/Tahini, 2 Tbsp, 1.1 oz	3
Sunflower kernels, $1/4$ cup, 1 oz	4.4
Teff Seeds, 1 oz	3.8

Fruit – Fresh

Apples: 1 medium, 6 oz (whole)	
with skin + core	5.5
with skin, no core	4.5
without skin, no core	3.7
Apricots, 2 medium, 4 oz	2
Avocado, average, $1/2$ medium	3
Banana, 1 medium, 6 oz (w. skin)	2
Blueberries, raw, $1/2$ cup, 4 oz	4.4
Cherries, sweet, raw, 10 fruits, $2^1/2$ oz	1.5
Grapefruit, average, $1/2$ fruit, $8^1/2$ oz	1
Grapes, 1 medium bunch, seedless, 7 oz	3
Kiwifruit, 1 medium, 3 oz	3
Mango, 1 medium, 11 oz (whole)	1.6
Melons, cantaloup, 4 oz (edible)	1
Nectarine, 1 medium, 4 oz	1.8
Olives, average all types, 7 jumbo, 2 oz	1.5
Oranges, 1 medium (7-8 oz w. skin)	
$5^1/2$ oz (peeled)	3.8
Passionfruit, 2 medium, $2^1/2$ oz	5
Peaches, 1 large, 6 oz	2
Pears, raw, 1 medium, 6 oz	4.5
Pineapple, 1 slice, 3 oz	1.8
Plums, 2 medium, 6 oz	2.8
Strawberries, 6 medium/3 large, 2 oz	1.5
Watermelon, 4 oz (edible)	0.5

Fruit – Dried, Juice — Fiber

	Fiber
Dried Fruit: Apricots, 8 halves, 1 oz	2.2
Dates (3 med); Raisins (2 Tbsp), 1 oz	1.5
Figs, 3 medium, $1^1/2$ oz	5
Prunes, 4 medium, 1 oz	2
Fruit Juice: Orange/Apple etc, 1 glass	<0.5
Prune Juice, 5 oz	1.4
Carrot Juice, 8 oz	1.8

Vegetables

Asparagus, 4 spears	2
Bean Sprouts, $1/2$ cup, $2^1/4$ oz	1.5
Beans: Snap/Green, $1/2$ cup, $2^1/2$ oz	2
Baked Beans in Tom Sce, $1/2$ c, $4^1/2$ oz	10
Dried Beans, ckd, average, $1/2$ cup	7
Beets, ckd, slices, $1/2$ cup, 3 oz	1.5
Broccoli, cooked, $1/2$ cup, 3 oz	2.2
Brussels Sprouts, ckd, $1/2$ cup, 3 oz	3.5
Cabbage: White, ckd, $1/2$ cup, $2^1/2$ oz	1
Red, ckd, $1/2$ cup, $2^1/2$ oz	2
Carrots, 1 medium ($7^1/2$"), $1/2$ cup, 3 oz	2.7
Cauliflower, cooked, $1/2$ cup, 3 oz	2.8
Celery, raw, diced, $1/2$ cup, 3 oz	1
Chick Peas (Garbanzos), ckd, $1/2$ c, $3^1/2$ oz	6
Corn, kernels, ckd, $1/2$ cup, $2^1/2$ oz	2.5
Cream-style, $1/2$ cup, $4^1/2$ oz	1.5
Cucumber/Lettuce/Mushrooms, 2 oz	0.5
Eggplant, raw, sliced, $1/2$ cup	2.5
Lentils, cooked, $1/2$ cup, $3^1/2$ oz	4
Onions, 1 medium, 4 oz	2
Spring Onions, chop., $1/4$ cup, 1 oz	1.5
Peas: Green, $1/2$ cup, 3 oz	3
Cowpeas (Black-eyed), ckd, $1/2$ cup	10
Split Peas, ckd, $1/2$ cup, $4^1/2$ oz	6.5
Peppers, sweet, raw, 1 large, $3^1/2$ oz	1.5
Potatoes: 1 medium, with skin, 5 oz	4
without skin	2
$1/2$ cup mashed, $3^1/2$ oz	1.5
French Fries, 3 oz serving	3
Spinach, cooked, $1/2$ cup, 3 oz	2
Squash: Summer, cookd, 3 oz	1.2
Winter, cooked, 3 oz	2.4
Tomatoes: 1 medium, 5 oz	2
Tomato Sauce, 1 cup	0.3
Frozen: Mixed Vegetables, ckd, $1/2$ cup	3
Soybean Products: Miso, $1/2$ c., 5 oz	7.7
Tempeh, 1 piece, 3 oz	2
Tofu, 4 oz	1.4
Salads: Side Salad, average	1
Bean Salad, $1/2$ cup	5
Coleslaw, $1/2$ cup	1
Potato Salad, $1/2$ cup	2

Protein Guide

General Notes

- **Protein has many important body functions.** It builds and repairs muscle, and is the basis of our body's organs, hormones, enzymes, and antibodies to fight infection.

- **Protein is also an emergency fuel** in the absence of sufficient carbohydrate and fats. For this reason, weight loss should be gradual so as to preserve protein levels in muscle, the heart and other body organs.

- **It is easy to obtain sufficient protein,** even if vegetarian. **Plant proteins are not inferior to animal proteins.** In fact, eating more soy and other plant proteins, and less animal protein, may help to build stronger bones and prevent osteoporosis; and may help to control blood cholesterol levels.

- **When changing to a vegetarian diet,** include soybeans, and other dried beans, soy milk drinks (calcium-enriched), lentils, tofu, tempeh, nuts, and wholegrain breads and cereals. Milk, yogurt, cheese and eggs may enhance nutrient intake.

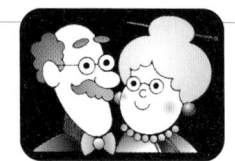

Elderly people (and dieters) must eat sufficient food to ensure adequate protein intake.

Inadequate protein leads to a drop in immune response with greater susceptibility to illness and infections. Muscle strength and muscle mass also drop.

Protein needs are easily met with sensible eating. Athletes who eat enough food for their energy needs, can obtain sufficient protein.

Protein & Muscle

- Although muscles are built of protein, protein is not a special fuel for working muscle cells - carbohydrates and fats are.

- In fact, a diet high in protein (and fat) and low in carbohydrate, can significantly reduce the performance of endurance sports athletes. **Carbohydrate** is the best fuel for muscles exercised for long periods.

- Any **extra protein** required by athletes and body-builders, can easily be obtained from the extra food eaten to satisfy hunger and energy needs - even allowing an excessive 120g protein daily for a 170 lb athlete (0.7g/lb body wt; twice the RDI).

- Remember, **excess protein** in food will not build bigger muscles. Any excess is converted and stored as fat. Excess protein can also strain the kidneys which excrete the waste products of protein metabolism.

PROTEIN
RECOMMENDED DAILY INTAKE (Grams)

(Figure in brackets - Recommended amount of protein per lb of ideal body weight.)

		Pro	
Infants:	0-6 mths	13g	(1g/lb)
	6-12 mths	14g	(0.7g/lb)
Children:	1-3 yrs	16g	(0.6g/lb)
	4-6 yrs	24g	(0.5g/lb)
	7-10	28g	(0.5g/lb)
Males:	11-14 yrs	45g	(0.45g/lb)
	15-18	59g	(0.4g/lb)
	19-24	58g	(0.36g/lb)
	25+	50g	(0.4g/lb)
Females:	11-14 yrs	46g	(0.45g/lb)
	15-18	44g	(0.37g/lb)
	19-24	46g	(0.36g/lb)
	25+	50g	(0.36g/lb)
Pregnancy:		60g	
Breastfeeding:		65g	

Note: Above figures allow for a large safety margin for most persons.

Iron & Anemia Guide

- **Iron deficiency** is one of the most common nutritional deficiencies in women. The risk is increased in dieters who do not eat well-balanced meals. Chronic shortage of iron leads to **anemia**.

- **Women** between 11 and 50 years of age are at greater risk because of the monthly loss of menstrual blood. Pregnancy, growth, and endurance sports also demand extra iron.

- **In red blood cells**, iron combines with protein to form **hemoglobin** - the red pigment which carries oxygen in the blood. A lack of iron limits the production of hemoglobin and hence the amount of vital oxygen delivered to body cells.

Note: A blood test will tell you if your Hb and Iron stores (ferritin) are adequate. (Iron stores can be low even when Hb is normal.)

- **Vitamin C** (in fruits/veges/salads) enhances absorption of 'non-heme' iron in bread, cereals, milk, vegetables, nuts, eggs and iron supplements. Small amounts of meat, fish or poultry also help. (They contain 'heme' iron.)

- **Iron absorption is lessened** by up to 60% when high calcium foods are consumed with iron-rich main meals. Tea, coffee, phytates (in bran) and oxalates lessen absorption of non-heme iron.

- **For infants to 1 year**, use iron-fortified milk/soy formula if not breast-feeding. Introduce iron-fortified baby cereals at 4-6 mths.

Note: Iron deficiency in children (even without anemia), can result in lethargy, irritability, repeated infections, and developmental problems.

Iron Supplements

- **Most people** can obtain adequate iron from their diet. **A wide variety** of animal and plant foods contain iron. (See Iron Counter)

- **Iron supplements** are only recommended for women with heavy menstrual blood losses, during pregnancy (if tests show a low-iron status), endurance athletes with low blood ferritin (iron stores) and for persons with diagnosed anemia. Check with your doctor.

- While the 5 mg of iron in multi-vitamin/mineral supplements is safe for most people, large amounts can be toxic, (especially in persons with hemochromatosis iron-overload condition).

ANEMIA SYMPTOMS

Anemia reduces the amount of oxygen carried in the blood. The body tissues become starved of oxygen. Symptoms include:

- **Pale skin; brittle finger nails (may turn up into spoon shape).**

- **Excessive tiredness or fatigue**

- **Breathlessness**

- **Feeling of malaise and irritability.**

- **Always feel cold.**

- **Decrease in attention span.**

Note: Other medical conditions may also cause similar symptoms. Check with your doctor.

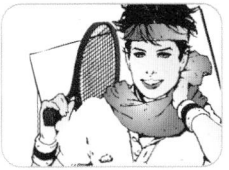

A nutritious diet with adequate iron is important - particularly for women and athletes.

RECOMMENDED DAILY IRON INTAKE (mg)

		Iron
Infants (0-6 mths):		
	Breastfed ~	0.5mg
	Bottlefed ~	3mg
	6-12 mths ~	9mg
Children: 1-11 yrs	~	6-8mg
Males: 12-18 yrs	~	10-13mg
	19+ yrs ~	7mg
Females: 12-50yrs	~	12-16mg
	51+ yrs ~	5-7mg
	Pregnancy ~	22-36mg
	Breastfeeding ~	12-16mg

Protein & Iron Counter

Pro ~ Protein (grams)   **Iron** ~ Iron (mg)

Meat

	Pro	Iron
Steak: Average all cuts, lean (no fat)		
Small (4 oz raw/3 oz ckd)	23	2.3
Medium (6 oz raw/4¼ oz ckd)	34	3.4
Large (10 oz raw/7¼ oz ckd)	57	5.7
Roast Beef, lean, 2 slices, 3 oz	24	2.5
Ground Beef patty, lean, ckd, 3 oz	21	2
Lamb chop, broiled, 3 oz	22	1.5
Liver, cooked, 3 oz	23	5.5
Veal cutlet, 1 medium	23	1
Pork, cooked, lean, 3 oz	24	1
Bacon, 3 medium slices	6	0.3
Ham, roasted, 2 pieces, 3 oz	18	1
Ham, luncheon, 2 slices, 1½ oz	7	0.3
Pastrami (Oscar Mayer), 3 sl., 1¾ oz	10	1.3
Sausages: Bologna, 2 sl., 2 oz	7	1
Braunschweiger, 2 sl., 2 oz	8	5.3
Pork link, thick, 2 oz	6	0.4
Frankfurter, 1⅓ oz	5	1
Salami, hard, 3 slices, 1 oz	7	0.5
Vegetarian (BocaBurger), 1 pattie	13	2

Chicken/Turkey

	Pro	Iron
Chicken, ckd; Breast portion, 3 oz	27	1
Leg/Thigh, lean, 3 oz	24	1
½ Whole Chicken	60	2.5
Drumstick, lean, 3 oz	12	0.6
Turkey, cooked: Light meat, 3 oz	24	2
Dark meat, lean, 3 oz	24	2

Fish

	Pro	Iron
Finfish: Per 4 oz, cooked		
Cod, Flounder/Sole, Pollock	28	0.5
Catfish, Haddock, Halibut, M/Mahi	28	1.3
Ocean Perch, Swordf., Orange Roughy	28	1.3
Canned Fish: Tuna, Light, 3 oz	25	1.5
White, 3 oz	23	0.5
Salmon, pink, 3 oz	17	0.7
Salmon, red, 3 oz	17	1
Sardines, 3 whole (3"), 1¼ oz	9	1
Anchovies, 1 can, 1½ oz	13	2
Shellfish: Crabmeat, 3 oz	17.5	0.7
Clams, raw, 4 large/9 sml, 3 oz	11	12
Crayfish, cooked, 3 oz	20	2.7
Lobster, cooked, 3 oz	17	0.5
Oysters, raw, 6 medium, 3 oz	7	5
Scallops, 2 lge/5 small, 1 oz	5	0.1
Shrimp, raw, 6 large, 1½ oz	8.5	1
Fish Products: Fish Sticks, 4 sticks	10	0.5
Fish Portions, in batter, 4 oz	13	0.6
Gefilte Fish, 1 medium ball, 2 oz	8	1

Eggs

	Pro	Iron
1 Large Egg, whole	6	0.7
Egg Yolk	3	0.7
Egg White	3	0
Omelet: Plain, 2 eggs	13	1.7
Ham & Cheese	17	3
Egg Substitutes (liquid):		
Eggbeaters, 1 egg equiv.	4.5	1
Scramblers, ¼ cup, 2 oz	6	0.7

Milk, Yogurt, Icecream

	Pro	Iron
Milk: Whole/Lowfat/Skim, 8 fl.oz cup	8	0.1
Protein Enriched, 1 cup	10	0.1
Chocolate Milk, 1 cup	8	0.6
Thick Shake, Chocolate, 10 oz	9	1
Vanilla, 10 oz	11	0.3
Soymilk (fortified), average, 1 cup	7	1
Yogurt: Plain, 6 oz	10	0.1
Fruit flavors: 6 oz	8	0.3
8 oz	11	0.5
Ice-Cream: Rich, ½ cup	2	0
Regular, Vanilla, ½ cup	2.5	0
Sherbet, ½ cup	1	0
Custard, baked, ½ cup	7	0.5

Cheese

	Pro	Iron
Hard Cheeses, average, 1 oz	7	0.2
4 oz piece	28	0.8
Cottage Cheese, ½ cup	13	0.3
Ricotta, part skim, ½ cup	14	1

Bread, Bagels, Biscuits

	Pro	Iron
Bread (w. enriched flour): 1 slice, 1 oz	2	1
4 slices, 4 oz	8	4
4 thick slices, 6 oz	1.2	6
Bagel, plain 2 oz	6	1.5
Biscuits, 1 oz	2	0.7
Pita Bread, 1 pita, 1½ oz	4	1
Pumpernickel, 1 slice, 1 oz	3	1

Infant/Baby Foods

	Pro	Iron
Infant Formula Milk:		
Enfamil/Gerber/Similac, 5 fl.oz		
Regular/Low Iron	2.2	0.2
With Iron	2.2	1.8
Isomil/Nursoy/ProSobee	3	1.8
Baby Cereals: *Average All Brands*		
Dry, 4 Tbsp, ½ oz	1	7
Jars (w. fruit), 4½ oz	1	7

Breakfast Cereals

	Pro	Iron
Hot Type, cooked:		
Bulgur, cooked, 1 cup, 5 oz	9	2
Oatmeal: Reg., non-fortified, 1 cup	6	1.5
Instant, fortified, average, 1 pkt	4	8
Quaker Extra, all flavors	4	18
Total, all types, 1 pkt	4	18
Corn/Hominy Grits: Reg., 1 cup	3	1.5
Quaker: Reg., 3 Tbsp, 1 oz	2	0.8
Instant White, 1 packet	2	8
Cream of Wheat, 1 cup	4	10
Ready-To-Eat: *Per 1 oz Serving Unless Shown*		
Arrowhead: Average, all varieties	3	1
General Mills: Basic 4, 1 cup, 2 oz	4	3.8
Cheerios, regular, 1 cup, 1 oz	3	6.8
Cocoa Puffs, 1 cup, 1 oz	1	3.9
Fiber One, 1/2 cup	2	3.8
Kix, 11/3 cups; 1 oz	2	6.8
Multi-Bran Chex, 1 cup, 2 oz	4	16
Total Corn Flakes, 11/3 cups, 1 oz	2	18
Total Raisin Bran, 1 cup, 2 oz	4	18
Wheaties Energy Crunch, 1 cup, 1.95 oz	6	18
Health Valley: 10 Bran O's, 3/4 cup	3	0.9
Amaranth Flakes, 3/4 cup	3	0.6
Bran Cereal w. Raisins, 3/4 cup	5	1.5
98% Fat Free Granola, 2/3 cup	5	1.2
Real Oat Bran, 1/2 cup	6	0.6
Golden Flax, 1/4 cup	6	1.2
Kashi GoLean: 3/4 cup, 1.5 oz	8	1.5
Crunch!, 1 cup, 1.9 oz	9	1.8
Kellogg's: All Bran, 1/2 cup	4	4.5
Complete Oatbran Flakes, 3/4 cup	3	8.5
Cocoa Krispies, 3/4 cup	2	1.8
Corn Flakes, 1 cup	2	8.4
Just Right, 1 cup	4	16
Nutrigrain Almond Raisin, 11/4 cup	4	1.4
Product 19, 1 cup, 1 oz	2	18
Raisin Bran, 1 cup, 2 oz	6	4.5
Rice Krispies, 11/4 cup	2	1.8
Special K, 1 cup	6	8
Post: Raisin Bran, 1/2 cup, 1 oz	3	4.5
Grape Nuts, 1/2 cup, 1 oz	3	1
Quaker: Crunchy Corn Bran, 1 cup, 1 oz	2	8
Oatmeal Squares, 1 cup, 1 oz	4	6
100% Natural Granola, 1/2 cup	3	1
Life, 1/4 cup, 1 oz	3	4.5
Puffed Rice/Wheat, 1 cup, 1/2 oz	1	0.5
Shreaded Wheat, 3 biscuits	4	1

Brans & Wheatgerm

	Pro	Iron
Oat Bran, raw, 1 Tbsp	2	0.5
Rice Bran, raw, 2 Tbsp	1	1
Wheat Bran, unprocessed, 2 Tbsp	1	1
Wheat Germ, 2 Tbsp, 1/2 oz	4	1.3

Grains & Flours

	Pro	Iron
Amaranth, 1 cup, 1/2 oz	10	3
Barley, 1/2 cup, 31/2 oz	8	2
Buckwheat Flour, dark, 1 cup	11.5	2.7
light, 1 cup	6	1
Carob Flour, 1 cup	5	3
Corn Flour, 1 cup, 4 oz	9	2
Corn Meal, enriched, 1 cup	11	3.5
Flour: White, enriched, 1 cup, 41/2 oz	13	6
Wholegrain, 1 cup, 41/4 oz	16	5
Millet, wholegrain, 1 cup, 31/2 oz	10	7
Rye Flour, dark, 1 cup, 41/2 oz	21	6
light, 1 cup, 31/2 oz	10	1
Soy Flour, full fat, 1 cup, 3 oz	32	5.5
Yeast: Brewer's, dry, 1 Tbsp	3	1.5

Rice, Spaghetti

	Pro	Iron
Rice: Brown/White, average		
1 cup cooked, 61/2 oz	5	1
Spaghetti/Macaroni/Noodles (enriched):		
Cooked, 1 cup, 41/2 oz	7	2
Canned: in Tomato Sauce, 1/2 cup	2	0.5
w. Meatballs, 1 cup, 8 oz	9	2

Soups

	Pro	Iron
With Noodles/Vegetables, 1 cup	3	0.5
With Meat/Beans/Peas, 1 cup	8	1.5

Fruit

	Pro	Iron
Fresh/Canned: Average, all types, 1 serving		
1 medium/2 small fruit	1	0.5
Avocado, 1/2 medium	2	1
Dried Fruit: Apricots, 8 halves, 1 oz	1	1.3
Dates, 6 dates, 2 oz	1.5	0.7
Figs, 4 medium figs, 2 oz	2	1.7
Prunes, 5 medium, 11/2 oz	1	1
Raisins, 1 oz	1	0.7
Fruit Juice: Average, 1 cup	0.5	0.5
Prune Juice, 6 fl.oz	1	2.5
Tomato Juice, 6 fl.oz	0.5	1

King Kong was a vegetarian!

Protein & Iron Counter

Vegetables	Pro	Iron
Beans: Snap/green, 1/2 cup	1	0.8
Dried: Average all types, cooked, 1/2 cup	7	2.5
Baked Beans, 1/2 cup 4 1/2 oz	5	2
Bean Sprouts, mung, 1 cup	3	1
Broccoli, 3/4 cup pieces, 4 oz	4	1.4
Cabbage; Cauliflower, 1 cup	1	0.6
Corn, 1/2 cup kernels, 3 oz	2.5	0.3
1 ear trimmed to 3 1/2"	2	0.4
Lentils, cooked, 1/2 cup, 3 1/2 oz	9	3.3
Mushrooms, raw, 1/2 cup, sliced	0.5	0.5
Peas: green, 1/2 cup, 3 oz	4	1.2
Split Peas, cooked, 1 cup	16	2.5
Potatoes, cooked:		
1 medium, with skin, 5 oz	3.3	2
without skin, 4 oz	2.3	1
French Fries, 3 oz	3	1
Potato Salad, 1/2 cup	3.5	2.5
Pumpkin, 1/2 cup mashed	1	2.5
Seaweed, kelp, 1 oz	<1	2.5
Spinach, cooked, 1/2 cup, 3 oz	2.7	2.5
Squash, ckd, all types, 1/2 cup	1	0.3
Tomatoes, 1 medium, 4 1/2 oz	1	0.6
Vegetables, mixed, ckd, 1 cup	2.5	0.7
Soybeans, cooked, 1/2 cup, 3 oz	14	4.4

Tofu, Tempeh, Miso		
Tofu, raw, firm, 1/2 cup, 4 1/2 oz	10	1.5
Tempeh, 1/2 cup, 3 oz	16	2
Miso, 1/2 cup, 5 oz	16	4
Miso Soup, 1 cup	3	0.4
Soybean Protein (TVP), 1 oz	18	3

Cakes, Pastries, Pies		
(Made with enriched flour)		
Carrot w. cream cheese frosting, 4 oz	4	1.3
Cheesecake, 1 piece, 3 1/2 oz	5	0.5
Chocolate, 1 piece, 2 oz	2	2
Fruitcake, 1 piece, 1 1/2 oz	2	1.2
Plain, 1 piece, 3 oz	4	1.2
Croissant, plain, 2 oz	5	2
Danish Pastry, 1 pastry, 2 1/4 oz	4	1.3
Donuts, average, 2 oz	4	1.2
Muffins, average, 1 medium, 1 1/2 oz	3	1
Pancakes, 4" diam., two, 2 oz	4	1
Pies: Fruit, 1 piece, 5 1/2 oz	4	1.5
Pecan, 1 piece, 5 oz	7	4.5
Puddings, average, 1/2 cup, 4 1/2 oz	4	0.3
Waffles, 1 large, 2 1/2 oz	7	1.5

Sugar, Honey, Jam	Pro	Iron
Sugar: White	0	0
Brown, 1 Tbsp	0	0.3
Molasses: Light/Medium, 1 Tbsp	0	1
Blackstrap, 1 Tbsp, 3/4 oz	0	3
Corn Syrup, 1 Tbsp, 3/4 oz	0	1
Honey, Jams, Jelly	0	0.2

Candy, Chocolate, Carob		
Candy, sugar-based	0	0
Chocolate: Plain, 2 oz bar	4	0.8
with nuts, 2 oz bar	6	0.8
Carob, plain, 2 oz	6	0.7

Cookies, Crackers, Chips		
Cookies, average, 4 cookies	2	1
Crackers: Graham, 2 1/2" sq., 2	1	0
Rice Cakes, average, one	1	0
Corn/Potato Chips, 1 oz	2	0.3

Nuts: Almonds, shelled, 20-25 nuts	6	1
Brazil Nuts, 7-8 medium nuts, 1 oz	4	1
Cashews, 12-16 nuts, 1 oz	5	1.5
Macadamias, 1 oz	2	0.5
Peanuts, dry roasted, 40 nuts, 1 oz	6	0.6
Pecans, 24 halves, 1 oz	2	0.5
Walnuts, 15 halves, 1 oz	4	0.7
Peanut Butter, 1 Tbsp	5	0.5

Seeds: Sesame Seeds, dry, 1 Tbsp	2	0.6
Pumpkin Kernels, dry, hulled, 1 oz	7	4.2
Sunflower Seeds, dried, hulled, 1 oz	6	1
Tahini, 1 Tbsp, 1/2 oz	2.5	1.4

Granola & Food/Protein Bars		
Granola Bars, average, 1 bar, 2 oz	2	0.5
Balance Oasis Bars, 1.76 oz	9	6.3
Bariatrix: Nutra Bars, 1.76 oz	11	3.6
Choice dm Bar, 1.23 oz	6	3.6
Dr Soy Protein Bars, 1.76 oz	11	18
Ensure Nutrition Energy Bar	9	3.6
Gatorade Bars, Chocolate, 2.3 oz	7	3.5
Genisoy Nature Grains, 2.3 oz	14	4.5
IDN: proGram-16, 65g	16	3.6
Jenny Craig Bars, 1.97 oz	10	3.6
Met-Rx Bar, 100g	27	7.2
Planters Peanut Bar, 1.6 oz	7	0.7
Power Bar, 1 bar, 2.3 oz	10	6.3
Slim-Fast Bar, 34g	6	4.5
SoBeBars (Mkt America), Peanut	18	6.3
Source One Bar, 2.2 oz	15	4.5
Sweet Success Snack Bar, 33g	2	2.7
Twin Lab Protein Fuel, 3 oz	35	4.5
High Energy Bars, 2 oz	15	1.5

Nutritional & High Protein Drinks

	Pro	Iron
Atkins Shakes, 11 fl.oz can	20	2.7
Bariatrix Shakes, dry, 1 oz	15	3.6
Proti-Max Meal Replacement, 67g	35	6.3
Boost Ready To Drink, 8 oz can	10	3.6
Carnation Instant Breakfast, 10 oz	12	4.5
Ensure High Protein, 8 oz can	12	2.3
GeniSoy Shake, 1 scoop, 35g	14	3.6
IDN Appeal, 1 pkg, 1 cup	16	2.7
Kashi GoLean Shake (RTD), 11 oz can	15	2.7
Kindercal, 8 fl.oz	7	2.5
Met-Rx Protein Shake, 11 oz	25	4.5
Myoplex (EAS), Nutrition Shake, 11 oz	20	5.4
Nature's Best, Protein Shake, 11 oz	20	4.5
Optifast 800, made-up, 8 oz	14	3.6
Resource (Novartis) Standard, 8 fl.oz	9	4.5
Revival Soy, Plain, 58g pkt	20	3.6
Slim Fast Shakes 325 ml can	10	3.6
Sweet Success (Nestle), 10 fl.oz can	10	4.5
Ultra Slim Fast, powder, 1 scoop, 33g	5	6.3
Usana Nutrimeal Mix, 2 scoops, 1¹/₂oz	12	6
Walgreens Slim For Less, 11 oz can	10	2.7
Weider: Muscle Builder, 2 scoops	18	9

Coffee, Tea, Soda

	Pro	Iron
Coffee, Coffee Substitutes, 1 cup	0	0.1
Tea (all types); Soft Drinks/Soda	0	0
Hot Chocolate, 6 fl.oz	2	2.2

Beer, Wine, Spirits

	Pro	Iron
Beer, 12 fl.oz	1	0
Wines, red/white, 1 glass	0	0.4
Spirits/Liquor	0	0

Fast-Foods/Burgers

Note: See Fast-Foods Section for comprehensive protein counts.

	Pro	Iron
Arby's: Roast Beef Sandwich, reg.	21	4
Giant Roast Beef S/wich	32	6
Italian Sub	29	2
Roast Chicken Club	29	3
Burger King: Whopper S/wich	29	2.5
Hamburger	19	1.5
Bacon Double Cheeseburger	24	2.5
Chicken Sandwich; Big Fish Sandwich	25	2
Carl's Jr: Famous Star Hamburger	24	2
Carl's Jr (Cont): Ranch Crispy Chicken	24	2
Super Star Hamburger	41	3
Charbroiled Chicken Club Sandwich	35	2

Fast Foods/Burgers (Cont)

	Pro	Iron
Domino's Pizza: Deep Dish (12"), 2 sl.		
Cheese, 2 slices	42	4
Pepperoni, Sausage, Ham	41	4
X-tra Cheese & Pepperoni	50	4.5
KFC: Original, Wing & Breast	35	0.4
3-Pce. Dinner, Original	51	0.4
Crispy Strips, 3	26	0.4
Original Recipe Sandwich	29	1.5
McDonald's: Big Mac	24	2.5
Cheeseburger	15	1.5
Chicken McNuggets (6)	15	0.6
Crispy Chicken Burger	23	1.5
Filet-O-Fish	15	1.5
Grilled Chicken Caesar Salad	17	1
Hamburger	12	1.5
Quarter Pounder w. Cheese	23	2.5
Sourdough Supreme Burger	21	2.5
French Fries: Small, 2.4 oz	3	0.2
Large, 6 oz	8	0.6
Breakfast: Egg McMuffin	17	1.5
Hotcakes w. Marg/Syrup	9	1.5
Sausage McMuffin w. Egg	19	1.5
Muffin, Lowfat, Apple Bran	6	1
Pancakes: 3 Pancakes	8	2
Pizza Hut: Per Medium, 2 slices		
Pan Pizzas, average	26	4
Thin 'n Crispy: Supreme	24	2
Hand Tossed: Pepperoni	26	3
Personal Pan Pizza: Beef	26	4
Shakes, Chocolate	12	0.4
Subway: 6" Subs, average	20	2
Meatball	-	-
Roast Chicken Breast	25	3.5
Steak & Cheese, 6"	23	6
Subway Club	22	3.5
Sundaes: Average all outlets	7	0.3
Taco Bell: Bean Burrito	13	3.5
Beef Burrito Supreme	17	3.5
Tostado	10	1.5
Enchirito; Chicken; Steak	22	3
Taco Supreme	10	2
Gordita Baja Beef	13	2.5
Chicken Quesadilla	25	3
Wendy's: Single w. Everything	25	3
Big Bacon Classic	34	3
Jr Hamburger Kid's Meal	14	2
Grilled Chicken Sandwich	24	1.5

High Blood Pressure

High Blood Pressure

Many American adults have hypertension (high blood pressure), and are unaware of it. It is generally symptomless, so **have your blood pressure checked annually** - particularly if there is a family history of hypertension.

Untreated hypertension overworks the heart, damages arteries and promotes atherosclerosis. This in turn greatly increases the risk of heart disease, stroke, blindness, kidney disease and impotence. The earlier hypertension is detected, the sooner it can be brought under control.

Treating Hypertension

If your blood pressure is high, consult your doctor about diet and medication. You may be referred to a dietitian for more detailed dietary advice and meal planning.

High-Normal and Stage 1 hypertension can often be treated by reducing sodium intake, losing weight if overweight, limiting alcohol to 2 drinks or less daily, exercising regularly, and dealing with stress.

Stages 2, 3 and 4 hypertension usually require drug therapy. However, salt restriction, abstaining from alcohol and the above lifestyle changes will improve the success of drug therapy, and enable smaller drug doses to be prescribed.

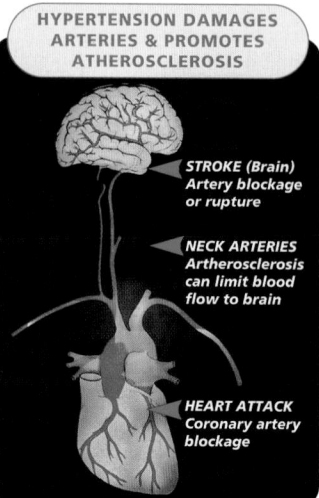

HYPERTENSION DAMAGES ARTERIES & PROMOTES ATHEROSCLEROSIS

STROKE (Brain) Artery blockage or rupture

NECK ARTERIES Artherosclerosis can limit blood flow to brain

HEART ATTACK Coronary artery blockage

BLOOD PRESSURE CLASSIFICATIONS

National High Blood Pressure Educ. Prog. (1993)

	DIASTOLIC	SYSTOLIC
Normal ►	80-84	120-129
High-Normal ►	85-89	130-139
Stage 1 ►	90-99	140-159
Stage 2 ►	100-109	160-179
Stage 3 ►	110-119	180-209
Stage 4 ►	120 or over	210 or over

STROKE
KNOW THE WARNING SIGNS!

If you notice one or more of these signs, **call your doctor immediately.** They may be signalling a possible stroke or transient ischemic attack:

- **Sudden weakness** or numbness in your face, arm or leg on one side of your body.
- **Sudden dimness,** blurring or loss of vision, particularly in one eye.
- **Loss of speech,** or trouble talking or understanding speech.
- **Sudden severe headache** - 'a bolt out of the blue' - with no apparent cause.
- **Unexplained dizziness,** unsteadiness or a sudden fall, especially if accompanied by any of the other symptoms.

Salt & Sodium

- **Sodium is a mineral element** most commonly found in salt (sodium chloride). It also occurs naturally in much smaller amounts in animal and plant foods, and water - normally sufficient for our needs without having to add salt.

- **Sodium is required** for nerve and muscle function as well as to balance the amount of fluid in our tissues and blood.
  Sodium acts like a sponge to attract and hold fluids in body tissues.

- **Excess sodium** can cause water retention, and increase the risk of developing hypertension. Very high salt intake may also increase the risk of stomach cancer.

- **Too little sodium** may cause low blood pressure (hypotension), and decrease blood flow to the heart, brain and kidneys - especially during exercise. (A certain blood volume is required to sustain the blood pressure needed for adequate blood flow in the capillaries).

Salt - Sensitive Persons

- **Normally, our kidneys** excrete excess dietary sodium. The thirst we feel after a salty meal is the body calling for water to dilute the sodium, and enable the kidneys to flush out excess sodium.

- **However, 'salt sensitive'** persons (perhaps 1 in 2-3 adults) tend to retain excess sodium (above approximately 3000mg daily) instead of excreting it. Such persons are more likely to develop hypertension and would most benefit from sodium restriction. Assume you are susceptible if there is a family history of hypertension.

- **Although not everyone will benefit**, all Americans are being asked to **moderate their salt and sodium intake** as a public health measure - particularly that so many do not know whether or not they have hypertension; and also because we do not know just who is salt-sensitive.

SAFE SODIUM LEVELS

The American Heart Association recommends a maximum sodium intake of **2400mg per day** for adults with normal blood pressure. Many Americans have double this amount.

Persons with hypertension and kidney ailments are usually restricted to as little as **1000mg sodium per day.** Your doctor will discuss the correct sodium level for you.

Persons engaged in prolonged strenuous work or exercise may lose sodium through heavy sweating - especially in hot, humid weather. Adequate salt (and fluids) is necessary to avoid dehydration. A little extra salt at mealtimes is usually sufficient to satisfy any extra need. Do not take salt tablets.

FINDING HIDDEN SODIUM

On average, only one third of our sodium intake comes from the salt shaker. The rest is hidden in processed foods that have salt added during manufacture.

Sodium compounds added to food or medicinals can also contribute significant sodium.

Sodium bicarbonate in particular is widely used in antacid tablets and powders, and saline drink powders (such as *Alka Seltzer*). Sodium bicarbonate contains 27% sodium by weight. Each gram contributes 270mg sodium. Large amounts of sodium can be unwittingly consumed.

Other sodium compounds include monosodium glutamate (MSG), sodium ascorbate, sodium nitrite, and sodium citrate.

ALCOHOL

Excess alcohol causes up to 20% of hypertension in America.
Susceptible persons should abstain to normalize their blood pressure.

Salt - Sodium Guide

Sodium accounts for only 40% of the weight of salt (sodium chloride). Examples:
1 gram (1000mg) Salt has 400mg Sodium

1 teasp. (5g) Salt has 2000mg Sodium

Hints to Reduce Sodium

- **Watch the salt shaker.** Start with an easy 50% cut in sodium by using Lite Salt (*Morton*). Then gradually cut back until you can leave the salt shaker off the table.

- **Taste your food before salting.** Use the pepper shaker (small holes) for more controlled sprinkling of salt.

- **Choose low sodium**, sodium free, and reduced sodium products in place of regular salted products.

- **Check labels for sodium levels.** The following sodium descriptors may appear on labels:

  Reduced Sodium: At least 75% less sodium than the original product.
  Low Sodium: 140 mg or less/serving.
  Very Low Sodium: 35mg or less/serving.
  Sodium Free: Less than 5mg per serving.

- **Use reduced-sodium breads**, butter and margarine. Regular varieties contain up to 2% salt. This is considered high in view of their significant contribution to our diet.

- **Go easy on condiments and sauces** such as tomato ketchup, mustard, soy sauce and spaghetti sauces, plus salad dressings. Use low sodium varieties.

- **Limit pizzas and salty fast-foods.** Check the *Fast-Food Restaurant* Section.

- **Avoid salty snack foods** such as potato chips, corn chips, salted nuts, pretzels and cheesy-flavoured snacks. **Choose unsalted** popcorn, nuts or seeds. Eat more fruit.

- **Don't salt children's food** to your taste.

- **Limit or avoid antacids and saline powders** with sodium bicarbonate (such as *Alka-Seltzer*). They are high in sodium.

FOODS HIGH IN SODIUM

- Cheese, Butter, Margarine
- Pickles, Sauerkraut, Olives
- Condiments, Sauces
- Salad Dressings
- Canned vegetables/salads/beans
- Deli Salads (with dressing)
- Frozen/Packaged Meals/Entrees
- Soups: Canned/dry; bouillon cubes
- Meats: Ham, bacon, sausage, luncheon meats, smoked meats
- Canned Fish (in brine)
- Seasoning Salts (e.g. garlic, celery)
- Snack Foods (potato chips, pretzels)
- Tomato Jce (Canned), V8 Vegetable Juice
- Fast Foods: Pizza, Burgers, Chicken
- *Alka-Seltzer* Antacid

MODERATE SODIUM

- Bread (Reduced Salt)
- Meat, Fish, Poultry - Unprocessed
- Milk, Yogurt, Soy Drinks, Eggs
- Peanut Butter
- Breakfast Cereals (<200mg/serving)
- Chocolate Candy, Fruit/Nut Bars
- *Reduced & Low-Sodium* Products

FOODS LOW IN SODIUM

- Products labelled *Very Low Sodium*, or *Sodium Free*
- Fresh fruits and vegetables
- Canned and Dried Fruits
- Potatoes, Rice, Pasta
- Dried Beans & Lentils, Tofu
- Nuts & Seeds (unsalted)
- Corn & Popcorn (unsalted)
- Pepper, Spices, Herbs
- Jam, Honey, Syrup
- Candy, Gum
- Hard & Jelly Candy
- Coffee, Tea, Alcohol
- Fresh Fruit Juices, Water

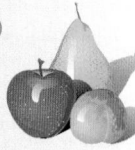

The American Heart Association recommends a sodium intake of **less than 2400mg/day**

Sod ~ Sodium (mg)

Milk & Dairy Products | **Sod**
Milk: Whole/lowfat/skim, average	
1 cup, 8 fl.oz	120
Whole, low sodium, 1 cup	5
Choc Milk (*Hershey's*), 1 cup	130
Human Milk, 8 fl.oz	40
Soy Milk, 8 fl.oz	30
Buttermilk, cultured, 8 fl.oz	250
Dry/Powder, skim, 1/4 cup, 1 oz	110
Yogurt: with fruit aver., 8 oz	130
Cheese:	
Blue, 1 oz	330
Parmesan, 1 oz	450
Kraft: Cheddar, 1 oz	180
Philadelphia Brand Cream Cheese	85
Process Cheese., average, 1 oz	430
Swiss, 1 oz	40
Cottage Cheese, 1/2 cup, 4 oz	450
Ricotta Cheese, 1/2 cup, 4 oz	150

Icecream, Frozen Yogurt
Icecream, average, 1/2 cup	50
Frozen Yogurt, 1/2 cup	50

Fats/Oils
Butter/Margarine:	
Regular, 2 Tbsp, 1 oz	230
Unsalted, reg., 2 Tbsp, 1 oz	5
Mayonnaise, aver., 2 Tbsp, 1 oz	160
Molly McButter, 1 tsp	120
Oils/Lard/Dripping	0
Cream, average, 1 Tbsp	6
Coffee-Mate: Powdered, 1 tsp	2
Liquid, 1 Tbsp	5

Eggs
Whole, 1 large	70
Omelet, 2 egg, plain	220
w. cheese	400
Egg Beaters (*Fleischmann's*), 1/4 cup	80

Meats
Meat, average all types, cooked	
(Beef/Lamb/Veal/Pork), 4 oz	80
Corned Beef, cooked, 3 oz	800
Bacon, cooked, 2 slices, 1/2 oz	270
Ham, 3 oz	1100

Chicken & Turkey
Chicken/Turkey, cooked, unsalted, 4 oz	80
Stuffing Mixes, average., 1/2 cup	500

Sausages & Meats | **Sod**
Bologna, 1 oz	280
Frankfurter, 2 oz	640
Ham, chopped, 3/4 oz slice	290
Liverwurst (Braunschweiger), 1 oz	320
Pepperoni, 5 slices, 1 oz	570
Salami, cooked, 1 oz	350
dry/hard, 1 oz	600
Sausage, 1 oz link	220
Pork, 2 oz patty	260
Turkey Roll, 1 oz	160

Fish: Fresh Fish, average, plain	
Cooked, 4 oz (no bone)	60
Broiled w. butter, 4 oz	150
Breaded & fried, 4 oz	320
Fish fillets, bat.-dipped 3 oz	350
Fish sticks, 1 oz stick	160
Gefilte Fish (w. broth), 1 pce, 1 1/2 oz	220
Herring, pickled, 2 pces, 1 oz	260
Lobster, meat only, 4 oz	180
Oysters, fresh, 6 med., 3 oz	95
Salmon, canned, 3 oz	460
No Salt Added, 3 oz	65
Smoked fish, average, 3 oz	650
Tuna, canned, 3 oz	330
No Added Salt, 3 oz	40

Entrees & Meals
Frozen Meals, average	600-900
Lean Cuisine, average	700
Stouffer's, average	580
Dinners, average	900-1200
Side Dishes, average	400-600
Pizza, frozen, 1/4 large, 6 oz	800-1200
Microwave Cup Meals	900-1200
Cup O'Noodles, average	1500

Fast-Foods & Restaurants
Cheeseburger	750
Chicken Dinner (3 piece)	2200
Chicken Nuggets w. Sauce	800
Fish/Chicken Sandwich	1000
French Fries, small, 2 1/2 oz	150
Hamburger: Regular	500
Large with cheese	1100
Hot Dog (Frankfurter)	800
Pizza, 2 medium slices	1200
Shake, chocolate	250
Taco	400

Sodium Counter

Sod ~ Sodium (mg) **Sod**

Soups: Condensed, 1 c., 8 oz — 800-1000
Low Sodium — 70
Chicken Noodle, 1 cup — 900
Bouillon Cube, average — 950
Cup-A-Soup, average — 850
Lite, average — 450
Soup Mixes, average, 1 cup — 900

Condiments, Sauces, Dressings
A-1 Sauce, 1 Tbsp — 270
Barbecue Sauce, 1 Tbsp — 130
Bragg Liquid Aminos, 1 tsp — 220
Chili Sauce, 1 Tbsp — 230
Ketchup: tomato, 1 Tbsp — 180
Low Sodium, 1 Tbsp — 20
Mayonnaise, 1 Tbsp — 80
Mustard, 1 tsp — 70
Pizza Sauce, $^1/_2$ cup — 700
Salad Dressings, 2 Tbsp, 1 oz — 160-400
Spaghetti Sauce, $^1/_2$ cup — 500
Soy Sauce, 1 Tbsp — 900
Lite *(Kikkoman)*, 1 Tbsp — 600
Sweet & Sour, $^1/_2$ cup — 250
Tabasco, 1 tsp — 25
Vinegar, Lemon Juice — 0
Worcestershire, 1 Tbsp — 200
Tomato: Sauce, 1 cup — 1200
Paste/Puree (salted), $^1/_2$ cup — 1000
No Salt Added, $^1/_2$ cup — 25

Salt & Salt Substitutes
Table Salt: 1 tsp, 6g — 2400
Single Serve packet, 1 g — 400
Lite Salt *(Morton)*, 1 tsp, 6g — 1200
No Salt Alternative, 1 tsp — 5
Garlic/Seasoned Salt 1 tsp, 4g — 1300
Sea Salt, 1 tsp, 5g — 2250

Seasonings, Herbs & Spices
Baking Powder, 1 tsp, 3g — 340
Baking Soda (Sodium bicarb), 1 tsp, 3g — 810
Accent (Flavor Enhancer), 1 tsp — 600
Chili Powder, 1 tsp, 3g — 25
Herbs/Spices: Curry Powder — 0
Lemon Pepper *(Lawry's)*, 1 tsp — 340
Meat Tenderizer, 1 tsp, 5g — 1750
MSG (Monosodium glutamate), 5g — 500
Mrs Dash (Herb/Spice Blend), 1 tsp — 0
Pepper, Mustard (dry), 1 tsp — 1
Yeast, Nutritional, 1 Tbsp — 10

Breakfast Cereals
Kellogg's:
All-Bran, $^1/_3$ cup, 1 oz — 260
Oatbran Flakes, $^3/_4$ cup, 1 oz — 220
Corn Flakes, 1 cup, 1 oz — 290
Just Right, $^1/_2$ cup, 1 oz — 200
Mini Wheats Frosted, $^3/_4$ cup, — -
Health Valley Cereals, 1 serving — 5
Quaker: Cap'n Crunch, $^3/_4$ cup, 1 oz — -
Crunchy Corn Bran, 1 cup, 1 oz — 320
100% Natural Granola, $^1/_2$ cup, 1 oz — 15
Puffed Rice/Wheat, 2 cups, 1 oz — 1
Total, 1 cup, 1 oz — 140
Oatmeal: Regular, $^3/_4$ cup — 1
Instant *(Quaker)*, $^2/_3$ cup (1 pkt) — 270

Breads, Bagels, Crackers
Bread: Average all types, 1 oz — 140
Low Sodium, 1 oz — 10
Bagels, plain, 2 oz — 200
Sara Lee, 3 oz — 500
Biscuits, average, 1 oz — 180
Bun/Roll, 1 medium, $1^1/_2$ oz — 200
Crackers: Saltine, 2 crackers — 70
Low Salt (Premium), 2 — 45
Graham, 2 regular — 50
Croissant, average, 2 oz — 280
Rice Cakes, average — 25
RyKrisp Crispbread, Sesame, 2 — 100

Cookies, Cakes, Desserts
Cookies, average, 2-3 cookies, 1 oz — 100
Mrs Fields', average, $2^1/_2$ oz — 180
Baked Custard, $^1/_2$ cup — 100
Brownie, $^1/_4$ oz piece — 75
Cake, average, 3 oz piece — 250
Cinnamon Sweet Roll, 2 oz — 250
Danish, Apple — 250
Donut, average — 150
Muffins, 1 medium, 2 oz — 150
Sara Lee, average, $2^1/_2$ oz — 300
Pancakes, 3 x 4" — 360
Pie, average $^1/_6$ of 9" pie — 300
Pudding, average, $^1/_2$ cup — 160
Jell-O (Mix), Instant, $^1/_2$ cup — 400
Waffles:
Home-made, 7", $2^1/_2$ oz — 350
Frozen, average, $1^1/_4$ oz — 260
Aunt Jemima, avg, $2^1/_2$ oz — 630

Fruit & Juices — Sod
Fresh Fruit, average all types, 1 serving	1
Dried/Canned Fruit, 1/2 cup	1
Fruit Juice: Fresh, sqz'd, 6 fl.oz	1
Commercial, aver., 6 fl.oz	20
Carrot Juice (*Ferraro's*), 8 fl.oz	230
Tomato Juice (*Campbell's*), 6 fl.oz	570
Low Sodium (No Salt Added)	20
V8 Vegetable (*Campbell's*), 6 fl.oz	600
(No Salt Added), 6 fl.oz	45

Vegetables
Fresh/Frozen (No Salt Added), 1/2 cup
Asparagus, Bean Sprouts, Corn	3
Beets, Carrots, Celery, 1/2 cup	40
Broccoli, Cabbage, Cauliflower	10
Cucumber, Green Beans, Mushroom, Okra	3
Onions, Peas, Potato, Pumpkin, Squash	3
Peppers, Hot Chili, raw, each	3
Spinach, Turnips, 1/2 cup, ckd	40
Tomato, 1 medium, 5 oz	10
Canned: Asparagus, 4 spears	300
Beans, baked in tomato sauce	450
Beets, 1/2 cup, 3 oz	240
Corn Kernels, 1/2 cup, 3 oz	190
Creamed, 1/2 cup, 4 1/2 oz	330
Mushrooms w. butter sce, 2oz	550
Peas, 1/2 cup, 3 oz	250
Sauerkraut, 1/2 cup, 4 oz	750

Pickles, Olives
Olives, pickled: Green, 1 large	90
Ripe/black, 1 large	40
Pickles: Bread & Butter, 4 sl., 1 oz	200
Dill, 1 pickle, 2 1/2 oz	900
Sweet, 1 gherkin, 1/2 oz	130

Soybean Products
Miso (Soy Paste), 1/4 c., 2 1/2 oz	2500
Soybean Protein Isolate, 1 oz	280
Tempeh, 1/2 cup, 3 oz	5
Tofu, average, 1/2 cup, 4 oz	5

Jam, Honey, Syrups
Jam/Jelly, 1 Tbsp	2
Honey/Maple Syrup, 1 Tbsp	1
Log Cabin Syrup, 1 fl.oz	35
Lite, 1 fl.oz	90

Peanut Butter
Peanut Butter, regular, 1 Tbsp	70
Unsalted, 1 Tbsp	1

Snacks, Nuts — Sod
Cheese Balls/Curls, 1 oz	280
Corn/Tortilla Chips, aver., 1 oz	220
Granola bars, aver., 1 bar	80
Nuts: Plain, unsalted, 1 oz	1
Lightly salted, 1 oz	80
Salted or Honey Roasted, 1 oz	160
Popcorn: Plain (unsalted), 1 cup	1
Flavored, average, 1 cup	60
Salt added, 1 cup	180
Potato Chips, plain, 1 oz	160
Flavored, average, 1 oz	250
Pretzels, regular, 3, 1 oz	450

Candy, Chocolate
Chocolate, milk, 1 oz	30
Carob Milk Bar, 1 oz	55
Fudge, chocolate, 1 oz	55
Candy Bars, average, 1 1/2 oz	60
Hard Candy, Jelly Beans, 1 oz	10
Licorice, 1 oz	30

Beverages, Alcohol
Coffee (& Substitutes), Tea, 1 cup	1
Cocoa, dry, plain, 1 Tbsp	0
Mix, average, 1 envelope	120
Quik (*Nestle*), 2 tsp	35
Soft Drinks, average, 8 fl.oz	20
Mineral Water, Perrier, 8 fl.oz	5
Gatorade Thirst Quencher, 8 fl.oz	110
Water, average, 1 cup, 8 fl.oz	5
Drier regions, 1 cup	20+
Alcohol: Beer, average, 12 fl.oz	15
Wines, average, 4 fl.oz	10
Spirits (distilled), 1 1/2 fl.oz	1

Antacids – Alka-Seltzer
Alka-Seltzer (Per Tablet): — Sod
Alka-Seltzer P.M., 1 tablet	500
Original (Light Blue Box)	570
Extra Strength (Dark Blue Box)	590
Flavored Lemon/Lime & Cherry	500
Antacid (yellow Box)	310
Gelatine Capsule, 1	0
Alka-Mints, chewable	0
Bromo Seltzer, 3/4 capful	760
Rolaids: All types	0
Tums: Regular/Extra Strength	0
Sodium Bicarbonate (27% sodium), 1g	270

Index A - C

Index E - H

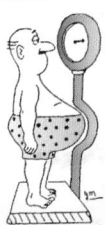

Index N - P

Index S - Z

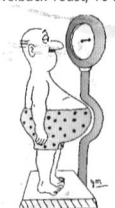

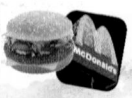

FAST-FOOD RESTAURANTS INDEX
~ SEE PAGE 175 ~